Lecture Notes in Computer Science   9006

Commenced Publication in 1973
Founding and Former Series Editors:
Gerhard Goos, Juris Hartmanis, and Jan van Leeuwen

More information about this series at http://www.springer.com/series/7412

Daniel Cremers · Ian Reid
Hideo Saito · Ming-Hsuan Yang (Eds.)

Computer Vision – ACCV 2014

12th Asian Conference on Computer Vision
Singapore, Singapore, November 1–5, 2014
Revised Selected Papers, Part IV

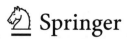 Springer

Editors

Daniel Cremers
Technische Universität München
Garching
Germany

Ian Reid
University of Adelaide
Adelaide, SA
Australia

Hideo Saito
Keio University
Yokohama, Kanagawa
Japan

Ming-Hsuan Yang
University of California at Merced
Merced, CA
USA

Videos to this book can be accessed at
http://www.springerimages.com/videos/978-3-319-16816-6

ISSN 0302-9743   ISSN 1611-3349 (electronic)
Lecture Notes in Computer Science
ISBN 978-3-319-16816-6   ISBN 978-3-319-16817-3 (eBook)
DOI 10.1007/978-3-319-16817-3

Library of Congress Control Number: 2015934895

LNCS Sublibrary: SL6 – Image Processing, Computer Vision, Pattern Recognition, and Graphics

Springer Cham Heidelberg New York Dordrecht London

Printed on acid-free paper

Springer International Publishing AG Switzerland is part of Springer Science+Business Media
(www.springer.com)

Preface

ACCV 2014 received a total of 814 submissions, a reflection of the growing strength of Computer Vision in Asia. We note, particularly, that a number of Area Chairs commented very positively on the overall quality of the submissions. The conference had submissions from all continents (except Antarctica, a challenge for the 2016 organizers perhaps) with 64 % from Asia, 20 % from Europe, and 10 % from North America.

The Program Chairs assembled a geographically diverse team of 36 Area Chairs who handled between 20 and 30 papers each. Area Chairs recommended reviewers for papers, and each paper received at least three reviews from the 638 reviewers who participated in the process. Paper decisions were finalized at an Area Chair meeting held in Singapore in September 2014. At this meeting, Area Chairs worked in triples to reach collective decisions about acceptance, and in panels of 12 to decide on the oral/poster distinction. The total number of papers accepted was 227, an overall acceptance rate of 28 %. Of these, 32 were selected for oral presentation.

We extend our immense gratitude to the Area Chairs and Reviewers for their generous participation in the process – the conference would not be possible if it were not for this huge voluntary investment of time and effort. We acknowledge particularly the contribution of 35 reviewers designated as "Outstanding Reviewers" (see page 14 in this booklet for a full list) who were nominated by Area Chairs and Program Chairs for having provided a large number of helpful, high-quality reviews.

The Program Chairs are also extremely grateful for the support, sage advice, and occasional good-natured prompting provided by the General Chairs. Each of them helped with matters that in other circumstances might have been left to the Program Chairs, so that it regularly felt as if we had a team of seven, not four Program Chairs. The PCs are very grateful for this.

Finally, we wish to thank the authors and delegates. Without their participation there would be no conference. The conference was graced with a uniformly high quality of presentations and posters, and we offer particular thanks to the three eminent keynote speakers, Stephane Mallat, Minoru Etoh, and Dieter Fox, who delivered outstanding talks.

Computer Vision in Asia is growing, and the quality of ACCV steadily climbing so that it is now, rightly, considered as one of the top conferences in the field. We look forward to future editions.

November 2014

Daniel Cremers
Ian Reid
Hideo Saito
Ming-Hsuan Yang

Organization

Organizing Committee

General Chairs

Michael S. Brown   National University of Singapore, Singapore
Tat-Jen Cham   Nanyang Technological University, Singapore
Yasuyuki Matsushita   Microsoft Research Asia, China

Program Chairs

Daniel Cremers   Technische Universität München, Germany
Ian Reid   University of Adelaide, Australia
Hideo Saito   Keio University, Japan
Ming-Hsuan Yang   University of California at Merced, USA

Organizing Chair

Teck Khim Ng   National University of Singapore, Singapore
Junsong Yuan   Nanyang Technological University, Singapore

Workshop Chairs

C.V. Jawahar   IIIT Hyderabad, India
Shiguang Shan   Institute of Computing Technology,
    Chinese Academy of Sciences, China

Demo Chairs

Bohyung Han   POSTECH, Korea
Koichi Kise   Osaka Prefecture University, Japan

Tutorial Chairs

Chu-Song Chen   Academia Sinica, Tawain
Brendan McCane   University of Otago, New Zealand

Publication Chairs

Terence Sim   National University of Singapore, Singapore
Jianxin Wu   Nanjing University, China

Industry Chairs

Hongcheng Wang   United Technologies Corporation, USA
Brian Price   Adobe, USA
Antonio Robles-Kelly   NITCA, Australia

Steering Committee

In-So Kweon	KAIST, Korea
Yasushi Yagi	Osaka University, Japan
Hongbin Zha	Peking University, China

Honorary Chair

Katsushi Ikeuchi	University of Tokyo, Japan

Area Chairs

Lourdes Agapito	Queen Mary University of London/University College London, UK
Thomas Brox	University of Freiburg, Germany
Tat-Jun Chin	University of Adelaide, Australia
Yung-Yu Chuang	National Taiwan University, Taiwan
Larry Davis	University of Maryland, USA
Yasutaka Furukawa	Washington University in St. Louis, USA
Bastian Goldluecke	University of Konstanz, Germany
Bohyung Han	POSTECH, Korea
Hiroshi Ishikawa	Waseda University, Japan
C.V. Jawahar	IIIT Hyderabad, India
Jana Kosecka	George Mason University, USA
David Kriegman	University of California, San Diego, USA
Shang-Hong Lai	National Tsing-Hua University, Taiwan
Ivan Laptev	Inria Rocquencourt, France
Kyoung Mu Lee	Seoul National University, Korea
Vincent Lepetit	École Polytechnique Fédérale de Lausanne, Switzerland
Jongwoo Lim	Hanyang University, Korea
Simon Lucey	CSIRO/University of Queensland, Australia
Ajmal Mian	University of Western Australia, Australia
Hajime Nagahara	Kyushu University, Japan
Ko Nishino	Drexel University, USA
Shmuel Peleg	The Hebrew University of Jerusalem, Israel
Imari Sato	National Institute of Informatics, Japan
Shin'ichi Satoh	National Institute of Informatics, Japan
Stefano Soatto	University of California, Los Angeles, USA
Jamie Shotton	Microsoft Research, UK
Ping Tan	Simon Fraser University, Canada
Lorenzo Torresani	Dartmouth College, USA
Manik Varma	Microsoft Research, India
Xiaogang Wang	Chinese University of Hong Kong, China
Shuicheng Yan	National University of Singapore, Singapore
Qing-Xiong Yang	City University of Hong Kong, Hong Kong
Jingyi Yu	University of Delaware, USA

Junsong Yuan	Nanyang Technological University, Singapore	
Hongbin Zha	Peking University, China	
Lei Zhang	Hong Kong Polytechnic University, Hong Kong, China	

Program Committee Members

Catherine Achard	Xun Cao	Jen-Hui Cheng
Hanno Ackermann	Gustavo Carneiro	Liang-Tien Chia
Haizhou Ai	Joao Carreira	Chen-Kuo Chiang
Emre Akbas	Umberto Castellani	Shao-Yi Chien
Naveed Akhtar	Carlos Castillo	Minsu Cho
Karteek Alahari	Turgay Celik	Nam Ik Cho
Mitsuru Ambai	Antoni Chan	Jonghyun Choi
Dragomir Anguelov	Kap Luk Chan	Wongun Choi
Yasuo Ariki	Kwok-Ping Chan	Mario Christoudias
Chetan Arora	Bhabatosh Chanda	Wen-Sheng Chu
Shai Avidan	Manmohan Chandraker	Albert C.S. Chung
Alper Ayvaci	Sharat Chandran	Pan Chunhong
Venkatesh Babu	Hong Chang	Arridhana Ciptadi
Xiang Bai	Kuang-Yu Chang	Javier Civera
Vineeth Balasubramanian	Che-Han Chang	Carlo Colombo
Jonathan Balzer	Vincent Charvillat	Yang Cong
Atsuhiko Banno	Santanu Chaudhury	Sanderson Conrad
Yufang Bao	Yi-Ling Chen	Olliver Cossairt
Adrian Barbu	Yi-Lei Chen	Marco Cristani
Nick Barnes	Jieying Chen	Beleznai Csaba
John Bastian	Yen-Lin Chen	Jinshi Cui
Abdessamad Ben Hamza	Kuan-Wen Chen	Fabio Cuzzolin
Chiraz BenAbdelkader	Chia-Ping Chen	Jeremiah D. Deng
Moshe Ben-Ezra	Yi-Ting Chen	Alessio Del Bue
AndrewTeoh Beng-Jin	Tsuhan Chen	Fatih Demirci
Benjamin Berkels	Xiangyu Chen	Xiaoming Deng
Jinbo Bi	Xiaowu Chen	Joachim Denzler
Alberto Del Bimbo	Haifeng Chen	Anthony Dick
Horst Bischof	Hwann-Tzong Chen	Julia Diebold
Konstantinos Blekas	Bing-Yu Chen	Thomas Diego
Adrian Bors	Chu-Song Chen	Csaba Domokos
Nizar Bouguila	Qiang Chen	Qiulei Dong
Edmond Boyer	Jie Chen	Gianfranco Doretto
Steve Branson	Jiun-Hung Chen	Ralf Dragon
Hilton Bristow	MingMing Cheng	Bruce Draper
Asad Butt	Hong Cheng	Tran Du
Ricardo Cabral	Shyi-Chyi Cheng	Lixin Duan
Cesar Cadena	Yuan Cheng	Kun Duan
Francesco Camastra	Wen-Huang Cheng	Fuqing Duan

Antony Lam
Francois Lauze
Duy-Dinh Le
Guee Sang Lee
Jae-Ho Lee
Chan-Su Lee
Yong Jae Lee
Bocchi Leonardo
Marius Leordeanu
Matt Leotta
Wee-Kheng Leow
Bruno Lepri
Frederic Lerasle
Fuxin Li
Hongdong Li
Rui Li
Jia Li
Yufeng Li
Yongmin Li
Yung-Hui Li
Cheng Li
Xin Li
Peihua Li
Xirong Li
Annan Li
Xi Li
Chia-Kai Liang
Shu Liao
T. Warren Liao
Jenn-Jier Lien
Joseph Lim
Ser-Nam Lim
Huei-Yung Lin
Haiting Lin
Weiyao Lin
Wen-Chieh (Steve) Lin
Yen-Yu Lin
RueiSung Lin
Yuanqing Lin
Yen-Liang Lin
Haibin Ling
Hairong Liu
Cheng-Lin Liu
Qingzhong Liu
Miaomiao Liu
Jingchen Liu
Ligang Liu

Haowei Liu
Guangcan Liu
Feng Liu
Shuang Liu
Shuaicheng Liu
Xiaobai Liu
Si Liu
Lingqiao Liu
Chen Change Loy
Feng Lu
Tong Lu
Zhaojin Lu
Le Lu
Huchuan Lu
Ping Luo
Lui Luoqi
Ludovic Macaire
Arif Mahmood
Robert Maier
Yasushi Makihara
Koji Makita
Yoshitsugu Manabe
Rok Mandeljc
Al Mansur
Gian-Luca Marcialis
Stephen Marsland
Takeshi Masuda
Thomas Mauthner
Stephen Maybank
Chris McCool
Xing Mei
Jason Meltzer
David Michael
Anton Milan
Gregor Miller
Dongbo Min
Ikuhisa Mitsugami
Anurag Mittal
Daisuke Miyazaki
Henning Müller
Thomas Moellenhoff
Pascal Monasse
Greg Mori
Bryan Morse
Yadong Mu
Yasuhiro Mukaigawa
Jayanta Mukhopadhyay

Vittorio Murino
Atsushi Nakazawa
Myra Nam
Anoop Namboodiri
Liangliang Nan
Loris Nanni
P.J. Narayanan
Shawn Newsam
Thanh Ngo
Bingbing Ni
Jifeng Ning
Masashi Nishiyama
Mark Nixon
Shohei Nobuhara
Vincent Nozick
Tom O'Donnell
Takeshi Oishi
Takahiro Okabe
Ryuzo Okada
Takayuki Okatani
Gustavo Olague
Martin Oswald
Wanli Ouyang
Yuji Oyamada
Paul Sakrapee
  Paisitkriangkrai
Kalman Palagyi
Hailang Pan
Gang Pan
Sharath Pankanti
Hsing-Kuo Pao
Hyun Soo Park
Jong-Il Park
Ioannis Patras
Nick Pears
Helio Pedrini
Pieter Peers
Yigang Peng
Bo Peng
David Penman
Janez Pers
Wong Ya Ping
Hamed Pirsiavash
Robert Pless
Dilip Prasad
Dipti Prasad Mukherjee
Andrea Prati

Xiao Wu	Jimei Yang	Cha Zhang
Yi Wu	Chih-Yuan Yang	Hong Hui Zhang
Xiaomeng Wu	Bangpeng Yao	Hui Zhang
Rolf Wurtz	Jong Chul Ye	Guofeng Zhang
Tao Xiang	Mao Ye	Xiao-Wei Zhao
Yu Xiang	Sai Kit Yeung	Rui Zhao
Yang Xiao	Kwang Moo Yi	Gangqiang Zhao
Ning Xu	Alper Yilmaz	Shuai Zheng
Li Xu	Zhaozheng Yin	Yinqiang Zheng
Changsheng Xu	Xianghua Ying	Zhonglong Zheng
Jianru Xue	Ryo Yonetani	Weishi Zheng
Mei Xue	Ju Hong Yoon	Wenming Zheng
Yasushi Yagi	Kuk-Jin Yoon	Lu Zheng
Koichiro Yamaguchi	Lap Fai Yu	Baojiang Zhong
Kota Yamaguchi	Gang Yu	Lin Zhong
Osamu Yamaguchi	Xenophon Zabulis	Bolei Zhou
Toshihiko Yamasaki	John Zelek	Jun Zhou
Takayoshi Yamashita	Zheng-Jun Zha	Feng Zhou
Pingkun Yan	De-Chuan Zhan	Feng Zhu
Keiji Yanai	Kaihua Zhang	Ning Zhu
Jie Yang	Tianzhu Zhang	Pengfei Zhu
Ruigang Yang	Yu Zhang	Cai-Zhi Zhu
Ming Yang	Zhong Zhang	Zhigang Zhu
Hao Yang	Yinda Zhang	Andrew Ziegler
Meng Yang	Xiaoqin Zhang	Danping Zou
Xiaokang Yang	Liqing Zhang	Wangmeng Zuo
Yi Yang	Xiaobo Zhang	
Yongliang Yang	Changshui Zhang	

Best Paper Award Committee

James Rehg	Georgia Institute of Technology, USA
Horst Bischof	Graz University of Technology, Austria
Kyoung Mu Lee	Seoul National University, South Korea

Best Paper Awards

1. Saburo Tsuji Best Paper Award

A Message Passing Algorithm for MRF inference with Unknown Graphs and Its Applications
Zhenhua Wang (University of Adelaide), Zhiyi Zhang (Northwest A&F University), Geng Nan (Northwest A&F University)

2. Sang Uk Lee Best Student Paper Award [Sponsored by Nvidia]

Separation of Reflection Components by Sparse Non-negative Matrix Factorization
Yasuhiro Akashi (Tohoku University), Takayuki Okatani (Tohoku University)

3. Songde Ma Best Application Paper Award [Sponsored by NICTA]

Stereo Fusion using a Refractive Medium on a Binocular Base
Seung-Hwan Baek (KAIST), Min H. Kim (KAIST)

4. Best Paper Honorable Mention

Singly-Bordered Block-Diagonal Form for Minimal Problem Solvers
Zuzana Kukelova (Czech Technical University, Microsoft Research Cambridge),
Martin Bujnak (Capturing Reality), Jan Heller (Czech Technical University),
Tomas Pajdla (Czech Technical University)

5. Best Student Paper Honorable Mention [Sponsored by Nvidia]

On Multiple Image Group Cosegmentation
Fanman Meng (University of Electronic Science and Technology of China),
Jianfei Cai (Nanyang Technological University), Hongliang Li (University of
Electronic Science and Technology of China)

6. Best Application Paper Honorable Mention [Sponsored by NICTA]

Massive City-scale Surface Condition Analysis using Ground and Aerial Imagery
Ken Sakurada (Tohoku University), Takayuki Okatani (Tohoku Univervisty),
Kris Kitani (Carnegie Mellon University)

ACCV 2014 – Outstanding Reviewers

Emre Akbas
Jonathan Balzer
Steve Branson
Sanderson Conrad
Marco Cristani
Alessio Del Bue
Anthony Dick
Bruce Draper
Katerina Fragkiadaki
Tatsuya Harada
Mehrtash Harandi
Nazli Ikizler-Cinbis

Catalin Ionescu
Suha Kwak
Junseok Kwon
Fuxin Li
Chen-Change Loy
Scott McCloskey
Xing Mei
Yasushi Makihara
Guy Rosman
Mathieu Salzmann
Pramod Sankar
Walter Scheirer

Bernt Schiele
Chunhua Shen
Sudipta Sinha
Deqing Sun
Yuichi Taguchi
Toru Tamaki
Dong Wang
Yu-Chiang Frank Wang
Paul Wohlhart
John Wright
Bangpeng Yao

ACCV 2014 Sponsors

Platnium   Singapore Tourism Board

Gold   Omron
Nvidia
Garena
Samsung

Silver   Adobe
ViSenze

Bronze   Lee Foundation
Morpx
Microsoft Research
NICTA

Contents – Part IV

Poster Session 2

Accelerating the Distribution Estimation for the Weighted Median/Mode Filters

Lu Sheng$^{(\boxtimes)}$, King Ngi Ngan, and Tak-Wai Hui

Department of Electronic Engineering, The Chinese University of Hong Kong,
Hong Kong, China
lsheng@ee.cuhk.edu.hk

Abstract. Various image filters for applications in the area of computer vision require the properties of the local statistics of the input image, which are always defined by the local distribution or histogram. But the huge expense of computing the distribution hampers the popularity of these filters in real-time or interactive-rate systems. In this paper, we present an efficient and practical method to estimate the local weighted distribution for the weighted median/mode filters based on the kernel density estimation with a new separable kernel defined by a weighted combinations of a series of probabilistic generative models. It reduces the large number of filtering operations in previous constant time algorithms [1,2] to a small amount, which is also adaptive to the structure of the input image. The proposed accelerated weighted median/mode filters are effective and efficient for a variety of applications, which have comparable performance against the current state-of-the-art counterparts and cost only a fraction of their execution time.

1 Introduction

A variety of popular image filters in computer vision are related to the local statistics of the input image. For example, the median filter outputs the point that reaches half of the local cumulative distribution [1,3,4]. The weighted mode filter [5–7] tries to find the global mode of the local distribution. Not only that, the widely popular bilateral filter [8], can be expressed as the mean of the local distribution that is estimated by a Gaussian kernel density estimator [9]. Provided a *guidance* feature map (*e.g.*, image intensity, patch and *etc.*), the weighted local distribution can be modified to jointly reflect the statistics of both the input image and the feature map, which in addition contributes to several kinds of structure- or style-transfer applications, like depth or disparity refinement in the stereo matching [1,5] and joint filtering [10].

Not explicitly estimating the local distribution, there are a certain number of approaches that are designed for accelerating the bilateral filter or similar weighted average filter, such as the domain transform filter [11], adaptive manifolds filter [12] and the guided filter [13]. However, efficient methods for immediate estimation of the local distributions need further attention because many

© Springer International Publishing Switzerland 2015
D. Cremers et al. (Eds.): ACCV 2014, Part IV, LNCS 9006, pp. 3–17, 2015.
DOI: 10.1007/978-3-319-16817-3_1

applications require direct operations on these distributions. Although the brute-force implementation is still adopted in many computer vision systems, its high complexity limits its popularity and hampers real-time systems and applications. Constant time algorithms for the estimation of the local distributions (or histograms) have been proposed in the literature. For instance, the constant time weighted median filter [1] and the smoothed local histogram filters [2]. The complexity of these methods relies on the *number of bins* to generate the histograms as well as the complexity of the *filtering operation* that calculates the value of each bin. Even though the complexity of filtering operations have been reported as $\mathcal{O}(1)$ in the literature, an 8-bit single channel gray-scale image usually needs 256 bins to produce a sufficiently accurate result, not to mention continuous or high-precision images.

Related to but different from these methods, in this paper we proposed a novel distribution estimation method for the sake of efficiency to accelerate various image filters. It is based on the kernel density estimation with a new separable kernel defined by a weighted combination of a series of probabilistic generative models. The resultant distribution has a much reduced number of filtering operations which are also independent of the values of the bins. The number of filtering operations is exactly the number of models used, and is usually smaller than the number of bins so as to abate the computational complexity. The required models can be the uniform quantization of the domain of the input image, or locally adaptive to the structures of the inputs. Since it is always the case that a local patch of an image can be decomposed into a limited number of distinct local structures, only a small amount of the locally adaptive models are necessary, thus the complexity is further reduced. We also accelerated the weighted mode filter and the weighted median filter by leveraging the proposed distribution estimation method. They own comparable performance in various applications but a faster speed in comparison with current state-of-art algorithms.

2   Related Work

Weighted average filters, like the bilateral filter [8,10], implicitly reflect properties of the local distribution. The brute-force implementation generally suffers the issue of inefficiency. In [14] an approximated solution was proposed by formulating the bilateral filtering as a high-dimensional low-pass filter, and can be accelerated by downsampling the space-range domain. Following this idea, different data structures have been proposed afterwards to further speedup the filters [12,15–17], in which the adaptive manifolds [12] caught our attention and inspired our research to construct the locally adaptive models. Guided filter [13] is a popular and efficient constant-time alternative. It can imitate a similar filter response as that of bilateral filter, but enforces local linear relationship between the filtering output and the guidance image. Domain transform filter [11] also produces a similar constant-time edge-preserving filter and earns real-time performance without quantization or coarsening.

Median filter might be the first image filter that explicitly applies the local histogram (a discretized distribution). Unlike the weighted median filter, which has no abundant work focusing on its acceleration, the unweighted counterpart receives several constant time solutions. One kind of these algorithms was present in the literature to lessen the histogram update complexity [3,4]. Another version introduced by Kass and Solomon [2] drawn the isotropic filtering into the construction of a so-called smoothed local histogram, which is a special case of the kernel density estimation, and the median and mode of this histogram are thus estimated by a look-up table.

The weighted median filter as well as the weighted mode filter, however, cannot directly duplicate the success in the previous discussion, since the weights are spatially varying for each local window. Min *et al.* [5] proposed a weighted mode filtering that adopts bilateral weights for the depth video enhancement, but it lacks an efficient implementations. The constant time weighted median filter [1] for disparity refinement is one of the most recent works that try to accelerate the local distribution construction. This method performs edge-preserving filtering to produce the probability of each bin in the local histogram. The number of bins determines the number of filtering operations applied. Thus it is less effective when hundreds of intensity levels are required, especially for the processing of the natural images.

3   Motivation

Estimating the probability distribution of each pixel is an essential element in various kinds of image filters like the weighted median filter [1], the weighted mode filter [5] and the bilateral filter [8] as a special case. A conventional way is to construct a weighted histogram of the target pixel in its local window, but a more flexible treatment is to exploit the kernel density estimation [7] so as to favor a smooth approximation [2].

Denote the probability distribution at pixel $\mathbf{x}$ as $h(\mathbf{x}, \cdot)$ and is specifically defined as

$$h(\mathbf{x}, g) = \frac{1}{Z(\mathbf{x})} \sum_{\mathbf{y} \in \mathcal{N}(\mathbf{x})} w(\mathbf{x}, \mathbf{y}) \phi_{\mathbf{x}}(g, f_{\mathbf{y}}), \tag{1}$$

where $f_{\mathbf{y}}$ is the input data of pixel $\mathbf{y}$. $\mathcal{N}(\mathbf{x})$ is a local window centered at $\mathbf{x}$, and the normalized factor $Z(\mathbf{x}) = \sum_{\mathbf{y} \in \mathcal{N}(\mathbf{x})} w(\mathbf{x}, \mathbf{y})$. The weight $w(\mathbf{x}, \mathbf{y})$ depends on the spatial relationship and the similarity of the guidance features between $\mathbf{x}$ and $\mathbf{y}$. The kernel $\phi_{\mathbf{x}}(g, f_{\mathbf{y}})$ varies in different applications. For discrete signals, a common kernel is the Kronecker delta function $\delta(\cdot)$, thus $h(\mathbf{x}, \cdot)$ becomes a weighted histogram [1]. An alternative common choice is the Gaussian kernel.

The approximated probability distribution immediately gets involved in the weighted median filter or the weighted mode filter since it replaces the value of a pixel by the median or the global mode of $h(\mathbf{x}, \cdot)$. The median is usually estimated by tracing the cumulative distribution [2]:

$$C(\mathbf{x}, \hat{g}) = \int_{-\infty}^{\hat{g}} h(\mathbf{x}, g) dg = \frac{1}{Z(\mathbf{x})} \sum_{\mathbf{y} \in \mathcal{N}(\mathbf{x})} w(\mathbf{x}, \mathbf{y}) \cdot \int_{-\infty}^{\hat{g}} \phi_{\mathbf{x}}(g, f_{\mathbf{y}}) dg \tag{2}$$

until it meets 0.5. Because it involves a high dimensional filtering operation in estimating $\mathcal{C}(\mathbf{x}, \hat{g})$ at each $\hat{g}$, too many samples of $\hat{g}$ will bring about heavy computational cost. On the other hand, typical ways to find the mode are the fixed-point iteration [6] or sampling by a look-up table and interpolation [2]. The key element in either method is the gradient of $h(\mathbf{x}, g)$ as

$$\frac{\partial h(\mathbf{x}, g)}{\partial g}\bigg|_{g=\hat{g}} = \frac{1}{\mathsf{Z}(\mathbf{x})} \sum_{\mathbf{y} \in \mathcal{N}(\mathbf{x})} w(\mathbf{x}, \mathbf{y}) \cdot \frac{\partial \phi_{\mathbf{x}}(g, f_{\mathbf{y}})}{\partial g}\bigg|_{g=\hat{g}}, \tag{3}$$

which is also the output after filtering. Similar problem occurs since the number of filtering operations depends on the number of iterations to converge or the sampling density of the look-up table.

To eliminate this issue, in the following sections we define a novel separable kernel as a weighted combination of a series of probabilistic generative models to decrease the number of filtering operations required to represent the distribution, and exploit the constant time filters [11,13] to reduce the complexity of the filtering operation.

4   Accelerating the Distribution Estimation

In this paper, we propose a novel approach to approximate the probability distribution by defining a new kernel based on a series of probabilistic generative models, which can be factorized explicitly so as to extract the filtering operations in advance before the distribution construction. With the proposed kernel, we introduce the accelerated versions of the weighted mode filter and the weighted median filter. We will show it later that they have excellent performance in terms of both quality and efficiency in various applications.

4.1   Kernel Definition

Assume the input image is modeled by several (*e.g.*, L) models throughout the whole pixel domain, each of which is governed by a distribution as $p(\eta_{\mathbf{x}}|l), l \in \mathcal{L} = \{1, 2 \ldots, L\}$ at each pixel $\mathbf{x}$. These models actually act as prior knowledge to represent *distinct local structures* in the input image. Two pixels $\mathbf{x}$ and $\mathbf{y}$ are similar if they both have high probabilities to agree with the lth model (see Fig. 1) as the following kernel:

$$\kappa^l(f_{\mathbf{x}}, f_{\mathbf{y}}) = p_{\mathbf{x}}(f_{\mathbf{x}}|l)p_{\mathbf{y}}(f_{\mathbf{y}}|l) \tag{4}$$

$$= \int_{\eta_{\mathbf{x}} \in \mathcal{H}_{\mathbf{x}}} p(f_{\mathbf{x}}|\eta_{\mathbf{x}})p(\eta_{\mathbf{x}}|l)d\eta_{\mathbf{x}} \cdot \int_{\eta_{\mathbf{y}} \in \mathcal{H}_{\mathbf{y}}} p(f_{\mathbf{y}}|\eta_{\mathbf{y}})p(\eta_{\mathbf{y}}|l)d\eta_{\mathbf{y}}, \tag{5}$$

where $p_{\mathbf{x}}(f_{\mathbf{x}}|\eta_{\mathbf{x}})$ is the data likelihood. $\mathcal{H}_{\mathbf{x}}$ and $\mathcal{H}_{\mathbf{y}}$ are the domains of $\eta_{\mathbf{x}}$ and $\eta_{\mathbf{y}}$, respectively. When all the L models are available, the overall kernel can be

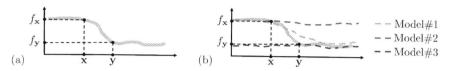

Fig. 1. Illustration of the proposed kernel. (a) shows a 1D signal and two pixels **x** and **y**. (b) represents the construction of $\kappa(f_\mathbf{x}, f_\mathbf{y})$, where the mean values of three models are shown in three different colors. It measures the similarity of $f_\mathbf{x}$ and $f_\mathbf{y}$ by evaluating the summation of the joint likelihood of them *w.r.t.* each model.

further defined as their weighted combination:

$$\kappa(f_\mathbf{x}, f_\mathbf{y}) = \sum_{l=1}^{L} \kappa^l(f_\mathbf{x}, f_\mathbf{y}) p_{\mathbf{x},\mathbf{y}}(l) = \sum_{l=1}^{L} p_\mathbf{x}(f_\mathbf{x}|l) p_\mathbf{y}(f_\mathbf{y}|l) p_{\mathbf{x},\mathbf{y}}(l), \tag{6}$$

where $p_{\mathbf{x},\mathbf{y}}(l)$ is the compatibility prior that measures the similarity between **x** and **y** on the lth model. This kernel is valid since it is an inner product in the L-dimensional feature space. What's more, it is able to reliably approximate some popular kernels like Gaussian kernel [12] or Kronecker delta kernel [1].

4.2   Probability Distribution Approximation

The approximated distribution can be written similarly as Eq. (1) by replacing $\phi_\mathbf{x}(g, f_\mathbf{x})$ with the proposed kernel as

$$\tilde{h}(\mathbf{x}, g) \propto \sum_{\mathbf{y} \in \mathcal{N}(\mathbf{x})} w(\mathbf{x}, \mathbf{y}) \sum_{l=1}^{L} p_\mathbf{x}(g|l) p_\mathbf{y}(f_\mathbf{y}|l) p_{\mathbf{x},\mathbf{y}}(l) = \sum_{l=1}^{L} p_\mathbf{x}(g|l) \cdot \psi_\mathbf{x}(l). \tag{7}$$

The filtering operation $\psi_\mathbf{x}(l) = \sum_{\mathbf{y} \in \mathcal{N}(\mathbf{x})} w(\mathbf{x}, \mathbf{y}) p_\mathbf{y}(f_\mathbf{y}|l) p_{\mathbf{x},\mathbf{y}}(l)$ is independent of g, and thus the approximated distribution becomes a mixture of L densities. Instead of immediately filtering $\phi_\mathbf{x}(g, f_\mathbf{y})$ for each g (*cf.*, Eq. (1)) to obtain $h(\mathbf{x}, g)$, the proposed method can precompute $\psi_\mathbf{x}(l)$ by merely L filtering operations in total and then estimate $\tilde{h}(\mathbf{x}, g)$ provided the priors $p(g|l)$. The proposed kernel approximates the distribution by extracting the filtering operations independent of g and therefore reduces the complexity of the distribution construction.

The cumulative distribution is hence $\tilde{\mathcal{C}}(\mathbf{x}, \hat{g}) \propto \sum_{l=1}^{L} \psi_\mathbf{x}(l) \int_{-\infty}^{\hat{g}} p(g|l) dg$ and the gradient $\frac{\partial \tilde{h}(\mathbf{x}, g)}{\partial g}|_{g=\hat{g}} \propto \sum_{l=1}^{L} \psi_\mathbf{x}(l) \frac{\partial p(g|l)}{\partial g}|_{g=\hat{g}}$, both of which do not contain additional filtering operations except those for $\psi_\mathbf{x}(l)$, and thus have the potential to accelerate the weighted median/mode filters.

Relationship with the Constant Time Weighted Median Filter [1] (CT-Median). Let the L models be equally quantized levels $\mu^l, l \in \mathcal{L}$ of the intensity space, and denote $p(\eta_\mathbf{x}|l) = \delta(\eta_\mathbf{x} - \mu^l), p(f_\mathbf{x}|\eta_\mathbf{x}) = \delta(f_\mathbf{x} - \eta_\mathbf{x}), p_{\mathbf{x},\mathbf{y}}(l) = 1/L$. We have the distribution as $\tilde{h}(\mathbf{x}, g) \propto \sum_{l=1}^{L} \delta(g - \mu^l) \cdot \sum_{\mathbf{y} \in \mathcal{N}(\mathbf{x})} w(\mathbf{x}, \mathbf{y}) \delta(f_\mathbf{y} - \mu^l)$, which is exact the form introduced in CT-median.

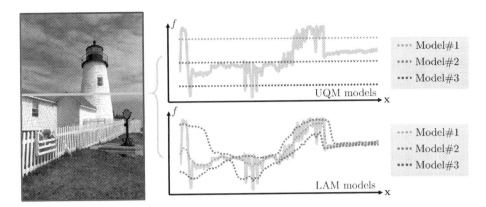

Fig. 2. Locally adaptive models (LAM) *v.s.* uniformly quantized models (UQM). A 1D signal is extracted from a gray-scale image shown in the left column and marked by orange. Both the LAM and UQM models ($L = 3$) are exploited to represent the signal, which are shown in the right column. The top row is by UQM models, the bottom one is by LAM models. The LAM models are adaptive to the local structures and own superior performance on representing the signal with limited number of models.

4.3   Accelerated Weighted Median/Mode Filters

In this section, we propose the accelerated versions of the weighted median/mode filters based on the kernel discussed previously. In particular, we apply the Gaussian model to define the probabilities for its efficiency in various image processing applications.

Kernel Definition. The *first* task is to define the L models that are suitable as the priors to represent the input image.

Case-I: *Uniformly Quantized Models* (UQM). A simple strategy is just to equally quantize the domain f, the mean of each model represents a quantization level μ^l and the diagonal elements in $\mathbf{\Sigma}^l$ is set as the square of half of the quantization interval. For a multi-dimensional image, each channel shares the same process. Specifically, $\mu_{\mathbf{x}}^l = \mu^l, \mathbf{\Sigma}_{\mathbf{x}}^l = \mathbf{\Sigma}^l$ at the lth model for all $\mathbf{x}$. It can well represent cartoon style images and disparity maps from frontal parallel stereos. However, more quantization levels are required to present a local complex structure under a sufficient accuracy, as shown in Fig. 2.

Case-II: *Locally Adaptive Models* (LAM). Locally adaptive models ought to be a superior idea since they tend to describe the local structures by fewer models. The idea behind it is that we assume a Gaussian mixture model in any local patch. Each model actually represents a local mean estimator. Therefore, we just need the number of *models* is a few more than the number of *modes* in the local distribution. For example, a natural image shown in Fig. 2 can be well represented by the LAM models. On the contrary, the UQM models cannot fit the local distribution if its number is insufficient.

The popular EM algorithm [18] is abandoned for the training of the LAM models due to its high complexity and instability to ensure a good estimation. In this paper, we exploit an alternative and more efficient way to train the required models. Similarly as [12], we also use a *hierarchical segmentation* approach to iteratively separate pixels from distinct structures, which act as local clusters, into different models. We set the segments as $\mathcal{S}_l, l \in \mathcal{L}$. This method involves simple low-pass filtering and fast PCA operations [12], thus is efficient in implementation. The mean and variance of the pixel $\mathbf{x}$ for the lth model are

$$\mu_{\mathbf{x}}^l = \frac{1}{\mathsf{W}_{\mathbf{x}}^l} \sum_{\mathbf{y} \in \mathcal{N}(\mathbf{x})} \theta_{\mathbf{y}}^l f_{\mathbf{y}}, \quad \Sigma_{\mathbf{x}}^l = \frac{1}{\mathsf{W}_{\mathbf{x}}^l} \sum_{\mathbf{y} \in \mathcal{N}(\mathbf{x})} \theta_{\mathbf{y}}^l f_{\mathbf{y}} f_{\mathbf{y}}^\top - \mu_{\mathbf{x}}^l {\mu_{\mathbf{x}}^l}^\top, \tag{8}$$

where $\theta_{\mathbf{y}} = 1_{[\mathbf{y} \in \mathcal{S}_l]}$ means the mask indicating pixels inside $\mathcal{S}_l$. $1_{[\cdot]}$ is the indicator function that equals to 1 when the input argument is true. The neighborhood $\mathcal{N}(\mathbf{x})$ is set as the same local window as Eq. (7). $\mathsf{W}_{\mathbf{x}}^l = \sum_{\mathbf{y} \in \mathcal{N}(\mathbf{x})} \theta_{\mathbf{y}}^l$ is the normalization factor.

Therefore, the prior probability for the lth model is $p(\eta_{\mathbf{x}}|l) = N(\eta_{\mathbf{x}}|\mu_{\mathbf{x}}^l, \Sigma_{\mathbf{x}}^l)$. Assume the data likelihood $p(f_{\mathbf{x}}|\eta_{\mathbf{x}}) = N(f_{\mathbf{x}}|\eta_{\mathbf{x}}, \Sigma_n)$, where Σ_n denotes the noise variance. Thus we have

$$\kappa^l(f_{\mathbf{x}}, f_{\mathbf{y}}) = N(f_{\mathbf{x}}|\mu_{\mathbf{x}}^l, \Sigma_n + \Sigma_{\mathbf{x}}^l) \cdot N(f_{\mathbf{y}}|\mu_{\mathbf{y}}^l, \Sigma_n + \Sigma_{\mathbf{y}}^l). \tag{9}$$

Given a prior tells the compatibility between pixel $\mathbf{x}$ and $\mathbf{y}$ for the lth model as $p_{\mathbf{x},\mathbf{y}}(l) = \exp(-\frac{1}{2}(\mu_{\mathbf{x}}^l - \mu_{\mathbf{y}}^l)^\top \Sigma_n^{-1}(\mu_{\mathbf{x}}^l - \mu_{\mathbf{y}}^l))$, the kernel $\kappa(f_{\mathbf{x}}, f_{\mathbf{y}})$ is therefore defined accordingly.

The proposed kernel otherwise needs two parameters Σ_n and L. For a highly complex image, L should be increased to fit the local structure to a large extent. Large Σ_n brings about smoother results but on the contrary, the necessary number of models can be reduced as well.

Probability Distribution Approximation. Based on the proposed kernel, the approximated probability distribution to each pixel $\mathbf{x}$ is

$$\tilde{h}(\mathbf{x}, g) = \frac{1}{\tilde{Z}(\mathbf{x})} \sum_{l=1}^{L} N(g|\mu_{\mathbf{x}}^l, \Sigma_n + \Sigma_{\mathbf{x}}^l)\psi_{\mathbf{x}}(l), \tag{10}$$

where $\psi_{\mathbf{x}}(l) = \sum_{\mathbf{y} \in N(\mathbf{x})} w(\mathbf{x}, \mathbf{y}) N(f_{\mathbf{y}}|\mu_{\mathbf{y}}^l, \Sigma_n + \Sigma_{\mathbf{y}}^l)p_{\mathbf{x},\mathbf{y}}(l)$ and $\tilde{Z}(\mathbf{x}) = \sum_{l=1}^{L} \psi_{\mathbf{x}}(l)$.

The *second* step of the weighted median/mode filters is to estimate $\psi_{\mathbf{x}}(l)$, $l \in \mathcal{L}$ by filtering $N(f_{\mathbf{y}}|\mu_{\mathbf{y}}^l, \Sigma_n + \Sigma_{\mathbf{y}}^l)$ characterized by the properties of $w(\mathbf{x}, \mathbf{y}) \times p_{\mathbf{x},\mathbf{y}}(l)$. This weight defines a joint filtering with the guidance of the guided feature map and the estimated models. Here we denote its parameters as $\boldsymbol{\omega}$. In this paper, we choose two kinds of filters: Guided filter (GF) [13] and Domain-transform filter (DF) [11]. They both have $\mathcal{O}(1)$ complexity and approximate the bilateral weight. GF has better performance on transferring local structures from the guided feature map to the target image while DF is natural to process higher dimensional images. Different applications exploit different weights.

The overall algorithm about the distribution approximation acceleration is summarized in Algorithm 1. The parameter setup refers to Sect. 5.1.

Algorithm 1. Distribution Approximation Acceleration

Input : Input image $\mathbf{F}_i$, guided image $\mathbf{F}_g$, parameter set $\{L^{\text{th}}, r, \sigma_n, \boldsymbol{\omega}\}$;

Output: Approximated distribution $\tilde{h}(\mathbf{x}, g)$;

`// 1. model generation`

1 **if** `model_type` *is* LAM **then**

2 $\quad$ $\{\mathcal{S}_l | \, l \in \mathcal{L}\} \leftarrow$ hierarchical segmentation [12] of $\mathbf{F}_i$ given L^{th} and r, σ_n;

3 $\quad$ **for** $l \leftarrow 1$ *to* L **do**

4 $\quad\quad$ $\theta_{\mathbf{y}}^l = 1_{[\mathbf{y} \in \mathcal{S}_l]}$, $\mathrm{W}_{\mathbf{x}}^l = \sum_{\mathbf{y} \in \mathcal{N}(\mathbf{x})} \theta_{\mathbf{y}}^l$;

5 $\quad\quad$ $\mu_{\mathbf{x}}^l \leftarrow \frac{1}{\mathrm{W}_{\mathbf{x}}^l} \sum_{\mathbf{y} \in \mathcal{N}(\mathbf{x})} \theta_{\mathbf{y}}^l f_{\mathbf{y}}$, $\boldsymbol{\Sigma}_{\mathbf{x}}^l = \frac{1}{\mathrm{W}_{\mathbf{x}}^l} \sum_{\mathbf{y} \in \mathcal{N}(\mathbf{x})} \theta_{\mathbf{y}}^l f_{\mathbf{y}} f_{\mathbf{y}}^{\top} - \mu_{\mathbf{x}}^l \mu_{\mathbf{x}}^{l \top}$;

6 $\quad$ $\mathcal{M}^l \leftarrow \{\mu_{\mathbf{x}}^l, \boldsymbol{\Sigma}_{\mathbf{x}}^l | \, \forall \mathbf{x}\}, l \in \mathcal{L}$ `// model parameters`

7 **else**

8 $\quad$ $\{\mu^l, \boldsymbol{\Sigma}^l | \, l \in \mathcal{L}\} \leftarrow$ quantize the image domain of $\mathbf{F}_i$ uniformly, given L^{th} ;

9 $\quad$ $\mathcal{M}^l \leftarrow \{\mu_{\mathbf{x}}^l = \mu^l, \boldsymbol{\Sigma}_{\mathbf{x}}^l = \boldsymbol{\Sigma}^l | \, \forall \mathbf{x}\}, l \in \mathcal{L}$ `// model parameters`

`// 2. distribution approximation`

10 $\psi_{\mathbf{x}}(l) \leftarrow \sum_{\mathbf{y} \in N(\mathbf{x})} w(\mathbf{x}, \mathbf{y}) \mathcal{N}(f_{\mathbf{y}} | \mu_{\mathbf{y}}^l, \boldsymbol{\Sigma}_n + \boldsymbol{\Sigma}_{\mathbf{y}}^l) p_{\mathbf{x}, \mathbf{y}}(l)$, $\psi_{\mathbf{x}}(l) \leftarrow \psi_{\mathbf{x}}(l) / \sum_{l=1}^{L} \psi_{\mathbf{x}}(l)$;

11 $\tilde{h}(\mathbf{x}, g) \leftarrow \sum_{l=1}^{L} N\left(g | \mu_{\mathbf{x}}^l, \sigma_n^2 \mathbf{I}^d + \boldsymbol{\Sigma}_{\mathbf{x}}^l\right) \psi_{\mathbf{x}}(l)$;

Weighted Median Filter. The weighted median filter wants to find the median value throughout the given probability distribution. Since the resultant distribution is actually a mixture of Gaussian models, an accelerated method is proposed by estimating the cumulative probability $\tilde{\mathcal{C}}(\mathbf{x}, \mu_{\mathbf{x}}^l)$ at the mean value $\mu_{\mathbf{x}}^l$ of each model. The median value is approximated by interpolating two adjacent cumulative probabilities $\tilde{\mathcal{C}}(\mathbf{x}, \mu_{\mathbf{x}}^k)$ and $\tilde{\mathcal{C}}(\mathbf{x}, \mu_{\mathbf{x}}^{k+1})$, where $\tilde{\mathcal{C}}(\mathbf{x}, \mu_{\mathbf{x}}^k) \leq 0.5$ and $\tilde{\mathcal{C}}(\mathbf{x}, \mu_{\mathbf{x}}^{k+1}) \geq 0.5$. In detail,

$$g_{\mathbf{x}}^{\text{med}} \approx \frac{0.5 - \tilde{\mathcal{C}}(\mathbf{x}, \mu_{\mathbf{x}}^k)}{\tilde{\mathcal{C}}(\mathbf{x}, \mu_{\mathbf{x}}^{k+1}) - \tilde{\mathcal{C}}(\mathbf{x}, \mu_{\mathbf{x}}^k)}(\mu_{\mathbf{x}}^{k+1} - \mu_{\mathbf{x}}^k) + \mu_{\mathbf{x}}^k. \tag{11}$$

In practice we find the proposed method is simple and effective after all. However, please notice that the median should be tracked per-channel for UQM models.

Weighted Mode Filter. The weighted mode filter is to find the global mode of $\tilde{h}(\mathbf{x}, g)$. Simple fixed-point iteration is sufficient for the proposed Gaussian models. Let the gradient $\partial \tilde{h}(\mathbf{x}, g) / \partial g = 0$, we have the fixed-point iteration as

$$g_{\mathbf{x}}^{n+1} = \left(\sum_{l=1}^{L} \mathcal{B}_{\mathbf{x}}^l(g_{\mathbf{x}}^n)\left(\boldsymbol{\Sigma}_n + \boldsymbol{\Sigma}_{\mathbf{x}}^l\right)^{-1}\right)^{-1}\left(\sum_{l=1}^{L} \mathcal{B}_{\mathbf{x}}^l(g_{\mathbf{x}}^n)\left(\boldsymbol{\Sigma}_n + \boldsymbol{\Sigma}_{\mathbf{x}}^l\right)^{-1}\mu_{\mathbf{x}}^l\right), \tag{12}$$

where $\mathcal{B}_{\mathbf{x}}^l(g_{\mathbf{x}}^n) = N(g_{\mathbf{x}}^n | \mu_{\mathbf{x}}^l, \boldsymbol{\Sigma}_n + \boldsymbol{\Sigma}_{\mathbf{x}}^l) \psi_{\mathbf{x}}(l)$. Equation (12) recursively goes to the closest mode and thus a good initialization $g_{\mathbf{x}}^0$ is necessary to avoid being stuck in wrong local mode. In practice, let $g_{\mathbf{x}}^0 = \mu_{\mathbf{x}}^{m^\star}$ where $m^\star = \arg\max_m \sum_{l=1}^{L} \mathcal{B}_{\mathbf{x}}^l(\mu_{\mathbf{x}}^m)$ is both effective and reasonable.

5   Experimental Results and Discussions

5.1   Implementation Notes

We have implemented the proposed weighted mode filter and the weighted median filter on a MATLAB platform. The results reported were measured on a 3.4 GHz Intel Core i7 processor with 16 GB RAM.

Parameter Definition. All input images and guidance images were normalized into $[0, 1]$ for the convenience of parameter definition. The data variance $\Sigma_n = \sigma_n^2 \mathbf{I}^d$, where σ_n is the standard variance of the noise, $\mathbf{I}^d$ is an identity matrix and d is the dimension of the input image. The guided filter (GF) and the domain transform filter (DF) share the same parameter setting, $i.e.$, $r = \sigma_s$ and $\varepsilon = \sigma_r^2$ ($\boldsymbol{\omega} = \{r, \varepsilon\}$ for GF, $\boldsymbol{\omega} = \{\sigma_s, \sigma_r\}$ for DF). r and σ_s was measured in pixels. For fair comparisons, the number of iterations in the weighted mode filter was set as 10 for all the experiments.

Number of Models. An automatic criterion [12] stops generating the LAM models when a high percentage of pixels are close to at least one model. In detail, the criterion of closeness is set as $\| f_\mathbf{x} - \mu_\mathbf{x}^l \|_{\Sigma_n} \leq 1$. Together with a user-given threshold L^{th}, the LAM models generation will be stopped when either the criterion or L^{th} is reached. In addition, the number of the UQM models shared the same threshold L^{th}, and no automatic stopping criterion was applied.

Compared Methods. In this paper, we compared our proposed filters with two popular filters: the constant time weighted median filter (CT-median) [1] and the bilateral weighted mode filter (BF-mode) [5]. The parameters of CT-median were given by the authors [1] and those of BF-mode were optimized by exhaustive search. The number of bins in the reference methods was fixed to 256 per-channel [1,2,5].

5.2   Performance Evaluation

Runtime Comparison. Figure 3 shows the execution time comparison between our method and the brute-force constant time algorithm ($cf.$ Eq. (1)) with GF weights to construct the distribution. Both LAM and UQM models were under evaluation. Related parameters were fairly configured. The y-axis is the ratio of runtime of the proposed method $w.r.t.$ the reference method, which assumed 256 discretized bins. L was defined manually without automatic stopping criterion. Both the two proposed methods only possess a fraction of the runtime against the reference one and are nearly proportion to the number of models. But the LAM spends a little bit more time because of additional filtering operations at the model generation step. Notice that when L is around 50, the execution time of the proposed methods becomes half of that of the reference one.

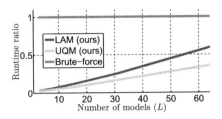

Fig. 3. Execution time comparison on the distribution construction $w.r.t.$ the number of models. The input is a 8-bit single-channel image and the guidance is a 3-channel image. The reference method is brute-force and traverses 256 discretized bins.

The Number of Necessary LAM Models. In fact, natural images, no matter color images or disparity/depth maps, are always locally smooth. There is little necessity to generate so many LAM models (*e.g.*, more than 60) to fit the local distribution. To validate this observation, we estimated the LAM models for all the color images in a published image dataset BSDS300 [19] with the threshold of $L^{\mathrm{th}} = 64$ and examined the distribution of necessary number of models. The automatic stopping criterion was triggered when no less than 99.9 % pixels were fulfilled the constraint in Sect. 5.1.

Results are illustrated in Fig. 4, where the left one was obtained by a window size 21×21 (*i.e.*, $r = 10$) and the right one was 11×11 (*i.e.*, $r = 5$). $\boldsymbol{\Sigma}_n = 0.01 \times \mathbf{I}^3$ for both cases. The majority of images generally required at most 50 models to meet the criterion. What's more, the smaller the window size is, the fewer number of necessary models are required, which verifies the discussions in Sect. 4.3. Based on these results, we conclude that for the general case, the number of LAM models required for a natural image merely exceeds a certain value under a given window size. As a typical case, let the window size be 21×21 or smaller, we can safely constrain the threshold to $L^{\mathrm{th}} = 64$, and the runtime on the probability distribution construction is always fewer than half of the brute-force implementation, as shown in Fig. 3.

As a conclusion, the gain of the proposed method is generally $2 \sim 3\times$ faster than the brute-force one for the gray-scale images. And it can be increased to $6 \sim 9\times$ for color images as the number of channels is increased. For disparity/depth

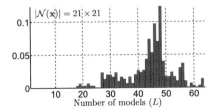
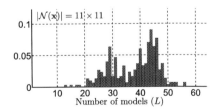

Fig. 4. The distribution of the number of necessary local adaptive models in BSDS300 dataset. *Left*: the window size is 21×21. *Right*: the window size is 11×11. The smaller the window size, the fewer number of locally adaptive models is necessary.

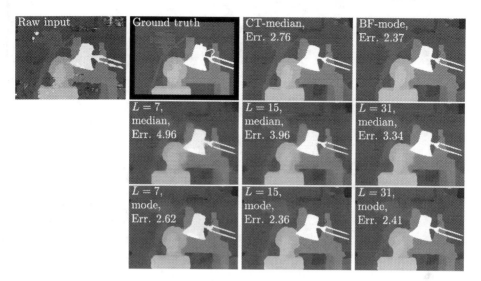

Fig. 5. Depth map enhancement on `tsukuba`. The first row shows the raw input disparity map, the ground truth, results by CT-median [1] and BF-mode [5] respectively, from left to right. Disparity maps in the 2nd and 3rd rows were obtained by the proposed weighted median filter and weighted mode filter, under different number of models. The models were generated by the LAM models. The error was evaluated on bad pixel ratio with the threshold 1. GF weights were chosen and related parameters were fairly configured.

maps and cartoon images, the number of necessary models can be reduced even further because of their high structure homogeneity.

5.3   Applications

Depth Map Enhancement. Depth maps with low resolution and poor quality, *e.g.*, structural outliers, depth holes, noise and *etc.*, can be enhanced with the guidance of the registered high resolution texture images [1,5]. It is a popular and practical post-processing for acquiring visual plausible and high accurate depth map from various depth acquisition techniques, like stereo, ToF-camera or Kinect. Two state-of-the art approaches that take advantage of the statistics information of the depth map are BF-mode [5] and CT-median [1]. Our methods, both the weighted mode filter and the weighted median filter, gain similar performance against them and require much less cost.

Figure 5 shows the results of a disparity map named `tsukuba`. The raw input was generated by a simple box-filter aggregation [20] followed by left-right check and hole-filling. LAM models were adopted for all these results and we fixed the number of models utilized. Small L (*e.g.*, $L = 7$) limits the LAM to define enough models to cover all the local structures, thus tended to output slightly blurred results or assign incorrect values in comparison with the referenced methods.

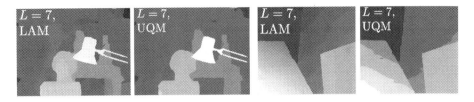

Fig. 6. Results of the weighted mode filter with 7 models.

Fortunately, by adopting a few more models, the results become stable and similar to the reference results. For instance, the BF-mode in our implementation required 15.09 s to process the `tsukuba` image, but the proposed weighted mode filter with 31 LAM models only cost 5.23 s. What's more, the bad pixel ratio of the proposed method (Err. 2.41) is similar as that (Err. 2.37) of BF-mode, but the PSNR is otherwise higher (25.28 dB) against that of the BF-mode (25.09 dB).

Although a small L of the LAM models cannot cover all the details of the input image, it still has a superior performance against the UQM models with the same L. As shown in Fig. 6, when $L = 7$, the LAM models captured more details of the two test disparity maps and produced smoother outputs than the UQM models. The staircase artifact of the UQM models also occurs at BF-mode and CT-median, since both of them are based on a discretized weighted histogram. When the bin number is not sufficient, the quantization artifact will happen around the smooth and slanted surfaces.

JPEG Artifact Removal. JPEG compression is a lossy compression scheme that usually brings about quantization noise and block artifact. CT-median has been proven effective in eliminating this compression artifact in clip-art cartoon images [1]. However, since CT-median encourages piecewise constant intensities/colors, its drawback is apparent when processing natural images.

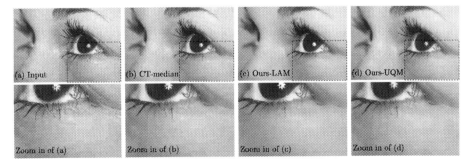

Fig. 7. JPEG compression artifact removal results by the weighted median filter. (a) The input degraded `eyes` image. (b) CT-median [1]. (c) The proposal weighted median filter with the LAM models and (d) is with the UQM models. The second row shows the corresponding zoomed-in patches. The DF weights were chosen and all the related parameters were fairly configured. Best viewed in electronic version.

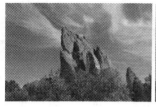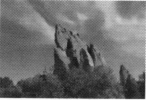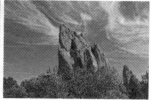

Fig. 8. Detail enhancement by the proposed weighted median filter under the LAM models. From left to right, the original `rock` image, after edge-preserving smoothing, and the detail enhanced image. GF weights were chosen.

As shown in Fig. 7(b) and its zoomed-in patch, CT-median forced the image eyes into several distinct layers, pixels inside one layer seemed constant everywhere. Contrary to it, exploiting the LAM models, our method represented a piecewise smooth result, as shown in Fig. 7(c). Not only the compression artifact was removal, but the structure of the input image was still preserved. The UQM models, unfortunately, had a slightly worse performance than that of LAM. The reason is straightforward as it also tried to recover piecewise constant colors. In terms of runtime comparison, both the LAM and UQM models only spent a small fraction of the runtime owned by CT-median (*i.e.*, 88.134 s) to obtain Fig. 7(b). The LAM models required $L = 15, \Sigma_n = 0.07^2 \times \mathbf{I}^3$ and $|\mathcal{N}(\mathbf{x})| = 11 \times 11$, it cost 16.74 s in total. The UQM models also owned $L = 15$, and the runtime was a little faster as 15.54 s.

More Applications. We show two additional applications to indicate the potential of the proposed weighted median filter and the weighted mode filter. Figure 8 shows the detail enhancement for a natural `rock` image by the proposed weighted median filter under the LAM models. The result is plausible for naked eyes without apparent artifact. Figure 9 presents the joint upsampling of a low-resolution and noisy disparity map with the guidance of a registered high-resolution image. Both of the proposed filters generated satisfactory results but the result by the weighted median filter tended to be smoother and introduced

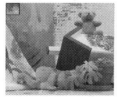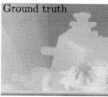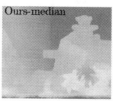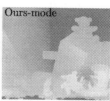

Fig. 9. Joint depth map upsampling. The input disparity map was 8× upsampled by the proposed weighted median filter and the weighted mode filter under the LAM models. The raw input diparity map is shown in the top-left corner of the leftmost image. GF weights were chosen.

a little blurring artifact, while that by the weighted mode filter was sharper and contained a slight of staircase artifact.

6   Conclusion and Future Work

In this paper, we propose a novel distribution construction method for accelerating the weighted median/mode filters by defining a new separable kernel based on the probabilistic generative models. Different from traditional methods that need quite a number of filtering operations to estimate a sufficiently accurate distribution, the proposed approach only requires a finite and a small amount of filtering operations based on the structure of the input image. The accelerated weighted median filter and weighted mode filter are thus introduced and utilized into various applications from depth map enhancement, joint depth upsampling, outlier removal, detail enhancement and so on.

As a part of the future work, the extension for video processing is interesting and meaningful. A more robust and efficient way to estimate the locally adaptive models shall be a great benefit. Moreover, increasing the efficiency on the median tracking and mode seeking can further accelerate the proposed filters.

References

1. Ma, Z., He, K., Wei, Y., Sun, J., Wu, E.: Constant time weighted median filtering for stereo matching and beyond. In: Proceedings of the IEEE International Conference Computer Vision (2013)
2. Kass, M., Solomon, J.: Smoothed local histogram filters. ACM Trans. Graph. **29**, 100 (2010)
3. Perreault, S., Hébert, P.: Median filtering in constant time. IEEE Trans. Image Process. **16**, 2389–2394 (2007)
4. Cline, D., White, K., Egbert, P.: Fast 8-bit median filtering based on separability. In: Proceedings of the IEEE International Conference Image Processing, vol. 5, pp. V-281–V-284 (2007)
5. Min, D., Lu, J., Do, M.: Depth video enhancement based on weighted mode filtering. IEEE Trans. Image Process. **21**, 1176–1190 (2012)
6. Van de Weijer, J., Van den Boomgaard, R.: Local mode filtering. In: Proceedings of the IEEE Conference on Computer Vision Pattern Recognition, vol. 2, pp. II-428–II-433 (2001)
7. Parzen, E.: On estimation of a probability density function and mode. Ann. Math. Stat. **33**, 1065–1076 (1962)
8. Tomasi, C., Manduchi, R.: Bilateral filtering for gray and color images. In: Proceedings of the IEEE International Conference on Computer Vision, pp. 839–846 (1998)
9. Barash, D., Comaniciu, D.: A common framework for nonlinear diffusion, adaptive smoothing, bilateral filtering and mean shift. Image Vis. Comput. **22**, 73–81 (2004)
10. Kopf, J., Cohen, M.F., Lischinski, D., Uyttendaele, M.: Joint bilateral upsampling. ACM Trans. Graph. **26**, 96:1–96:10 (2007)
11. Gastal, E.S.L., Oliveira, M.M.: Domain transform for edge-aware image and video processing. ACM Trans. Graph. **30**, 69:1–69:12 (2011)

12. Gastal, E.S., Oliveira, M.M.: Adaptive manifolds for real-time high-dimensional filtering. ACM Trans. Graph. **31**, 33 (2012)
13. He, K., Sun, J., Tang, X.: Guided image filtering. In: Daniilidis, K., Maragos, P., Paragios, N. (eds.) ECCV 2010, Part I. LNCS, vol. 6311, pp. 1–14. Springer, Heidelberg (2010)
14. Paris, S., Durand, F.: A fast approximation of the bilateral filter using a signal processing approach. In: Leonardis, A., Bischof, H., Pinz, A. (eds.) ECCV 2006. LNCS, vol. 3954, pp. 568–580. Springer, Heidelberg (2006)
15. Chen, J., Paris, S., Durand, F.: Real-time edge-aware image processing with the bilateral grid. ACM Trans. Graph. **26** (2007) Article 103
16. Adams, A., Gelfand, N., Dolson, J., Levoy, M.: Gaussian kd-trees for fast high-dimensional filtering. ACM Trans. Graph. **28**, 21:1–21:12 (2009)
17. Adams, A., Baek, J., Davis, M.A.: Fast high-dimensional filtering using the permutohedral lattice. Comput. Graph. Forum. **29**, 753–762 (2010)
18. Bishop, C.M., Nasrabadi, N.M.: Pattern Recognition and Machine Learning, vol. 1. Springer, New York (2006)
19. Martin, D., Fowlkes, C., Tal, D., Malik, J.: A database of human segmented natural images and its application to evaluating segmentation algorithms and measuring ecological statistics. In: Proceedings of the IEEE International Conference on Computer Vision, vol. 2, pp. 416–423 (2001)
20. Scharstein, D., Szeliski, R.: A taxonomy and evaluation of dense two-frame stereo correspondence algorithms. Int. J. Comput. Vis. **47**, 7–42 (2002)

Saliency Aggregation: Does Unity Make Strength?

Olivier Le Meur[1(✉)] and Zhi Liu[1,2]

[1] IRISA, University of Rennes 1, Rennes, France
olemeur@irisa.fr
[2] School of Communication and Information Engineering,
Shanghai University, Shanghai, China

Abstract. In this study, we investigate whether the aggregation of saliency maps allows to outperform the best saliency models. This paper discusses various aggregation methods; six unsupervised and four supervised learning methods are tested on two existing eye fixation datasets. Results show that a simple average of the TOP 2 saliency maps significantly outperforms the best saliency models. Considering more saliency models tends to decrease the performance, even when robust aggregation methods are used. Concerning the supervised learning methods, we provide evidence that it is possible to further increase the performance, under the condition that an image similar to the input image can be found in the training dataset. Our results might have an impact for critical applications which require robust and relevant saliency maps.

1   Introduction

In 1985, Koch and Ullman proposed the first plausible architecture for modelling the visual attention [1]. This seminal paper has motivated much of the following work of computational models of attention. Today there exist a number of saliency models for predicting the most visually salient locations within a scene. A taxonomy composed of 8 categories has been recently proposed by Borji and Itti [2]. The two main categories, encompassing most existing models, are termed as *cognitive models* and *information theoretic models*. The former strives to simulate the properties of our visual system whereas the latter is grounded in the information theory. Although all existing models follow the same objective, they provide results which could be, to some extent, different. The discrepancies are related to the quality of the prediction but also to the saliency map representation. Indeed some models output very focused saliency maps [3–5] whereas the distribution of saliency values is much more uniform in other models [6,7]. Others tend to emphasize more on the image edges [8], the color or luminance contrast. This saliency map manifold contains a rich resource that should be used and from which new saliency maps could be inferred. Combining saliency maps generated using different models might enhance the prediction quality and the robustness of the prediction. Our goal is then to take saliency maps from this manifold and to produce the final saliency map.

© Springer International Publishing Switzerland 2015
D. Cremers et al. (Eds.): ACCV 2014, Part IV, LNCS 9006, pp. 18–32, 2015.
DOI: 10.1007/978-3-319-16817-3_2

To the best of our knowledge, there is no study dealing with the fusion of saliency maps. In the context-of-object of interest detection, we can mention two related studies. Borji et al. [9] combined the results of several models and found out that the simple average method performs well. Mai et al. [10] combined results of models detecting object-of-interest on simple images (mainly composed of one object-of-interest with simple background). They use simple methods as well as the trained methods. The main drawback of the aforementioned studies concerns the choice of the tested models, which are not The best-in-class. Consequently, the room for improvement is still important and can be obtained, to some degree, by aggregating different results. However, we draw attention to a crucial difference between our work and the two aforementioned studies [9,10]. The saliency maps that are aggregated in this study are computed using computational models of visual attention for eye fixation prediction. In [9,10], the saliency maps are the outputs of saliency models which aim to completely highlight salient objects such as [11].

Keeping all these points in mind, we investigate whether we could improve on the prediction quality by aggregating a set of saliency maps or not. Eye fixation datasets will be used as the ground truth.

The paper is organized as follows. Section 2 presents the methods we use for aggregating saliency maps. Section 3 shows the performance of the saliency models, taken alone, and the performance of the aggregation functions. Finally, we draw some conclusions in Sect. 4.

2 Saliency Aggregation

2.1 Context and Problem

As illustrated by Fig. 1, the predicted saliency maps do not exhibit similar characteristics. Figure 1(b), which plots the distribution of saliency values for four models, clearly shows the discrepancy that exists between saliency maps. Some are very focused whereas others are much more uniform. We can also notice that the contrast between salient and non-salient areas can be either high or very low. This discrepancy between maps can be considered as noise but also as an important cue that needs to be exploited. Combining saliency models may enhance the similarity between human and the predicted saliency maps. Human saliency maps, as we will see in Sect. 3, will be inferred from publicly-available eye fixation datasets.

To investigate this point, we select 8 state-of-the-art models (GBVS [3], Judd [12], RARE2012 [13], AWS [5], Le Meur [4], Bruce [7], Hou [8] and Itti [6]) and aggregate their saliency maps into a unique one. The following subsections present the tested aggregation methods. Two categories of methods have been tested. The methods in the first category are unsupervised, meaning that there is neither optimization nor prior knowledge on saliency maps. The methods in the second category are supervised. Different algorithms are used to train the best way to combine together saliency maps.

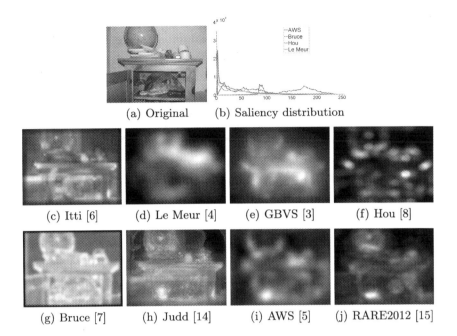

Fig. 1. (a) Original picture; (b) saliency distribution obtained using 4 models (AWS, Bruce, Hou and Le Meur); (c) to (j) the predicted saliency maps from the 8 state-of-the-art saliency models considered in this study.

2.2   Unsupervised Methods

Six aggregation methods are tested here. The first 4 functions are based on a simple weighted linear summation:

$$p(x|M_1, \cdots, M_K) = \sum_{k=1}^{K} w_k \times p(x|M_k) \tag{1}$$

where $p(x|M_1, \cdots, M_K)$ is the probability of an image pixel x ($x \in \Omega$, with $\Omega \subset \mathcal{R}^2$) to be salient after the combination; $p(x|M_1, \cdots, M_K)$ is positive or null. M_k is the saliency map produced by model k. $p(x|M_k)$ is the probability of an image pixel x from the saliency map M_k to be salient. w_k is the weighting coefficient, given that $\sum_{k=1}^{K} w_k = 1$ and $w_k \geq 0, \forall k$. K is the number of saliency maps ($K = 8$ in our case).

The main goal is to compute the weighting coefficients in order to improve the degree of similarity between the ground truth and the aggregated saliency map. These weights are computed thanks to the following methods:

– Uniform: weights w are uniform and spatially invariant, $w_k = \frac{1}{K}$;
– Median: weights w are locally deduced from the saliency values. All weights are null, except for the one which corresponds to the median value of the saliency values for a given location. In this case, weights are spatially variant;

– M-estimator: weights w are computed by a weight function commonly used for robust regression. The weight function aims to limit the influence of outlier data by decreasing their contributions. We consider three weight functions. They are defined by the second derivatives of the Welsh, the $L_1 L_2$ and the Geman-McClure functions. The first one requires a parameter whereas the other two functions are non-parametric:

$$g_{Welsh}(e(x|M_k)) = exp\left(-\frac{e(x|M_k)^2}{\sigma^2}\right) \tag{2}$$

$$g_{L_1 L_2}(e(x|M_k)) = \frac{1}{\sqrt{1 + e(x|M_k)^2/2}} \tag{3}$$

$$g_{Geman}(e(x|M_k)) = \frac{1}{(1 + e(x|M_k)^2)^2} \tag{4}$$

where, the error $e(x|M_k)$ for a location x and model k represents the deviation between the current location and the average saliency value computed locally over all saliency maps:

$$e(x|M_k) = p(x|M_k) - \frac{1}{Z}\sum_{y \in \nu}\sum_{k=1}^{K} p(y|M_k) \tag{5}$$

where ν is a 3×3 local neighbourhood centred on x. Z is a normalization factor. Functions g_{Welsh} and g_{Geman} further reduce the effect of large errors compared to function $g_{L_1 L_2}$. Weights of equation (1) are finally given by $w_k = g_{Welsh}(e(x|M_k))$, $w_k = g_{L_1 L_2}(e(x|M_k))$ and $w_k = g_{Geman}(e(x|M_k))$ for Welsh, $L_1 L_2$ and the Geman-McClure function, respectively. For the function g_{Welsh}, the standard deviation is locally estimated using the K saliency maps.

– The last tested method is based on a global minimization of an energy function. Let $\mathcal{I}$ be the set of pixels in the final saliency map and $\mathcal{L}$ be the finite set of labels. The labels correspond to the final saliency values (coming from one given model) that we want to estimate at each pixel. A labeling f assigns a label $f_x \in \mathcal{L}$ to each pixel x of image $\mathcal{I}$. The best labeling minimizes the energy given below

$$E(f) = \sum_{p \in \mathcal{L}} D(p) + \lambda \sum_{(x,y) \in \mathcal{N}} V(f_x, f_y) \tag{6}$$

where $\mathcal{N}$ is a 3×3 square neighbourhood, λ is a positive constant that controls the trade-off between $D(p)$ and $V(f_x, f_y)$. $D(p)$ is the data cost and $V(f_x, f_y)$ is the smoothness term. They are defined as

$$D(p) = \sum_{n \in \mathcal{L}}\sum_{u \in \nu}(p(x + u|M_p) - p(x + u|M_n))^2$$

$$V(n, m) = \| p(x|M_n) - p(y|M_n) \|^2 + \| p(x|M_m) - p(y|M_m) \|^2 \tag{7}$$

The minimization of the energy E is achieved using loopy belief propagation [14], and the number of iterations is set to 10.

2.3 Supervised Learning Methods

In this section, the weights w_k are computed by minimizing the residual r between the actual and the predicted saliency values:

$$r(x) = \|p(x) - \sum_{k=1}^{K} w_k p(x|M_k)\|^2 \tag{8}$$

where $p(x)$ is the actual saliency deduced from the eye fixation dataset and $p(x|M_k)$ is the saliency at location x for model M_k. The actual saliency map which represents the ground truth is classically obtained by convolving the fixation map (considering all visual fixations of all observers) by a 2D Gaussian function, having a standard deviation of one degree of visual angle. More details can be found in [15].

For a given image $\mathcal{I}$ defined over $\Omega \subset \mathcal{R}^2$, and given that the number of unknowns, i.e. K, which is much smaller than the number of locations in $\mathcal{I}$, the optimal vector of weights W^* can be computed by the least-squares method as follows:

$$W^* = \arg\min \sum_{x \in \Omega} r(x) \tag{9}$$

In this study, W^* is computed by the following methods: The first one is the classical least-squares method, noted as LS, which minimizes the residual error between the actual and the aggregated saliency maps. One drawback is that the weights do not sum to 1 and can be positive or negative. This makes the interpretation difficult. This is the reason why three other methods have been tested. Two methods are constraint least-squares problems. Adding constraints aims to ease the interpretation of the computed weights. However, it is important to keep in mind that introducing constraint will reduce the solution space. The first constraint is that the weights have to sum to one. The sum-to-one constraint of the weights moves the LS problem onto the Locally Linear Embedding (LLE) [16]. Another constraint is that the weights are positive; this problem is similar to the problem of Non-negative Matrix Factorization (NMF) [17]. Finally, we also test a robust least-squares problem, noted as LSR. Instead of minimizing a sum of squares of the residuals, we use a Huber-type M-estimator [18] to reduce the influence of outliers. The algorithm simply consists in re-weighting iteratively the residuals according to the Cauchy weighting function given that a higher residual leads to a lower weight.

3 Performance

The performance of the aggregation functions have been evaluated on Bruce's [7] and Judd's [12] eye fixation datasets. Four metrics were used: linear correlation coefficient, Kullback-Leibler divergence, normalized scanpath saliency and hit rate. The linear correlation coefficient, noted as CC, computes the linear relationship between the ground truth saliency map and the predicted saliency

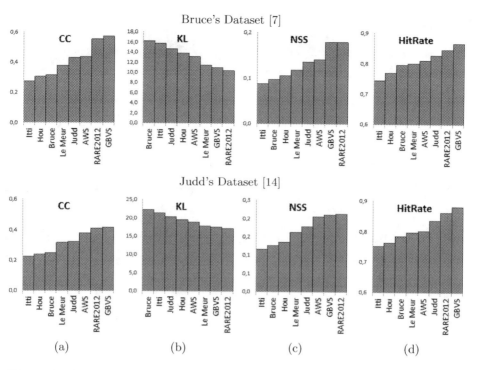

Fig. 2. Ranking visual saliency models over two datasets. Top row: Bruce's dataset; Bottom row: Judd's dataset. Four metrics are used. From left to right: correlation coefficient (CC), Kullback-Leibler divergence (KL), NSS (normalized scanpath saliency) and HitRate. Models are ranked in the increasing order according to their performance.

map. There is a perfect linear relationship when $CC = 1$. The Kullback-Leibler divergence, noted as KL, computes an overall dissimilarity between two distributions. The first step is to transform the ground truth saliency map and the predicted saliency maps into 2D distributions. The KL-divergence is positive or null. The perfect similarity ($KL = 0$) is obtained when the two saliency maps are strictly equal. The normalized scanpath saliency (NSS) proposed by [19] involves a saliency map and a set of fixations. It aims at evaluating the saliency values at fixation locations. The higher the NSS value, the better the predicted saliency maps. The hit rate measure used in this study is similar to the measure used in [12]. It involves a binarized saliency map and a set of fixations. It aims at counting the number of fixations falling within the binarized salient areas. By varying the binarization threshold, a hit rate curve is plotted. The hit rate measure is simply the area under the curve. The chance level is given by 0.5, whereas the highest similarity is given by 1. More details can be found in [15].

3.1   Performance of State-of-the-Art Models

Figure 2 illustrates the performance of the 8 selected models (GBVS [3], Judd [12], RARE2012 [13], AWS [5], Le Meur [4], Bruce [7], Hou [8] and Itti [6]) over Bruce

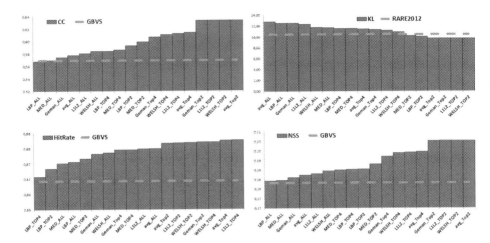

Fig. 3. Performance on Bruce's dataset of the six aggregation functions: Avg (for average), Geman (for g_{Geman}), L1L2 (for $g_{L_1L_2}$), Welsh (for g_{Welsh}), LBP (for Loopy Belief Propagation) and MED (for Median operator). These functions are tested when considering the top 2, top 4 and all models. For each metric, namely CC, KL, HitRate and NSS, the aggregation functions are ranked from the lowest to the highest performance. The orange bar indicates the performance of the best saliency model. For instance, GBVS model achieves the best results on Bruce's dataset for CC, KL and NSS metrics (Color figure online).

and Judd datasets. According to our results, we find that the top 2 models are GBVS and RARE2012, the top 4 models are GBVS, RARE2012, Judd and AWS. This result is consistent with the recent benchmark of Borji et al. [20].

3.2 Performance of Saliency Aggregation

The aggregation functions described in Sect. 2 are applied on the top 2 (GBVS and RARE2012), top 4 (GBVS, RARE2012, Judd, AWS) and the 8 saliency models. Figure 3 gives the performance of the saliency aggregation on Bruce's dataset. The performance of the best saliency model (out of the 8 models) for each metric is also indicated by the orange bar. From these results, we can draw several conclusions.

1. Except for the KL-divergence, the aggregation of saliency map outperforms the best saliency models in all cases. For instance, in terms of HitRate, the best aggregation function, i.e. L1L2 TOP4 (meaning that the function $g_{L_1L_2}$ is applied on the top 4 saliency models) performs at 0.878 whereas the best saliency model performs at 0.864 (note that this gain is statistically significant (paired t-test, $p < 0.01$)). For the KL-divergence, only the *LBP TOP2*, *avg TOP2*, *L1L2 TOP2* and *WELSH TOP2* aggregation function perform better than the best saliency model, i.e. RARE2012 model;

2. The second observation is related to the number of saliency models required to get the good performance. It is indeed interesting to notice that the aggregation functions using all saliency maps get the lowest scores. At the opposite, the best performances are obtained when the top 2 models are used for the CC, KL and NSS metrics. For the hit rate metric, the aggregation of the top 4 models is ranked first. However, the performances between the aggregation of the top 2 and top 4 models are not statistically significant. Considering more models tend to decrease the performances, the worst case occurring when all models are considered;

3. The third observation is related to the aggregation functions. The average, L1L2 and Welsh functions perform similarly and better than the median and LBP functions (considering the top 4 and top 2 models). The low performance of the LBP method can be explained by the obvious difference and the lack of spatial coherency between saliency maps as illustrated in Fig. 1.

To conclude, a simple aggregation function, such as the average function, operating on the top 4 or top 2 models is a good candidate to improve significantly the performance of saliency models. For the sake of simplicity, we could only consider GBVS and RARE2012 models and average their saliency maps. Note that on Judd's dataset, we get similar trends (results are not presented here due to the page limit). The best performance is given by the average of the top 4 and the top 2 models.

Figure 4(a) presents some results of the aggregation methods for a given image. For this example, it is difficult to see a significant difference between the average, Welsh and L1L2 methods. This is consistent with our previous findings (see Fig. 3). However, concerning the LBP method, we notice a lack of spatial consistency, especially when all saliency maps are taken into account.

3.3   Performance of Supervised Methods

The optimal weights for aggregating the saliency maps are learned on Bruce's dataset. The different methods, namely LS, LSR, LLE and NMF, are evaluated for the top 2, top 4 and all models. Figure 5 illustrates the results on Bruce's dataset. The orange bar indicates the performance of the best saliency model.

As expected, the performance increases when the weights are learned. This is perfectly normal since we seek for the weights minimizing the prediction error (error between the ground truth and the aggregated saliency maps). Whatever the regression methods, the learning process outperforms the best saliency model, taken alone, in most of the tested configurations. There are only 3 cases out of 48 for which the weight optimization does not bring any improvement. Compared to the average of the top 2 models (performances were presented in the previous section), results are more contrasted (see the green horizontal line in Fig. 5): only the simple least-squares method involving all models (noted as LS ALL) performs significantly better than the average of the top 2 models (except for the KL metric).

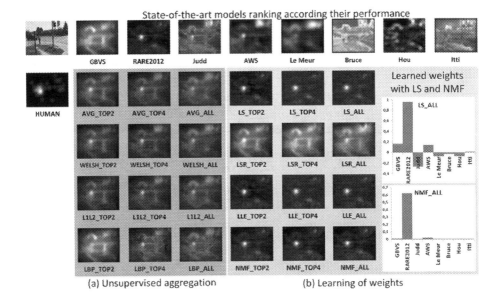

Fig. 4. Results of the aggregation obtained by (a) unsupervised and (b) supervised approaches. The original image and the human saliency map (i.e. the ground truth) are given on the top-left corner. On the top, the predicted saliency maps, obtained with the 8 tested saliency models, are illustrated. Results of the average, Welsh, L1L2 and LBP functions are shown in the green box (a) when the top 2, top 4 and all models are considered. Results of the LS, LSR, LLE and NMF learning methods are shown in the light blue box (b). On the right hand-side of the light blue box, the weights computed by the LS and NMF methods (considering all the maps of saliency models) are given. As we can see, RARE2012 model gets, for this particular example, the highest weights. Notice that for the NMF method, weights are positive (Color figure online).

As soon as a constraint is added, such as the sum-to-one constraint of the weights (LLE) or the positivity of the weights (NMF), performance tends to decrease. This observation is valid when we consider the top 2, top 4 and all models. Figure 4(b) presents some results of the supervised aggregation methods for a given image.

Similar results have been observed on Judd's dataset. The best learning function is the simple least-squares method involving all saliency maps; for instance, in terms of HitRate, it achieves 0.91, whereas the average of the top 2 models and the best model (Judd in this case) achieves 0.88. Figure 6 presents the results on Judd's dataset.

The learning results presented so far in Figs. 5 and 6 have to be considered as the upper-bound on the performance we can achieve by using a learning method. Obviously, in practice, we do not know the ground truth represented by the human saliency map, which is exactly what we want to predict.

To overcome this problem, we learn the weights for all pictures of Bruce's and Judd's datasets. The method chosen is the simple least-squares method which

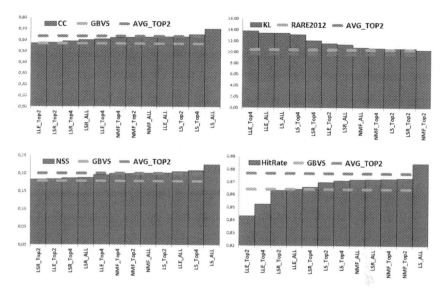

Fig. 5. The performance for the four methods (LS, LSR, LLE and NMF) in terms of (a) CC, (b) KL, (c) NSS and (d) HitRate on Bruce's dataset. We combine all saliency maps coming from the top 4 models (GBVS, RARE2012, Judd, AWS) and maps coming from the top 2 models (GBVS and RARE2012). Methods are ranked from the lowest to the highest performance.

is applied on the 8 saliency maps. This strategy is called LS ALL, in previous paragraphs. As illustrated by Figs. 5 and 6, this method provides the best results.

Once all the weights have been computed (8 weights per image), we compute the aggregated saliency map of an input image by using the pre-computed weights corresponding to the nearest neighbor image of the input image. In other words, we assume that the discrepancy between weights of two similar images is not significant. Figure 7(a) presents the synoptic of the proposed method.

Given an input image, the first thing to do is to retrieve its nearest image from the dataset. This problem can be efficiently handled by using the VLAD (Vector of Locally Aggregated Descriptors) method introduced by Jégou et al. [21]. VLAD is an image descriptor which has been designed to be very low dimensional: only 16 bytes are required per image. The computation of VLAD descriptor is based on the vector quantizing a locally invariant descriptor such as SIFT. From the weights of the most similar image, the aggregated saliency map is computed. We call this method WMSI, for Weight of Most Similar Image.

Figure 6 presents the results of the WMSI method (see the rightmost red column). Whatever the metrics, the WMSI method gets the lowest performance compared to the best saliency model, taken alone, the average of the two best saliency maps and, as expected, the learning method *LS ALL*. These results suggest that the initial assumption does not hold, i.e. similar images do not have the same distribution of weights. However, it is necessary to tone down this conclusion. Figure 8 illustrates this point. Two pairs of images ((a)–(b) and

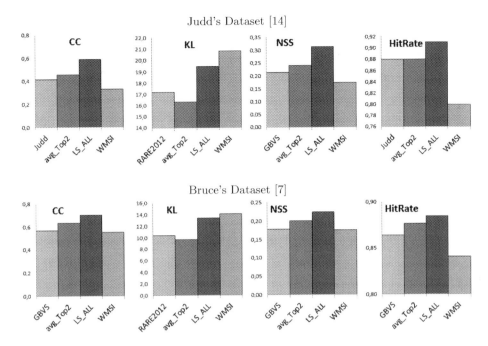

Fig. 6. Performance of LS and WMSI methods on Bruce's and Judd's dataset. To ease the comparison, the performance of the best saliency model and the performance of the best aggregated method (average of the top 2 models) are displayed. The color code is the same as Fig. 5: orange for the best saliency model, green for the best aggregation method (*avg Top2*) and blue for the learning method (*LS ALL*). The red bar, called WMSI (Weight of Most Similar Image), indicates the performance of the aggregation method when the weights of the most similar image in the dataset are used (Color figure online).

(c)–(d)) are given: the image (b) is the most similar image to the image (a). The VLAD score is equal to 0.22. The second pair of images (c)–(d), for which image (d) is the image which is the most similar to image (c) presents a low VLAD score, i.e. 0.06.

In the first case, when the VLAD score is high, the two sets (optimal versus weights of the similar image) of weights are strongly correlated $r = 0.94$. The difference between the method *LS ALL* (which represents the upper-bound of performance) and the WMSI method is limited: -0.012 and -0.015 for the metrics CC and HitRate, respectively. For this case, the WMSI method provides better results than GBVS and *avg TOP2* methods.

The loss of performance is much more significant when the similarity score is low. For image (c) and (d) in Fig. 8, the gap between *LS ALL* and WMSI becomes much more significant: -0.237 and -0.144 for the metrics CC and HitRate, respectively. The two sets of weights are here not well correlated, $r = -0.42$, and are negatively correlated. To go one step further on this point, Fig. 7(b) plots the relationship between performance loss and VLAD score on

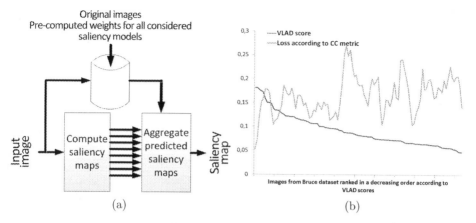

Fig. 7. (a) From a dataset composed of a number of still color images for which the vector of weights W^* is known, we compute the aggregated saliency map for any input image. The first step is to compute the 8 saliency maps according to the 8 saliency models. We search into the dataset the image which is the most similar to the input image. This search is performed by using the VLAD method. The result of this search query is a set of optimal weights. They are used to combine the 8 saliency maps. (b) Loss of performance for the metric CC in function of VLAD score on Bruce's dataset. We ranked these images in the decreasing order according to the similarity score VLAD.

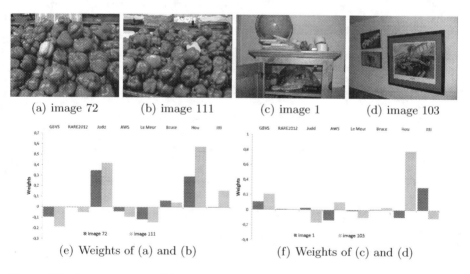

Fig. 8. Weights differences: (a) to (d) represent four images extracted from Bruce's dataset. (b) is the nearest neighbors of (a) and (d) is the nearest neighbors of (c) according to the VLAD score. (e) and (f) are the weights for the pair of images (a) and (b) and the pair of images (c) and (d), respectively.

Bruce's dataset. The Y-axis displays the loss of performance when considering the CC metric. To display the trend line, we smooth the raw data with a sliding average window using the two past and two next values. We observe that the loss of performance in terms of CC metric is correlated to the similarity score VLAD (the correlation coefficient is $r = -0.41$). The more similar the two images, the less important is the loss.

These results suggest that a supervised method might improve the quality of saliency map, provided that we succeed in finding an image similar to the input one. However, regarding the trade-off quality of prediction versus complexity, our study suggests that the simple average of the two best saliency maps is already a good candidate.

4   Conclusion

In this paper, we investigate whether the aggregation of saliency maps can improve the quality of eye fixation prediction or not. Simple aggregation methods are tested as well as the supervised learning methods. Our experiments, requiring the computation of more than 100,000 saliency maps, show that saliency aggregation can consistently improve the performance in predicting where observers look within a scene. Among the 6 tested unsupervised methods, the best method is the simple average of the saliency maps from the top 2 best models. Considering more saliency maps do not allow to further improve the performance. Concerning the supervised learning approaches, they do not succeed in improving the performance on average. This is mainly due to the image matching: if the similarity score between the input image and its most similar image is low, the trained weights for combining the predicted saliency maps are not appropriate. However, when the similarity score is high, we provide evidence that the loss is limited, compared to the upper bound for which the weights are estimated by minimizing the prediction error.

For critical applications for which the relevance and robustness of the saliency map are fundamental such as video surveillance [22], object detection [23], clinical diagnostic [24], implementation of traffic sign [25], the conclusion of this study is interesting; the robustness of the prediction can be indeed enhanced by either averaging the saliency maps of the top 2 models or by considering a dedicated training dataset.

Future works will deal with the improvement of the learning methods as well as other retrieval methods, given a query image. In this context, it will be also required to define and build a very large database of eye tracking data.

Acknowledgment. This work is supported in part by a Marie Curie International Incoming Fellowship within the 7th European Community Framework Programme under Grant No. 299202 and No. 911202, and in part by the National Natural Science Foundation of China under Grant No. 61171144. We thank Dr. Wanlei Zhao for his technical assistance for computing the VLAD scores.

References

1. Koch, C., Ullman, S.: Shifts in selective visual attention: towards the underlying neural circuitry. Human Neurobiol. **4**, 219–227 (1985)
2. Borji, A., Itti, L.: State-of-the-art in visual attention modeling. IEEE Trans. Pattern Anal. Mach. Intell. **35**, 185–207 (2013)
3. Harel, J., Koch, C., Perona, P.: Graph-based visual saliency. In: Proceedings of Neural Information Processing Systems (NIPS) (2006)
4. Le Meur, O., Le Callet, P., Barba, D., Thoreau, D.: A coherent computational approach to model the bottom-up visual attention. IEEE Trans. PAMI **28**, 802–817 (2006)
5. Garcia-Diaz, A., Fdez-Vidal, X.R., Pardo, X.M., Dosil, R.: Saliency from hierarchical adaptation through decorrelation and variance normalization. Image Vis. Comput. **30**, 51–64 (2012)
6. Itti, L., Koch, C., Niebur, E.: A model for saliency-based visual attention for rapid scene analysis. IEEE Trans. PAMI **20**, 1254–1259 (1998)
7. Bruce, N., Tsotsos, J.: Saliency, attention and visual search: an information theoretic approach. J. Vis. **9**, 1–24 (2009)
8. Hou, X., Zhang, L.: Saliency detection: A spectral residual approach. In: CVPR (2007)
9. Borji, A., Sihite, D.N., Itti, L.: Salient object detection: A benchmark. In: Fitzgibbon, A., Lazebnik, S., Perona, P., Sato, Y., Schmid, C. (eds.) ECCV 2012, Part II. LNCS, vol. 7573, pp. 414–429. Springer, Heidelberg (2012)
10. Mai, L., Niu, Y., Feng, L.: Saliency aggregation: a data-driven approach. In: CVPR (2013)
11. Liu, Z., Zou, W., Le Meur, O.: Saliency tree: A novel saliency detection framework. IEEE Trans. Image Process. **23**, 1937–1952 (2014)
12. Judd, T., Ehinger, K., Durand, F., Torralba, A.: Learning to predict where people look. In: ICCV (2009)
13. Riche, N., Mancas, M., Duvinage, M., Mibulumukini, M., Gosselin, B., Dutoit, T.: Rare 2012: A multi-scale rarity-based saliency detection with its comparative statistical analysis. Sig. Process. Image Commun. **28**, 642–658 (2013)
14. Boykov, Y., Kolmogorov, V.: An experimental comparison of min-cut/max-flow algorithms for energy minimization in vision. IEEE Trans. PAMI **26**, 1124–1137 (2004)
15. Le Meur, O., Baccino, T.: Methods for comparing scanpaths and saliency maps: strengths and weaknesses. Behav. Res. Method **1**, 1–16 (2012)
16. Roweis, S., Saul, L.: Nonlinear dimensionality reduction by locally linear embedding. Science **5500**, 2323–2326 (2000)
17. Lee, D.D., Seung, H.S.: Algorithms for non-negative matrix factorization. In: Advances in Neural Information Processing System, (NIPS) (2000)
18. Huber, P.: Robust regression: Asymptotics, conjectures and monte carlo. Ann. Stat. **1**, 799–821 (1973)
19. Peters, R.J., Iyer, A., Itti, L., Koch, C.: Components of bottom-up gaze allocation in natural images. Vis. Res. **45**, 2397–2416 (2005)
20. Borji, A., Sihite, D.N., Itti, L.: Quantitative analysis of human-model agreement in visual saliency modeling: A comparative study. IEEE Trans. Image Process. **22**, 55–69 (2012)
21. Jégou, H., Perronnin, F., Douze, M., Sánchez, J., Pérez, P., Schmid, C.: Aggregating local image descriptors into compact codes. IEEE Trans. Pattern Anal. Mach. Intell. **34**, 1704–1716 (2012)

22. Yubing, T., Cheikh, F., Guraya, F., Konik, H., Trémeau, A.: A spatiotemporal saliency model for video surveillance. Cogn. Comput. **3**, 241–263 (2011)
23. Liu, Z., Zhang, X., Luo, S., Le Meur, O.: Superpixel-based spatiotemporal saliency detection. IEEE Trans. Circuits Syst. Video Technol. **24**, 1522–1540 (2014)
24. Mamede, S., Splinter, T., van Gog, T., Rikers, R.M.J.P., Schmidt, H.: Exploring the role of salient distracting clinical features in the emergence of diagnostic errors and the mechanisms through which reflection counteracts mistakes. BMJ Qual. Saf. **21**, 295–300 (2012)
25. Won, W.J., Lee, M., Son, J.W.: Implementation of road traffic signs detection based on saliency map model. In: Intelligent Vehicles Symposium, pp. 542–547 (2008)

Spontaneous Subtle Expression Recognition: Imbalanced Databases and Solutions

Anh Cat Le Ngo[1]([✉]), Raphael Chung-Wei Phan[1], and John See[2]

[1] Faculty of Engineering, Multimedia University (MMU), Cyberjaya, Malaysia
lengoanhcat@gmail.com, raphael@mmu.edu.my
[2] Faculty of Computing and Informatics,
Multimedia University (MMU), Cyberjaya, Malaysia
johnsee@mmu.edu.my

Abstract. Facial expression analysis has been well studied in recent years; however, these mainly focus on domains of posed or clear facial expressions. Meanwhile, subtle/micro-expressions are rarely analyzed, due to three main difficulties: inter-class similarity (hardly discriminate facial expressions of two subtle emotional states from a person), intra-class dissimilarity (different facial morphology and behaviors of two subjects in one subtle emotion state), and imbalanced sample distribution for each class and subject. This paper aims to solve the last two problems by first employing preprocessing steps: facial registration, cropping and interpolation; and proposes a person-specific AdaBoost classifier with Selective Transfer Machine framework. While preprocessing techniques remove morphological facial differences, the proposed variant of AdaBoost deals with imbalanced characteristics of available subtle expression databases. Performance metrics obtained from experiments on the SMIC and CASME2 spontaneous subtle expression databases confirm that the proposed method improves classification of subtle emotions.

1 Introduction

Emotion recognition is an ability which human beings learn through observations of facial expressions. Recognizing normal expressions tends to be easy; however, recognizing subtle or micro-expressions proves to be more elusive for untrained eye. Recognizing subtle facial expressions is a difficult task because of their very brief durations ($1/3$ s to $1/25$ s); moreover, they usually happen suddenly and involuntarily. Frank et al. [1] sets up psychological experiments to quantify how accurate untrained and trained people can recognize five different subtle emotions of unseen subjects. It reported that a naive group achieved 32 % accuracy while even a trained group can only achieve 47 % accuracy. While these small expressions are easily misinterpreted, psychological studies [2,3] show that subtle expressions sometimes convey vital information such as a brief glimpse into concealed and suppressed feelings. Therefore, affective computer

---

This work was funded by TM under UbeAware project.

D. Cremers et al. (Eds.): ACCV 2014, Part IV, LNCS 9006, pp. 33–48, 2015.
DOI: 10.1007/978-3-319-16817-3_3

vision-based recognition systems could improve emotion-related activities. For instance, police could have non-intrusive means for monitoring suspects' abnormal and subtle emotions, doctors could use the system for identifying patients' responses through their subtle expressions; mediators could understand whether their offers would satisfy other parties, etc. These scenarios would be unrealistic without extremely accurate systems which could even outperform highly trained human experts.

Like any other developments of machine learning systems, the first important step is the preparation of training and testing samples. Though posed or normal expression databases are popular and highly accessible, subtle expressions databases are not easy to build due to complex collecting procedures. Video samples need to be recorded spontaneously while subjects are told to conceal their emotions after viewing short video clips. Ground-truths and duration of video samples are identified by human-experts who have undergone intensive Micro Expression Training Tools (METT) courses [4]. Due to these high requirements, their availability are scarce. So far, there are only three publicly released datasets: SMIC [5], CASME1 [6], and CASME2 [7]. As CASME2 is the latest extension of CASME1 from the same group of researchers, utilization of CASME2 alone will be sufficiently thorough. While both CASME2 and SMIC are recommended databases for evaluating subtle expression recognition systems, their imbalanced nature of the data distribution across expression classes and subjects, would be a challenging ordeal for generic classifiers. This problem needs careful consideration in the development of any subtle expression recognition system.

This paper aims to analyze the imbalances of spontaneous micro-expression databases (CASME2 and SMIC) as well as to propose an effective and robust subtle expression recognition scheme. Section 2 shows statistical composition of CASME2 and SMIC across different classes and subjects, notably high skewness of the databases especially when leave-one-subject-out is the main cross-validation approach. Furthermore, variety in frame lengths of video samples, another imbalanced characteristic of the databases, directly affects feature-extraction stage. Section 3 proposes a robust system toward addressing those imbalances. At first preprocessing steps like facial cropping and registration in Sect. 3.1 are employed to remove morphological facial differences. Then, temporal interpolation (TIM) is utilized for equalizing frame lengths among samples in Sect. 3.2, and LBP-TOP extracts spatial-temporal texture features from these samples in Sect. 3.3. Finally, a person-specific AdaBoost filter, a combination of general adaBoost classifier and selective transfer machine (STM) framework, is introduced for solving imbalanced natures of spontaneous subtle expression databases in Sects. 3.4, 3.5, and 3.6. Experimental results are shown and discussed in Sect. 4 for CASME2 and SMIC databases to verify robustness and usefulness of the proposed solutions. Section 5 summarizes aims and achievements of this paper.

2   Statistical Study of CASME2 and SMIC

Before SMIC and CASME2 databases are chosen as main data of spontaneous subtle expression for training, testing and evaluating the recognition system, they have to be statistically studied throughly. The CASME2 database has 257 video samples with frame rate of 60 frame per seconds (*fps*) and collected from 26 subjects. The SMIC database has 16 subjects and 164 samples with frame rate of 100 *fps*. Besides these differences in number of subjects and frame rates, CASME2 and SMIC also differ in terms of the distribution of samples with respect to expression classes. The CASME2 database has five different subtle-expression classes: happiness, disgust, repression, surprise and tense, labeled from C1 to C5 accordingly. The distribution of video samples across these classes is rather non-uniform, and this is reflected by the number of samples for each expression shown in Table 1. Meanwhile, SMIC has only three classes of subtle emotions: positive, negative and surprise, of which labels given are S1, S2 and S3 respectively.

As leave-one-subject-out cross validation (LOSOCV), which take test samples from only single subject and use sample from the other subjects as training samples, is recommended by several facial macro-expression recognition works [8,9], it is necessary to analyze how video samples are distributed according to both subjects and expression classes. Tables 2a and b show frequency of samples according to a particular subject and expression type in CASME2 and SMIC respectively. In Table 2, only a few highlighted subjects, e.g. Subject 17 in CASME2 and Subjects 03, 04, 11, etc. in SMIC have samples for all expression classes. The rest of the subjects have no samples in at least one expression class. Furthermore, the number of samples is not distributed equally among available classes as well, e.g. Subject 17 of CASME2 database has 14 samples in C2 class but only 1 sample in C4 class. By this observation, it is clear that samples are non-uniformly distributed to each class and subject.

Table 1. Distribution of samples in CASME2 and SMIC databases

CASME2			SMIC		
Emotion	Label	# samples	Emotion	Label	# samples
Happiness	C1	33	Positive	S1	51
Disgust	C2	60	Negative	S2	70
Repression	C3	25	Surprise	S3	43
Surprise	C4	27			
Tense	C5	102			

Distribution of databases also depends on whether video frame or video samples are considered as a basic unit. For examples, if each C# class has a video sample, each class occupies 20 % of the database according to video samples. However, if the C1 sample has 60 frames, the rest has 10 frames each sample, the distribution according to video frames are 60 % for C1, 10 % for C2, C3, C4, C5. As CASME2 and SMIC samples are recorded at various frame rates and durations, each sample has different frame lengths. Therefore, distributions of video samples and frames are unnecessarily and rarely identical. Furthermore,

Table 2. Numbers of samples and frames according to subjects and emotions

(a) CASME2

	# samples					# frames				
	C1	**C2**	**C3**	**C4**	**C5**	**C1**	**C2**	**C3**	**C4**	**C5**
01	1	2			6	41	177			279
02	1		5	3	4	100		459	193	344
03		1		1	5		61		41	370
04		2			3		142			158
05	1	1		5	12	61	55		305	805
06	1	1		2	1	56	58		101	46
07		6			3		383			198
08			1		2			78		193
09	6		5		3	481		490		268
10					13					934
11		4			6		314			450
12	2	5		4	1	173	354		318	66
13	2				6	157				305
14	3				1	203				76
15	1			1	1	61			91	58
16	2		1		1	182		24		113
17	7	14	9	1	3	453	876	605	91	126
18					3					144
19	3	3		5	3	272	178		275	143
20		2			9		82			578
21			1		1			96		31
22			2					203		
23	1	4	3		4	95	303	232		254
24		3		1	4		181		36	162
25		3		2	2		153		154	145
26	2	9			5	171	602			328

(b) SMIC

	# samples			# frames		
	S1	**S2**	**S3**	**S1**	**S2**	**S3**
01	1	3	2	33	95	53
02	5		1	168		29
03	6	22	11	159	627	308
04	5	10	4	146	268	117
05	1	1		43	30	
06	2	2		66	75	
07						
08		9	4		313	138
09	3		1	108		42
10						
11	1	3	3	32	93	141
12	1		8	38		313
13			10			409
14	5	3	2	199	147	99
15	2	1	1	74	50	49
16						
17						
18	5	2		173	85	
19	1		1	50		35
20	5	14	3	174	433	115

note that each sample video clip is the result of clipping a long continuous video footage of each subject over time based on detected onset and offset points, i.e. when an expression is first spotted and when it is no longer observed, respectively. The number of times a subject could exhibit a particular expression would vary from across subjects and across types of expressions.

Figures 1 and 2 show normalized distributions of samples and frames for databases CASME2 and SMIC with respect to expression classes and a single selected subject. Subject indexes are shown in horizontal axes and there are a number of columns with various colors representing amount of samples available at each expression class of the subject. In general, the distributions of samples and frames in both databases are slightly different from each other. This discrepancy becomes more apparent when a single subject is considered; for example, Subject 25 of CASME2 in Fig. 1 (left side) and Subject 11 of SMIC in Fig. 2 (left side).

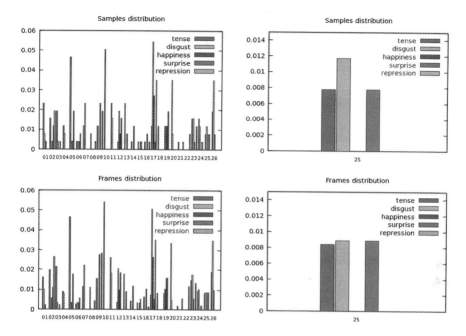

Fig. 1. CASME2 database analysis

3   Subtle Expression Recognition

As unevenly distributed databases can cause significant problems to any machine learning system, this paper proposes robust techniques to tackle this imbalance in subtle expression recognition. As biases in the two spontaneous subtle expression databases were previously analyzed, this section focuses on describing the techniques used in our robust system to mitigate the imbalance. The solution follows the common 3-stage framework: preprocessing, feature extraction and classification. The first stage standardizes samples spatially by cropping faces according to eye positions using a Haar eye detector and registers faces of multiple subjects to a common facial model with fiducial points from Active Shape Model (ASM) [10]. Temporally, it also ensures the same number of frames are uniform for all samples by applying temporal interpolation model (TIM) [5]. In the second stage, Local Binary Pattern with Three Orthogonal Planes (LBP-TOP) [11], a spatio-temporal local texture descriptor, is used to extract the main features for the learning and classification stage. As leave-one-subject-out cross-validation (LOSOCV) is adopted in the evaluation process, we propose a person-specific AdaBoost classifier with Selective Transfer Machine (STM) framework to deal with the person-specific bias and imbalanced training and testing datasets.

3.1   Face Cropping and Local Weighted Mean Transformation

As expressions are only caused by facial muscles, other background visual information is deemed to be irrelevant; therefore, it is filtered out from input data.

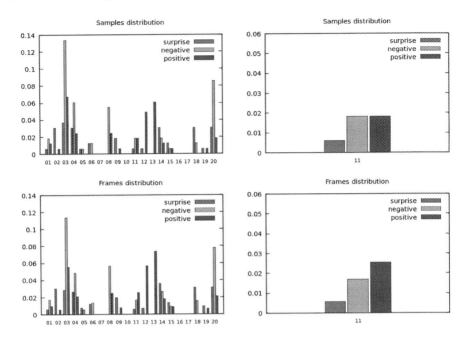

Fig. 2. SMIC database analysis

In addition, facial structures of each subject are distinguished from each other, which is helpful in recognizing subjects' identity but obstructive towards generalizing classifiers for expressions (intra-class dissimilarity). Therefore, faces of multiple subjects need standardizing into a single common facial model M.

Let $S = [s_i | i = 1, \ldots, N]$ be a set of N subtle expression samples and each ith sample be $s_i = [f_{i,j}, j = 1, \ldots, n_i]$, where n_i is the number of video frames for each ith sequence s_i. A model face M is built from 68 facial landmark points $\psi(M)$, detected by ASM from a frontal face of a chosen subject in the database. Facial coordinates of the first frame $f_{i,1}$, i.e. $\psi(f_{i,1})$, are then used to estimate parameters of Local Weighted Mean (LWM) [12] transformation.

$$T = LWM(\psi(M), \psi(f_{i,i}))$$

This T can linearly transform faces from the rest of the sequence s_i according to the model face M. Finally, eye coordinates localized by a standard Haar feature-based cascaded eye detector are checked against the ASM coordinates and used to crop the transformed faces.

3.2   Temporal Interpolation Model

Video samples with different frame lengths may cause biases in the feature extraction and classification stages. Therefore, the temporal interpolating model (TIM) presented in [5,13] is used for standardizing the number of frames in each sequence. This technique is able to produce the same number of frames for each sequence to reduce the bias effected upon the later stages. Previously, Zhou et al. [13] employed the TIM for synthesizing a talking mouth while Pfister et al. [5] applied it to micro-expression recognition to increase frame lengths before feature extraction. In this paper, we use TIM to balance the frame lengths across all samples in a database to provide temporal standardization. TIM operates on the assumption that frames of subtle expression samples form a continuous function, a curve in a low-dimensional manifold. In other words, a sequence of frames can be represented by a path graph P_n with n vertices, corresponding to n frames. Edges of P_n form an adjacency matrix $\mathbf{W} \in \{0,1\}^{n,n}$ whereof $W_n = 1$ means direct connection between two vertices and $W_n = 0$ means otherwise. Mathematically, edges are defined as follows.

$$W_{i,j} = \begin{cases} 1, & \text{if } |i - j| = 1 \\ 0, & \text{otherwise} \end{cases} \tag{1}$$

Parameters of manifolds, for n embedded vertices, can be found by mapping P_n to a line such that it minimizes distances between connected vertices.

$$\underset{\mathbf{y}}{\arg\min} \sum_{i,j} (y_i - y_j)^2 W_{i,j}, \quad i, j = 1, 2, \ldots, n \tag{2}$$

where $\mathbf{y} = (y_1, y_2, \ldots, y_n)$ are projections of video frames on the manifold of the graph path P_n. Obtaining $\mathbf{y}$ is equivalent to calculating the eigenvectors of the Laplacian graph of P_n such that it has eigenvectors $\mathbf{y_1}, \mathbf{y_2}, \ldots, \mathbf{y_{n-1}}$. Linear extension of graph embedding [14] allows finding linear projection w from zero-mean vectorized image x such that the objective function (2) is satisfied.

$$\underset{w}{\arg\min} \sum_{i,j} (\mathbf{w}^\mathbf{T}\mathbf{x_i} - \mathbf{w}^\mathbf{T}\mathbf{x_j})^2 W_{i,j}, \quad i, j = 1, 2, \ldots, n \tag{3}$$

He et al. [15] solves the resulting eigenvalue problem

$$\mathbf{XLX^Tw} = \lambda' \mathbf{XX^Tw} \tag{4}$$

by using the singular value decomposition with $\mathbf{X} = \mathbf{U \Sigma V^T}$. In [13], Zhou et al. show that the interpolated images can be computed as follows:

$$x = \mathbf{UM}\mathcal{F}^n(t) \tag{5}$$

where $\mathbf{M}$ is a square matrix and $\mathcal{F}^n(t)$ is a resulting curve of the Laplacian graph P_n. Let $\theta \in \{10, 15, 20\}$ be the number of interpolated frames for each video sample. The best value for θ is determined empirically by experiments for each evaluated database.

3.3   Local Binary Pattern with Three Orthogonal Planes

Local Binary Pattern (LBP) [16] is a popular texture operator that thresholds the local neighborhoods of each pixel in an image and converts them into a binary value. The binary values are then counted to form a histogram of different binary patterns. Zhao et al. [11] extended the LBP to LBP-TOP for use with dynamic spatio-temporal textures. LBP-TOP performs the classic LBP on all three orthogonal planes (XY, XY, YT) lying in a volumetric neighborhood. As a result, three sets of descriptors along the three orthogonal planes— LBP_{XY}, LBP_{YZ}, and LBP_{XZ}, are then concatenated into a single histogram to extract the features for each sample clip. Owing to its robustness towards illumination and noise, LBP-TOP is our choice of feature extractor in our proposed scheme.

3.4 Selective Transfer Machine

In Sect. 3.2, the proposed system utilizes TIM before LBP-TOP feature extraction to solve imbalances of datasets caused by differences in frame lengths between video samples. This section focuses on imbalances caused by leave-one-subject-out cross-validation (LOSOCV) approach. It is due to infrequent distribution of training and testing video samples among subjects, as shown in Table 3a for the CASME2 corpus and Table 3b for the SMIC corpus and thoroughly described in Sect. 2. Though this imbalance is apparent, it is unavoidable due to practical difficulties in psychological experiments of collecting and evaluating spontaneous subtle emotion databases [6,7,17]. In these experiments, after stimuli are shown to subjects, their facial responses are recorded continuously in a long video, which is then post-processed into several short clips according to particular expressions exhibited at different moments. Subjects respond differently to the same stimuli; for instances, females express wider and more intense emotions than males do [18]. These differences would affect judgments of METT experts about types, numbers, on/off-set frames of subtle emotions samples.

As both released corpora of spontaneous subtle expressions suffer from biases while the existence of perfectly unbiased databases is highly improbable, it is necessary to develop domain adapted learning algorithms which can cope with such modern biased datasets [19]. Aytar and Zisserman [20] suggest utilization of pre-learned models in regularizing the training of new object class. Khosla et al. [21] integrate a specific and a common discriminative model to remove biases. These techniques are supervised solutions requiring one or more labeled test samples in advance. This requirement is unrealistic for some subjects in CASME2 and SMIC corpora since there is only one sample for one expression. Moreover, it is infeasible to identify subtle emotions of unseen subjects without METT trained experts.

Therefore, our proposed recognition system employs Selective Transfer Machine (STM), an unsupervised approach that re-samples weights for each training sample in order to fill up gaps or mismatches between distributions of training and testing samples. The STM framework jointly optimizes weights of training samples as well as losses of any classifiers; thus, preserving the discriminative property of decision boundaries on the re-weighted dataset. Furthermore, performances of any classifier trained on this dataset should improve since its model would more likely fit better to the testing dataset. As STM is a classifier-independent technique, there exists a single general formulation regardless of the

Table 3. Training and Testing Sample Distribution

(a) CASME2   (b) SMIC

	# samples									
	training					testing				
	C1	C2	C3	C4	C5	C1	C2	C3	C4	C5
01	32	58	27	25	96	1	2	0	0	6
02	32	60	22	22	98	1	0	5	3	4
03	33	59	27	24	97	0	1	0	1	5
04	33	58	27	25	99	0	2	0	0	3
05	32	59	27	20	90	1	1	0	5	12
06	32	59	27	23	101	1	1	0	2	1
07	33	54	27	25	99	0	6	0	0	3
08	33	60	26	25	100	0	0	1	0	2
09	27	60	22	25	99	6	0	5	0	3
10	33	60	27	25	89	0	0	0	0	13
11	33	56	27	25	96	0	4	0	0	6
12	31	55	27	21	101	2	5	0	4	1
13	31	60	27	25	96	2	0	0	0	6
14	30	60	27	25	101	3	0	0	0	1
15	32	60	27	24	101	1	0	0	1	1
16	31	60	26	25	101	2	0	1	0	1
17	26	46	18	24	99	7	14	9	1	3
18	33	60	27	25	99	0	0	0	0	3
19	30	57	27	20	99	3	3	0	5	3
20	33	58	27	25	93	0	2	0	0	9
21	33	60	26	25	101	0	0	1	0	1
22	33	60	25	25	102	0	0	2	0	0
23	32	56	24	25	98	1	4	3	0	4
24	33	57	27	24	98	0	3	0	1	4
25	33	57	27	23	100	0	3	0	2	2
26	31	51	27	25	97	2	9	0	0	5

	# samples					
	training			testing		
	S1	S2	S3	S1	S2	S3
01	49	67	42	2	3	1
02	50	70	38	1	0	5
03	40	48	37	11	22	6
04	47	60	38	4	10	5
05	51	69	42	0	1	1
06	51	68	41	0	2	2
07	51	70	43	0	0	0
08	47	61	43	4	9	0
09	50	70	40	1	0	3
10	51	70	43	0	0	0
11	48	67	42	3	3	1
12	43	70	42	8	0	1
13	41	70	43	10	0	0
14	49	67	38	2	3	5
15	50	69	41	1	1	2
16	51	70	43	0	0	0
17	51	70	43	0	0	0
18	51	68	38	0	2	5
19	50	70	42	1	0	1
20	48	56	38	3	14	5

choice of classifiers or classifiers' parameters. Let a training set be denoted as $\mathcal{D}^{tr} = \{\mathbf{x}_i, y_i\}_{i=1}^{n^{tr}}, y_i \in \{+1, -1\}$, STM can be formulated as:

$$(\mathbf{w}, \mathbf{s}) = \arg\min_{\mathbf{w},\mathbf{s}} R_{\mathbf{w}}(\mathcal{D}^{tr}, \mathbf{s}) + \lambda \Omega_{\mathbf{s}}(\mathbf{X}^{tr}, \mathbf{X}^{te}) \qquad (6)$$

where $R_{\mathbf{w}}(\mathcal{D}^{tr}, \mathbf{s})$ is the classifier loss on $\mathcal{D}^{tr}$ with vector of weights for each instance $\mathbf{s} \in \mathbb{R}^{n^{tr}}$, and learning coefficients $\mathbf{w}$. $\Omega_{\mathbf{s}}(\mathbf{X}^{tr}, \mathbf{X}^{te})$ measures dissimilarity between training and testing distribution. λ is a trade-off constant to balance the loss and distribution dissimilarity. As STM simultaneously optimizes a classifier loss and shifts a model such that it fits a subject's testing samples better, the final model can effectively remove biases caused by the person-specific bias.

3.5   AdaBoost Classifier

A boosted classifier is a linear combination of several weak classifiers in the form $\mathbf{H}(\mathbf{x}) = \sum_t w_t \mathbf{h}_t(\mathbf{x})$. It can be trained by greedily minimizing a loss function ϵ or optimizing scalar w_t and weaker learners $\mathbf{h_t}()$. Initially, a non-negative weight w_i derived from loss function ϵ is assigned to each sample $\mathbf{x_i}$ at the beginning. After each iteration, misclassified samples are weighted more heavily; thereby, losses of getting the same samples misclassified become severe in the next iterations. This is the basic principle of boosting algorithms (AdaBoost,LogitBoost, or L2Boost). They all need to iteratively classify samples given the sample weights.

In this paper, shallow trees are chosen as weak learners. The decision trees h_{TREE}, composed of a stump $h_j(\mathbf{x})$ at every non-leaf nodes j, are quickly trained in the manner proposed by Appel et al. [22]. Each stump generates a binary decision given an input $\mathbf{x} \in R^K$, polarity parameter $p \in \{\pm 1\}$, a threshold $\tau \in R$ and a feature index $k \in \{1, 2, \ldots, K\}$.

$$h_j(\mathbf{x}) = p_j \text{sign}(\mathbf{x}[k_j] - \tau_j) \tag{7}$$

Decision stump training can be used for classification if the goal at each stage is minimizing the weighted classification error ϵ.

$$\epsilon = \frac{1}{Z} \left[\sum_{\mathbf{x_i}[k] \leq \tau} w_i \mathbf{1}_{\{y_i = +p\}} + \sum_{\mathbf{x_i}[k] > \tau} w_i \mathbf{1}_{\{y_i = -p\}} \right], \quad Z = \sum w_i \tag{8}$$

This error is minimized by selecting a single best feature k^* from all features K at each iteration. Determining the optimal threshold τ^* is costly due to $\mathcal{O}(N, K)$ accumulation of N weights, corresponding to N samples $\mathbf{x_i}[k]$, into discrete bins of feature values and indexes histogram. Appel et al. proves a bound on error of a decision stump given its preliminary errors on a subset of training data, which helps to identify and prune unpromising features early. In this paper, a fast AdaBoost training algorithm [22] is utilized to exploit this bound which reduces training time by an order of magnitude without any loss in performances.

3.6   Person-Specific AdaBoost Classifier

AdaBoost, a generic classifier, is regarded as a versatile algorithm in machine learning. However, it is not designed to accommodate person-specific bias, which often occurs in the LOSOCV approach. Moreover, AdaBoost neglects individual marked variety in facial morphology and behavior so it does not cope well with imbalanced data and generalize well to unseen faces well. Therefore, this paper proposes Person-specific AdaBoost classifier, which integrates AdaBoost with STM framework to transfer knowledge of testing samples onto distribution of training samples. Based on the generic classifier with STM defined by Eq. 6, the AdaBoost classifier with STM is formulated as,

$$(\mathbf{w}, \mathbf{s}) = \underset{\mathbf{w}, \mathbf{s}}{\arg \min} \, \epsilon_{\mathbf{w}}(\mathcal{D}^{tr}, \mathbf{s}) + \lambda \Omega_{\mathbf{s}}(\mathbf{X}^{tr}, \mathbf{X}^{te}) \tag{9}$$

where $\epsilon_{\mathbf{w}}$ is the loss function of AdaBoost classifier (Eq. 8). To minimize Eq. 9 requires Alternate Convex Search method [23] since the STM objective function in Eq. 9 is biconvex, i.e. convex in $\mathbf{w}$ when $\mathbf{s}$ is fixed, and convex in $\mathbf{s}$ when $\mathbf{w}$ is fixed. A biconvex problem is guaranteed to converge with alternated optimization approach since its objective function monotonically converged to a critical point. The optimization process is shown in Algorithm 1.

Algorithm 1. AdaBoost with Selective Transfer Machine

Input: $\mathbf{X}^{tr}$, $\mathbf{X}^{te}$, number of weak classifiers N , λ
Output: instance-wise weights $\mathbf{w}$ of modified adaBoost and $\mathbf{s}$ of STM
    Initialize training loss $\epsilon_{\mathbf{w}} \leftarrow 0$;
    for i = 1:N **do**
        Find $\mathbf{s}$ of STM by solving the QP in Eq. 10.
        Find $\mathbf{w}$ of AdaBoost by solving the modified AdaBoost in Eq. 11
    end for

Fixing w and Minimizing over s: Denote training losses as $\epsilon_w = \epsilon_w(D^{tr}, \mathbf{s})$. The optimization over $\mathbf{s}$ $\Omega_s(X^{tr}, X^{te})$ in Eq. 6 can be re-written as a quadratic programming (QP) problem.

$$\min_s \frac{1}{2}\mathbf{s}^T\mathbf{K}\mathbf{s} + \left(\frac{C}{\lambda}\epsilon - \kappa\right) \tag{10}$$

$$\text{s.t. } 0 \leq s_i B, n_{tr}(1 - \epsilon) \leq \sum_{i=1}^{n_{tr}} s_i \leq n_{tr}(1 + \epsilon)$$

where $\mathbf{K}$ is a nonlinear kernel matrix of training samples, κ measures closeness between training and each test sample, and B defines upper bound of weights $\mathbf{s}$. This can be solved efficiently by interior point methods or Alternating Direction Method of Multipliers (ADMM) [24]. Further details on how this problem is optimized can be found in [25].

Fixing s and Minimizing over w: As STM is formulated regardless of the types of classifier, the objective function (Eq. 6) can take on a modified AdaBoost loss function (Eq. 8) instead of a general loss function $R_{\mathbf{w}}(\mathcal{D}^{tr}, \mathbf{s})$:

$$\epsilon_s(\mathcal{D}^{tr}, \mathbf{w}) = \frac{1}{Z}\left[\sum_{\mathbf{x_i}[k]\leq\tau} s_i w_i \mathbf{1}_{\{y_i=+p\}} + \sum_{\mathbf{x_i}[k]>\tau} s_i w_i \mathbf{1}_{\{y_i=-p\}}\right], \quad Z = \sum s_i w_i \tag{11}$$

where s_i is a weight assigned to the ith sample for matching distributions of training and testing data, and w_i is an instance-wise weight identifying risks of misclassifying the ith sample. Beside additional weights s_i, the optimization processes strictly follow proposals by Appel et al. [22].

4   Experiments and Discussion

In Sects. 2 and 3.4, CASME2 and SMIC databases, two most comprehensive spontaneous subtle expressions databases, are statistically analyzed for their imbalance in a leave-one-subject-out cross-validation setting. Hence, these databases are suitable for evaluating the effectiveness of the proposed method in dealing with such imbalances. The experiments are set up with the following common parameters: number of interpolated frames for TIM and learning method AdaBoost with or without STM. Results demonstrate that rebalancing the number of frames in each sample by TIM interpolation can improve classifier performances and show the effectiveness of STM in personalizing a generic classifier AdaBoost while partly reducing person-specific bias during classification.

There are specific settings for CASME2 and SMIC due to different composition in each database. For instance, 5-class classification of subtle emotions (happiness, disgust, repression, tense, surprise) is performed on the CASME2 while SMIC is a 3-class classification problem (positive, negative and surprise). Furthermore, LBP-TOP extracts features from CASME2 and SMIC using different sets of parameters. Let us denote $R = (R_X, R_Y, R_T)$ as the radii of three orthogonal planes, and $S = (S_X, S_Y, S_T)$ as the number of block partitions used along the X, Y and T dimensions. More details on these LBP-TOP parameters can be found in [11]. In CASME2 database, LBP-TOP is used with the parameters $R = (1, 1, 4)$, $S = (5, 5, 1)$ while the LBP-TOP parameters for SMIC database are fixed to $R = (1, 1, 4)$, $S = (8, 8, 1)$. These values are suggested by the authors of each respective database [5, 7].

Besides the usage of commonly used parameters, fairness in evaluation also depends on the choice of performance metrics. For machine learning problems and classification tasks on highly skewed databases (like CASME2 and SMIC), the *accuracy* rate is an inadequate measure of the effectiveness of a classifier despite its popularity in literature. This is due to its susceptibility of inaccuracies due to heavily skewed data, i.e. unequal number of samples per class. The accuracy metric shows the average "hit rate" of all classes; therefore, it does not reflect how well a machine learning method performs for each class. Therefore, additional metrics such as *precision, recall* and *f-measure* are necessary to provide a better measure of a classifier's performance [26].

For a multi-class classification task, confusion matrices proved to be more informative about behaviors of the evaluated classifier. The confusion tables are well-summarized by precision, recall and f-measure if a correctly retrieved positive data is the only important target. Each measure is the average of the same measures calculated for each class to evaluate unbalanced classes fairly regardless of the number of samples they have. In a binary or one-versus-all multi-class classification, precision is the number of true positive samples divided by the number of classified positive samples. Recall is the number of true positive samples divided by the number of ground-truth positive samples. F-measure is the overall combination of precision and recall which reflects relations between classified positive examples and ground-truth positive examples. As the leave-one-subject-out cross-validation (LOSOCV) approach is employed, evaluating the

Table 4. Performance evaluation of subtle expression classification with leave-one-subject-out cross-validation

(a) CASME2 - 5-class recognition

No	Learning Method	TIM	Accuracy	Precision	Recall	F_measure
1	AdaBoost		0.3945	0.212	0.5095	0.2609
2	AdaBoost + STM		0.3876	0.2104	0.4824	0.2593
3	AdaBoost	TIM10	0.4015	0.2416	0.5242	0.2908
4	AdaBoost + STM	TIM10	0.4216	0.2587	0.5729	0.3077
5	AdaBoost	TIM15	0.422	0.2472	0.5455	0.3089
6	AdaBoost + STM	TIM15	**0.4378**	**0.291**	**0.532**	**0.3337**
7	AdaBoost	TIM20	0.365	0.2184	0.4414	0.2563
8	AdaBoost + STM	TIM20	0.3887	0.2257	0.4585	0.2672

(b) SMIC - 3-class recognition

No	Learning Method	TIM	Accuracy	Precision	Recall	F_measure
1	AdaBoost		0.4453	0.3424	0.6844	0.3994
2	AdaBoost + STM		0.4446	0.2947	0.6341	0.3611
3	AdaBoost	TIM10	0.4343	0.3706	0.7209	0.4356
4	AdaBoost + STM	TIM10	**0.4434**	**0.4009**	**0.7393**	**0.4731**
5	AdaBoost	TIM15	0.3677	0.2394	0.5392	0.2993
6	AdaBoost + STM	TIM15	0.3651	0.2955	0.7251	0.3703
7	AdaBoost	TIM20	0.3855	0.3244	0.6607	0.4036
8	AdaBoost + STM	TIM20	0.4285	0.3093	0.6937	0.3848

datasets produces N measurement sets where N is a number of subjects. Thus, the final value of each measure is an average of the same measures across N subjects so that performance of classifiers are fairly evaluated and independent from imbalances in the sample distribution across subjects. Tables 4a and b show the experimental results on CASME2 and SMIC databases. Experiments 1 and 2 of both tables contain results of subtle emotions classification without equalization of frame length in each video sample; while the remaining experiments are carried out with TIM## (TIM10,TIM15,TIM20), interpolating a video sample into a fixed number {10, 15, 20} of frames. Performances on both CASME2 and SMIC show a marked improvement with deployment of TIM; for instance, experiments 3–6 in Table 4a show better classifier performance on the CASME2 corpus, especially when TIM15 is used. Meanwhile, experiments 3–4 in Table 4b demonstrate that classifiers with TIM10 outperform those without TIM, giving the best performances among all experiments on the SMIC database. These results indicate the important role of TIM in rebalancing frame lengths of video samples across the entire corpus, reducing the effect of biases on the LBP-TOP feature extraction stage. Moreover, experimental results also highlight appropriate choices in the number of interpolated frames; for instance, TIM15 for the CASME2 corpus and TIM10 for the SMIC corpus shown in Tables 4a and b. Interestingly, over-interpolation does not help but harm the performance of classifiers due to an increase in artificial noises inherited from the interpolation process. The effects of that can be observed in experiments 7–8 of Table 4a and experiments 5–8 of Table 4b.

Furthermore, experimental results also proved the importance of utilizing the Selective Transfer Machine (STM) framework in reducing the effects of person-specific biases on the overall performance of AdaBoost classifiers used. Highlighted results in the Table 4a and b demonstrate that AdaBoost classifiers with STM (on the best TIM setting discussed earlier) outperform those without STM in all four metrics, when all other parameters and conditions are identical. In general, superiority of classifiers with STM can be observed from the pair-wise results of experiments 3–4 and 5–6 on both tables; while it appears to be less obvious in experiments 7–8. Again, the unprecedented results in experiments 7, 8 may be caused by a seemingly more prominent issue of TIM over-interpolation.

5   Conclusion

Imbalanced datasets are unavoidable practical problems in developing spontaneous subtle expression classification solution especially when a leave-one-subject-out cross-validation is the main evaluation approach. This paper proposes the use of TIM and STM to tackle the imbalances in the frames and sample levels. While TIM uses interpolation techniques to equalize frame lengths for all video samples, STM helps to personalize AdaBoost classifier, attenuate person-specific bias and reduce effects of imbalanced sample distribution in training and testing datasets. Experiments and performance validation are carefully designed to quantify the effectiveness of the proposed solution. Most importantly, the experimental results confirm that the solutions improve the overall classification performance for all evaluation metrics. Future work will include further comparisons with other solutions for imbalaned datasets e.g. TrAdaBoost [27].

References

1. Frank, M., Herbasz, M., Sinuk, K., Keller, A., Nolan, C.: I see how you feel: training laypeople and professionals to recognize fleeting emotions. In: The Annual Meeting of the International Communication Association, Sheraton New York, New York City (2009)
2. Ekman, P.: Lie catching and microexpressions. In: Martin, C. (ed.) The Philosophy of Deception, pp. 118–133. Oxford University, Oxford (2009)
3. Gottman, J.M., Levenson, R.W.: A two-factor model for predicting when a couple will divorce: exploratory analyses using 14-year longitudinal data*. Fam. Process 41, 83–96 (2002)
4. Ekman, P.: Microexpression Training Tool (METT). University of California, San Francisco (2002)
5. Pfister, T., Li, X., Zhao, G., Pietikainen, M.: Recognising spontaneous facial microexpressions. In: 2011 IEEE International Conference on Computer Vision (ICCV), pp. 1449–1456. IEEE (2011)

6. Yan, W.J., Wu, Q., Liu, Y.J., Wang, S.J., Fu, X.: Casme database: a dataset of spontaneous micro-expressions collected from neutralized faces. In: 2013 10th IEEE International Conference and Workshops on Automatic Face and Gesture Recognition (FG), pp. 1–7. IEEE (2013)

7. Yan, W.J., Li, X., Wang, S.J., Zhao, G., Liu, Y.J., Chen, Y.H., Fu, X.: CASME II: an improved spontaneous micro-expression database and the baseline evaluation: an improved spontaneous micro-expression database and the baseline evaluation. PloS one **9**, e86041 (2014)

8. Lucey, P., Cohn, J.F., Kanade, T., Saragih, J., Ambadar, Z., Matthews, I.: The extended cohn-kanade dataset (ck+): a complete dataset for action unit and emotion-specified expression. In: 2010 IEEE Computer Society Conference on Computer Vision and Pattern Recognition Workshops (CVPRW), pp. 94–101. IEEE (2010)

9. Shan, C., Gong, S., McOwan, P.W.: Facial expression recognition based on local binary patterns: a comprehensive study. Image Vis. Comput. **27**, 803–816 (2009)

10. Cootes, T.F., Taylor, C.J., Cooper, D.H., Graham, J.: Active shape models-their training and application. Comput. Vis. Image Underst. **61**, 38–59 (1995)

11. Zhao, G., Pietikainen, M.: Dynamic texture recognition using local binary patterns with an application to facial expressions. IEEE Trans. Pattern Anal. Mach. Intell. **29**, 915–928 (2007)

12. Goshtasby, A.: Image registration by local approximation methods. Image Vis. Comput. **6**, 255–261 (1988)

13. Zhou, Z., Zhao, G., Pietikainen, M.: Towards a practical lipreading system. In: 2011 IEEE Conference on Computer Vision and Pattern Recognition (CVPR), pp. 137–144. IEEE (2011)

14. Yan, S., Xu, D., Zhang, B., Zhang, H.J., Yang, Q., Lin, S.: Graph embedding and extensions: a general framework for dimensionality reduction. IEEE Trans. Pattern Anal. Mach. Intell. **29**, 40–51 (2007)

15. He, X., Cai, D., Yan, S., Zhang, H.J.: Neighborhood preserving embedding. In: Tenth IEEE International Conference on Computer Vision, ICCV 2005, vol. 2, pp. 1208–1213. IEEE (2005)

16. Ojala, T., Pietikäinen, M., Mäenpää, T.: A generalized local binary pattern operator for multiresolution gray scale and rotation invariant texture classification. In: Singh, S., Murshed, N., Kropatsch, W.G. (eds.) ICAPR 2001. LNCS, vol. 2013, p. 397. Springer, Heidelberg (2001)

17. Li, X., Pfister, T., Huang, X., Zhao, G., Pietikainen, M.: A spontaneous micro-expression database: Inducement, collection and baseline. In: 2013 10th IEEE International Conference and Workshops on Automatic Face and Gesture Recognition (FG), pp. 1–6. IEEE (2013)

18. Brody, L.R., Brody, L.R.: On understanding gender differences in the expression of emotion. In: Ablon, S.L., Brown, D., Khantzian, E.J., Mack, J.E. (eds.) Human feelings: Explorations in Affect Development and Meaning. Analytic Press, Hillsdale (1993)

19. Torralba, A., Efros, A.A.: Unbiased look at dataset bias. In: 2011 IEEE Conference on Computer Vision and Pattern Recognition (CVPR), pp. 1521–1528. IEEE (2011)

20. Aytar, Y., Zisserman, A.: Tabula rasa: model transfer for object category detection. In: 2011 IEEE International Conference on Computer Vision (ICCV), pp. 2252–2259. IEEE (2011)

21. Khosla, A., Zhou, T., Malisiewicz, T., Efros, A.A., Torralba, A.: Undoing the damage of dataset bias. In: Fitzgibbon, A., Lazebnik, S., Perona, P., Sato, Y., Schmid, C. (eds.) ECCV 2012, Part I. LNCS, vol. 7572, pp. 158–171. Springer, Heidelberg (2012)

22. Appel, R., Fuchs, T., Dollár, P., Perona, P.: Quickly boosting decision trees-pruning underachieving features early. In: JMLR Workshop and Conference Proceedings, vol. 28, pp. 594–602 (2013). (JMLR)

23. Gorski, J., Pfeuffer, F., Klamroth, K.: Biconvex sets and optimization with biconvex functions: a survey and extensions. Math. Methods Oper. Res. **66**, 373–407 (2007)

24. Boyd, S., Parikh, N., Chu, E., Peleato, B., Eckstein, J.: Distributed optimization and statistical learning via the alternating direction method of multipliers. Found. Trends Mach. Learn. **3**, 1–122 (2011)

25. Chu, W.S., Torre, F.D.L., Cohn, J.F.: Selective transfer machine for personalized facial action unit detection. In: 2013 IEEE Conference on Computer Vision and Pattern Recognition (CVPR), pp. 3515–3522. IEEE (2013)

26. Sokolova, M., Lapalme, G.: A systematic analysis of performance measures for classification tasks. Inf. Process. Manag. **45**, 427–437 (2009)

27. Dai, W., Yang, Q., Xue, G.R., Yu, Y.: Boosting for transfer learning. In: Proceedings of the 24th International Conference on Machine Learning, pp. 193–200. ACM (2007)

EPML: Expanded Parts Based Metric Learning for Occlusion Robust Face Verification

Gaurav Sharma[1]([✉]), Frédéric Jurie[2], and Patrick Pérez[1]

[1] Technicolor, Cesson-Sévigné, France
grvsharma@gmail.com
[2] GREYC CNRS UMR 6072, University of Caen Basse-Normandie, Caen, France

Abstract. We propose a novel Expanded Parts based Metric Learning (EPML) model for face verification. The model is capable of mining out the discriminative regions at the right locations and scales, for identity based matching of face images. It performs well in the presence of occlusions, by avoiding the occluded regions and selecting the next best visible regions. We show quantitatively, by experiments on the standard benchmark dataset Labeled Faces in the Wild (LFW), that the model works much better than the traditional method of face representation with metric learning, both (i) in the presence of heavy random occlusions and, (ii) also, in the case of focussed occlusions of discriminative face regions such as eyes or mouth. Further, we present qualitative results which demonstrate that the method is capable of ignoring the occluded regions while exploiting the visible ones.

1 Introduction

Face verification technology is critical for many modern systems. Handling occlusions is a major challenge in its real world application. In the present paper, we propose a novel Expanded Parts based Metric Learning (EPML) model which is capable of identifying many discriminative parts of the face, for the task of predicting if two faces are of the same person or not, especially in the presence of occlusions.

Metric Learning approaches [1–3] have recently shown promise for the task of face verification. However the face representation is usually fixed and is separate from the task of learning the model. The faces are usually represented as either features computed on face landmarks [3] or over a fixed grid of cells [4]. Once such fixed representations are obtained, a discriminative metric learning model is learned, with annotated *same* and *not-same* faces, for comparing faces based on identity. Since the representation is fixed, it is completely the model's responsibility to tackle the challenge of occlusions that might occur in-the-wild applications. In the present, the proposed EPML model learns a collection of discriminative parts (of the faces) along with the discriminative model to compare faces with such a collection of parts. The collection of discriminative parts is automatically mined from a large set of randomly sampled candidate parts, in the learning phase. The distance function used considers the distances between

© Springer International Publishing Switzerland 2015
D. Cremers et al. (Eds.): ACCV 2014, Part IV, LNCS 9006, pp. 49–63, 2015.
DOI: 10.1007/978-3-319-16817-3_4

all the n different parts in the model and computes the final distance between the two faces with the closest (small number of) $k < n$ parts. Such `min` operation lends non-linearity to the model and allows it to selectively choose/reject parts at runtime, which is in contrast to the traditional representation where the model has no choice but to consider the whole face. This capability is specially useful in case of occlusion: while the traditional method is misguided by the occluded part(s), the proposed method can simply choose to ignore significantly occluded parts and use only the visible parts. We discuss this further later, along with qualitative results, in Sect. 3. In the following, we first set the context by briefly describing the traditional metric learning approaches (Sect. 1.1). We then motivate our method (Sect. 2) and present it in detail (Sect. 2.1) and finally we give experimental results (Sect. 3) and conclude the article (Sect. 4).

1.1   Background: Face Verification Using Metric Learning

Given a face image dataset $\mathcal{X}$ of positive (of the same person) pairs of images and negative pairs of images, represented with some feature vectors i.e.,

$$\mathcal{X} = \{(\mathbf{x}_i, \mathbf{x}_j, y_{ij}) | i = 1, \ldots, l, j = 1, \ldots, m\}, \tag{1}$$

with $\mathbf{x}_i \in \mathbb{R}^D$ a face feature vector and $y_{ij} \in \{-1, +1\}$, the task is to learn a function to predict if two unseen face images, potentially of unseen person(s), are of the same person or not.

Metric learning approaches, along with standard image representations, have been recently shown to be well suited to this task [1–3]. Such approaches learn from $\mathcal{X}$ a Mahalanobis-like metric parametrized by matrix $M \in \mathbb{R}^{D \times D}$, i.e.,

$$d^2(\mathbf{x}_i, \mathbf{x}_j) = (\mathbf{x}_i - \mathbf{x}_j)^\top M(\mathbf{x}_i - \mathbf{x}_j). \tag{2}$$

To be a valid metric, M needs to be symmetric and positive semi-definite (PSD) and hence can also be factorized as

$$M = L^\top L, \tag{3}$$

with $L \in \mathbb{R}^{d \times D}$ and $d \leq D$. The metric learning can then be seen as an embedding learning problem: To compare two vectors, first project them on the d-dim row-space of L and then compare them with their ℓ^2 distance in the projected space, i.e.,

$$\begin{aligned} d^2(\mathbf{x}_i, \mathbf{x}_j) &= (\mathbf{x}_i - \mathbf{x}_j)^\top M(\mathbf{x}_i - \mathbf{x}_j) \\ &= (\mathbf{x}_i - \mathbf{x}_j)^\top L^\top L(\mathbf{x}_i - \mathbf{x}_j) \\ &= (L(\mathbf{x}_i - \mathbf{x}_j))^\top (L(\mathbf{x}_i - \mathbf{x}_j)) \\ &= ||L\mathbf{x}_i - L\mathbf{x}_j||_2^2. \end{aligned} \tag{4}$$

Many regularized loss minimization algorithms have been proposed to learn such metrics with the loss functions arising from probabilistic (likelihood) or margin-maximizing motivations [1–3].

1.2   Related Work

The recognition of face under occlusions has a long history in computer vision literature. One of the pioneering work was that of Leonardis et al. [5] who proposed to make the *Eigenface* method more robust to occlusion by computing the coefficients of the eigenimages with a hypothesize-and-test paradigm using subsets of image points. Since then, more efficient face matching algorithms have been proposed, raising the question of how to make them more robust to occlusions. The best performing state-of-the-art methods (e.g. [6,7]) are holistic in the sense that they represent the whole face by a single vector and are, hence, expected to be sensitive to occlusions.

The impact of occlusions on face recognition has been studied by Rama et al. [8], who evaluated three different approaches based on Principal Component Analysis (PCA) (i.e., the eigenface approach, a component-based method built on the eigen-features and an extension of the Lophoscopic Principal Component Analysis). They analysed the three different strategies and compared them when used for identifying partially occluded faces. The paper also explored how prior knowledge about occlusions, which might be present, can be used to improve the recognition performance.

Generally speaking, two different methodologies have been proposed in the literature. One consists of detecting the occlusions and reconstructing occluded parts prior to doing face recognition, while the other one relies on integrated approaches (of description and recognition together) i.e., those that are robust to occlusions by construction.

Within the family of *detect and reconstruct* approaches, one can mention the works of Colombo et al. [9,10], who detect occlusions by doing a comparison of the input image with a generic model of face and reconstruct missing part with the Gappy Principal Component Analysis (GPCA) [11]. Lin et al. [12], propose another approach for automatically detecting and recovering the occluded facial regions. They consider the formation of an occluded image as a generative process which is then used to guide the procedure of recovery. More recently, Oh et al. [13] proposed to detect occluded parts by dividing the image into a finite number of disjoint local patches coded by PCA and then using 1-NN threshold classifier. Once detected, only the occlusion-free image patches are used for the later face recognition stage, where the matching is done with a nearest neighbor classifier using the Euclidean distance. Wright et al. [14] and Zhou et al. [15] explored the use of sparse coding, proposing a way to efficiently and reliably identify corrupted regions and exclude them from the sparse representation. Sparse coding has also been used efficiently by Ou et al. [16], while Morelli et al. [17] have proposed using compressed sensing. Min et al. [18] proposed to detect the occlusion using Gabor wavelets, PCA and support vector machines (SVM), and then do recognition with the non-occluded facial parts, using block-based Local Binary Patterns of Ojala et al. [19]. Tajima et al. [20] suggested detecting occluded regions using Fast-Weighted Principal Component Analysis (FW-PCA) and using the occluded regions for weighting the blocks for face representation. Alyuz et al. [21] proposed to deal with occlusions by using fully automatic 3-D face recognition system in which face alignment is done through an adaptively selected model based registration scheme (where only the valid non-occluded patches are utilized), while during the classification stage, they proposed a masking strategy to enable the use of subspace analysis techniques with incomplete data. Min et al. [22] proposed to compute an occlusion mask indicating which pixel in a face image is occluded and to use a variant of local Gabor binary pattern histogram sequences (LGBPHS) to represent occluded faces by excluding features extracted from the occluded pixels. Finally, different from previous approaches, Colombo et al. [23] addressed the question of detection and reconstruction of faces using 3D data.

The second paradigm for addressing the recognition of occluded faces, which is to develop method that are intrinsically robust to occlusion, has received less attention in the past. Liao et al. [24] developed an alignment-free face representation method based on Multi-Keypoint Descriptors matching, where the descriptor size of a face is determined by the actual content of the image. Any probe face image (holistic or partial) can hence be sparsely represented by a large dictionary of gallery descriptors, allowing partial matching of face components. Weng et al. [25] recently proposed a new partial face recognition approach by aligning partial face patches to holistic gallery faces automatically, hence being robust to occlusions and illumination changes. Zhao [26] used a robust holistic feature relying on stable intensity relationships of multiple point pairs, being intrinsically invariant to changes in facial features, and exhibiting robustness to illumination variations or even occlusions.

Face verification in real world scenarios has recently attracted much attention, specially fueled by the availability of the excellent benchmark: Labeled Faces in the Wild (LFW) [27]. Many recent papers address the problem with novel approaches, e.g. discriminative part-based approach by Berg and Belhumeur [28], probabilistic elastic model by Li et al. [29], Fisher vectors with metric learning by Simonyan et al. [2], novel regularization for similarity metric learning by Cao et al. [30], fusion of many descriptors using multiple metric learning by Cui et al. [31], deep learning by Sun et al. [32], method using fast high dimensional vector multiplication by Barkan et al. [33]. Many of the most competitive approaches on LFW combine different features, e.g. [3,34,35] and/or use external data, e.g. [36,37].

The works of Liao et al. [24] and Weng et al. [25] are the most closely related and competing works to the proposed EPML. They are based on feature set matching (via dictionaries obtained with sparse representation). Like in image retrieval, there are two ways of doing occlusion robust face matching: (i) match local features detected around keypoints from the two faces or (ii) aggregate the local features to make a global (per cell) feature vector and then match two image vectors. These works fall in the first category while the proposed method falls in the second. The first type of methods are robust to occlusions due to the matching process, while for the second type, the model and aggregation together have to account for the occlusion. Also, the first type of methods claim that they don't need alignment of faces. If a face detector is used then by the statistical properties of the detector the faces will be already approximately aligned (LFW is made this way and strong models already give good results without further alignment). So the first type of methods are arguably more useful when an operator outlines a difficult 'unaligned' face manually and gives it as an input. In that case, we could also make her approximately align the faces as well. And in the case when the face detector is trained to detect faces in large variations in pose, then probably the pose will come out as a latent information from the detector itself, which can then be used to align the face approximately. In summary, we argue that both the approaches have merit and the second type, which is the subject of this paper, has the potential to be highly competitive when used with recently developed strong features with a model-and-aggregation designed to be robust to occlusion like the proposed EPML.

Our work could also be contrasted with feature selection algorithms, e.g. Viola and Jones [38], and many other works in similar spirit, where a subset of features (in a cascaded fashion) are selected from a very large set of features. The proposed method is similar to feature selection methods as we are selecting a subset of parts from among a large set of potential candidate parts. However, it is distinctly different as it performs a dynamic test time selection of most reliable parts, from among the parts selected at training, which are available for the current test pair.

Finally, our work is also reminiscent of the mid-level features stream of work, e.g. see Doersch et al. [39] and the references within, which aim at extracting visually similar recurring and discriminative parts in the images. In a similar spirit, we are interested in finding parts of faces which are discriminative for verification, after the learnt projection.

2 Motivation and Approach

A critical component in computer vision applications is the image representation. The state-of-the-art image representation methods first compute local image statistics (or features as they are usually called) and then *aggregate* them to form a fixed length representation of the images. This aggregation/pooling step reduces a relatively large number of local features to a smaller fixed length vector and there is a trade-off involved here, specially at a spatial level; it is now commonly accepted, e.g. for image classification, that, instead of a global image level aggregation, including finer spatial partitions of the image leads to better results [40]. Learning such partitions does better still [41,42].

In the present paper, we would like to draw attention to some issues related to the fixed grid based spatial aggregation aspect in the context of facial verification tasks with metric learning algorithms. While the metric learning algorithms are expected to find and exploit (absence of) correlations between the various facial regions (or *parts*), they can only do so effectively if local features from different regions are not aggregated into the same (or a very small number of) dimension(s) of the final representation. Towards this issue of aggregation, there are two closely related points:

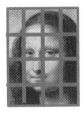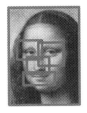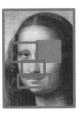

Fig. 1. While the uniform grid might aggregate features from two discriminative regions, e.g. nose and mouth (left) and thus make the final representation less effective, the proposed Expanded Parts based Metric Learning (EPML) model can optimally mine out the spatial bins required for the task (middle) leading to the most discriminative full representation. Further, in case a part of the face is occluded (marked gray in the figure), EPML can ignore the occluded part and take the decision based on the other visible parts (right) and hence be robust to occlusions.

(i) At *what resolutions and locations* such parts should appear?
(ii) *How many* of such parts are optimal for the task?

The current face verification methods usually split the face using uniform grids, possibly at multiple scales, and leave the rest to the metric learning stage. We, instead, propose a novel Expanded Parts based Metric Learning (EPML) model, inspired by the recently proposed Expanded Parts Model for image classification [43], for the task of face verification. The proposed method is capable of mining out the parts from a set of large number of randomly sampled candidate parts. The distance function used in EPML is a non-linear function which uses a subset of best matching parts from among all the parts present in the model. Hence, in the case of occlusions, while the traditional metric learning methods have no choice but to use the fixed full image representation, the proposed EPML can choose to ignore the occluded parts and select the next best matching visible parts. Figure 1 illustrates the points.

2.1   Proposed Method

The goal of the algorithm is to learn a collection of n parts and match a pair of face images using only $k < n$ best matching parts.

In contrast to the metric learning approaches, discussed above, we define the distance between a pair of face images as

$$d_e^2(\mathbf{x}_i, \mathbf{x}_j) = \frac{1}{k} \min_{\boldsymbol{\alpha}_{ij} \in \{0,1\}^n} \sum_{p=1}^{n} \alpha_{ij}(p) \| L_p \mathbf{x}_{i|p} - L_p \mathbf{x}_{j|p} \|^2 \tag{5}$$

$$\text{s.t. } \|\boldsymbol{\alpha}_{ij}\|_1 = k \text{ and } O_v(\boldsymbol{\alpha}_{ij}) < \theta,$$

where, $\boldsymbol{\alpha}_{ij} = (\alpha_{ij}(1), \ldots, \alpha_{ij}(n)) \in \{0,1\}^n$ is the binary indicator vector specifying which of the parts are being used and which are not, L_p is the projection matrix for the pth part and $\mathbf{x}_{i|p}$ is the feature vector of the region corresponding

---

Algorithm 1. Stochastic gradient descent for learning EPML

```
1: Given: Number of candidate parts (N), rate (r), parameters k, β_p, d'
2: parts ← Randomly sample N candidate parts
3: for p = 1, ..., N do
4:     L_p ← Whitened-PCA({x_{i|p}, ∀x_i in training set}, d')
5: end for
6: for iter = 1, 2, 3, ..., 10^6 do
7:     Randomly sample a pos or neg training pair (x_i, x_j, y_{ij}), with equal probability
8:     Compute distance (Eq. 5) to get d_e^2(x_i, x_j) and α_{ij}
9:     if y_{ij}(b − d_e^2(x_i, x_j)) < 1 then
10:        for all p such that α_{ij}(p) = 1 do
11:            L_p ← L_p − rL_p(x_{i|p} − x_{j|p})(x_{i|p} − x_{j|p})^⊤
12:        end for
13:        b ← b + ry_{ij}
14:    end if
15:    parts_image_map ← note_used_parts (α_{ij})
16:    if mod(iter, 10^5) = 0 then
17:        (parts, {L_p}) ← prune_parts (parts_image_map, β_p, parts, {L_p})
18:    end if
19:    Output: (parts, {L_p}, b)     // n parts left after pruning
20: end for
```

---

to the part p for face image i. We also ensure that the parts do not overlap more than a threshold θ, captured by the second constraint based on the overlap function O_v, to encourage coverage of the faces. To mine out the parts and learn the parameters $\{L_p|p = 1, \ldots, n\}$, we propose to solve the following margin maximization problem:

$$\min_{\{L_p\}, b} F(\mathcal{X}; \{L_p\}, b) = \sum_{\mathcal{X}} \max\left(0, 1 − y_{ij}\{b − d_e^2(x_i, x_j)\}\right), \qquad (6)$$

$$\text{where,} \quad \mathcal{X} = \{(x_i, x_j, y_{ij})|i = 1, \ldots, l, j = 1, \ldots, m\} \qquad (7)$$

is the given (annotated) training set, and the b parameter is an offset/threshold to which the distances between the two examples x_i and x_j is to be compared (to decide same or not-same) and is learnt (Algorithm 1, more below).

Computing the Distance. We solve the distance computation (5) by resorting to an approximate greedy forward selection. We first compute the distances between each of the parts in the two images and then recursively (i) select the best matching parts and (ii) discard the remaining parts which overlap more than a threshold with the combined area of the already selected parts.

Solving the Optimization with SGD. The optimization (6) is non-convex due to the presence of the min function in the distance (5). We use stochastic gradient descent to solve it. The analytical subgradients of the objective function, w.r.t. a single training pair (x_i, x_j, y_{ij}), are given by

$$\nabla_{L_p} F = y_{ij} L_p(x_{i|p} − x_{j|p})(x_{i|p} − x_{j|p})^⊤. \qquad (8)$$

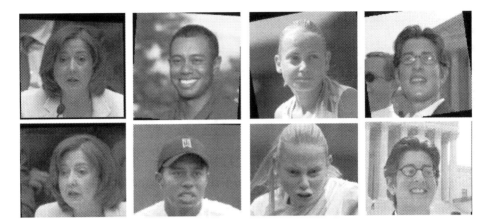

Fig. 2. Example positive image pairs from the LFW [27,34] dataset.

The algorithm we use for learning is given in Algorithm 1. We use no regularization and a small step size (rate r) with a fixed number of one million iterations.

Parts Mining. We divide the whole set of one million learning iterations into 10 sets and after each set (i.e., 100 thousand iterations), we prune the parts by removing those parts which were used for less than β_p fraction of iterations in that set. So, if there are T iterations after which pruning happens, a part has to be utilized in at least $\lceil \beta_p T \rceil$ iterations. Such pruning helps in removing redundant and/or non-discriminative parts. We start with N candidate parts, which are randomly sampled, and prune them to n parts in the final model. N, β_p are free parameters of the algorithm.

Initialization with WPCA. We use Whitened Principal Component Analysis (WPCA) to initialize the projection matrices for each part. For each part, we crop all the faces, in the training set, corresponding to that part and perform WPCA on them, which is used to initialize the projection matrix L_p for the respective part.

3   Experimental Results

Database Used. We use the aligned version [34] of the Labeled Faces in the Wild (LFW) database by Huang et al. [27]. The dataset has more than 13000 images of over 4000 persons. The evaluation is done on the task of face verification in the unrestricted setting. The test set of LFW contains 10 folds of 300 positive and 300 negative pairs, Fig. 2 shows some example positive pairs. The evaluation is done by using 1 fold for testing and remaining 9 folds for training and reporting the average of the accuracies obtained for 10 folds. The identities of the persons in the training set are used to make positive pairs (of same person) and negative pairs (of different persons) of face images, for training. The training is done with unoccluded images and the testing is done with one of the test pair images occluded by one of the methods discussed below. The evaluation simulates the case when the database has unoccluded images of the known persons and the test images come with unexpected occlusions.

Image Description. To describe the face (part) images, we resort to the Local Binary Pattern (LBP) descriptors of Ojala et al. [19]. We use grayscale images and centre crop them to size 150×100 pixels and do not do any other preprocessing. We utilize the publicly available vlfeat [44] library for LBP, with cell size of 10 pixels, resulting in $D = 9860$.

Baseline Method (ML). The baseline metric learning method, denoted ML in the following, is a max margin optimization similar to Eq. 6 with the distance function as explained in Sect. 1.1. The training is done with stochastic gradient based algorithm, same as that of the proposed EPML.

Parameters. We fixed the projection dimension for the baseline method to be 64 after doing preliminary experiments and observing saturation of performance for large values of the projection dimension. The number of randomly generated candidate parts was fixed to $N = 500$. The parts were sampled randomly, to have between 20 % to 80 % of the widths and heights of the face image with random locations. Other parameters were fixed to as $k = 20, d = 20$, because of diminishing returns for higher values of these parameters which makes learning and testing slower. Each candidate part was itself represented by LBP similar to the baseline method.

Horizontal Train/Test-Time Flipping. Since the face images are taken 'in the wild' and have highly varied expressions, poses and appearances, we average out some of the variations by replacing every face pair by four pairs through horizontal flip of each image. Doing this at training should ideally make the system invariant to such variations and make such flipping redundant at test time. However, as the training set is limited, we investigate test time flipping as well.

Random Occlusions. To test the robustness of the system to occlusions, we overlay uniform rectangular patches at randomly sampled locations *on one of the faces* (randomly selected) of a test pair. This simulates the case when an unoccluded image is present in the dataset and an occluded image, captured by a system on the field, has to be matched to it. Such cases can happen when there is natural occlusion due to damage or dust on the camera lens or front glass, especially in the case of surveillance cameras. We sample such patches with areas ranging from 20 % to 80 % of the face area. Figure 3 (top row) shows examples of such randomly occluded faces used in the experiments.

Focussed Occlusions. To stress the system further, we manually mark the parts which are frequently found discriminative, e.g. eyes, central part of the face around the nose and the mouth. We then occlude these regions, one at a time and in combinations, by overlaying uniform patches. As with the random occlusions above, we do it for one of the, randomly selected, faces in the pair.

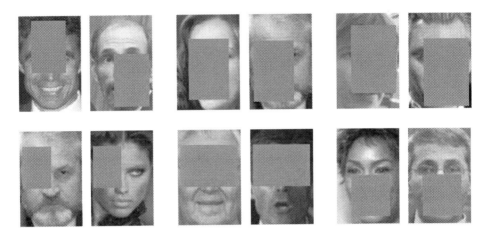

Fig. 3. Examples images showing the kind of occlusions used in the experiments. The top row shows random occlusions while the bottom row shows focussed, and fixed, occlusion of eyes (one, both) and mouth+nose.

We test the system for robustness to occlusion of (i) left/right eye, (ii) both eyes, (iii) central face part around the nose, (iv) mouth and (v) nose and mouth. Figure 3 (bottom row) shows examples of such occlusions.

3.1   Quantitative Results

Figure 4 shows the results for the proposed Expanded Parts based Metric Learning (EPML) method vs. the baseline Metric Learning (ML), in the case of random occlusions. The four graphs correspond to the cases when the horizontal flipping is used, or not, for train and test image pairs (marked 'train flip' and 'test flip' in the graph titles). We observe that the proposed EPML model clearly outperforms the metric learning (ML) method with fixed grid image representation. The improvements are significant, from 2 % to 6 % absolute across the range of occlusions. The standard error on the mean are always relatively small (less than 0.5 %) and hence the improvements are statistically significant.

Table 1 gives the results of the proposed EPML model vs. ML, in the case of focussed occlusions. We find again that the proposed method is robust to occlusions especially for the discriminative parts, e.g. the performance drops much more significantly (to 61.7, for ML) when the eyes are occluded, compared to when the nose and mouth are occluded (to 73.5, for ML) and the gain in such cases is larger for the proposed method, e.g. +7.5 absolute for both eyes occluded vs. only +2 for nose and mouth both occluded. The method, thus, seems to recover gracefully from the occlusion of highly discriminative face regions compared to the traditional ML methods.

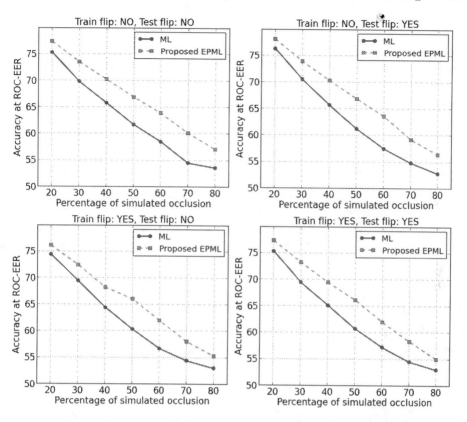

Fig. 4. The performance of the proposed EPML vs. the traditional metric learning methods in the presence of different level of random occlusions. The image pairs are flipped or not during training and/or testing. See Sect. 3 for discussion.

Hence we conclude that the proposed method is more robust to occlusion and learning a localized parts based model instead of a model based on a global face representation is beneficial for obtaining occlusion robustness.

3.2   Qualitative Results

Figure 5 shows the visualization of the scoring by the proposed EPML model in the presence of significant occlusions. We can see that the model is capable of ignoring the occluded parts and using the visible regions for scoring the face images. Based on the part occurrences, it may be inferred that the discriminative regions are mostly around the eyes and mouth of the faces. Note that there appears to be a preference by the model to the left region of the face, particularly the left eye, while it seems that it is ignoring the right part of the face. Since the scoring is done by averaging over the four possible pairs formed by horizontally flipping the two images, every part should be perceived along with its horizontally mirror version (about the centre vertical axis) and hence,

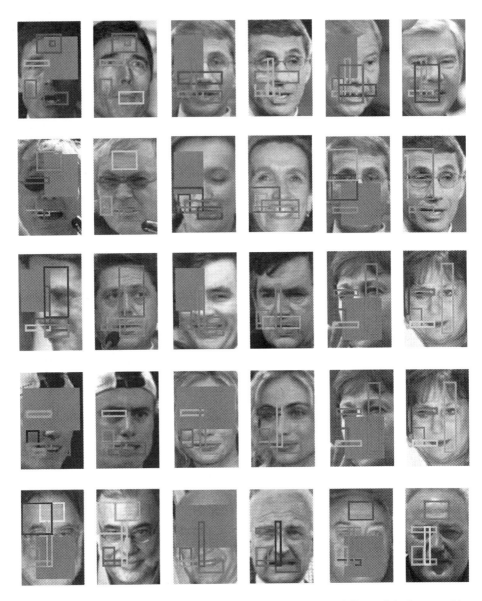

Fig. 5. Visualization of the parts used by the proposed EPML model, for matching pairs of faces in the presence of significant occlusions. The top 5 parts out of 20 (with randomly selected colors for better visibility) selected by the model for scoring the face image pairs are shown. We observe that the method quite successfully ignores the occluded parts. The parts used are also quite diverse and have good coverage as ensured by the model. See Sect. 3.2 for discussion.

Table 1. Results with focussed occlusion on the LFW dataset. See Sect. 3.1 for discussion.

	Left eye	Right eye	Both eyes	Nose	Mouth	Nose + mouth
ML	75.5	73.4	61.7	78.0	77.3	73.5
EPML	78.9	77.0	69.2	79.1	78.5	75.5

there is no such preference by the model. We conclude that the model seems to counter occlusions well.

3.3 Discussion w.r.t. State-of-the-Art Methods

The focus of this paper was to propose a novel method based on localized parts and to evaluate it specially in the context of occlusion robust face verification. Face verification is a very active topic and many features have been proposed obtaining from about around 70 % to up to 93 % performance on the LFW dataset without using external data and a near perfect 99 % while using large amounts of external data[1]. Our implementation with Local Binary Pattern (LBP) features obtains 86 % on the test set of LFW (ROC-EER without occlusion) which is competitive with other methods using similar features.

The EPML algorithm localizes parts and mines them out from a large set of candidate parts. It uses only a subset of parts to match a given pair of images, which allows it to be robust to occlusion. We demonstrated the benefits of the model for the highly popular and lightweight LBP features and we believe that the proposed EPML model will similarly benefit other strong, but global, image representations as well, especially in the case of occlusions.

4   Conclusion

We proposed a novel Expanded Parts based Metric Learning algorithm. The proposed method is capable of mining out the discriminative parts, from among a large set of randomly sampled candidate parts, at the appropriate locations and scales. While the traditional metric learning algorithms use a fixed grid based image representation and are strongly misguided by occlusions, the proposed method has the flexibility to be able to ignore the occluded parts and work with the next best matching visible parts and hence has better robustness to occlusions. The effectiveness of the proposed method w.r.t. the traditional metric learning methods was verified by experiments on the challenging Labeled Faces in the Wild (LFW) dataset with a single feature channel. In the future we would like to use the method with multiple channels of features and perhaps use similar principle to do feature selection as well.

---

[1] http://vis-www.cs.umass.edu/lfw/results.html.

Acknowledgement. This work was partially supported by the FP7 European integrated project AXES and by the ANR project PHYSIONOMIE.

References

1. Mignon, A., Jurie, F.: PCCA: a new approach for distance learning from sparse pairwise constraints. In: CVPR (2012)
2. Simonyan, K., Parkhi, O.M., Vedaldi, A., Zisserman, A.: Fisher vector faces in the wild. In: BMVC (2013)
3. Guillaumin, M., Verbeek, J., Schmid, C.: Is that you? Metric learning approaches for face identification. In: ICCV (2009)
4. Chen, D., Cao, X., Wen, F., Sun, J.: Blessing of dimensionality: high-dimensional feature and its efficient compression for face verification. In: CVPR (2013)
5. Leonardis, A., Bischof, H.: Dealing with occlusions in the eigenspace approach. In: CVPR (1996)
6. Simonyan, K., Vedaldi, A., Zisserman, A.: Deep fisher networks for large-scale image classification. In: NIPS (2013)
7. Taigman, Y., Yang, M., Ranzato, M., Wolf, L.: Deepface: closing the gap to human-level performance in face verification. In: CVPR (2014)
8. Rama, A., Tarres, F., Goldmann, L., Sikora, T.: More robust face recognition by considering occlusion information. In: FG (2008)
9. Colombo, A., Cusano, C., Schettini, R.: Detection and restoration of occlusions for 3d face recognition. In: ICME (2006)
10. Colombo, A., Cusano, C., Schettini, R.: Recognizing faces in 3d images even in presence of occlusions. In: BTAS (2008)
11. Everson, R., Sirovich, L.: Karhunen-loeve procedure for gappy data. JOSA A **12**, 1657–1664 (1995)
12. Lin, D., Tang, X.: Quality-driven face occlusion detection and recovery. In: CVPR (2007)
13. Oh, H.J., Lee, K.M., Lee, S.U.: Occlusion invariant face recognition using selective local non-negative matrix factorization basis images. IVC **26**, 1515–1523 (2008)
14. Wright, J., Yang, A.Y., Ganesh, A., Sastry, S.S., Ma, Y.: Robust face recognition via sparse representation. PAMI **31**, 210–227 (2009)
15. Zhou, Z., Wagner, A., Mobahi, H., Wright, J., Ma, Y.: Face recognition with contiguous occlusion using markov random fields. In: CVPR (2009)
16. Ou, W., You, X., Tao, D., Zhang, P., Tang, Y., Zhu, Z.: Robust face recognition via occlusion dictionary learning. PR **47**, 1559–1572 (2014)
17. Andrés, A.M., Padovani, S., Tepper, M., Jacobo-Berlles, J.: Face recognition on partially occluded images using compressed sensing. PRL **36**, 235–242 (2014)
18. Min, R., Hadid, A., Dugelay, J.: Improving the recognition of faces occluded by facial accessories. In: FG (2011)
19. Ojala, T., Pietikainen, M., Maenpaa, T.: Multiresolution gray-scale and rotation invariant texture classification with local binary patterns. PAMI **24**, 971–987 (2002)
20. Tajima, Y., Ito, K., Aoki, T., Hosoi, T., Nagashima, S., Kobayashi, K.: Performance improvement of face recognition algorithms using occluded-region detection. In: ICB (2013)
21. Alyuz, N., Gokberk, B., Akarun, L.: 3-d face recognition under occlusion using masked projection. IEEE Trans. Inf. Forensics and Secur. **8**, 789–802 (2013)

22. Min, R., Hadid, A., Dugelay, J.L.L.: Efficient detection of occlusion prior to robust face recognition. Sci. World J. **2014**, 10 (2014). 519158
23. Colombo, A., Cusano, C., Schettini, R.: Three-dimensional occlusion detection and restoration of partially occluded faces. J. Math. Imaging Vis. **40**, 105–119 (2011)
24. Liao, S., Jain, A.K., Li, S.Z.: Partial face recognition: alignment-free approach. PAMI **35**, 1193–1205 (2013)
25. Weng, R., Lu, J., Hu, J., Yang, G., Tan, Y.P.P.: Robust feature set matching for partial face recognition. In: ICCV (2013)
26. Zhao, X., He, Z., Zhang, S., Kaneko, S., Satoh, Y.: Robust face recognition using the GAP feature. PR **46**, 2647–2657 (2013)
27. Huang, G.B., Ramesh, M., Berg, T., Learned-Miller, E.: Labeled faces in the wild: a database for studying face recognition in unconstrained environments. Technical report 07–49, University of Massachusetts, Amherst (2007)
28. Berg, T., Belhumeur, P.N.: POOF: part-based one-vs.-one features for fine-grained categorization, face verification, and attribute estimation. In: CVPR (2013)
29. Li, H., Hua, G., Lin, Z., Brandt, J., Yang, J.: Probabilistic elastic matching for pose variant face verification. In: CVPR (2013)
30. Cao, Q., Ying, Y., Li, P.: Similarity metric learning for face recognition. In: ICCV (2013)
31. Cui, Z., Li, W., Xu, D., Shan, S., Chen, X.: Fusing robust face region descriptors via multiple metric learning for face recognition in the wild. In: CVPR (2013)
32. Sun, Y., Wang, X., Tang, X.: Hybrid deep learning for face verification. In: ICCV (2013)
33. Barkan, O., Weill, J., Wolf, L., Aronowitz, H.: Fast high dimensional vector multiplication face recognition. In: ICCV (2013)
34. Wolf, L., Hassner, T., Taigman, Y.: Similarity scores based on background samples. In: Zha, H., Taniguchi, R., Maybank, S. (eds.) ACCV 2009, Part II. LNCS, vol. 5995, pp. 88–97. Springer, Heidelberg (2010)
35. Nguyen, H.V., Bai, L.: Cosine similarity metric learning for face verification. In: Kimmel, R., Klette, R., Sugimoto, A. (eds.) ACCV 2010, Part II. LNCS, vol. 6493, pp. 709–720. Springer, Heidelberg (2011)
36. Kumar, N., Berg, A.C., Belhumeur, P.N., Nayar, S.K.: Attribute and simile classifiers for face verification. In: ICCV (2009)
37. Berg, T., Belhumeur, P.N.: Tom-vs-pete classifiers and identity-preserving alignment for face verification. In: BMVC (2012)
38. Viola, P., Jones, M.J.: Robust real-time face detection. Intl. J. Comput. Vis. **57**, 137–154 (2004)
39. Doersch, C., Gupta, A., Efros, A.A.: Mid-level visual element discovery as discriminative mode seeking. In: NIPS (2013)
40. Lazebnik, S., Schmid, C., Ponce, J.: Beyond bags of features: Spatial pyramid matching for recognizing natural scene categories. In: CVPR (2006)
41. Sharma, G., Jurie, F.: Learning discriminative representation image classification. In: BMVC (2011)
42. Jiang, L., Tong, W., Meng, D., Hauptmann, A.G.: Towards efficient learning of optimal spatial bag-of-words representations. In: ICMR (2014)
43. Sharma, G., Jurie, F., Schmid, C.: Expanded parts model for human attribute and action recognition in still images. In: CVPR (2013)
44. Vedaldi, A., Fulkerson, B.: VLFeat: an open and portable library of computer vision algorithms (2008). http://www.vlfeat.org/

Pixel-Level Hand Detection with Shape-Aware Structured Forests

Xiaolong Zhu$^{(\boxtimes)}$, Xuhui Jia, and Kwan-Yee K. Wong

Department of Computer Science, The University of Hong Kong,
Pokfulam Road, Hong Kong, China
{xlzhu,xhjia,kykwong}@cs.hku.hk

Abstract. Hand detection has many important applications in HCI, yet it is a challenging problem because the appearance of hands can vary greatly in images. In this paper, we propose a novel method for efficient pixel-level hand detection. Unlike previous method which assigns a binary label to every pixel independently, our method estimates a probability shape mask for a pixel using structured forests. This approach can better exploit hand shape information in the training data, and enforce shape constraints in the estimation. Aggregation of multiple predictions generated from neighboring pixels further improves the robustness of our method. We evaluate our method on both ego-centric videos and unconstrained still images. Experiment results show that our method can detect hands efficiently and outperform other state-of-the-art methods.

1 Introduction

In recent years, we have witnessed great progress in object detection in the field of computer vision. Successful applications can be found in face detection [1], pedestrian detection [2], *etc.* Nevertheless, hand detection is still a challenging problem as the appearance of hands can vary greatly in images. For instances, the shape of a hand can change dramatically due to the articulation of fingers as well as changes in viewpoint. A hand can be (partially) occluded while interacting with other objects. The color of a hand can vary greatly under different illuminations, and a hand can even appear to be textureless under extreme illuminations. Generic object detection methods [3] based on gradients often have difficulties in representing the varying appearance of hands. Heuristic skin-color detection methods [4] may also fail in practice when skin color is not discriminative enough from the background.

Recently, ego-centric cameras have become more and more popular. Images captured by such cameras often have a dynamic background, which makes hand detection even more difficult. A pixel labeling approach recently proposed by Li and Kitani [5] has shown to be quite successful in hand detection in ego-centric videos. In this paper, we extend such a pixel labeling approach to a structured image labeling problem. Instead of assigning a binary label to every pixel independently, our method estimates a probability shape mask for a pixel using structured forests. As shown in Fig. 1, our method can detect hand regions more

© Springer International Publishing Switzerland 2015
D. Cremers et al. (Eds.): ACCV 2014, Part IV, LNCS 9006, pp. 64–78, 2015.
DOI: 10.1007/978-3-319-16817-3_5

robustly than the previous method which predicts pixel labels independently. In summary, our proposed approach has the following advantages:

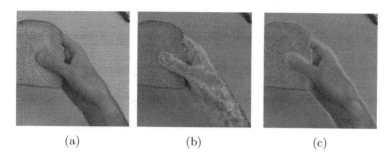

(a)   (b)   (c)

Fig. 1. Introduction to our method. (a) Original image. (b) Pixel-level hand detection by single pixel prediction. (c) Pixel-level hand detection by structured label prediction.

- As hand pixel labels are not independent, our method explicitly models a pixel using a probability shape mask. This allows our method better utilize hand shape information in the training data and enforce shape constraints in the estimation.
- Since a probability shape mask is determined for a pixel, pixels in its neighborhood would also benefit from this prediction. Aggregation of multiple predictions generated from neighboring pixels further improves the robustness of our method.
- Our method is extremely efficient in generating a probability map of hands using random forest scheme.

2   Literature Review

Hand detection has been studied as part of human layout parsing and gesture analysis for many years. Hand detection methods can be categorized into three main approaches, namely (1) color-based methods, (2) model-based methods and (3) motion-based methods.

Methods based on skin color usually build a skin model in a color space for detecting hand regions. Mixture of Gaussians [4] is commonly used to model colors of skin and non-skin regions for hand localization [6] and hand tracking [7,8]. Color-based methods often require a prior knowledge of skin color, extracted either from training data or from face detection, to build the skin model. These methods, however, often fail in unconstrained images and ego-centric videos where changes in illuminations cause a large variation in skin color.

Model-based methods usually model the appearance of hands using a hand template. They can be implemented as a Viola & Jones like boosted detector [1], or as a HOG detector built from a large number of images [3], or learned as an ensemble of edges [9, 10] from a set of $2D$ projections of a $3D$ synthetic hand model.

Color information can also be used to further create more proposals to improve the detection performance [11]. However, their applications are often limited to a small number of hand configurations. To overcome this problem, these methods often exploit more training data in order to cover a larger configuration space. It is also possible to detect hands as part of human pictorial structure [12], which may bring more context information and allow inferring hand position via optimization. This is a common practice for still images, but usually it requires at least the upper body being visible for the inference of human layout.

Motion-based methods are mostly used for *ad-hoc* applications, *e.g.*, activity analysis and gesture recognition. They segment foreground hands from background by motion and appearance cues [13–15]. Hands can usually be tracked easily and it does not require a strong appearance model in most cases. However, motion-based methods are often not suitable for moving cameras which produce images with lots of background motion.

Recently, ego-centric cameras, *e.g.*, Google Glasses and GoPro cameras, have become more and more popular. A local-appearance-based pixel labeling method recently proposed by Li and Kitani [5] has shown to be quite successful in dealing with dynamic background and varying appearance of hands in ego-centric videos. However, their method only predicts the label of every pixel independently without considering any shape constraint. In this paper, we are going to investigate how local hand shape information can improve hand detection.

3   Shape-Aware Structured Forests

In this section, we first briefly review the pixel-level hand detection using random forests. We then extend this framework by introducing a shape mask to represent the structure information. We refer to our method as *Shape-aware Structured Forests*. We also present an intermediate mapping that can accelerate the calculation of information gain during the training process. Finally, a multi-scale hand detection method will be illustrated in details.

3.1   Random Forests

Given a patch $\mathbf{I}_p \in \mathbb{R}^{w \times w \times 3}$ with a size of $w \times w$ centered at pixel p in a color image $\mathbf{I}$, we first extract a feature vector $\mathbf{x}_p \in \mathcal{X}$ using channel features [16]. A decision tree $f_{\Theta}(\mathbf{x}_p)$, parameterized by Θ, is learned to map $\mathbf{x}_p$ to a binary label $y_p \in \{0, 1\}$, which indicates whether p is a hand pixel (i.e., $y_p = 1$) or not (i.e., $y_p = 0$). A random forest is a collection of such decision trees, each with an independent parameter Θ_i. The output of the random forest $F(\mathbf{x}_p)$ is the final class label y_p^*, which is obtained as the ensemble of the posterior distribution $P_i(y_p|\mathbf{x}_p)$ in the leaf node of tree i as,

$$y_p^* = \arg\max_{y_p} \frac{1}{T} \sum_{i=1}^{T} P_i(y_p|\mathbf{x}_p), \tag{1}$$

where T is the number of trees in the forest.

During the training process, each decision tree is constructed independently from a randomly sampled subset of the training data $S = \{(\mathbf{x}_p, y_p)\}$. For each decision node in a tree, one element of the feature vector $\mathbf{x}_p$ is selected for a binary test. Based on the binary test, a split function with parameter $\boldsymbol{\theta}$ is defined as

$$\Phi(\mathbf{x}_p, \boldsymbol{\theta}) = \begin{cases} 1, & \text{if } \boldsymbol{\theta}^\top [\mathbf{x}_p^\top \ 1]^\top \leq 0 \\ 0, & \text{otherwise} \end{cases}, \tag{2}$$

where only the last element and one other element of θ are non-zero values. This function splits the training data in the current node into two subsets for its children. Usually the candidates of $\boldsymbol{\theta}$ are randomly generated and our goal is to find a candidate that maximizes the information gain, $\mathbf{G}(\boldsymbol{\theta})$, of the current split test. The information gain is defined as

$$\mathbf{G}(\boldsymbol{\theta}) = H(S_j) - \sum_{k \in \{L,R\}} \frac{|S_j^k|}{|S_j|} H(S_j^k), \tag{3}$$

where S_j denotes the set of training data in node j, $S_j^L = \{(\mathbf{x}_p, y_p) \in S_j | \Phi (\mathbf{x}_p, \boldsymbol{\theta}) = 1\}$ denotes the set of training data to be assigned to its left child and $S_j^R = S_j \setminus S_j^L$ denotes the set of training data to be assigned to its right child, $|\cdot|$ denotes the size of a set and $H(\cdot)$ denotes purity measurement $w.r.t.$ y_p. As in our formulation, y_p is a binary variable, the purity can be measured by Shannon Entropy or Gini impurity [17]. A decision tree is constructed by splitting its nodes repeatedly until either the minimum number of training data in a leaf node or the maximum depth of a tree has been reached.

During the test phase, each tree will be evaluated on an input patch according to the split function in Eq. (2) iteratively until a leaf node is reached. The posterior distribution stored in that node will then be used for MAP estimation according to Eq. (1).

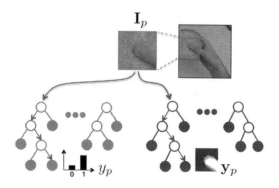

Fig. 2. The main difference between random forests and structured forests.

3.2   Learning Shape Masks via Intermediate Mapping

For each pixel p' in the patch $\mathbf{I}_p$, similarly, a binary label can be determined by the random forests based on the feature vector $\mathbf{x}_{p'}$ extracted from the patch $\mathbf{I}_{p'}$. If these labels are considered as a whole, they form a shape mask of the hand for the patch $\mathbf{I}_p$. Obviously, pixel labels within such a shape mask should not be independent of each other. This suggests that it will be logical to learn a shape mask rather than just a single pixel label for an image patch. Learning a shape mask allows shape information from the training data be exploited to enforce shape constraints on hand detection. More precisely, the original output space $y_p \in \{0, 1\}$ can be extended to a shape mask $\mathbf{y}_p \in \mathcal{Y} = \{0, 1\}^{w \times w}$. Accordingly, the posterior of the shape mask is stored instead of that of the central pixel in the leaf nodes of the random forest (see Fig. 2). In this way, shape information is considered explicitly and represented as a local binary pattern in the new output space $\mathcal{Y}$. For a set of patches sharing similar appearance features in $\mathcal{X}$, our goal becomes to predict similar binary shape mask in $\mathcal{Y}$.

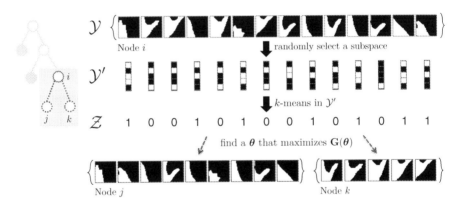

Fig. 3. Intermediate mapping during node splitting. In the parent node, all mask images are firstly grouped into two clusters. Next, θ for $\mathcal{X}$ is selected to maximize $G(\theta)$ calculated from cluster labels in $\mathcal{Z}$.

However, it will be extremely time consuming to calculate information gain in the new shape mask space as we need to enumerate all possible states. For instance, there will be $2^{16 \times 16}$ possible states for a patch with a size of 16×16. In order to speedup the calculation of information gain, an intermediate mapping is used during training to approximate the mask space by a lower dimensional space as illustrated in Fig. 3. In each node splitting, a subspace $\mathcal{Y}'$ is first randomly selected from the original mask space $\mathcal{Y}$ so that additional randomness can be injected into forest training to ensure the diversity of trees. This can be done by randomly selecting m elements from the mask $\mathbf{y}_p$. Next, k-means algorithm can be performed over the subspace $\mathcal{Y}'$ to group the training masks into 2 clusters. Either Shannon Entropy or Gini Impurity can then be used to compute information gain of a candidate split test. Finally, a standard procedure like in decision forest training can be applied to find an optimal split parameter θ for the current node.

3.3   Implementation Details

Similar to [18], we apply the structured forest to the input image of multiple scales as illustrated in Fig. 4. We first rescale the input image $\mathbf{I}$ into several copies to form an image pyramid. In each level, color and gradient features are extracted as channel features. In particular, we extract *CIELUV* channels as color features, which have been shown to be the most discriminative color features in many applications [2,5,19]. As for gradient features, we simply extract the magnitude and the orientation for each pixel and bin its orientation into a histogram followed by Gaussian smoothing among all bins. In order to describe the texture of a hand, we also include self-similarity features [20], which are pairwise differences between different cells that subdivide a patch like tiles. This will also help to differentiate the hand and non-hand regions in the patches. As all features are either channel features of order 1 or pairwise features of order 2, a lookup table can be built so that feature extraction can be done very efficiently during the test phase.

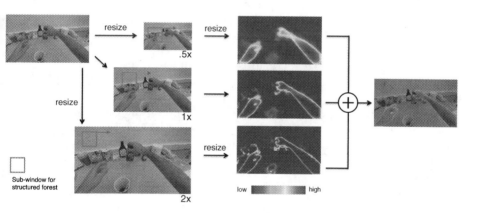

Fig. 4. Hand detection in multiple scales.

After features are extracted, a sliding window of width w can be used to apply our structured forests. For each tree i, the patch will pass through several binary tests until a leaf node is reached. In the leaf node, a posterior distribution of a mask is stored as a per-pixel posterior $m_i(x,y)$ at (x,y) as illustrated in Fig. 2 along with a per-pixel variance $\sigma_i(x,y)$. The output of the structured forest is defined as the weighted average of all these posteriors,

$$m^*(x,y) = \frac{1}{Z} \sum_{i=1}^{T} e^{-k\sigma_i(x,y)} m_i(x,y). \tag{4}$$

where $Z = \sum_i e^{-k\sigma_i(x,y)}$ is a normalization term, and k is a parameter for tuning the weights. If $k = 0$, Z will become the total number of trees T and $m^*(x,y)$ will simply be the average of all the posteriors.

The final probability map of pixel-level hand detection is obtained by averaging the results over different scales and sub-windows.

4   Experimental Results

We evaluate our structured hand detector on two types of data. The first type is characterized as the hands in ego-centric videos, where fine shape is always needed for further high-level analysis, such as action analysis or object recognition. The second type contains the hands in still images where the environment is much more unconstrained so the hand recall rate is always low using traditional object detection approaches. We first compare our methods with the state-of-the-art methods and analyze different factors that may affect the detection performance. We then conclude our observations for each type of data.

4.1   Hands in Ego-Centric Videos: GTEA and EDSH Dataset

We first test our approach on Geogia Tech Ego-centric Activity dataset (GTEA) [14]. The GTEA dataset involves little camera motion and is taken under the same environment as it is primarily recorded for activity recognition. Similar to the experimental setup in [5], all video clips are firstly down-sampled to 720p. There are 7 actions for 4 subjects, one of which the ground truth labels are available for evaluation. The original hand masks are quite noisy and sometimes confused with the objects in hand due to unsatisfactory segmentation. We turned to the masks made available in [5] obtained using GrabCut [21]. We performed three experiments that use Coffee sequence for training and Tea and Peanut sequences for testing, and use Tea sequence for training and Coffee sequence for testing.

We also test our approach on publicly available EDSH dataset[1], which involves more illumination changes and camera motion. EDSH1 and EDSH2 record both hands of a subject walking through different indoor and outdoor scenes in order to capture the changes in skin color. EDSH-Kitchen records a subject performing different activities in a kitchen, where there are great ego-motion and hand deformations. These are typical scenarios for hand detection in daily life and all these videos are recorded in 720 p, and 442 labeled frames are used for training our shape-aware structured forests.

As far as evaluation is concerned, the F-score, *i.e.* harmonic mean of precision-recall rate, is used to measure the detection performance. We compare our result with [5] which uses a random forest of depth 10 for single pixel prediction.

Comparison. We perform the same experiment using the public code [5] extracting 9×9 patches using color and HOG features and also include their reported

---

[1] http://www.cs.cmu.edu/~kkitani/perpix/.

Table 1. Comparison on F-score.

	Li et al. [5]	Li et al. (Color+HOG) [5]	Ours
GTEA-Coffee	88.8	78.05	$90.19_{\pm 1.07}$
GTEA-Tea	88.0	72.53	$84.30_{\pm 1.12}$
GTEA-Peanut	76.4	74.71	$84.37_{\pm 2.11}$
EDSH2	76.8	72.31	$80.43_{\pm 3.10}$
EDSH-Kitchen	80.5	74.37	$92.11_{\pm 1.41}$

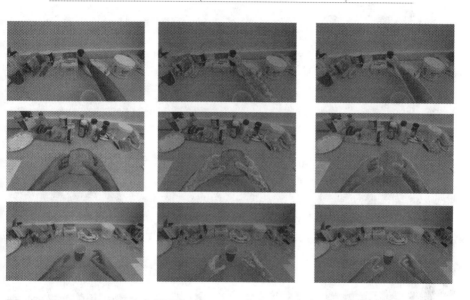

Fig. 5. Sample Images of GTEA dataset: (left column) original images, (second column) results of Li's Method [5], and (last column) our results. From top to bottom: GTEA-Coffee, GTEA-Peanut and GTEA-Tea. Best view in color.

best results for all 5 experiments. The F-scores are shown in Table 1. Our approach outperforms the results produced by their code in all 5 experiments by a large scale. The improvement mainly happens in some cluttered regions because our method can filter out the noise and also smooth the prediction of hand region by averaging.

Figures 5 and 6 show some sample images overlaid by per-pixel probabilities produced by their public code and our method in GTEA and EDSH dataset.

In Fig. 5, we find that single pixel hand prediction always fails at the edge of hand and fingers. This is because the local neighborhood of these pixels vary a lot when the hand is moving and deforming. Therefore it cannot collect a strong evidence saying that the central pixel belongs to a hand. On the contrary, our method can provide partial support from the neighborhood of edge pixels via structured label predictions because these partial contributions will aggregate into the edge pixel such that the ambiguity along the edge can be removed.

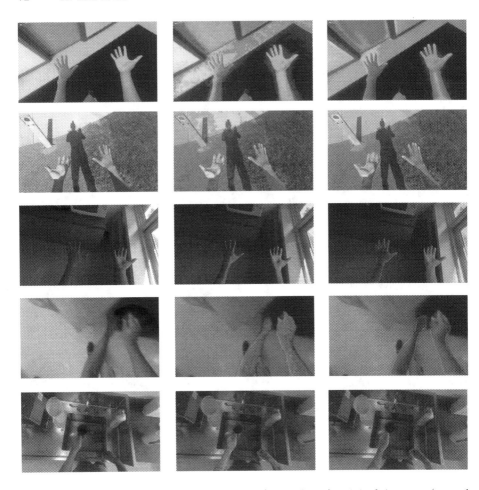

Fig. 6. Sample Images of EDSH data set: (left column) original images, (second column) results of Li's Method [5], and (last column) our results. From top to bottom: confusion with the door in EDSH1; shade on the hand in outdoor in EDSH2; poor light condition in EDSH2; motion blur in EDSH-Kitchen; confusion with sink in EDSH-Kitchen. Best view in color.

In Fig. 6, both our method and single pixel prediction may cause confusion with certain textureless objects, $e.g.$, doors in 1st row. However, our method smooths these regions so that it could be easily removed by post-processing. Meanwhile, our method is more robust to the incorrect labels in training samples due to improper segmentation. These labels often appear along edges of hand or suppose to be the objects in hand. For single pixel prediction, these incorrect labels will be directly treated as negative samples during training, so they will affect the prediction in a fundamental way. However, it is not common in our approach as ours is based on patch observation that is robust to pixel-level noise.

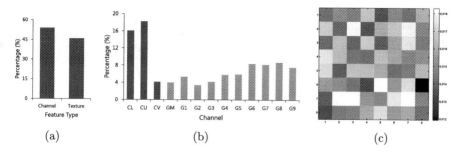

(a)   (b)   (c)

Fig. 7. Usage of features in the structured forest. (a) Feature of channel and similarity features. (b) Feature in different channels. The first 3 channels are $CIELUV$ color channels, the 4th are magnitude of gradient and the rest are gradients in different orientations. (c) Spatial distribution of the features rasterized in a 8×8 grid.

Feature. We investigate the contribution of different features by checking its usage in the structured forests. All selected features are aggregated from all of non-leaf nodes in the forests. First in Fig. 7(a), we show the ratio of channel features and texture features. They are almost equally important so the pairwise texture descriptor is essential in mask prediction. If we remove these features, the overall F-score will generally drop by 5 %. Figure 7(b) shows that the color features (first 3 channels) are the mostly used ones among all channel features. This means that color is still the most discriminative feature for hand detection. Moreover, the orientations of the gradients are more often used than their magnitudes, which suggests that the edge orientation of a hand is more informative in determining its shape mask. Figure 7(c) shows the spatial distribution of selected channel features in a 32×32 patch, we can see that most of the places are used for predicting the hand shape mask.

Size. We next examine the effect of increasing the size of patches used for our structured forests. In order to examine the hand in different resolution for egocentric videos, we down-sample the EDSH dataset from 720 p to 320 p. For both datasets, we increase the size of training patches from half the finger size to twice the palm size. Both in Figs. 8 and 9, there are two phases in the F-score curve. During the increasing phase, it brings more spatial context for shape mask prediction so the F-score will increase dramatically. In the decreasing phase, the

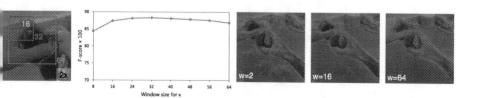

Fig. 8. Performance of our structured forests of different patch sizes for GTEA dataset.

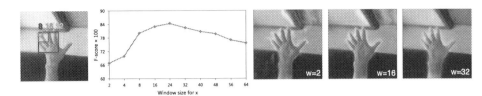

Fig. 9. Performance of our structured forests of different patch sizes for EDSH dataset.

structured forests will suffer from two limitations. First, it will over-smooth along the hand contour which makes it sensitive to the threshold for detection. Second, there will not be sufficient training samples for the exponentially increased output space. Thus the forests will probably overfit the training data. From our observation, more than half the palm size is suitable for a robust hand detector.

Number of Trees. As for the common smoothing effect introduced by our structured forests, we further examine the contribution of different number of trees to shape detection. Figure 10(a) shows the performance of structured forests of different number of trees. We use a forest trained from 16×16 patches to observe the shape mask prediction. In Fig. 10(c), we can see that a single tree can outline the shape but the shape contour is not smooth enough. This can be improved either by increasing the number of trees T as shown in Fig. 10(d) or reducing the stride width d as shown in Fig. 10(e). Both can accumulate more spatial context in order to obtain a better shape mask.

Timing. Table 2 records the time cost for evaluating a 720×405 image. We compare the public code provided by the author [5] with our MATLAB implementation. We use 9×9 patch to train the single pixel predictor, and use the same size in our implementation. s and m stands for single and multiple scale detection. d is the stride width. Most of their time is spent on feature extraction compared with ours. Moreover, the time cost can be reduced greatly for multiscale implementation by increasing the stride width with a little performance drop.

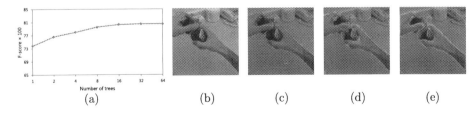

Fig. 10. Performance of different number of trees and stride width. (a) Overall F-score $w.r.t.$ different number of trees. (b) Original image. (c) Prediction by forest ($d = 16$, $T = 1$). (d) Prediction by forest ($d = 1$, $T = 16$) (e) Prediction by forest ($d = 1$, $T = 1$).

Table 2. Comparison on time cost.

	Li *et al.* [5]	Ours (*s*, *d*=1)	Ours (*m*, *d*=1)	Ours (*m*, *d*=2)
Time (ms)	2138	664	3277	1129
F-Score (100×)	–	79.84	81.83	80.27

4.2   Hands in Still Images: BMVC Dataset

We evaluate our approach on a publicly available image dataset for hand detection in still images. All images are collected from various sources as cataloged in [11], of different resolution and imaging condition. Since there is only a bounding box available for a hand in each image, we manually annotated 3904 hands, of which 2806 are large instances. All hand images are rescaled to 128 × 128 size for sampling positive patches during training. Additional negative patches are sampled from the rest non-skin area and the images from natural scenes. Finally, our implementation is evaluated on 100 test images.

Hand Orientation. As the number of training samples is much bigger for training, we adopt a heuristic training method. All the hand images are rotated to the same orientation, and then the structured forests are trained from the samples of each orientation. Next, all predictions are merged by averaging the probability map over different orientations similar to Eq. (4).

Figure 11 shows the performance of final ensemble model *w.r.t.* the number of orientations of samples used for training. We can find the more orientations we use, the better it performs. This is because the hands in still images appear in arbitrary directions, so we need to enumerate all possible orientations during training. Otherwise, this has to be done in testing phase, which becomes a drawback in [11] which predicts an image in a long time.

Figure 12 shows several sample images predicted by single direction and 16 orientations. The later can predict hands with stronger confidence than the former. Meanwhile, the overall F-score is quite low in this dataset, as the face regions

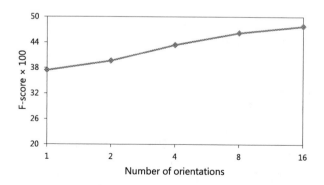

Fig. 11. Performance of F-Score *w.r.t.* different orientations used for prediction.

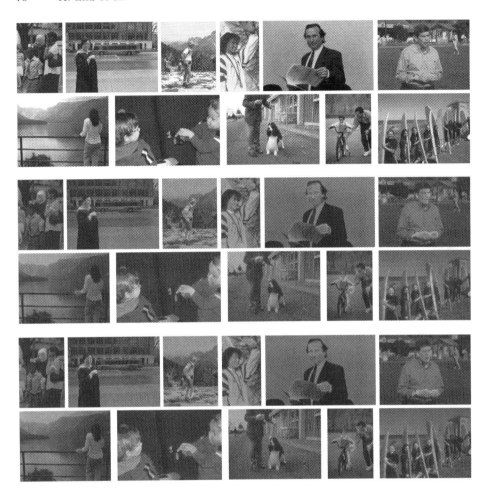

Fig. 12. Sample Images. From top to bottom: original images, predictions by a detector training from the samples with orientation downwards, predictions by a detector training from the samples with 16 orientations.

and other skin-like regions are also confused in both experiments. Thus higher-level analysis is required in differentiating hands from other parts of human body in still images.

5   Conclusions

Our approach can detect a hand up to pixel-level accuracy in an efficient way while achieving the state-of-the-art performance. The structured output considers the information of neighboring labels so actually each pixel is evaluated much more than once during testing. Through the experimental results, we also find that the color information is critical in predicting the patch while the gradient and texture information are also relevant to the shape of the mask. This suggests that further work can be done to explore the relation between gradients, hand shapes and hand postures, which bridges the appearance with the semantic meaning of the hand.

References

1. Viola, P., Jones, M.: Robust Real-time Object Detection. Int. J. Comput. Vis. **57**, 137–154 (2004)
2. Dollár, P., Wojek, C., Schiele, B., Perona, P.: Pedestrian Detection: An Evaluation of the State of the Art. IEEE Trans. Pattern Anal. Mach. Intell. **34**, 743–761 (2012)
3. Dalal, N., Triggs, B., Europe, D.: Histograms of oriented gradients for human detection. In: Proceedings of the IEEE International Conference on Computer Vision and Pattern Recognition. vol. 1, pp. 886–893. IEEE (2005)
4. Jones, M., Rehg, J.: Statistical color models with application to skin detection. Int. J. Comput. Vis. **46**, 81–96 (2002)
5. Li, C., Kitani, K.: Pixel-level hand detection in ego-centric videos. In: Proceedings of the IEEE Conference on Computer Vision and Pattern Recognition (2013)
6. Sigal, L., Sclaroff, S., Athitsos, V.: Skin Color-Based Video Segmentation under Time-Varying Illumination. IEEE Trans. Pattern Anal. Mach. Intell. **26**, 862–877 (2004)
7. Kolsch, M., Turk, M.: Hand tracking with flocks of features. In: Proceedings of the IEEE Conference on Computer Vision and Pattern Recognition (2005)
8. Pérez, P., Hue, C., Vermaak, J., Gangnet, M.: Color-based probabilistic tracking. In: Heyden, A., Sparr, G., Nielsen, M., Johansen, P. (eds.) ECCV 2002, Part I. LNCS, vol. 2350, pp. 661–675. Springer, Heidelberg (2002)
9. Thayananthan, A., Torr, P.H.S., Member, S., Stenger, B., Cipolla, R.: Model-based hand tracking using a hierarchical Bayesian filter. IEEE Trans. on Pattern Anal. Mach. Intell. **28**, 1372–1384 (2006)
10. Oikonomidis, I., Kyriazis, N., Argyros, A.A.: Markerless and efficient 26-DOF hand pose recovery. In: Kimmel, R., Klette, R., Sugimoto, A. (eds.) ACCV 2010, Part III. LNCS, vol. 6494, pp. 744–757. Springer, Heidelberg (2011)
11. Mittal, A., Zisserman, A., Torr, P.: Hand detection using multiple proposals. In: Proceedings of the British Machine Vision Conference, pp.75.1–75.11. British Machine Vision Association (2011)
12. Buehler, P., Everingham, M., Huttenlocher, D.P., Zisserman, A.: Upper Body Detection and Tracking in Extended Signing Sequences. Int. J. Comput. Vis. **95**, 180–197 (2011)
13. Sheikh, Y., Javed, O., Kanade, T.: Background subtraction for freely moving cameras. In: Proceedings of the IEEE 12th International Conference on Computer Vision, pp. 1219–1225. IEEE (2009)
14. Fathi, A., Ren, X., Rehg, J.M.: Learning to recognize objects in egocentric activities. In: Proceedings of the IEEE Conference on Computer Vision and Pattern Recognition, pp. 3281–3288. IEEE (2011)
15. Trinh, H., Fan, Q., Gabbur, P., Pankanti, S.: Hand tracking by binary quadratic programming and its application to retail activity recognition. In: Proceedings of the IEEE Conference on Computer Vision and Pattern Recognition (2012)
16. Dollár, P., Tu, Z., Perona, P., Belongie, S.: Integral channel features. In: Proceedings of the British Machine Vision Conference, pp. 1–11 (2009)

17. Breiman, L., Friedman, J., Stone, C.J., Olshen, R.A.: Classification and Regression Trees. Chapman and Hall/CRC, New York (1984)
18. Felzenszwalb, P.F., Girshick, R.B., McAllester, D., Ramanan, D.: Object detection with discriminatively trained part-based models. IEEE Trans. Pattern Anal. Mach. Intell. **32**, 1627–1645 (2010)
19. Sagonas, C., Tzimiropoulos, G., Zafeiriou, S., Pantic, M.: 300 faces in-the-wild challenge: the first facial landmark localization challenge. In: IEEE International Conference on Computer Vision Workshops, pp. 397–403. IEEE (2013)
20. Bagon, S., Brostovski, O., Galun, M., Irani, M.: Detecting and sketching the common. In: Proceedings of the IEEE Conference on Computer Vision and Pattern Recognition, pp. 33–40. IEEE (2010)
21. Rother, C., Kolmogorov, V., Blake, A.: Grabcut: Interactive foreground extraction using iterated graph cuts. ACM Trans. Graph. **23**, 309–314 (2004)

Beyond Procedural Facade Parsing: Bidirectional Alignment via Linear Programming

Mateusz Koziński[(✉)], Guillaume Obozinski, and Renaud Marlet

LIGM (UMR CNRS 8049), ENPC, Université Paris-Est,
77455 Marne-la-Vallée, France
mateusz.kozinski@enpc.fr

Abstract. We propose a novel formulation for parsing facade images with user-defined shape prior. Contrary to other state-of-the-art methods, we do not explore the procedural space of shapes derived from a grammar. Instead we formulate parsing as a linear binary program which we solve using Dual Decomposition. The algorithm produces plausible approximations of globally optimal segmentations without grammar sampling. It yields state-of-the-art performance on standard datasets.

1 Introduction

The goal of facade parsing is to segment rectified building images into regions corresponding to architectural elements, like windows, balconies and doors. The resulting segments have to satisfy structural constraints, e.g., alignment of windows on the same floor, or requirement that a balcony is associated to a window and right below it. Applications include creating 3D models of urban scenes.

A common approach to this problem is to let the user specify a shape prior encoding the structural constraints. It often takes the form of a shape grammar and proposed algorithms try to find a sequence of instantiated grammar rules yielding an optimal segmentation [1–3]. But the dimension of the search space is very large. Consequently, these algorithms suffer from the 'curse of structural exploration'. They search the solution space randomly [1,2], which does not guarantee optimality or repeatability, or severely subsample the image [3].

In this paper we lift the curse of structural exploration by proposing an alternative formulation of priors, which can be mapped to a linear binary program and solved efficiently, yielding state-of-the-art performance on standard datasets.

1.1 Related Work

Most proposed priors that are complex enough to model constraints of building facades rely on shape grammars [4]. The concept has been introduced by Stiny et al. [5] in the 70's, and the idea of representing image contents in a hierarchical

---

Electronic supplementary material The online version of this chapter (doi:10. 1007/978-3-319-16817-3_6) contains supplementary material, which is available to authorized users.

D. Cremers et al. (Eds.): ACCV 2014, Part IV, LNCS 9006, pp. 79–94, 2015.
DOI: 10.1007/978-3-319-16817-3_6

and semantized manner traces back to the work of Ohta et al. [6,7]. Practical applications to image segmentation and interpretation are more recent [8–11].

A grammar is typically given by a set of nonterminal symbols $\mathcal{N}$, a set of terminal symbols $\mathcal{T}$, a start symbol in $\mathcal{N}$, and a set of production rules of the form $A_0 \to A_1 \ldots A_n$ where $A_0 \in \mathcal{N}$ and $A_i \in \mathcal{N} \cup \mathcal{T}$ for $1 \leq i \leq n$.

In the grammar of Han and Zhu [8], terminal symbols are rectangles and production rules combine them into rows, columns or grids, allowing rectangle nesting. The authors resort to a greedy algorithm for constructing the parse tree, which illustrates the difficulty of optimizing over a grammar derivation.

Drawing ideas from architectural modeling [12], where facade generation is analogous to string derivation in formal languages, the top-down parser of Teboul et al. [1,2] is one of the first attempts to parse facades using 'split grammars'. The input image is recursively split into rectangular subregions which are assigned a class label. Splitting directions as well as the number and class of subrectangles are non-deterministically chosen according to a predefined set of production rules. The process continues until all rectangles have a terminal class. The parser actually samples a number of possible derivations, exploring only a small part of the structural space. Even with a 'smart' sampling strategy [2], it does not produce repeatable results: as reported in [13], inference consists in independently running the exploration five times and keeping the best solution.

To counter the drawbacks of sampling, Riemenschneider et al. [3] propose an adaptation of the Cocke-Younger-Kasami (CYK) algorithm for parsing string grammars to two-dimensional split grammars. Its complexity is $O(w^2 h^2 N)$, where w and h are image dimensions and N is the number of possible combinations of production rule attributes (including splitting positions). This limits practical applications of the algorithm to grids of about 60 by 60 cells. To circumvent this limitation the authors test different methods of image subsampling.

An attempt to fight the curse of procedural exploration was proposed by Koziński and Marlet [14], using graph grammars and MRF optimization. In contrast to parsers like [2] whose combinatorial search explores both the nature of splits and their position at the same time, sampling here concerns structure only; optimal positions for a given sampled structure are found with a principled and efficient method. The space to explore, which now does not depend on image size, is considerably smaller, but the curse of the procedural space is not eliminated completely as graph-grammar sampling remains.

Some facade segmentation methods [15,16] do not use any user-defined shape prior. The bottom-up method proposed by Martinovic et al. [15] applies 'soft' architectural principles as a postprocessing step after image segmentation, but cannot accommodate 'hard' structural constraints. It can produce artifacts, like windows extending further than their balconies. A more recent work by Cohen et al. [16] uses a sequence of dynamic programs to recover a segmentation that respects a set of hard-coded constraints and attains state-of-the-art performance on the standard datasets. In our experiments, our method matches the performance of this algorithm while offering full flexibility with respect to shape prior specification.

In this paper we formulate the problem of finding an optimal segmentation as a binary linear program. We solve this program using the Dual Decomposition

(DD) approach [17,18]. Similar techniques include Alternating Direction of Multipliers Method (ADMM) [19]. We chose DD because ADMM, although known to feature better convergence properties, requires solving quadratic subproblems. The experiments confirm that DD behaves well in our application.

1.2 Contributions

Our approach for image parsing does not suffer from the curse of procedural exploration. It is based on a shape prior formalism that allows efficient parsing.

Instead of expressing a shape prior using grammar rules, we propose to represent the structural decomposition of a scene as a hierarchy of classes, complemented by a specification of forbidden configurations of neighboring elements.

The parsing problem can then be turned into a linear binary program, which we solve efficiently using Dual Decomposition, eliminating the need for a procedural exploration of the solution space. As shown in the experiment section, our algorithm features the accuracy of methods using hard-coded structural constraints [15,16] while retaining the flexibility of grammar-based methods [2,3]. The comparison to state of the art is summarized in Table 1.

Table 1. Comparison of with state-of-the-art facade parsing methods.

Property	[2]	[15]	[16]	[3]	Ours
User-defined shape prior	✓	–	–	✓	✓
Approximation of global optimum	–	–	–*	✓	✓
No need of image subsampling (for tractability)	✓	✓	✓	–	✓
Simultaneous alignment in two dimensions	✓	✓	–	✓	✓

* Cohen et al. [16] can issue a certificate of optimality if the found solution is optimal.

2 Proposed Model

Although it departs from the grammar-based methods, our approach to structural segmentation is inspired by the process of hierarchical image subdivision into rectangular regions, which we will refer to as rectangles in the rest of the paper. The shape prior consists of a tree of rectangle classes and a specification of pairwise potentials penalizing unlikely or invalid configurations of adjacent rectangles. In the tree, child nodes represent classes of rectangles resulting from splitting a rectangle of a parent class. We require that a rectangle of a class resulting from a vertical split can only be split horizontally, and vice versa. Consequently, all non-leaf nodes at a given tree depth are split along the same direction. Each nonterminal is assigned a table of pairwise potentials penalizing pairs of child classes assigned to neighboring rectangles. Our algorithm can handle infinite values of the potentials and in our experiments we only use binary potentials that take the value of zero or infinity, preventing some configurations of neighbors and allowing the others.

In contrast to split grammars, which are context-free and cannot be used to express simultaneous alignment in two dimensions (other than with implementation tricks that introduce some context dependency [2]), we require rectangles of the same class to be aligned both vertically and horizontally. This requirement can be enforced by constraining all rectangles of the same class that are aligned along the splitting direction to be split in the same positions into subrectangles of the same classes. A tree example and corresponding segmentations are presented in Fig. 1. Note the bidirectional alignment of windows (class g).

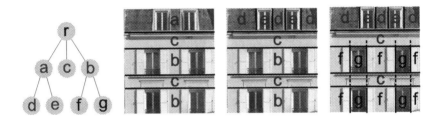

Fig. 1. A shape prior consists of a hierarchy of classes (image 1) and a table of pairwise potentials for each nonterminal node (not shown here). Each image (2–4) shows substitution of all rectangles of a particular class with rectangles of child classes.

2.1 Optimal Segmentation as a Binary Linear Program

We denote the set of indices of image pixels by $\mathcal{I} = \{(i,j)|i \in I, j \in J\}$, $I = \{1, \ldots, h\}$ and $J = \{1, \ldots, w\}$, where h is image height and w is image width. We denote the set of rectangle classes by $\mathcal{C} = K \cup L$, where K denotes the set of classes that result from a horizontal split, also called row-classes, and L is the set of classes that result from a vertical split, called column-classes, and $K \cap L = \emptyset$. The root of the tree r is a 'starting class', corresponding to the whole image. Without loss of generality we assume that r is split horizontally and by convention we consider $r \in L$. We recall that nodes in K can only have children in L and vice versa. In consequence, all nodes at a given level of the tree are either col-classes or row-classes. We denote the set of children of class $n \in \mathcal{C}$ by $Ch(n)$ and the set of descendants of n, including n, by $Desc(n)$. Similarly, we denote the set of ancestors of n, including n, by $Anc(n)$, and its parent by $Pa(n)$. The set of siblings of n is denoted $Sib(n)$. We call $t \in \mathcal{C}$ corresponding to the leaves of the tree terminal classes and denote their set by T.

A sequence of vertical and horizontal splits assigns a sequence of rectangle class labels to every pixel of the image. For any row i, it is thus possible to list all the classes that are assigned to at least one pixel on the row. Below we show that a segmentation consistent with a prior of the proposed form can be encoded in terms of the sets of classes assigned to each image row and column. This row- and column-based formulation enables global alignment of distant rectangles of the same class. We define variables $y_{ik}, y_{il}, x_{jk}, x_{jl} \in \{0,1\}$ such that $y_{ik} = 1$ if k is present in row i and $x_{jl} = 1$ if l appears in column j. We make a distinction

Table 2. Illustration of the splitting process and interpretation of the variables x_{jl} and y_{ik}. The splitting process is just a concept that helps us to introduce our formulation and not a mode of operation of the proposed algorithm.

	Example sequence of splits	Specific constraints for the example	General constraints
First split $r \rightarrow \{A, B\}$	A / B / A	$x_{jA} = 1$ $x_{jB} = 1$ $y_{iA} + y_{iB} = 1$	$\forall k \in Ch(r),\ x_{jk} = 1$ $\sum_{k \in Ch(r)} y_{jk} = 1$
Vertical splits $A \rightarrow \{C, D\}$ $B \rightarrow \{E, F\}$	C D / E F / C D	$x_{jC} + x_{jD} = x_{jA}$ $x_{jE} + x_{jF} = x_{jB}$ $y_{iA} = y_{iC} = y_{iD}$ $y_{iB} = y_{iE} = y_{iF}$	$\forall k \in K,\ \sum_{l \in Ch(k)} x_{jl} = x_{jk}$ $\forall k \in K, \forall l \in Ch(k),\ y_{jl} = y_{jk}$
Horiz. splits $C \rightarrow \{G, H\}$ $D \rightarrow \{P, Q\}$	G P / H Q / E F / H P / G Q	$x_{jC} = x_{jG} = x_{jH}$ $x_{jD} = x_{jP} = x_{jQ}$ $y_{iC} = y_{iG} + y_{iH}$ $y_{iD} = y_{iP} + y_{iQ}$	$\forall l \in L, \forall k \in Ch(l),\ x_{jk} = x_{jl}$ $\forall l \in L,\ \sum_{k \in Ch(l)} y_{ik} = y_{il}$

between the variables encoding assignment of row-classes $k \in K$ and column-classes $l \in L$, because they behave differently for horizontal and vertical splits.

In Table 2 we present how the process of shape derivation changes the sets of row- and column-classes present in image rows and columns, and formulate constraints on y_{ik}, y_{il}, x_{jk} and x_{jl} that reflect this behaviour. As shown in the second row of the table, a vertical split of a rectangle of parent class results in a number of rectangles of child classes. Because the split is along the vertical axis, only one child rectangle is going to appear in each image column previously occupied by the parent. However, all children are going to occur in each image row where the parent was present. We emphasize that all vertically aligned rectangles of the same class are split simultaneously along the same lines, so that the child rectangles are aligned and their classes are consistent along the splitting axis. The same reasoning applies to horizontal splits.

The corresponding constraints on x_{jl}, x_{jk}, y_{il} and y_{ik} are presented in the third column of Table 2. We note that for vertical splits the state of each y_{il} for $l \in Ch(k)$ is determined by y_{ik} and that the same holds for horizontal splits, x_{jk} and x_{jl}, as shown in the fourth column of Table 2. We therefore eliminate the redundant variables x_{jk} and y_{il}. This will result in a formulation where row-classes are assigned to image rows and col-classes are assigned to image columns. We combine the two first equations and the two second ones from rows two and three of the table to get

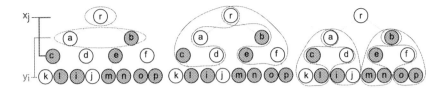

Fig. 2. Visualization of the state of variables y_{ik} and x_{jl} for some pixel i, j. The white nodes correspond to classes k and l for which $y_{ik} = 1$ and $x_{jl} = 1$. The gray nodes correspond to classes with $y_{ik} = 0$ or $x_{jl} = 0$. The domains of constraints (1) on y_{ik} are circled in blue and the domains of constraints on x_{jl} are circled in red. Left: the domains of (1b). Middle and right: the domains of (1a). Note that only one leaf is connected to the root by a path of white nodes. This illustrates the uniqueness of pixel class given the state of variables corresponding to its row and column (Color figure online).

$$\forall i \in I, \forall l \in \mathring{L}, \quad \sum_{k' \in Ch(l)} y_{ik'} = y_{iPa(l)}, \quad \forall j \in J, \forall k \in \mathring{K}, \quad \sum_{l' \in Ch(k)} x_{jl'} = x_{jPa(k)},$$
(1a)

where $\mathring{L} = L \backslash (T \cup \{r\})$ and $\mathring{K} = K \backslash T$. We visualize the domain of the constraints in Fig. 2.

In the interest of maintaining the convention of assigning row-classes $k \in K$ to rows and column-classes $l \in L$ to columns, we modify the constraint from the first row of the table. We require that the root class is assigned to each column and that the first horizontal split assigns a unique class to each row:

$$\forall j \in J, \ x_{jr} = 1 \ , \quad \forall i \in I, \quad \sum_{k \in Ch(r)} y_{ik} = 1 \ .$$
(1b)

From Table 2 it is evident that at each stage of the splitting process each pixel is assigned a unique class. Below we show that constraints (1) also capture this property and that the class assigned to pixel (i, j) is unambiguously determined by vectors (y_{ik}) for given i and (x_{jl}) for a fixed j.

Lemma 1. *Consider a hierarchy of classes given as a tree, as defined earlier. Denote the depth of the tree by M, the set of column-classes at the m-th level of the tree by L^m and the set of row-classes at the m-th level of the tree by K^m. Note that L^m is nonempty only for even m and K^m for odd m. Denote the vectors of y_{ik} and x_{jl} by $\mathbf{y}$ and $\mathbf{x}$. Denote the set of $\mathbf{y}$ and $\mathbf{x}$ satisfying constraint (1) by C_h. Then*

$$(\mathbf{y}, \mathbf{x}) \in C_h \implies \forall (i, j) \in \mathcal{I} \quad \forall m \in \{0, \dots, M\},$$

$$\exists! l_j^m \in L^m : \quad \forall n \in Anc(l_j^m), \quad (x_{jn} = 1) \vee (y_{in} = 1) \quad \text{if } m \text{ is even} \quad (2)$$

$$\exists! k_i^m \in K^m : \quad \forall n \in Anc(k_i^m), \quad (x_{jn} = 1) \vee (y_{in} = 1) \quad \text{if } m \text{ is odd} \ . \quad (3)$$

In words, for any pixel $(i,j) \in \mathcal{I}$, for any values of variables y_{ik} and x_{jl}, that satisfy constraints (1), at any depth of the tree there exists exactly one row-class, or one column-class such that the variables x_{jl} and y_{ik} corresponding to the class and all its ancestors are equal to one.

Proof. We prove the lemma by induction on the depth of the tree.

The root r is the only node at depth $m = 0$ of the tree and, by constraint (1b), it holds that $x_{jr} = 1$ for all $j \in J$. Therefore the lemma holds for $m = 0$.

For depth $m = 1$ the tree is formed of the root and its children. By constraints (1b), we have that for each i there exists a single $k_i \in Ch(r)$ such that $y_{ik_i} = 1$ and $y_{ik} = 0$ for $k \neq k_i$. This proves the lemma for the case of a tree of depth 1.

Assume Lemma 1 holds at depth m. If the m is even, then by assumption for each j we have a single l_j^m such that the variables associated to all its ancestors are equal one. By constraint (1), exactly one child of l_j^m will have its associated variable $y_{ik_i^m}$ equal to one. Similar reasoning applies to odd levels of the tree. $\square$

We model the assignment of terminal classes to pixels by variables $z_{ijt} \in \{0,1\}$, where $z_{ijt} = 1$ if pixel (i,j) is of class $t \in T$ and $z_{ijt} = 0$ otherwise. A single terminal class has to be assigned to each pixel

$$\forall (i,j) \in \mathcal{I}, \quad \sum_{t \in T} z_{ijt} = 1 . \tag{4}$$

By Lemma 1, all ancestors of the class assigned to pixel (i,j) have the variables y_{ik} and x_{jl} equal to one, which leads to the inequalities

$$\forall (i,j) \in \mathcal{I}, \forall k \in K, \quad \sum_{t \in Desc(k)} z_{ijt} \leq y_{ik}, \quad \forall (i,j) \in \mathcal{I}, \forall l \in L, \quad \sum_{t \in Desc(l)} z_{ijt} \leq x_{jl}. \tag{5}$$

Each nonterminal class has a table of pairwise potentials defined on its children. The potentials determine the likelihood of observing neighboring rectangles of the child classes. We implement the potentials with variables $y_{ikk'}$ and $x_{jll'}$

$$\forall i \in \{1, \ldots, h-1\}, \forall k \in K \quad \sum_{k' \in Sib(k)} y_{ikk'} = y_{ik} , \tag{6a}$$

$$\forall i \in \{1, \ldots, h-1\}, \forall k' \in K \quad \sum_{k \in Sib(k')} y_{ikk'} = y_{i+1k'} , \tag{6b}$$

$$\forall j \in \{1, \ldots, w-1\}, \forall l \in L \quad \sum_{l' \in Sib(l)} x_{jll'} = x_{jl} , \tag{6c}$$

$$\forall j \in \{1, \ldots, w-1\}, \forall l' \in L \quad \sum_{l \in Sib(l')} x_{jll'} = x_{j+1l'} . \tag{6d}$$

We denote the cost of assigning type t to pixel (i,j) by c_{ijt}, and the pairwise cost for column- and row-classes by $c_{kk'}$ and $c_{ll'}$. We define the sets of pairs of row- and column-classes that are siblings in the tree by $Iiblings$ and $Jiblings$. The segmentation task can be formulated as minimizing the following objective

Algorithm 1. Dual Decomposition

$\forall_m \lambda_m^0 \leftarrow 0, \quad n \leftarrow 1$
while not converged **do**
$\quad \forall_m \quad \hat{x}_m^n \leftarrow \arg \min E_m(x_m) + (\lambda_m^{n-1})^\mathsf{T} x_m$
$\quad \forall_m \quad \lambda_m^n \leftarrow \lambda_m^{n-1} + \alpha_n(\hat{x}_m^n - \frac{1}{m} \sum_m \hat{x}_m^n)$
$\quad n \leftarrow n + 1$
end while
$\hat{x} \leftarrow \text{GETFINALX}(\hat{x}_m, \lambda_m)$

$$E = \sum_{(i,j)\in\mathcal{I}} \sum_{t\in T} z_{ijt}c_{ijt} + \sum_{i=1}^{h-1} \sum_{(k,k')\in SK} y_{ikk'}c_{kk'} + \sum_{j=1}^{w-1} \sum_{(l,l')\in SL} x_{jll'}c_{ll'} \quad (7)$$

subject to constraints (4) to (6).

3   Inference

The formulated problem is linear and has a large number of binary variables. We relax the binary domain constraint and let the variables take values within the range $[0, 1]$. We apply dual decomposition to the resulting continuous problem.

3.1   The Dual Decomposition Algorithm

The dual decomposition algorithm is based on the idea of decomposing a difficult problem into a number of 'slave' subproblems that are easy to solve. Given an original problem $\hat{x} = \arg \min \sum_m E_m(x)$, $x \in C$, where C is a feasible set, we construct a number of copies of the variable x, denoted x_m, and couple them by means of a new constraint $x_m = x$. We formulate the dual problem $\max_{\lambda_m} \min_{x,x_m} \sum_m (E_m(x_m) + \lambda_m^\mathsf{T}(x - x_m))$, subject to $x_m \in C$, where λ_m is a vector of Lagrange multipliers. The problem is solved using a projected subgradient algorithm. Calculating the subgradient of the dual objective requires solving $\hat{x}_m = \arg \min E_m(x_m) + \lambda_m^\mathsf{T} x_m$, subject to $x_m \in C$, separately for each m. The latter minimizations are called slave problems. We present Dual Decomposition in Algorithm 1 and refer the reader to [17,18] for a detailed derivation. We denote the values of variables in iteration n by a superscript and the stepsize by α. The algorithm is run with decaying step size. The values of $\hat{x}_m$ eventually converge and heuristics, represented in Algorithm 1 by procedure GETFINALX, can be used to decide on the components of $\hat{x}$ on which $\hat{x}_m$ disagree [17].

The main design decision to be made when applying dual decomposition is how to decompose the original objective function into slave objectives. The main criterion is the ability to efficiently solve the slave problems. Below we present a decomposition of the objective (7) into subproblems that can be solved by means of dynamic programming in time linear in the number of pixels.

3.2   Application of Dual Decomposition to the Problem

To make the slave problem tractable we need to decouple the variables y_{ik} from the variables x_{jl} corresponding to columns. The resulting slaves would assign sets of classes to rows or columns of the image, and terminal classes to pixels.

This decoupling is however not sufficient since feasible configurations of the sets, encoded by vectors (y_{ik}) and (x_{jl}), are determined by constraints (1), that have a complex structure. We propose a further decomposition, that results in a larger number of slaves with simpler constraints. The slaves assign a single class to each pixel and each image row or column.

Each instantiation of constraints (1) can be transformed by recursively plugging its left-hand side to a left-hand side of another equation of type (1) until the resulting sum equals one. Consequently, we get

$$\forall l \in L\backslash T \quad \sum_{k \in H_l} y_{ik} = 1 , \quad \forall k \in K\backslash T \quad \sum_{l \in V_k} x_{jl} = 1 , \tag{8}$$

where $V_k = Ch(k) \cup [L \cap (Ch(A_k)\backslash A_k)]$, $A_k = Anc(k)$ and $Ch(A_k)$ is the set of all children of all elements of A_k. Informally, V_k is the smallest set containing all children of k and such that if l belongs to V_k, then all siblings of its grandparent do as well. The structure of V_k is illustrated in Fig. 3. H_k is defined similarly. Note that (8) can be transformed back to (1). It is enough to subtract from constraint (8) for some $l \in L\backslash T$ a constraint of the same type for $l' = Pa(Pa(l))$ to get a constraint of type (1). The reader can verify that on the example from Fig. 3. Thus, constraints (8) are equivalent to their original form (1).

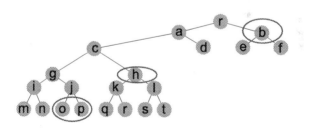

Fig. 3. The structure of set H_l, for $l = j$, visualized on a tree of classes. Elements of the set are outlined in red. Exactly one of them has to be assigned to each image row (Color figure online).

The advantage of constraint (8) is that it is an intersection of simplex constraints, which entails that the problem can be naturally decomposed into a number of subproblems, one for each $l \in L\backslash T$ and each $k \in K\backslash T$.

3.3   Structure of Slave Subproblem

We create one slave for each $l \in L\backslash T$ and one for each $k \in K\backslash T$. Below we present the structure of a slave subproblem for some l. The slaves for k are created symmetrically. We denote by SH_l the set of pairs of sibling row classes k, k' such that $k, k' \in H_l$. Copies of variables that appear in many slaves are denoted with a superscript l. By $n_{kk'}$ we denote the number of times the pair k, k' appears in different slaves. The cost coefficients of a slave: $\tilde{c}_{ijt} = \frac{c_{ijt}}{\left(|L\backslash T|+|K\backslash T|\right)}$ and $\tilde{c}_{kk'} = \frac{c_{kk'}}{n_{kk'}}$, sum to the costs of the original objective. The slave objective is

$$\min_{z^l_{ijt}, y^l_{ik}, y^l_{kk'}} \sum_{\substack{(i,j)\in\mathcal{I} \\ t\in T}} (\tilde{c}_{ijt} + \lambda^l_{ijt})z^l_{ijt} + \sum_{\substack{i\in I \\ k\in H_l}} \lambda^l_{ik}y^l_{ik} + \sum_{\substack{i\in\{1,\dots,h-1\} \\ k,k'\in SH_l}} \tilde{c}_{kk'}y^l_{ikk'} \quad , \qquad (9)$$

where λ^l_{ijt} is a Lagrange multiplier corresponding to a constraint coupling the variables z^l_{ijt} for different slaves and λ^l_{ik} is a Lagrange multiplier coupling y^l_{ik} for different slaves. The derivation of the slave objective from the original objective (7) is straightforward and is omitted here but detailed in the supplementary material. The feasible set of each slave problem is a projection of the original feasible set, defined by constraints (4) to (6), to the space of the slave variables:

$$\forall(i,j)\in\mathcal{I}, \ \forall t\in T, \ z^l_{ijt} \geq 0 \ , \qquad \forall(i,j)\in\mathcal{I}, \ \sum_{t\in T}z^l_{ijt} = 1 \ , \qquad (10\text{a})$$

$$\forall i\in I, \ \forall k\in H_l, \ y^l_{ik} \geq 0 \ , \qquad \forall i\in I, \ \sum_{k\in H_l}y^l_{ik} = 1 \ , \qquad (10\text{b})$$

$$\forall(i,j)\in\mathcal{I}, \quad \forall k\in H_l \qquad \sum_{t\in Desc(k)}z^l_{ijt} \leq y^l_{ik} \ , \qquad (10\text{c})$$

$$\forall i\in J\backslash\{h\}, \quad \forall k\in H_l, \qquad \sum_{k'\in Sib^l(k)}y^l_{ikk'} = y^l_{ik} \ , \qquad (10\text{d})$$

$$\forall i\in J\backslash\{h\}, \quad \forall k'\in H_l, \qquad \sum_{k\in Sib^l(k')}y^l_{ikk'} = y^l_{i+1k'} \ , \qquad (10\text{e})$$

where $Sib^l(k)$ denotes the set of sibling of class k that belong to the set H_l. The nonnegativity constraints (10a) and (10b) are introduced due to the relaxation of the variables from binary to continuous domain. Constraints (10c) to (10e) have the same form as the corresponding constraints (4) to (6) in the original problem. The constraint (10b) represents constraints (1) of the original problem, transformed according to (8). Summarizing, an intersection of the feasible sets of the slaves is equivalent to the feasible set of the original problem, in the sense that if for all i, j, k, l, t we have $z_{ijt} = z^k_{ijt} = z^l_{ijt}$ and $y_{ik} = y^l_{ik}$, $x_{jl} = x^k_{jl}$, then $(z, y, x) \in C \iff \forall l\in L\backslash T, \ (z^l, y^l) \in C^l \wedge \forall k\in K\backslash T, \ (z^k, x^k) \in C^k$, where C, C^k and C^l denote the feasible sets of the original problem and of the slaves, respectively.

3.4   Solving the Slave Subproblem

It can be proven that the feasible set of the slave problem has integral vertices. A proof can be found in the appendix. In consequence, each slave can be seen as a labelling problem where we assign a label $k \in H_l$ to each row i and a label t to each pixel $(i, j) \in \mathcal{I}$. We find the optimal labelling by dynamic programming.

Given row-class k assigned to row i by slave l, it is easy to determine for each pixel in the row the optimal class t_{ij}^{lk}. Constraint (10c) restricts the set of classes that can be used in a row labelled k to descendants of k or to ones that do not descend from any $k \in H_l$. We denote the latter set by $\tilde{T}_l = T \backslash \bigcup_{k \in H_l} Desc(k)$. The class assigned by the slave to pixel (i, j) is

$$t_{ij}^{lk} = \arg\min_{t \in Desc(k) \cup \tilde{T}_l} (\tilde{c}_{ijt} + \lambda_{ijt}^l) \quad . \tag{11}$$

From objective (9) we derive the optimal cost of assigning row class k to image row i, which is the sum of costs for each pixel and the per-row cost

$$c_{ik}^l = \sum_{j=1}^{w} (\tilde{c}_{ijt_{ij}^{lk}} + \lambda_{ijt_{ij}^{lk}}^l) + \lambda_{ik}^l \quad . \tag{12}$$

The optimal cost of assigning classes for the i first rows, denoted $\phi^l(i, k)$, where k is the row class assigned to row i, can be recursively defined as

$$\phi^l(i, k) = \begin{cases} c_{1k}^l & \text{if } i = 1 \\ \min_{k' \in H_l} \phi^l(i - 1, k') + c_{ik}^l + \tilde{c}_{k'k} & \text{otherwise.} \end{cases} \tag{13}$$

We use the recursive structure of the subproblem to formulate Algorithm 2 for finding its optimal solution. First, for each row and each candidate row label $k \in H_l$, optimal pixel classes t_{ij}^{lk} are determined for each pixel in the row according to (11). They are then used for determining costs c_{ik}^l of assigning classes $k \in H_l$ to image rows according to (12). Finally we run the Viterbi algorithm according to (13) to retrieve the optimal labelling of all rows.

4   Experiments

We tested the performance of our algorithm on two datasets. For each of them, we created a shape prior consisting of a tree hierarchy of classes and a table of pairwise potentials for each nonterminal node. We used binary potentials to penalize invalid pairs of neighboring classes, like sky under wall, with infinite cost. For each image, we run the DD algorithm for 100 iterations, with a fixed sequence of decaying step size $\alpha_n = a/\sqrt{n}$, where n is iteration number and a is a constant. The average running time was about 4 min per image.

The ECP dataset [2] consists of about 100 rectified images of Haussmannian building facades with annotations of 7 classes: sky, roof, wall, window, balcony, shop and door. The ground-truth annotations are consistent with the grammar used in [2], which models facade structure as a grid of windows with balconies

---

Algorithm 2. Dynamic program solving the slave subproblem.

for all $k \in H_l, i \in I$ **do**   ▷ dyn. prog. on t_{ij}
    for all $j \in J$ **do**
        $t_{ij}^{lk} \leftarrow \arg\min_{t \in Desc(k) \cup \tilde{T}_l}(\tilde{c}_{ijt} + \lambda_{ijt}^l)$
    end for
    $c_{ik}^l \leftarrow \sum_j (\tilde{c}_{ijt_{ij}^{lk}} + \lambda_{ijt_{ij}^{lk}}^l) + \lambda_{ik}^l$
end for
for all $k \in H_l$ **do**   ▷ dyn. prog. on k_i
    $\phi^l(1,k) \leftarrow c_{1k}^l$
end for
for $i = 2, \ldots, h$ **do**
    for $k \in H_l$ **do**
        $\phi^l(i,k) \leftarrow \min_{k' \in H_l} \phi^l(i-1,k') + c_{ik}^l + \tilde{c}_{k'k}$
        $k^l(i-1,k) \leftarrow \arg\min_{k' \in H_l} \phi^l(i-1,k') + c_{ik}^l + \tilde{c}_{k'k}$ ▷ store opt. prev. class
    end for
end for
$k_i, t_{ij} \leftarrow \text{BACKTRACK}(\phi^l, k^l)$ ▷ extract optimal k_i and t_{ij} from recorded info

---

Table 3. Performance on the ECP dataset. The rows corresponding to classes present class accuracy (the diagonal entries of confusion matrices, or recall). The bottom rows contain average class accuracy and total pixel accuracy. Starting from left, we present the performance of three layers of Martinovic's solution [15], and the results of Cohen et al. [16], using 'raw' per-pixel energies, and with SVM scores on top of the energies.

	[15]-L1	[15]-L2	[15]-L3	[16]	[16]-SVM	Ours	Our confusion matrix							
roof	70	73	74	93	90	91	91	0	0	2	2	0	5	roof
shop	79	86	93	96	94	95	0	95	0	0	0	0	4	shop
balcony	74	71	70	92	91	90	1	0	90	0	4	0	5	balc.
sky	91	91	97	96	97	96	4	0	0	96	0	0	0	sky
window	62	69	75	87	85	85	3	1	4	0	85	0	5	wind.
door	43	60	67	82	79	74	0	22	0	0	0	74	4	door
wall	92	93	88	88	90	91	1	3	2	0	3	0	91	wall
class aver.	73.0	77.6	80.6	90.6	89.4	88.8								
pixel accur.	82.6	85.1	84.2	90.3	**90.8**	**90.8**								

Table 4. Results of the experiment on the Graz50 dataset. The second and third columns of the table show diagonal entries of the confusion matrices for results reported by Riemenschneider et al. [3] and our results. The right-hand side of the table contains the confusion matrix for our results. Example result is shown on the right hand side.

	[3]	Ours	conf. mat.				
sky	91	93	93	0	0	6	sky
window	60	82	0	82	0	17	window
door	41	50	0	14	50	36	door
wall	84	96	0	3	0	96	wall
class average	69.0	80.3					
total pixel accur.	78.0	**91.8**					

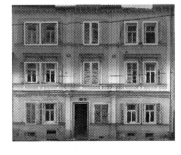

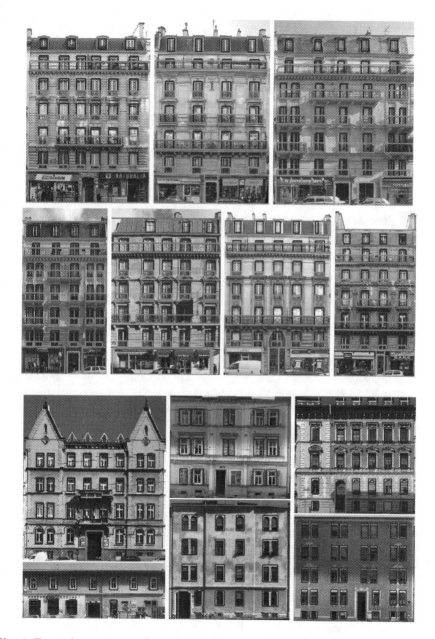

Fig. 4. Example parsing results on the ECP dataset (top) and on the Graz50 dataset (bottom). Green lines separate sky from roof and roof from facade. Balconies are outlined in magenta, shops in yellow, and doors in cyan. Note the variety of alignment patterns supported by the algorithm (top right). Typical errors are missed doors and missed roof windows (Color figure online).

constrained to individual windows or extending over the width of the facade. In consequence the ground truth is incorrect on a number of images. We use the annotations provided by [15], which do not respect semantic constraints (balconies and windows can be misaligned, small pieces of doors may float above the ground), but are more accurate in terms of pixel classification.

The Graz50 dataset [3] is composed of 50 rectified images of facades of different architectural styles. They feature more structural variation than the ones of the ECP dataset. The labels include four classes: sky, wall, window and door.

Performance on the ECP Dataset has been tested using per-pixel energies that follow the description from [16]. We use a multi-feature extension of Texton-Boost, implemented by the authors of [20]. We use SIFT and Color SIFT, Local Binary Patterns and location features. Features of each type are clustered using K-means into 512 clusters. The final feature vector is a concatenation of histograms of appearance of cluster members in a neighborhood of 200 randomly sampled rectangles. The per-pixel costs c_{ijt} are output by a multi-class boosting classifier [21]. We follow the protocol of [15,16] in performing experiments on five folds with 80 training and 20 testing images. The results are presented in Table 3. Our method attains the same performance as [16]. However, our algorithm can accept a user-defined shape prior as input, which makes it more general. The shape prior can express constraints on alignment of architectural elements in two dimensions, which is beyond the expressive power of [16].

Performance on the Graz50 dataset has been tested using the same type of pixel costs as for the ECP dataset. Five folds were used, each time the dataset was split into 40 training and 10 test images. The results are presented in Table 4. One reason why our results are superior to those in [3] is that their method requires severe subsampling of the image to be tractable. Our method is more computationally efficient and can be run on full-resolution images (Fig. 4).

5   Conclusion and Future Work

We presented a novel approach to shape prior-based facade analysis in which the task of parsing is formulated as a binary linear program. Our formulation does not suffer from the curse of procedural exploration, that is typical for existing split grammar parsers. It enables approximating globally optimal segmentations by means of efficient optimization algorithms. We established a new state-of-the-art level of performance on the ECP and Graz50 facade datasets.

As a direct extension of this work, we are considering learning the pairwise potentials using the approach presented in [22]. In longer perspective, due to increasingly good results reported recently on rectified images, we see the relevance of addressing difficulties arising from the use of real life images, like modeling projection of three-dimensional geometry of buildings on the image plane and handling occlusions (e.g., by cars, vegetation, pedestrians or other buildings).

Acknowledgements. This work was carried out in IMAGINE, a joint research project between Ecole des Ponts ParisTech (ENPC) and the Scientific and Technical Centre for Building (CSTB). It was partly supported by ANR project Semapolis ANR-13-CORD-0003.

References

1. Teboul, O., Simon, L., Koutsourakis, P., Paragios, N.: Segmentation of building facades using procedural shape priors. In: CVPR, pp. 3105–3112 (2010)
2. Teboul, O., Kokkinos, I., Simon, L., Koutsourakis, P., Paragios, N.: Shape grammar parsing via reinforcement learning. In: CVPR, pp. 2273–2280 (2011)
3. Riemenschneider, H., Krispel, U., Thaller, W., Donoser, M., Havemann, S., Fellner, D., Bischof, H.: Irregular lattices for complex shape grammar facade parsing. In: CVPR (2012)
4. Zhu, S.C., Mumford, D.: A stochastic grammar of images. Found. Trends Comput. Graph. Vis. **2**, 259–362 (2006)
5. Stiny, G.N.: Pictorial and Formal Aspects of Shape and Shape Grammars and Aesthetic Systems. PhD thesis, University of California, Los Angeles (1975). AAI7526993
6. Ohta, Y., Kanade, T., Sakai, T.: An analysis system for scenes containing objects with substructures. In: Proceedings of the Fourth International Joint Conference on Pattern Recognitions, pp. 752–754 (1978)
7. Ohta, Y., Kanade, T., Sakai, T.: A production system for region analysis. In: Proceedings of the Sixth International Joint Conference on Artificial Intelligence, pp. 684–686 (1979)
8. Han, F., Zhu, S.C.: Bottom-up/top-down image parsing with attribute graph grammar. IEEE Trans. Pattern Anal. Mach. Intell. **31**, 59–73 (2009)
9. Wang, W., Pollak, I., Wong, T.S., Bouman, C.A., Harper, M.P.: Hierarchical stochastic image grammars for classification and segmentation. IEEE Trans. Image Process. **15**, 3033–3052 (2006)
10. Jin, Y., Geman, S.: Context and hierarchy in a probabilistic image model. In: CVPR (2), pp. 2145–2152 (2006)
11. Ahuja, N., Todorovic, S.: Connected segmentation tree - a joint representation of region layout and hierarchy. In: CVPR (2008)
12. Müller, P., Wonka, P., Haegler, S., Ulmer, A., Van Gool, L.: Procedural modeling of buildings. ACM Trans. Graph. **25**, 614–623 (2006)
13. Teboul, O.: Shape Grammar Parsing: Application to Image-based Modeling. PhD thesis, Ecole centrale Paris (2011)
14. Koziński, M., Marlet, R.: Image parsing with graph grammars and Markov random fields. In: WACV (2014)
15. Martinovic, A., Mathias, M., Weissenberg, J., Van Gool, L.: A three-layered approach to facade parsing. In: Fitzgibbon, A., Lazebnik, S., Perona, P., Sato, Y., Schmid, C. (eds.) ECCV 2012 Part VII. LNCS, vol. 7578, pp. 416–429. Springer, Heidelberg (2012)
16. Cohen, A., Schwing, A., Pollefeys, M.: Efficient structured parsing of facades using dynamic programming. In: CVPR (2014)
17. Komodakis, N., Paragios, N., Tziritas, G.: MRF energy minimization and beyond via dual decomposition. IEEE Trans. PAMI **33**, 531–552 (2011)

18. Sontag, D., Globerson, A., Jaakkola, T.: Introduction to dual decomposition for inference. In: Sra, S., Nowozin, S., Wright, S.J. (eds.) Optimization for Machine Learning. MIT Press, Cambridge (2011)
19. Boyd, S., Parikh, N., Chu, E., Peleato, B., Eckstein, J.: Distributed optimization and statistical learning via the alternating direction method of multipliers. Found. Trends Mach. Learn. **3**, 1–122 (2011)
20. Ladický, L., Russell, C., Kohli, P., Torr, P.H.S.: Associative hierarchical random fields. IEEE Trans. Pattern Anal. Mach. Intell. **99**, 1 (2013)
21. Shotton, J., Winn, J.M., Rother, C., Criminisi, A.: TextonBoost: joint appearance, shape and context modeling for multi-class object recognition and segmentation. In: Leonardis, A., Bischof, H., Pinz, A. (eds.) ECCV 2006, Part I. LNCS, vol. 3951, pp. 1–15. Springer, Heidelberg (2006)
22. Komodakis, N.: Efficient training for pairwise or higher order CRFs via dual decomposition. In: CVPR, pp. 1841–1848 (2011)

Shape Matching Using Point Context and Contour Segments

Christian Feinen, Cong Yang, Oliver Tiebe, and Marcin Grzegorzek$^{(\boxtimes)}$

Research Group for Pattern Recognition, Department ETI, University of Siegen,
Hoelderlinstr. 3, 57076 Siegen, Germany
marcin.grzegorzek@uni-siegen.de

Abstract. This paper proposes a novel method to generate robust contour partition points and applies them to produce point context and contour segment features for shape matching. The main idea is to match object shapes by matching contour partition points and contour segments. In contrast to typical shape context method, we do not consider the topological graph structure since our approach is only considering a small number of partition points rather than full contour points. The experimental results demonstrate that our method is able to produce correct results in the presence of articulations, stretching, and contour deformations. The most significant scientific contributions of this paper include (i) the introduction of a novel partition point extraction technique for point context and contour segments as well as (ii) a new fused similarity measure for object matching and recognition, and (iii) the impressive robustness of the method in an object retrieval scenario as well as in a real application for environmental microorganism recognition.

1 Introduction

Shape is a powerful feature for recognition as psychophysical studies [1] have shown. As an important feature carrier, shape contour is widely used in object detection and matching methods [2,3]. This is because shape contour is invariant to lighting conditions and variations in object colour and texture. More importantly, it can efficiently represent image structures with large spatial extents [3].

Since shape contour is sensitive to object deformation, developing robust contour-based shape descriptors invariant to shape rotation, translation, scaling, and transformation is still a challenge task. Although skeleton-based descriptors contain both shape features and topological structures of original objects, they require heavy calculation for skeleton pruning [4]. Moreover, the following matching process is highly dependent on the quality of branch pruning. Recently, researchers have tried to employ contour segment [2,5,6] for shape matching since contour segments are invariant to shape deformation. However, in order to generate applicable contour segments, appropriate partition points are required. Traditionally, skeleton endpoints can be used as partition points since they are stable and covering most visual parts of original shapes. Nevertheless, as we discussed previously, it heavily relies on skeleton pruning.

© Springer International Publishing Switzerland 2015
D. Cremers et al. (Eds.): ACCV 2014, Part IV, LNCS 9006, pp. 95–110, 2015.
DOI: 10.1007/978-3-319-16817-3_7

The main goal of this paper is to present a method that extracts the exact contour partition points and its related robust descriptors for shape matching. Our proposed method is easy to implement and can be computed efficiently. To achieve this, we propose a novel method for generating contour partition points which is robust and stable for shape deformation. Based on these points, we generate point context and contour segments as shape descriptor. For object matching, we apply the point context-based matching and the contour segments-based matching independently. By fusing two matching results with an integrated Gradient Hill Climbing [7] and Simulated Annealing [8] method, we calculate the shape distance and apply it for a shape retrieval scenario. Finally, we employ a modified mutual kNN graph on the distance matrix to improve the accuracy of shape retrieval. The advantages of our proposed approach include (i) low computational complexity as well as (ii) the inclusion of only a limited number of sampling points instead of all contour points with point context, and (iii) the impressive robustness of the method in an object retrieval scenario.

2   Related Work

Contour-Based Shape Matching: For contour-based approaches, many methods achieve state-of-the-art performance by only utilising contour information. For example, Shotton et al. [9] present a categorical object detection scheme that uses only local contour-based features and is realised in a partly supervised learning framework. Nguyen et al. [10] propose a shape-based local binary descriptor for object detection that has been tested in the task of detecting humans from static images. In [11], an algorithm for partial shape matching with mildly non-rigid deformations using Markov chains and the Monte Carlo method is introduced. Based on contour points, Belongie et al. proposed shape context [12] descriptor for object matching. Shape context appears to be one of the best performing shape descriptor and definitely the most popular one. With the same basic geometric units of shape context, Ma and Latecki [6] proposed a shape descriptor that is particularly suitable for shape matching of edge fragments in images to model contours of target objects. Inspired by the Bag of Words model, Wang et al. [13] introduced the Bag of contour fragments as a higher level shape descriptor. Combining it with an linear SVM the authors were able to achieve impressive results on existing Datasets.

Skeleton-Based Shape Matching: Though skeleton (or medial axis) can be generated by shape contour with maximal disk model [14], comparing to contour matching methods, skeleton matching approaches feature lower sensitivity to occlusion, limb growth and articulation [15]. However, they are computationally more complex [16] and still have not yet been fully successfully applied to real images. Baseski et al. [17] present a tree-edit-based shape matching method that uses a recent coarse skeleton representation. Their dissimilarity measure gives a better understanding within group versus between group separation which mimics the asymmetric nature of human similarity judgements. To the best of our knowledge, the best performing skeleton-based object matching algorithm has been proposed by Bai et al. [18]. Their main idea is to match skeleton graphs by comparing the geodesic paths between skeleton endpoints.

Shape Matching by Skeletons and Contours: Besides the utilisation of only contour or skeleton features for shape matching, some fused shape descriptors with contours and skeletons have been proposed. Bai et al. [5] combine the object contour and skeleton properties for shape classification. They extract contour segments using the Discrete Curve Evolution [4]. However, their approach works in a supervised pattern recognition mode and multiple training examples of an object class are necessary for modelling. Zeng et al. [19] combine properties of skeletons and boundaries for general shape decomposition. Unfortunately, this method is rotation variant and highly sensitive to shape deformation. Yang et al. [2] proposed an approach for object retrieval that uses contour segment and skeleton matching for shape similarity computation. They employ skeleton endpoints for contour partition. For contour segment, they proposed a new feature extraction technique for contour segments. Though this method achieved excellent results, however, it still highly relies on skeleton pruning.

3 Shape Representation

Partition Point: Here we describe the contour partitioning approach employed for separating the shape of an arbitrary object Ω into a set of sub-parts. This subset as well as the partition points p_i are required to perform the matching described below. The general idea is to detect contour regions with a high curvature toward the overall shape trend. Therefore, either a single or multiple *reference points* (x_i) inside the shape are selected to compute distances between all contour points $\partial\Omega$ and their closest x_i. By sampling the contour clockwise and arranging these values linearly, a signal s is generated that can be used to detect peaks in its second-order derivative. By backtracking these peaks, the desired partition points are obtained.

Therefore, first the contour is extracted and subsequently converted to a polygon $\mathcal{P}$. For the purpose of polygonisation the well-known *Douglas-Peucker* technique is recursively applied to $\partial\Omega$. Here, only a small tolerance value $\epsilon^{(DP)}$ is taken which drastically reduces the noise-to-signal ratio without removing significant characteristics of the shape. Figure 1 illustrates this on the example image of the bird by using two different tolerance values.

Next, the reference points x_i have to be located inside the shape in order to sample the contour. They are detected by utilising a high accurate *fast marching*

Fig. 1. The original image and two versions created by different tolerance values.

method proposed by the authors Hassouna et al. in [20]. The result is a distance map whose values are generated based on a given initialisation (seed point(s)). In this context, $\mathcal{P}$ is taken as initialisation with the result of a distance or rather a time-crossing map T. The values in T can also be interpreted as contour contraction or expansion, respectively. This is illustrated in Fig. 2.

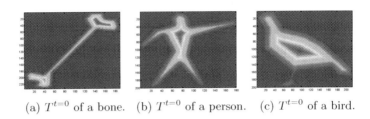

(a) $T^{t=0}$ of a bone.   (b) $T^{t=0}$ of a person.   (c) $T^{t=0}$ of a bird.

Fig. 2. The figures shows the time-crossing maps of a bone, a person and a bird. They can also be interpreted as distance maps initialised with the objects' contours.

The actual reference points are then discovered at maximum value locations in T. Therefore, a detection procedure is localising iteratively candidate regions and validates them in terms of being a new reference point. This is done based on a dynamically adapting threshold $\mu^{(BG)}$, that is applied to T in order to remove background values to emphasise these candidate regions:

$$\mu^{(BG)} = \phi(T(\Omega)) - 2 \cdot \psi(T(\Omega)), \tag{1}$$

where $\phi(\cdot)$ is a function returning the maximum value with $\{v^\star \mid v^\star \in T, \forall v \in T : v^\star > v\}$ inside Ω. In contrast to this, $\psi(\cdot)$ indicates the standard derivation. Once the background pixels are removed, the remaining ones are clustered to disjoint regions $\boldsymbol{A}_i$ which are subsequently used to determine *weighted centroids*, respectively. The first iteration ($t = 0$) is then completed with storing all $\boldsymbol{A}_i^{t=0}$ inside a binary mask $\boldsymbol{B}$ having the same size as the input image $\boldsymbol{I}$ and the weighted centroids are collected in a set, depicted by $\mathcal{C}^{t=0}$. The next iterations are processing the same way, but differ as follows: In each further iteration t, the algorithm loops only over the reference points found previously ($\mathcal{C}^{t-1}$), where each of them is used as seed point for the fast marching method. The resulting T_i^t (where $i = [1, 2, \ldots, \otimes(\mathcal{C}^{t-1})]$ with $\otimes(\cdot)$ being a function that returns the number of elements) is then applied (here multiplied) to $T^{t=0}$. The effect of $T^t \circ T^{t=0}$ is illustrated in Fig. 3 based on the example of a glass. As shown, the method would not return a reference point for the lower part by only using $T^{t=0}$.

On the basis $T^t \circ T^{t=0}$ the threshold $\mu^{(BG)}$ is adapted and new candidate regions $\boldsymbol{A}_i^t$ are located. Subsequently, the centroids ($\boldsymbol{x}_i^t$) are calculated for all $\boldsymbol{A}_i^t$. If one of these $\boldsymbol{x}_i^t$ is residing in an already processed area, which means $\boldsymbol{B}(\boldsymbol{x}_i^t) = 1$, the point is rejected, otherwise $\boldsymbol{x}_i^t \in \mathcal{C}^t$ and $\boldsymbol{B}$ is updated. It terminates if the current iteration returns an empty set of newly detected reference points ($\mathcal{C}^t = \emptyset$). The final set, in turn, is generated by $\boldsymbol{P} = \bigcup_{j=0}^t \mathcal{C}^{t=j}$. Finally, all reference points have to pass two further constraints. First, none of the reference points

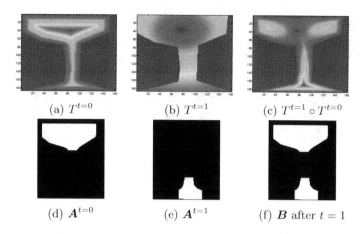

(a) $T^{t=0}$ (b) $T^{t=1}$ (c) $T^{t=1} \circ T^{t=0}$

(d) $\boldsymbol{A}^{t=0}$ (e) $\boldsymbol{A}^{t=1}$ (f) $\boldsymbol{B}$ after $t = 1$

Fig. 3. The figure illustrates the working principle to detect reference points iteratively. As shown, the lower point inside the glass would not be found by only using $T^{t=0}$.

are allowed to be too close to the centroid of the shape, which is ensured with the threshold $\mu^{(cog)}$. If only one x_i is violating this constraint, all reference points are discarded except of the responsible one. Second, in presence of multiple reference points, the contour has to be split into sub-parts. During that separation the algorithm monitors that each x_i has only one assignment. If two contour parts get assigned to one x_i, the point will be removed. Once the validation is completed, the fast marching approach has to be invoked a last time initialised by the final set of reference points. From the resulting time-crossing map $T^{(final)}$ only the values corresponding to the object's contour are extracted. Afterwards, they are arranged in a vector s where the number of elements equals the number of pixels belonging to $\partial\Omega$. Actually, this data is responsible for the final contour partitioning. For this purpose, s is regarded as 1D signal in the following content. The goal is now to derive the second-order derivative of s to determine maximum and minimum points. By backtracking these turning points, contour pixel can be selected as partition points p_i for the object's contour. Figure 4 shows both, the $T^{(final)}$ values corresponding to the contour as well as their signal plots. Since the bone structure yields two reference points, the contour has to be separated into two parts, which are shown in the first and the second column.

It is obvious that the noise-to-signal ratio exacerbates the peak detection with the result of an imprecise and noisy contour partitioning set. Thus, all subsequent matching methods are faced with unnecessarily challenging input data. In order to alleviate artifacts and to increase the robustness of the proposed approach, the signal is smoothed at first. Therefore, the *Fast Fourier Transform (FFT)* is employed with the intention to implement a *low pass filter (LPF)*. The FFT is applied, since it is capable to transform a periodic signal that is defined in the time or spatial domain toward its frequency spectrum as vice-versa. Therefore, the signal is approximated as a sum of sine and cosine functions, where the coefficients describe the power of the corresponding frequency in the input signal.

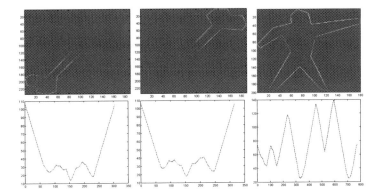

Fig. 4. The figure shows the 1D signal that has been derived from the contour depicted on the image above. The colours on the contour line encode the distance from a pixel to its closest reference point.

Since noise (and only detail information) usually manifests in high frequencies, thus, one can easily suppress noisy information without losing characteristic properties of the signal. This is shown in Fig. 5, where the signals of Fig. 4 are plotted once again, but this time after applying a LPF to them. Here, the LPF is established by a Gaussian filter that is directly applied to the zero-shifted frequency domain.

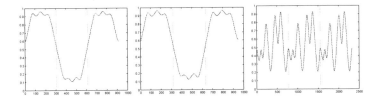

Fig. 5. From left to right, one can observe the smoothed signal of the lower left, upper right part of the bone as well as of the person. These smoothed versions are achieved by applying all LPF established in the frequency domain of the signals. It has to be noted, that the signals have been padded at start and end to alleviate border artifacts.

Two things have to be noted here: First, before the signal is passed to the LPF, it has to be padded at the start and at the end to alleviate border artifacts. Second, the padding process reacts in different ways depending on the number of reference points. This means, in the case of only a single reference, the signal is doubled at its start and its end, since the contour was not separated and thus forms a circle. If there are more than one x_i (with $i > 1$), the contour parts should not be repeated in the signal, since it would lead to a fake peak. Hence, the start and the end are only extended by flipping s. Finally, the first ($\hat{s}'$) and the second-order ($\hat{s}''$) derivative of the smoothed (and discretised) signal

$\hat{s}$ is calculated to determine all zero locations in $\hat{s}'$ with positive or negative curvature in $\hat{s}''$. Figure 6 shows the second-order derivatives for the signal plots in Fig. 5. Please note, that the computation of the second-order derivative only considers a signed binary version of the first-order derivative ($\text{sign}(\hat{s}')$, where $\text{sign}(\cdot)$ returns 0 if $\hat{s}'_i = 0$, the value 1 if $\hat{s}'_i > 0$ and -1 otherwise).

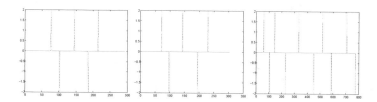

Fig. 6. Second-order derivatives that correspond to the smoothed versions of the signals shown in Fig. 4. Please note, that for the computation of the second-order derivative only a signed binary version of the first-order derivative is taken.

Theoretically, the desired partition points p_i can now be easily detected by localising all positions in $\hat{s}''$ which are not equal to zero. Practically, this naive approach might still encompass limited amount of false-positives generated by noise. The problem is, that it is not possible to find one Gaussian filter that is fitting for all object instances caused by the varying degree of deformation. In order to tackle this problem, the second-order derivative is analysed in terms of neighbours whose distance is too close to each other. Figure 7 demonstrates such a situation, where the red circle indicates the problem. To detect such cases in $\hat{s}''$, a threshold, $\mu^{(sdiff)}$, is applied, defined as the half of the standard derivation of all distances between adjacent peaks in $\hat{s}''$.

If the distance between adjacent peaks is below $\mu^{(sdiff)}$, the difference of their heights (taken from $\hat{s}$) is compared to a threshold $\mu^{(hdiff)}$ which has to be chosen close to zero. If this threshold is also greater than the height difference, the sigma of the Gaussian filter is decreased by 0.1 and the smoothing procedure is repeated with the original s. Experiments showed, that it only requires one to

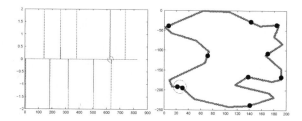

Fig. 7. The figure illustrates a situation, where the sigma of the Gaussian filter has not been chosen appropriately. It is obvious, that these artifacts can be easily determined by analysing the second-order derivative. The red circles indicate the problem.

two iterations if the algorithm starts with a sigma = 1. Finally, based on this validated set of peaks, the corresponding contour partition points are determined. Figure 8 shows the final results of the bone, the person and the bird.

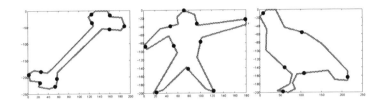

Fig. 8. Final contour partitioning set of the bone, bird and the person.

Point Context: For each partition point $p_i, i = 1, 2, ..., N$, we propose a point descriptor, *Point Context*, which has the same basic geometric unit as shape context [12]. Considering the set of vectors originating from a partition point to all other points on a shape, these vectors express the configuration of the entire shape relative to the reference point. However, different from the proposed matching method from [12], we only consider the feature vectors from partition points instead of roughly uniform spacing for selecting sample points. Moreover, during object shape matching, we calculate the shape distance by corresponding matrix between pairs of partition points without any modelling transformation process. We employ a diagram of log-polar histogram bins used in computing the point context. More specifically, as has been defined in [12], for a partition point p_i on the shape contour, we compute a coarse histogram p_i of the relative coordinates of the remaining contour points,

$$p_{i,m} = \#\{q \neq p_i : (q - p_i) \in bin(m)\}, \qquad (2)$$

where $\#\{\cdot\}$ is the function that extracts feature values for log-polar histogram and $q = \partial\Omega \setminus \{p_i\}$. We use five bins for $\log r$ and 12 bins for θ. This histogram is defined to be the point context of p_i. To achieve scale invariance we normalise all radial distances by the mean distance between the contour point pairs in the shape. Thereafter, for each partition point p_i, it can be represented as a 60 dimension feature vector:

$$p_i = (p_{i,1}, p_{i,2}, \ldots, p_{i,60})^{\mathrm{T}}. \qquad (3)$$

The whole partition points can be represented as a set of feature vectors describing its points context:

$$P = \{p_1, p_2, \ldots, p_i \ldots, p_N\}. \qquad (4)$$

Contour Segment: Based on partition points, the object contour is divided into N Contour Segments (CS). For each CS a 10-dimensional meaningful feature vector c'_n is extracted, whereas its first element is equal to Euclidean distance of contour segment two partition points $c'_{n,1}$. The total number of pixels in a CS determines $c'_{n,2}$. These two features are able to express how much a CS differs from a straight line. In order to distinguish contour segments of the type presented in [2], the area between the straight line connecting the CS endpoints and the contour segment itself is used as the third feature ($c'_{n,3}$). Moreover, the ratio between $c'_{n,1}$ and $c'_{n,2}$ is applied as $c'_{n,4}$ to evaluate the path variation.

Before computing remaining features, each CS is transformed into a normalised vertical orientation (i.e., so that its endpoints are vertically aligned) to ensure rotation invariance of the object contour representation (see Fig. 9). From the two possible results of such a normalising transformation, the CS with the majority of points lying on the right side of the straight line connecting its endpoints is selected for further processing. For computing further features $c'_{n,5}, c'_{n,6}, \ldots, c'_{n,10}$, we use the bounding box of the whole CS as well as the three equally high sub-boxes shown in Fig. 9:

$$c'_{n,5} = \frac{h_n}{w_n} \qquad c'_{n,6} = \frac{h_{n,1}}{w_{n,1}} \qquad c'_{n,7} = \frac{h_{n,2}}{w_{n,2}}$$
$$c'_{n,8} = \frac{h_{n,3}}{w_{n,3}} \qquad c'_{n,9} = \frac{w_{n,3}h_{n,3}}{w_{n,1}h_{n,1}} \qquad c'_{n,10} = \frac{w_{n,2}h_{n,2}}{w_{n,1}h_{n,1}} . \qquad (5)$$

Finally, we divide the elements of the feature vector by a half of the bounding box perimeter for scale invariance:

$$c_n = \frac{c'_n}{w_n + h_n} = (c_{n,1}, \ldots, c_{n,10})^{\mathrm{T}} \qquad (6)$$

The object contour can now be represented as a set of feature vectors describing its contour segments:

$$C = \{c_1, c_2, \ldots, c_n \ldots, c_N\}. \qquad (7)$$

Finally, we fuse the partition point vectors and the contour segment vectors as the descriptor for the whole object shape contour $\partial \Omega$:

$$\partial \Omega = \{P, C\}. \qquad (8)$$

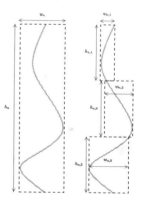

Fig. 9. CS bounding box and equally high sub-boxes ($h_{n,1} = h_{n,2} = h_{n,3}$) used for feature extraction.

4   Shape Matching

The matching of two objects including the computation of their similarity is performed separately for their partition points and contour segments representations. After matching, we estimated shape distances as the weighted sum of two terms: partition points dissimilarity, contour segments dissimilarity. For query-by-example shape retrieval, we built our approach by considering the underlying structure of the shape manifold, which is estimated from the shape distance scores between all the shapes within a database.

Point Context-Based Matching: Let $\partial\Omega$ and $\partial\Omega'$ denote two shape contours to be matched, and let $\boldsymbol{p}_n$ and $\boldsymbol{p}'_k$ be some partition points in $\boldsymbol{P}$ and $\boldsymbol{P}'$, respectively. Let the numbers of the partition points in $\partial\Omega$ and $\partial\Omega'$ be N and K, respectively, and $N \leq K$. As point contexts are distributions represented as histograms, the dissimilarity $d(\boldsymbol{p}_n, \boldsymbol{p}'_k)$ between $\boldsymbol{p}_n$ and $\boldsymbol{p}'_k$ is estimated based on the χ^2 test statistic:

$$d(\boldsymbol{p}_n, \boldsymbol{p}'_k) = \frac{1}{2} \sum_{m=1}^{M} \frac{[p_{n.m} - p_{k.m}]^2}{p_{n.m} + p_{k.m}}. \tag{9}$$

where $M = 60$ is the dimensionality of the feature space. $h_n(m)$ and $h_k(m)$ denote the M-bin normalised histogram at $\boldsymbol{p}_n$ and $\boldsymbol{p}'_k$, respectively. For two shapes contour, $\partial\Omega$ and $\partial\Omega'$, we use the lists of feature vectors for the clockwise ordered partition points. We compute all the dissimilarity between partition points and obtain a matrix:

$$D(\boldsymbol{P}, \boldsymbol{P}') = \begin{pmatrix} d(\boldsymbol{p}_1, \boldsymbol{p}'_1) & d(\boldsymbol{p}_1, \boldsymbol{p}'_2) & \ldots & d(\boldsymbol{p}_1, \boldsymbol{p}'_K) \\ d(\boldsymbol{p}_2, \boldsymbol{p}'_1) & d(\boldsymbol{p}_2, \boldsymbol{p}'_2) & \ldots & d(\boldsymbol{p}_2, \boldsymbol{p}'_K) \\ \vdots & \vdots & \vdots & \\ d(\boldsymbol{p}_N, \boldsymbol{p}'_1) & d(\boldsymbol{p}_N, \boldsymbol{p}'_2) & \ldots & d(\boldsymbol{p}_N, \boldsymbol{p}'_K) \end{pmatrix}. \tag{10}$$

Based on (10), we find the best matched points from $\boldsymbol{P}$ to $\boldsymbol{P}'$ by Hungarian algorithm [12]. For each partition point $\boldsymbol{p}_i$ in $\boldsymbol{P}$, the Hungarian algorithm can find its corresponding partition point $\boldsymbol{p}'_j$ in $\boldsymbol{P}'$. Since $\partial\Omega$ and $\partial\Omega'$ may have different numbers of partition points, the total dissimilarity value should include the penalty for end nodes that didn't find any partner. To achieve this, we simply add additional rows with a constant value const to (10) so that $\boldsymbol{D}(\boldsymbol{P}, \boldsymbol{P}')$ becomes a square matrix. The constant value const is the average of all the other values in $\boldsymbol{D}(\boldsymbol{P}, \boldsymbol{P}')$.

The resulting dissimilarity values of the matched partition points can be denoted as $d_1, d_2, \ldots, d_N$ and the global partition point-based dissimilarity between $\boldsymbol{P}$ and $\boldsymbol{P}'$ is calculated as follows:

$$d_{\text{points}}(\boldsymbol{P}, \boldsymbol{P}') = \frac{1}{N} \sum_{n=1}^{N} d_n. \tag{11}$$

Contour Segment-Based Matching: Similar to point context-based matching, Let $\partial\Omega$ and $\partial\Omega'$ denote two shape contours to be matched, and let $\boldsymbol{c}_n$ and $\boldsymbol{c}'_k$ be some contour segments in $\boldsymbol{C}$ and $\boldsymbol{C}'$, respectively. The numbers of contour segments is equal to the number of partition points in $\partial\Omega$ and $\partial\Omega'$, be N and K, respectively, and $N \leq K$.

We introduce a matching cost measure for contour segments $\boldsymbol{c}_n$ and $\boldsymbol{c}'_k$ belonging to different shape contour $\partial\Omega$ and $\partial\Omega'$:

$$d(\boldsymbol{c}_n, \boldsymbol{c}'_k) = \frac{1}{M} \sum_{m=1}^{M} \frac{\sigma_m |c_{n,m} - c'_{k,m}|}{\sum_{j=1}^{K} |c_{n,m} - c'_{k,m}|}, \tag{12}$$

where $M = 10$ is the dimensionality of the feature space and σ_m is the weight for each feature achieved in an optimisation process explained in [2]. As one can see, the dissimilarity value between c_n and c'_k does not only depend on these two contour segments. All CS of C are taken into consideration, whereby (12) does not fulfil the symmetry property $d(c_n, c'_k) \neq d(c'_k, c_n)$. However, it behaves in accordance to human perception. If the matching cost of c_n to the neighbours of c'_k in C' decreases, $d(c_n, c'_k)$ increases.

We arrange the contour segments of both objects in a clockwise way so that the objects can be represented by ordered lists of feature vectors:

$$C = (c_1, c_2, \ldots, c_n, \ldots, c_N)$$
$$C' = (c'_1, c'_2, \ldots, c'_k, \ldots, c'_K). \tag{13}$$

Using (12) we generate a matrix of matching cost between all CS in C and in C':

$$D(C, C') = \begin{pmatrix} d(c_1, c'_1) & d(c_1, c'_2) & \ldots & d(c_1, c'_K) \\ d(c_2, c'_1) & d(c_2, c'_2) & \ldots & d(c_2, c'_K) \\ \vdots & \vdots & \vdots \\ d(c_N, c'_1) & d(c_N, c'_2) & \ldots & d(c_N, c'_K) \end{pmatrix}. \tag{14}$$

The next steps are the same as partition points. In order to find an optimum match of contour segments from C to CS from C', we apply the Hungarian algorithm for the matrix expressed in (14). Then we can find the resulting dissimilarity values of the matched contour segments denoted as $d_1, d_2, \ldots, d_N$ and the global dissimilarity $d_{\text{contours}}(C, C')$ is calculated by the same method in (11).

Shape Distance and Retrieval: In this paper, we defined the distance between two shapes with a fused scheme between partition points and contour segments:

$$d(\Omega, \Omega') = \alpha d_{\text{points}}(P, P') + (1 - \alpha)d_{\text{contours}}(C, C'). \tag{15}$$

The weight α in (15) has been optimised by an integrated Gradient Hill Climbing [7] and Simulated Annealing [8] method on the Kimia216 dataset. By experiment, the optimised weight is $\alpha = 0.7$ and we employ it for all experiments in Sect. 5.

For the task of shape retrieval, given a set of H shapes, a shape matching algorithm (15) can be applied to obtain a $H \times H$ distance matrix to describe the pairwise relations between all shapes in terms of a dissimilarity measure. Such an approach ignores the fact that also distances to all other shapes contain important information about the overall shape manifold. Therefore, in this paper, we employ a method proposed by [21] that allows to improve retrieval results by analysing the underlying structure of the shape manifold. This method captures the manifold structure of the data by defining a neighbourhood for each data point in terms of a modified version of a mutual kNN graph which yields improved performance on all experiment databases in Sect. 5.

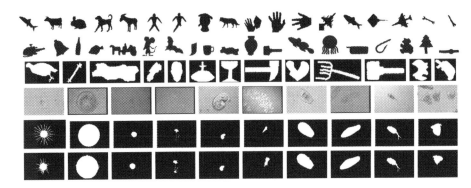

Fig. 10. Example shapes from the experimental datasets: Kimia-99 (first row), MPEG-400 (second row), Kimia-216 (third row) and EM-200 (fourth row with original, fifth row with manually- and the sixth row with semi-automatically segmented images).

5   Experiments and Results

Correspondence Matching: In Fig. 11 (left), we match a dog to another dog with legs and backside deformation. Since the articulations of the query dog is similar to the deformed one, our matching process finds the correct correspondences between partition points as well as contour segments. Figure 11 (right) shows the correspondence between two tools. Based on human perception there are two mismatched partition points. This is due to their symmetric silhouette and there are many similar contour segments and partition points in one object which could affect the performance of matching approach. However, in terms of the geometry, the correspondences are correct since the matched partition points and contour segments have the same geometrical location among their objects. Therefore, the final similarity between two objects is not affected. Figure 12 are taken from Kimia-99's person dataset, whereas the silhouette on the right side is manually modified. It demonstrates that the proposed method is able to establish a correct correspondence if parts are substantially deformed. The obtained correspondence in Kimia-99 [22] illustrates that our matching process has strong performance in the presence of occlusion.

Application Independent Experiments: We tested our algorithm on two shape databases provided by Kimia-216 [18] (the fourth row in Fig. 10) and MPEG-400 [2] (the third row in Fig. 10). We compare our method to the Path Similarity Skeleton Graph Matching (PSSGM) [18] and the Contour Segments-based Matching [2] in which contour segments are generated by the endpoints of skeletons. To compare our partition point extraction technique against existing methods, we also tested our algorithm with partition points gained from Discrete Curve Evolution [23]. To get the best results we set the stop parameter at 4. For each of the shapes used as a query, we have checked whether the retrieved results are correct, i.e., belong to the same class as the query. In order to enable

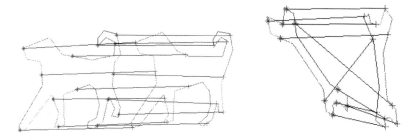

Fig. 11. The corresponding partition points (linked with lines) and contour segments (linked with colours) between two dogs (left) and tools (right) from Kimia99 dataset.

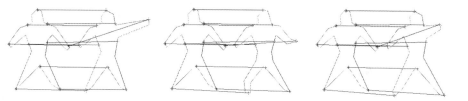

Fig. 12. Example correspondence between articulating persons.

quantitative comparison, we have kept the experimental convention proposed in [18] and considered the 10 best matches for each query. Results achieved for the Kimia-216 and the MPEG-400 datasets can be found in Table 1, whereas in [24] the PSSGM algorithm had been re-evaluated without any preliminary assumptions regarding the object skeletonisation. For these two databases, it is important to observe that the fused point context and contour segment outperforms skeleton-based methods [18] and contour segments-based methods [2] while the complexity of feature generation and matching has been reduced.

Environmental Microorganism Retrieval: EMs and their species are very important indicators to evaluate environmental quality, but their manual recognition is very time-consuming [25]. Thus, automatic analysis techniques for microscopic images of EMs would be very appreciated by environmental scientists. We have tested our methodology for this application using a real dataset acquired in environmental laboratories of the University of Science and Technology Beijing. We segmented the images manually and semi-automatically with the method introduced in [26]. Examples of EM original images as well as manually segmented and semi-automatically segmented EM images can be seen in Fig. 10. The impressive results for the EM-200 [27] dataset (see Table 1) confirm the high descriptive power of our new feature extraction technique for contours and prove the applicability of our shape retrieval algorithm to real-world applications.

Table 1. Experimental comparison of our methodology to the most related algorithm using the MPEG-400, Kimia216 datasets as well as the proof of applicability of our approach to real world problems using the EM-200 dataset. Results are summarised as the number of shapes from the same class among the first top 1–10 shapes.

Object Retrieval for MPEG-400

Algorithm	1st	2nd	3rd	4th	5th	6th	7th	8th	9th	10th
PSSGM [24]	380	371	361	351	344	339	332	320	330	309
Contours [2]	375	348	333	325	317	311	300	295	276	275
DCE [23] + CS [2]	375	368	346	337	338	323	308	297	286	276
Our method	**389**	**374**	**368**	**368**	**358**	**347**	**344**	**339**	**346**	**330**

Object Retrieval for Kimia-216

Algorithm	1st	2nd	3rd	4th	5th	6th	7th	8th	9th	10th
PSSGM [24]	205	208	202	199	200	192	184	167	161	130
Contours [2]	216	215	206	204	200	186	172	163	130	124
DCE [23] + CS [2]	216	204	197	185	175	162	154	154	142	131
Our method	**216**	**214**	**207**	**204**	**201**	**204**	**191**	**188**	**192**	**185**

Object Retrieval for EM-200

Algorithm	1st	2nd	3rd	4th	5th	6th	7th	8th	9th	10th
Manually	200	183	175	167	166	156	154	146	156	153
Semi-Automatically	200	180	174	163	160	160	150	143	153	147

6   Conclusion and Future Work

In this paper, we proposed a method for 2D shape similarity measure based on contour segment matching and, after fusion with a partition point matching, use it for object retrieval. The most innovative part of our approach is the robust and stable partition point generation and the comparison and matching of contour segments. The algorithm can be easily implemented to real applications. In the future, we will investigate possibilities of weighting properties on contour segment feature, which could be applied for dataset adopting with a supervised optimisation scheme.

Acknowledgement. Research activities leading to this work have been supported by the China Scholarship Council, the German Research Foundation (DFG) within the Research Training Group 1564. We greatly thank M.Sc Chen Li from the University of Siegen for providing us with the Environmental Microorganism image dataset for experiments. We are also very grateful to Dr. Kimiaki Shirahama from University of Siegen for his guiding on significant technologies.

References

1. Biederman, I., Ju, G.: Surface versus edge-based determinants of visual recognition. Cogn. Psychol. **20**, 38–64 (1988)
2. Yang, C., Tiebe, O., Pietsch, P., Feinen, C., Kelter, U., Grzegorzek, M.: Shape-based object retrieval by contour segment matching. In: International Conference on Image Processing (ICIP). IEEE Computer Society (2014, to appear)
3. Shotton, J., Blake, A., Cipolla, R.: Multiscale categorical object recognition using contour fragments. IEEE Trans. Pattern Anal. Mach. Intell. **30**, 1270–1281 (2008)
4. Bai, X., Latecki, L., Yu Liu, W.: Skeleton pruning by contour partitioning with discrete curve evolution. PAMI **29**, 449–462 (2007)
5. Bai, X., Liu, W., Tu, Z.: Integrating contour and skeleton for shape classification. In: 2009 IEEE 12th International Conference on Computer Vision Workshops (ICCV Workshops), pp. 360–367 (2009)
6. Ma, T., Latecki, L.: From partial shape matching through local deformation to robust global shape similarity for object detection. In: 2011 IEEE Conference on Computer Vision and Pattern Recognition (CVPR), pp. 1441–1448 (2011)
7. Russell, S., Norvig, P.: Artificial Intelligence: A Modern Approach, 3rd edn. Prentice Hall Press, Englewood Cliffs (2009)
8. Kirkpatrick, S., Gelatt, C.D., Vecchi, M.P.: Optimization by simulated annealing. Science **220**, 671–680 (1983)
9. Shotton, J., Blake, A., Cipolla, R.: Contour-based learning for object detection. ICCV **1**, 503–510 (2005)
10. Nguyen, D.T., Ogunbona, P.O., Li, W.: A novel shape-based non-redundant local binary pattern descriptor for object detection. Pattern Recognit. **46**, 1485–1500 (2013)
11. Cao, Y., Zhang, Z., Czogiel, I., Dryden, I., Wang, S.: 2d nonrigid partial shape matching using mcmc and contour subdivision. In: CVPR, pp. 2345–2352 (2011)
12. Belongie, S., Malik, J., Puzicha, J.: Shape matching and object recognition using shape contexts. IEEE Trans. Pattern Anal. Mach. Intell. **24**, 509–522 (2002)
13. Wang, X., Feng, B., Bai, X., Liu, W., Latecki, L.J.: Bag of contour fragments for robust shape classification, pp. 2116–2125 (2014)
14. Yang, X., Bai, X., Yang, X., Zeng, L.: An efficient quick algorithm for computing stable skeletons. In: 2nd International Congress on Image and Signal Processing, CISP 2009, pp. 1–5 (2009)
15. Goh, W.B.: Strategies for shape matching using skeletons. CVIU **110**, 326–345 (2008)
16. Sebastian, T., Kimia, B.: Curves vs skeletons in object recognition. ICIP **3**, 22–25 (2001)
17. Baseski, E., Erdem, A., Tari, S.: Dissimilarity between two skeletal trees in a context. Pattern Recognit. **42**, 370–385 (2009)
18. Bai, X., Latecki, L.: Path similarity skeleton graph matching. PAMI **30**, 1282–1292 (2008)
19. Zeng, J., Lakaemper, R., Yang, X., Li, X.: 2d shape decomposition based on combined skeleton-boundary features. In: Bebis, G., et al. (eds.) Advances in Visual Computing. LNCS, vol. 5359. Springer, Heidelberg (2008)
20. Hassouna, M.S., Farag, A.A.: MultiStencils fast marching methods: a highly accurate solution to the eikonal equation on cartesian domains. IEEE Trans. Pattern Anal. Mach. Intell. **29**, 1563–1574 (2007)

21. Kontschieder, P., Donoser, M., Bischof, H.: Beyond pairwise shape similarity analysis. In: Zha, H., Taniguchi, R., Maybank, S. (eds.) Computer Vision - ACCV 2009. LNCS, pp. 655–666. Springer, Heidelberg (2010)
22. Sebastian, T., Klein, P., Kimia, B.: Recognition of shapes by editing their shock graphs. IEEE Trans. Pattern Anal. Mach. Intell. **26**, 550–571 (2004)
23. Latecki, L., Lakamper, R.: Convexity rule for shape decomposition based on discrete contour evolution. Comput. Vis. Image Underst. **73**, 441–454 (1999)
24. Hedrich, J., Yang, C., Feinen, C., Schaefer, S., Paulus, D., Grzegorzek, M.: Extended investigations on skeleton graph matching for object recognition. In: Burduk, R., Jackowski, K., Kurzynski, M., Wozniak, M., Zolnierek, A. (eds.) CORES 2013. AISC, vol. 226, pp. 371–381. Springer, Heidelberg (2013)
25. Li, C., Shirahama, K., Grzegorzek, M., Ma, F., Zhou, B.: Classification of environmental microorganisms in microscopic images using shape features and support vector machines. In: ICIP, pp. 2435–2439. IEEE Computer Society (2013)
26. Li, C., Shirahama, K., Czajkowska, J., Grzegorzek, M., Ma, F., Zhou, B.: A multistage approach for automatic classification of environmental microorganisms. In: IPCV, pp. 364–370. CSREA Press (2013)
27. Yang, C., Li, C., Tiebe, O., Shirahama, K., Grzegorzek, M.: Shape-based classification of environmental microorganisms. In: International Conference on Pattern Recognition (ICPR), pp. 3374–3379. IEEE Computer Society (2014)

A+: Adjusted Anchored Neighborhood Regression for Fast Super-Resolution

Radu Timofte[1]($\boxtimes$), Vincent De Smet[2], and Luc Van Gool[1,2]

[1] CVL, D-ITET, ETH Zürich, Zürich, Switzerland
{radu.timofte,vangool}@vision.ee.ethz.ch
[2] VISICS, ESAT/PSI, KU Leuven, Leuven, Belgium
vincent.desmet@esat.kuleuven.be

Abstract. We address the problem of image upscaling in the form of single image super-resolution based on a dictionary of low- and high-resolution exemplars. Two recently proposed methods, Anchored Neighborhood Regression (ANR) and Simple Functions (SF), provide state-of-the-art quality performance. Moreover, ANR is among the fastest known super-resolution methods. ANR learns sparse dictionaries and regressors anchored to the dictionary atoms. SF relies on clusters and corresponding learned functions. We propose A+, an improved variant of ANR, which combines the best qualities of ANR and SF. A+ builds on the features and anchored regressors from ANR but instead of learning the regressors on the dictionary it uses the full training material, similar to SF. We validate our method on standard images and compare with state-of-the-art methods. We obtain improved quality (*i.e.* 0.2–0.7 dB PSNR better than ANR) and excellent time complexity, rendering A+ the most efficient dictionary-based super-resolution method to date.

1 Introduction

Single-image super-resolution (SR) is a branch of image reconstruction that concerns itself with the problem of generating a plausible and visually pleasing high-resolution (HR) output image from a low-resolution (LR) input image. As opposed to the similar branch of image deblurring, in SR it is generally assumed that the input image, while having a low resolution in the sense of having a low amount of pixels, is still sharp at the original scale. SR methods are mainly concerned with upscaling the image without losing the sharpness of the original low-resolution image.

SR is an ill-posed problem because each LR pixel has to be mapped onto many HR pixels, depending on the desired upsampling factor. Most popular single-image SR methods try to solve this problem by enforcing natural image priors based on either intuitive understanding (*e.g.* natural images consist mainly of flat regions separated by sharp edges) or statistical analysis of many natural images [2–5]. Some recent approaches try to shift the focus from finding good image priors to finding an appropriate blur kernel [6,7]. In both cases the authors usually work on the level of small image patches. These provide a good basis for finding effective local image priors and can be combined in different ways ranging

© Springer International Publishing Switzerland 2015
D. Cremers et al. (Eds.): ACCV 2014, Part IV, LNCS 9006, pp. 111–126, 2015.
DOI: 10.1007/978-3-319-16817-3_8

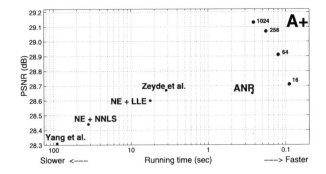

Fig. 1. Our proposed A+ method (*red*, operating points for 16, 64, 256, and 1024 sized dictionaries) provides both the best quality and the highest speed in comparison with state-of-the-art example-based SR methods. A+ preserves the time complexity of ANR (*green*) [1]. See Table 1 and Fig. 2 for more details (Color figure online).

from simple averaging of overlapping patches to finding maximum-a-posteriori patch candidate combinations using belief propagation or graph cuts [8]. Very recently, convolutional neural networks were applied to this problem [18].

Patch-based SR methods tend to require a large database of many image patches in order to learn effective priors and to super-resolve general classes of natural images. Both the resulting time-complexity and memory requirements can be strong limiting factors on the practical performance of these methods. One class of SR approaches that tries to solve this bottleneck are the neighbor embedding approaches [9,10]. These have the nice feature of compensating for the lack of density in the patch feature space by assuming that all patches lie on manifolds in their respective LR and HR spaces, which allows for an input patch to be approximated as an interpolation of existing database patches, with one set of interpolation coefficients being applied to both spaces. Another class of methods is focused on creating sparse representations of large patch databases [4,11], which can reduce overfitting to training data and is a good way of avoiding the need for a large patch database.

Two recent neighbor embedding approaches, ANR [1] and SF [12], have been successful in reducing the time complexity of single-image super-resolution significantly without sacrificing the quality of the super-resolved output image. They show results which are qualitatively and quantitatively on par with other state-of-the-art methods, while improving execution speed by one or two orders of magnitude. We take these approaches (specifically ANR) as a starting point to introduce a novel SR method, which we have dubbed A+, that makes no sacrifices on the computational efficiency and achieves an improved quality of the results which surpasses current state-of-the-art methods. Figure 1 shows the performance of our method compared to other neighbor embedding and sparsity-based methods and shows our improvement over the original ANR approach.

In the following section we will first give some background on other neighbor embedding approaches and sparse coding approaches and review the SF method. In Sect. 3 we introduce our A+ approach and explain it in detail. Section 4 describes our experiments, where we compare the performance of our approach to other state-of-the-art methods based on quality and processing time. Finally in Sect. 5 we conclude the paper.

2 Dictionary-Based Super-Resolution

Our proposed approach builds on theories from neighbor embedding and sparse coding super-resolution methods. Both of these are dictionary-based approaches, which means they rely on a dictionary of patches or patch-based atoms that can be trained to form an efficient representation of natural image patches. This gives them the potential to drastically reduce the computational complexity of patch-based single-image super-resolution methods and enhance their representational power.

2.1 Neighbor Embedding Approaches

One way to add more generalization ability to the basic patch-based super-resolution scheme is to allow LR input patches to be approximated by a linear combination of their nearest neighbors in the database. Neighbor embedding (NE) approaches assume that the LR and HR patches lie on low-dimensional nonlinear manifolds with locally similar geometry. Assuming this, the same interpolation coefficients that are used between LR patches to approximate an input patch can be used in HR space to estimate an output patch. Chang et al. [9] assume that the manifolds lie on or near locally linear patches and use Locally Linear Embedding (LLE) [13] to describe LR patches as linear combinations of their nearest neighbors, assuming the patch space is populated densely enough. The same coefficients can then be used to perform linear interpolation of the corresponding HR patches:

$$\mathbf{x} = \sum_{i=1}^{K} w^{\star}{}_i \mathbf{x}'_i. \qquad (1)$$

We use $\mathbf{x}$ to refer to the HR output patch, $\mathbf{x}'_i$ is the i'th candidate HR patch corresponding to the i'th nearest neighbor of the input patch in LR space, $w^{\star}{}_i$ is the weight of the i'th candidate, and we limit our search to K nearest neighbors. Bevilacqua et al. [10] also use neighbor embedding for SR. They use a nonnegative least-squares decomposition to find weights that can be used in LR and HR space.

2.2 Sparse Coding Approaches

Instead of using a dictionary consisting of a collection of patches taken from natural images, as neighbor embedding methods typically do, one could try to create an efficient representation of the patch space by training a codebook of dictionary atoms. Yang et al. [4] start from a large collection of image patches and use a sparsity constraint to jointly train the LR and HR dictionaries so that they are able to represent LR patches and their corresponding HR counterparts using one sparse representation. Once the dictionaries are trained, the algorithm searches for a close sparse representation of each input patch as a combination of dictionary atoms:

$$\min_{\alpha} \|\mathbf{D}_l \alpha - \mathbf{y}\|_2^2 + \lambda \|\alpha\|_1, \tag{2}$$

where $\mathbf{D}_l$ is the LR dictionary, α is a weight matrix that functions as a sparse selector of dictionary atoms, and λ is a weighing factor to balance the importance of the sparsity constraint. Other approaches, most notably Zeyde *et al.* [11], build on this work and reach significant improvements both in speed and output quality.

2.3 Simple Functions

The neighbor embedding approaches use a database of patches and represent each LR input patch as a combination of its nearest neighbors, whereas the sparse coding approaches explicitly enforce sparsity to create a coupled LR-HR dictionary which is used to map an LR patch to HR space. Another approach would be to cluster the LR patch space and to learn a separate mapping from LR to HR space for each cluster. This is what Yang and Yang [12] propose. They collect a large amount of natural images to harvest patches. These are clustered into a relatively small number of subspaces (*e.g.* 1024 or 4096) for which a simple mapping function from LR to HR is then learned. The authors compare three different functions for this mapping: an affine transformation learned for each cluster using a least squares approximation, and a support vector regressor with either a linear kernel or a radial basis function kernel. Because of the visual similarity of the resulting images for all of these, the authors propose to use the affine transformation, as it is by far computationally the fastest. The mapping coefficients can be learned offline and stored for each cluster. LR patches are then super-resolved by finding the closest cluster center and applying the corresponding transformation,

$$\mathbf{x} = \mathbf{C}_i^\star \begin{bmatrix} \mathbf{y} \\ 1 \end{bmatrix}, \; with \; \mathbf{C}_i^\star = \arg\min_{\mathbf{C}_i} \left\| \mathbf{Y}_i - \mathbf{C}_i \begin{bmatrix} \mathbf{X}_i \\ 1 \end{bmatrix} \right\|_2^2. \tag{3}$$

We denote with $\mathbf{y}$ and $\mathbf{x}$ an LR input patch that is matched to cluster i and its estimated HR output patch, with $\mathbf{C}_i$ the transformation matrix and $\mathbf{Y}_i$ and $\mathbf{X}_i$ the training patches for cluster i. 1 is a vector with the same number of elements as the amount of training patches in $\mathbf{X}_i$, filled entirely with ones. Storing the mapping coefficients results in a big boost in performance speed.

2.4 Anchored Neighborhood Regression

The Anchored Neighborhood Regression approach proposed by Timofte *et al.* [1] has a similar strategy to boost performance speed but shares more properties with sparse coding than the simple functions approach. It relies on precalculating and storing transformations to dramatically improve execution speed at test-time. Starting from the same dictionaries as Zeyde *et al.* [11], which are efficiently trained for sparsity, ANR reformulates the patch representation problem from Eq. (2) as a least squares regression regularized by the l_2-norm of the coefficient matrix (which we refer to as β to avoid confusion with the sparse methods described in Sect. 2.2):

$$\min_{\beta}\|\mathbf{y} - \mathbf{N}_l\beta\|_2^2 + \lambda\|\beta\|_2. \tag{4}$$

Instead of considering the whole dictionary like the sparse encoding approach in Sect. 2.2, the authors propose to work in local neighborhoods $\mathbf{N}_{l,h}$ of the dictionary. The main advantage of working with the l_2-norm is that this turns the problem into Ridge Regression [14] and gives it a closed solution, which means they can precalculate a projection matrix based on the neighborhood that is considered. An LR input patch $\mathbf{y}$ can be projected to HR space as

$$\mathbf{x} = \mathbf{N}_h(\mathbf{N}_l^T\mathbf{N}_l + \lambda\mathbf{I})^{-1}\mathbf{N}_l^T\mathbf{y} = \mathbf{P}_j\mathbf{y}, \tag{5}$$

with $\mathbf{P}_j$ the stored projection matrix for dictionary atom $\mathbf{d}_{lj}$. Each dictionary atom has its own neighborhood $\mathbf{N}_l$ of dictionary atoms assigned to it. The SR process for ANR at test time then becomes mainly a nearest neighbor search followed by a matrix multiplication for each input patch. On the extreme part of the spectrum the neighborhoods could be made the size of the entire dictionary $\mathbf{D}_{l,h}$. In this case each atom has the same transformation matrix and there is no need to perform a nearest neighbor search through the dictionary. This is called Global Regression (GR), and at test time the global transformation can be applied, reducing the process to the application of a simple stored projection. This makes the process lose a lot of flexibility and results in a lower output quality for the benefit of greatly enhanced speed.

3   Adjusted Anchored Neighborhood Regression (A+)

We propose a method based on the ANR approach [1]. We name our method A+ due to the fact that it inherits and adjusts the ANR key aspects such as the anchored regressors, the features, and the test time complexity, while at the same time significantly improving over its performance. We will first explain the insights that lead to A+, then we will provide its general formulation and then discuss the influence of the different model parameters.

3.1   Insights

Most neighbor embedding methods (exceptions are ANR [1] and SF [12]) rely on extracting a neighborhood of LR training patches for each LR test patch, followed by solving the HR patch reconstruction problem, usually through some optimization process. ANR instead places this computation at the training stage, leaving at test time only the search of a neighboring anchor followed by a projection to HR space. The anchoring points are the atoms of a sparse dictionary trained to span the space of LR patch features and to provide a uniform coverage, while at the same time being optimized to have a low decomposition error for the LR patch features available in the training database. On these anchoring points ANR learns offline regressors to the local neighborhood of correlated atoms from the same sparse dictionary.

We make the following observations related to the ANR formulation:

(i) the atoms are rather sparsely sampling the space, while the training pool of samples is (or can be) practically infinite, as long as enough training images are available to harvest patches;

(ii) the local manifold around an atom, which is the associated hypercell of an atom, is more accurately spanned by dense samples interior to the hypercell than by a set of external neighboring atoms.

Therefore, we can expect that the more samples we use from the interior of the anchor hypercell the better the approximation of that subspace or manifold will be, both on the unit hypersphere where the atom lies and on any translation of it along the atom's direction.

For this purpose we will consider the neighborhood of training samples that may cover both the hypercell of the anchoring atom and part of its adjacent atom hypercells. This is one of the key ideas exploited in our A+ method. Another one is the assumption that in the neighborhood of an atom one can regress linearly to a solution that accommodates all the local neighborhood training samples and moreover, can interpolate to samples from the space spanned by them. The bigger the neighborhood of LR patches, the stronger the linearity imposed not only on LR patches but on their corresponding HR patches. The one LR patch to many HR patches problem is tackled by the power of linear LR patch decomposition over many close to unit norm patches from anchored neighborhoods. Having a dictionary of anchors of unit l_2 norm reduces the general clustering of the whole LR space to a clustering around the unit hypersphere, where the atoms are definitive and the correlation of a sample to the atom can determine its adherence to the atom's spanned space of LR patches. Therefore, for a new LR patch, we first find its most correlated atom and then we apply the sample-based regression stored by that atom to reconstruct the HR patch in the same fashion as ANR.

The SF [12] method differs from A+ (and ANR) in at least 3 main aspects: SF uses different LR patch features, follows the Euclidean space clustering assumption and its functions are bounded to the cluster samples. Since a sample can be found on the boundary area between clusters, we consider that either the number of clusters should be consistently large or the functions should be anchored on clusters but learned using also the neighboring clusters. Therefore, while we formulate our insight using the ANR framework, a derivation inside the SF framework could also be possible.

3.2 Formulation

We adopt the dictionary training method of Zeyde *et al.* and ANR, which first optimizes over LR patches to obtain a sparse dictionary $\mathbf{D}_l$ to then reconstruct its corresponding $\mathbf{D}_h$ by enforcing the coefficients in the HR patch decompositions over $\mathbf{D}_h$ to be the same coefficients from the corresponding LR patch decompositions over $\mathbf{D}_l$.

ANR and the other sparse coding approaches have no need for the training samples anymore after the dictionary is trained, but for A+ they are still crucial, as the neighborhood used for regression (calculated during training and used at test time) is explicitly taken from the training pool of samples. We reuse the ridge regression formulation of ANR as shown in Eq. (4) to regress at train time, but redefine the neighborhood in terms of the dense training samples rather than the sparse dictionary atoms. Our optimization problem then looks like this,

$$\min_{\boldsymbol{\delta}} \|\mathbf{y} - \mathbf{S}_l \boldsymbol{\delta}\|_2^2 + \lambda \|\boldsymbol{\delta}\|_2. \tag{6}$$

We have replaced the neighborhood of atoms $\mathbf{N}_l$ (of which each dictionary atom has its own version) with a matrix $\mathbf{S}_l$, containing the K training samples that lie closest to the dictionary atom to which the input patch $\mathbf{y}$ is matched. We set K to 2048 in our experiments. The distance measure used for the nearest neighbor search is the Euclidean distance between the anchor atom and the training samples. More details on the sampling can be found in the next section.

3.3 Sampling Anchored Neighborhoods

In order to have a robust regressor anchored to an atom, we need to have a neighborhood of samples (in a Euclidean sense) centered on the atom, or brought to unit l_2 norm, on the surface of the unit hypersphere. When the l_2 norm of the LR patch feature is below a small threshold (0.1 in our case) we do not l_2-normalize it, as we want to avoid enhancing the potential noise of a flat patch. The local manifold on the unit hypersphere can be approximated by the set of neighboring samples, even if they are not all lying on the hypersphere. However, due to our choice of LR patch features (the same as ANR and the approach of Zeyde *et al.*) we do have a uniform scaling factor between the LR feature and its HR patch. Therefore, when we bring the LR patch features to the hypersphere by l_2 normalization we also transform the corresponding HR patches linearly by scaling them with the same factor (the l_2-norm of the original LR patch features) to preserve the relation between LR and HR spaces.

We propose that if more samples are closer to the anchoring atom the local manifold approximation through regression on these samples will improve. Therefore, we retrieve for each atom as many training samples as a given neighborhood size. The same samples can be shared among different atom centered neighborhoods. This ensures that the regressors are learned robustly even in extreme cases where either the number of atoms is very small with respect to the number of training samples or where we only have few samples around certain atoms.

4   Experiments

In this section we analyze the performance of our proposed A+ method in relation to its design parameters and benchmark it in quantitative and qualitative comparison with ANR and other state-of-the-art methods.[1]

4.1   Benchmarks

We adopt the testing benchmarks of the original ANR algorithm [1] and in addition we use the 100 test images from the BSDS300 Berkeley dataset which is widely used as a benchmark for various computer vision tasks including super-resolution.

Training Dataset. We use the training set of images as proposed by Yang et al. [4] and used, among others, by Timofte et al. [1] and by Zeyde et al. [11].

Set5 and Set14. 'Set5' [10] and 'Set14' [11] contain 5 and respectively 14 commonly used images for super-resolution evaluation. They are used in the same settings as in [1]. In order to compare with ANR as fairly as possible, we conduct most of our experiments related to the internal parameters of our A+ method on Set14. This is similar to ANR, its internal parameters being first evaluated on Set14.

B100 Aka Berkeley Segmentation Dataset. The Berkeley Segmentation Dataset (BSDS300) [15] is a dataset of natural images which was originally designed for image segmentation but has been widely used in many image restoration approaches such as super- resolution and denoising to test performance [17]. We will use its 100 testing images (named here 'B100') to compare our method more thoroughly to the closely related ANR and GR methods.

Compared Methods. We compare with all the methods of [1] under the same conditions as originally compared with ANR. Where applicable, we use a shared sparse dictionary among the methods, or at least the methods use similar sized dictionaries and share the training material, which is the same from [1,11,16]. The methods are as follows: NE+LS (Neighbor Embedding with Least Squares), NE+LLE (Neighbor Embedding with Locally Linear Embedding, similar to Chang et al. [9]), NE+NNLS (Neighbor Embedding with Non-Negative Least Squares, similar to Bevilacqua et al. [10]), GR (Global Regression) and ANR (Anchored Neighborhood Regression) of Timofte et al. [1]; the sparse coding method of Yang et al. [16], the efficient sparse coding method of Zeyde et al. [11], and the Simple Functions (SF) method of Yang and Yang [12]. In addition we briefly report to the very recent Convolutional Neural Network method (SRCNN) of Dong et al. [18] which uses the same benchmark as us (training data, Set5, Set14, as in [1]).

---

[1] All the codes are publicly available at: http://www.vision.ee.ethz.ch/~timofter.

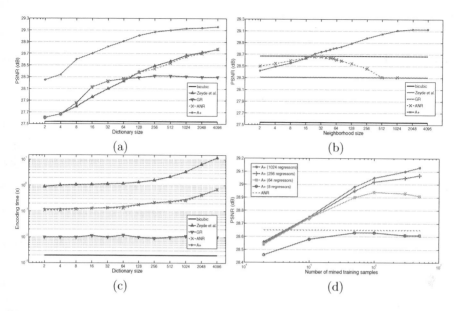

Fig. 2. Parameters influence on performance on average on Set14. (a) Dictionary size for $A+$, ANR, GR, and $Zeyde$ et al. versus PSNR; (b) Neighborhood size for $A+$ and ANR versus PSNR, with dictionary size fixed to 1024; GR, $Zeyde$ et al. and $Bicubic$ interpolation are provided for reference. (c) Dictionary size for $A+$, ANR, GR, and $Zeyde$ et al. versus encoding time; $Bicubic$ is for reference. (d) Number of mined training samples versus PSNR for $A+$ with different number of regressors (aka dictionary size); ANR with a dictionary of 1024 is provided for reference.

Features. We use the same LR patch features as Zeyde *et al.* [11] and Timofte *et al.* [1]. Therefore, we refer the reader to their original works for a discussion about features.

4.2 Parameters

In this subsection we analyze the main parameters of our proposed method, and at the same time compare on similar settings with other methods, especially with ANR since it is the closest related method. The standard settings we use are upscaling factor $\times 3$, 5000000 training samples of LR and HR patches, a dictionary size of 1024, and a neighborhood size of 2048 training samples for A+ and 40 atoms for ANR, or the best or common parameters for the other methods as reported in their respective original works. Figure 2 depicts the most relevant results of the parameter settings.

Dictionaries. There is a whole discussion concerning what are the best dictionaries of pairs of LR and HR patches (or pair samples hereafter). Some NE methods prefer to keep all the training samples, leaving the task of sublinear retrieval of relevant neighboring samples to a well-chosen data structuring. The sparse coding methods, the recent NE methods (SF, ANR) and the parameter study of Timofte *et al.* [1] argue that learning smaller dictionaries is beneficial, greatly reducing the search complexity and even improving in speed or quality. We adhere to the setup from [1] and we vary the size of the learned dictionary from 2 up to 4096 atoms. The training pool of samples extracted from the same training images as used also in [1] or [16] is in the order of 0.5 million. The results are depicted in the Fig. 2(a) for quantitative Peak Signal-to-Noise Ratios (PSNRs) and (c) for encoding time. We refer the reader to [1] for a study about NE+LS, NE+LLE and NE+NNLS. We focus mainly on ANR (with a neighborhood size of 40 atoms) and A+ (with a neighborhood size of 2048 samples), and provide results also for bicubic interpolation, Zeyde *et al.* and GR as comparison. Both A+ and ANR have the same time complexity, the running times are almost identical for the same learned dictionary size. The difference is in the quantitative PSNR performance, where A+ is clearly ahead of ANR. In fact A+ is ahead of all compared methods regardless of the dictionary size.

Neighborhoods. The size of the neighborhood that is used by the neighboring embedding methods to compute the regression of the LR input patch in order to reconstruct the HR output patch is usually a critical parameter of most NE methods. Timofte *et al.* [1] already show how sensitive this parameter is for NE+LS, NE+NNLS or NE+LLE. In the experiment from Fig. 2(b) we compare the behavior of A+ and ANR over the same dictionary, while varying the neighborhood size. Note that while A+ forms the neighborhoods from the closest training LR patches in Euclidean distance, ANR builds the local neighborhoods from the other atoms in the learned dictionary using the correlation as similarity measure. As we see, ANR peaks at a neighborhood size of 40, while our A+ faces a plateau above 1024. We had 5 million samples in the training pool, and this is a possible explanation why A+ with 1024 atoms faces a plateau above 1024 neighborhood sizes, as we will investigate in the next subsection. From now on, unless mentioned otherwise, A+ will always use neighborhoods of size 2048 for each of its atoms.

Training Samples and Dictionary Size. In the previous subsection we found that A+ seems to face a plateau in relation with the available pool of training samples from where it can pick its neighborhoods. In Fig. 2(d) we present the results of an experiment showing the relation between the amount of training samples mined from the training set of images and the dictionary size of our method. Since for each atom we learn one regressor from its neighborhood, we decide to evaluate A+ with 8, 64, 256, and 1024 regressors respectively (or in other words, its dictionary size or number of anchoring points/atoms). For reference we also plot the ANR result with a 1024 dictionary and its optimal neighborhood size of 40 atoms. The result of the experiment is relevant in that we can see that the larger we make the training pool, the better the performance of the regressors becomes, even if the number of regressors is very small. This is

Table 1. PSNR and running time for upscaling factor ×3 for Set14. All methods are trained on the same images and, with the exception of Yang et al. (1022 atoms), share a dictionary of 1024 atoms; A+ trained with 5000000 samples. A+ and ANR are 5 times faster than Zeyde et al. If we consider only the encoding time, our A+ takes 0.23 s on average, being 14 times faster than Zeyde et al., and 10 times faster than NE+LS.

Set14 images	Bicubic PSNR	Time	Yang et al. [16] PSNR	Time	Zeyde et al. [11] PSNR	Time	GR [1] PSNR	Time	ANR [1] PSNR	Time	NE+LS PSNR	Time	NE+NNLS PSNR	Time	NE+LLE PSNR	Time	A+ PSNR	Time
baboon	23.2	0.0	23.5	138.7	23.5	4.1	23.5	0.5	**23.6**	0.7	23.5	2.8	23.5	28.1	23.6	5.4	**23.6**	0.7
barbara	26.2	0.0	26.4	146.6	**26.8**	7.4	26.8	1.0	26.7	1.4	26.7	5.3	26.7	48.7	26.7	9.4	26.5	1.3
bridge	24.4	0.0	24.8	169.5	25.0	4.3	24.9	0.5	25.0	0.8	24.9	3.1	24.9	30.2	25.0	5.8	**25.2**	0.8
coastguard	26.6	0.0	27.0	39.9	27.1	1.7	27.0	0.2	27.1	0.3	27.0	1.1	27.0	12.0	27.1	2.2	**27.3**	0.3
comic	23.1	0.0	23.9	59.8	24.0	1.5	23.8	0.2	24.0	0.3	23.9	1.0	23.8	10.3	24.0	1.9	**24.4**	0.3
face	32.8	0.0	33.1	22.6	33.5	1.3	33.5	0.1	33.6	0.2	33.5	0.9	33.5	8.4	33.6	1.6	**33.8**	0.2
flowers	27.2	0.0	28.2	88.6	28.4	3.1	28.1	0.4	28.5	0.5	28.3	2.1	28.2	21.4	28.4	4.0	**29.0**	0.6
foreman	31.2	0.0	32.0	30.4	33.2	1.7	32.3	0.2	33.2	0.3	33.2	1.2	32.9	11.5	33.2	2.1	**34.3**	0.3
lenna	31.7	0.0	32.6	76.7	33.0	4.4	32.6	0.6	33.1	0.8	33.0	3.0	32.8	30.5	33.0	5.8	**33.5**	0.8
man	27.0	0.0	27.8	120.9	27.9	4.2	27.6	0.5	27.9	0.8	27.9	3.0	27.7	28.9	27.9	5.9	**28.3**	0.8
monarch	29.4	0.0	30.7	128.0	31.1	6.5	30.4	0.8	31.1	1.2	30.9	4.7	30.8	46.1	30.9	8.6	**32.1**	1.2
pepper	32.4	0.0	33.3	78.9	34.1	4.3	33.2	0.5	33.8	0.7	33.9	2.9	33.6	28.8	33.8	5.8	**34.7**	0.8
ppt3	23.7	0.0	27.8	106.6	25.2	5.4	25.0	0.7	25.0	1.1	25.1	4.0	24.8	35.3	24.9	7.6	**26.1**	1.0
zebra	26.6	0.0	28.0	122.9	28.5	3.7	27.9	0.4	28.4	0.7	28.3	2.6	28.1	25.7	28.3	4.9	**29.0**	0.7
average	27.54	0.01	28.31	95.00	28.67	3.83	28.31	0.47	28.65	0.69	28.59	2.68	28.44	26.15	28.60	5.08	**29.13**	**0.69**
avg.encoding		0.01		~90.00		3.37		0.01		0.23		2.22		25.69		4.62		**0.23**

due to the fact that by having a larger training pool of samples, the density of points favorably placed near the anchoring atoms increases and the regression can better fit a manifold in the proximity of the unit hypersphere of the atoms. Nevertheless, for better performance the neighborhood size (here fixed at 2048) should be adjusted as well to the number of mined training samples. And this especially when the number of training samples is much larger or smaller than the number of regressors times the neighborhood size. Our assumption of the space spanned by anchored neighborhoods on atoms on the unit hypersphere seems to hold.

Our experiment, which we stopped after harvesting 5 million training samples, shows surprisingly that we are able to learn sufficiently accurate as low as 8 regressors to the high resolution space to get close to the 1024 regressors used in the ANR method, but algorithmically we are up to 128× faster! Also, we reach 29.13 dB on Set14 with 1024 regressors and 5 million extracted samples (with 0.5 million samples we get only 28.97 dB).

Noteworthy is that the performance of A+ does not seem to saturate with the number of extracted samples, which allows better performance at the price of increasing the training time which is only about 15 min for 1024 regressors and 5 millions extracted patches on our tested setup (Intel i7-4770K with 16 GBytes of RAM).

4.3   Performance

In order to assess the quality of our proposed A+ method, we tested it on 3 datasets (Set5, Set14, B100) for 3 upscaling factors (×2, ×3, ×4). We report quantitative PSNR results, as well as running times for our bank of methods

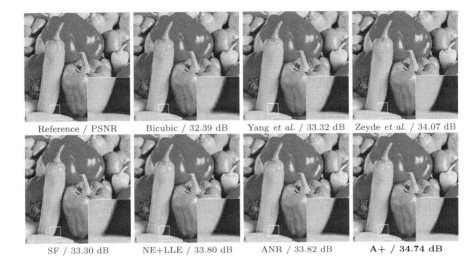

Fig. 3. 'Pepper' image from Set14 with upscaling ×3.

run under the same testing conditions. In Table 3 we summarize the quantitative results, while in Figs. 3, 4, and 5 we provide a visual assessment on three images.[2]

Quality. Timofte *et al.* [1] show that most of the current neighbor embedding methods are able to reach comparable performance quality for the right sets of parameters, such as dictionary size, training choices, features, and internal regulatory parameters. The critical difference among most methods (including neighborhood embedding, sparse coding methods, and not only these) is the time complexity and the running time during testing (and training). In Table 1 we evaluate on the same trained dictionary, with their best parameters, a set of methods (as proposed in [1]) on Set14 dataset. Yang *et al.* [16] uses a different dictionary, but of comparable size (1022 vs 1024) and learned on the same training images. In Table 2 we show results for upscaling factor ×3, and in Table 2 we report results for ×2, ×3, and ×4 upscaling factors. As repeatedly shown, our proposed method is the best method quality-wise, improving on average 0.26 dB (B100,×4) up to 0.72 dB (Set5,×2) over the next top methods, Zeyde *et al.* or ANR. The very recent SRCNN method [18] is 0.2 dB behind A+ on Set5 and more than 0.13 dB on Set14 according to its published results. At the same time, A+ is very efficient, has the time complexity of ANR and except for bicubic interpolation and the Global Regression (GR) method [1], which are clearly outperformed in quality, A+ is the fastest method for a given target in quality of the SR result (see Fig. 2(a) and (c) for PSNR and time vs. dictionary size for different methods). In Figs. 3, 4, and 5 we show how A+ has a visual quality comparable or superior to the other compared methods on a couple of images.

---

[2] For more results: http://www.vision.ee.ethz.ch/~timofter/.

Table 2. PSNR and running time for upscaling factors ×2, ×3 and ×4 for Set5. All methods are trained on the same images and share a dictionary of 1024 atoms; A+ trained with 5000000 samples. For upscaling factor 3, A+ and ANR are 5 times faster than Zeyde *et al.* 120 times faster than Yang *et al.* and 4 times faster than NE+LS.

Set5 images	Scale	Bicubic PSNR	Time	Yang et al. [16] PSNR	Time	Zeyde et al. [11] PSNR	Time	GR [1] PSNR	Time	ANR [1] PSNR	Time	NE+LS PSNR	Time	NE+NNLS PSNR	Time	NE+LLE PSNR	Time	A+ PSNR	Time
baby	x2	37.1	0.0	-		38.2	9.9	38.3	0.8	38.4	1.3	38.1	6.5	38.0	71.1	38.3	12.9	**38.5**	1.3
bird	x2	36.8	0.0	-		39.9	3.0	39.0	0.2	40.0	0.4	39.9	2.0	39.4	22.0	40.0	3.9	**41.1**	0.4
butterfly	x2	27.4	0.0	-		30.6	2.4	29.1	0.2	30.5	0.3	30.4	1.7	30.0	17.9	30.4	3.2	**32.0**	0.3
head	x2	34.9	0.0	-		35.6	2.9	35.6	0.2	35.7	0.4	35.5	1.9	35.5	20.8	35.6	3.8	**35.8**	0.4
woman	x2	32.1	0.0	-		34.5	2.9	33.7	0.2	34.5	0.4	34.3	2.1	34.2	21.0	34.5	3.8	**35.3**	0.4
average	x2	33.66	0.00	-		35.78	4.25	35.13	0.33	35.83	0.54	35.66	2.83	35.43	30.56	35.77	5.51	**36.55**	0.55
baby	x3	33.9	0.0	34.3	89.6	35.1	4.3	34.9	0.6	35.1	0.8	35.0	3.1	34.8	29.9	35.1	5.8	**35.2**	0.8
bird	x3	32.6	0.0	34.1	35.4	34.6	1.3	33.9	0.2	34.6	0.3	34.4	0.9	34.3	9.1	34.6	1.8	**35.5**	0.2
butterfly	x3	24.0	0.0	25.6	32.9	25.9	1.1	25.0	0.1	25.9	0.2	25.8	0.7	25.6	7.0	25.8	1.4	**27.2**	0.2
head	x3	32.9	0.0	33.2	25.3	33.6	1.3	33.5	0.2	33.6	0.2	33.5	0.9	33.5	8.4	33.6	1.7	**33.8**	0.2
woman	x3	28.6	0.0	29.9	31.1	30.4	1.3	29.7	0.2	30.3	0.2	30.2	0.9	29.9	8.4	30.2	1.7	**31.2**	0.2
average	x3	30.39	0.00	31.42	42.86	31.90	1.86	31.41	0.24	31.92	0.34	31.78	1.29	31.60	12.56	31.84	2.46	**32.59**	0.35
baby	x4	31.8	0.0	-		33.1	2.7	32.8	0.4	33.0	0.6	32.9	1.9	32.8	16.5	33.0	3.5	**33.3**	0.6
bird	x4	30.2	0.0	-		31.7	0.8	31.3	0.1	31.8	0.2	31.6	0.6	31.5	4.9	31.7	1.0	**32.5**	0.2
butterfly	x4	22.1	0.0	-		23.6	0.6	23.1	0.1	23.5	0.1	23.4	0.4	23.3	3.8	23.4	0.8	**24.4**	0.1
head	x4	31.6	0.0	-		32.2	0.7	32.1	0.1	32.3	0.2	32.2	0.5	32.1	4.7	32.2	1.0	**32.5**	0.2
woman	x4	26.5	0.0	-		27.9	0.7	27.4	0.1	27.8	0.2	27.6	0.5	27.6	4.6	27.7	1.0	**28.6**	0.2
average	x4	28.42	0.00	-		29.69	1.12	29.34	0.17	29.69	0.25	29.55	0.78	29.47	6.89	29.61	1.45	**30.28**	0.24

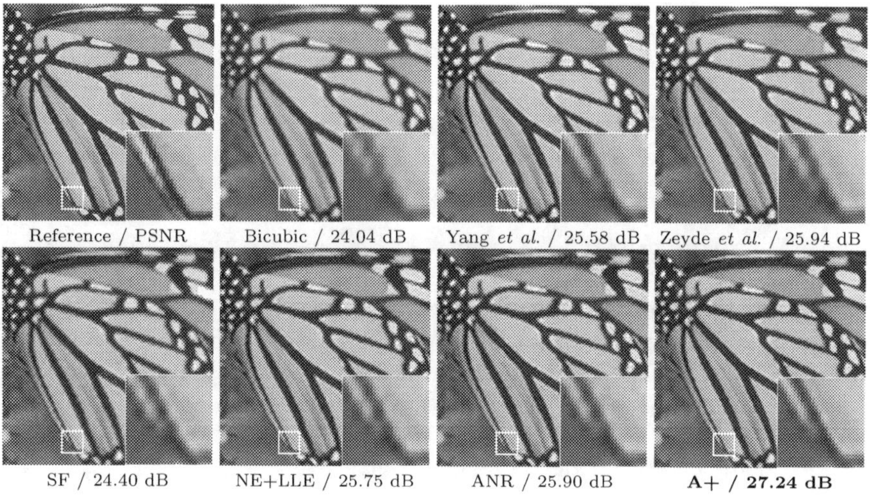

Reference / PSNR   Bicubic / 24.04 dB   Yang *et al.* / 25.58 dB   Zeyde *et al.* / 25.94 dB

SF / 24.40 dB   NE+LLE / 25.75 dB   ANR / 25.90 dB   **A+ / 27.24 dB**

Fig. 4. 'Butterfly' image from Set5 with upscaling ×3.

Table 3. PSNR and running time for upscaling factors ×2, ×3 and ×4 for Set14, Set5, and B100. All methods are trained on the same images and share a dictionary of 1024 atoms, except for SF, which is trained with 1024 clusters and corresponding functions.

Dataset	Scale	Bicubic PSNR	Time	SF [12] PSNR	Time	Zeyde et al. [11] PSNR	Time	GR [1] PSNR	Time	ANR [1] PSNR	Time	NE+LS PSNR	Time	NE+NNLS PSNR	Time	NE+LLE PSNR	Time	A+ PSNR	Time
Set5	x2	33.66	0.00	35.63	20.46	35.78	4.25	35.13	0.33	35.83	0.54	35.66	2.83	35.43	30.56	35.77	5.51	**36.55**	0.55
Set5	x3	30.39	0.00	31.27	11.89	31.90	1.86	31.41	0.24	31.92	0.34	31.78	1.29	31.60	12.56	31.84	2.46	**32.59**	0.35
Set5	x4	28.42	0.00	28.94	6.42	29.69	1.12	29.34	0.17	29.69	0.25	29.55	0.78	29.47	6.89	29.61	1.45	**30.29**	0.24
Set14	x2	30.23	0.00	31.04	39.11	31.81	8.58	31.36	0.73	31.80	1.15	31.69	5.69	31.55	60.53	31.76	11.27	**32.28**	1.20
Set14	x3	27.54	0.00	28.20	24.59	28.67	3.83	28.31	0.47	28.65	0.69	28.59	2.68	28.44	26.15	28.60	5.08	**29.13**	0.69
Set14	x4	26.00	0.00	26.25	11.99	26.88	2.42	26.60	0.42	26.85	0.57	26.81	1.68	26.72	14.49	26.81	3.07	**27.33**	0.56
B100	x2	29.32	0.00	30.35	10.15	30.40	5.80	30.23	0.45	30.44	0.73	30.36	3.79	30.27	39.83	30.41	7.50	**30.78**	0.76
B100	x3	27.15	0.00	27.76	4.94	27.87	2.54	27.70	0.31	27.89	0.45	27.83	1.81	27.73	17.57	27.85	3.47	**28.18**	0.46
B100	x4	25.92	0.00	26.19	2.75	26.51	1.53	26.37	0.25	26.51	0.35	26.45	1.09	26.41	2.04	26.47	2.01	**26.77**	0.35

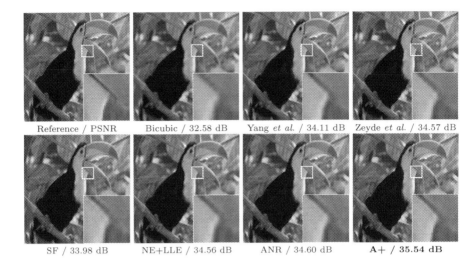

Fig. 5. 'Bird' image from Set5 with upscaling ×3.

Running Time. The time complexity of A+ for encoding LR input patches to HR output patches is linear in the number of input image patches and linear in the number of anchoring atoms. One can easily get sub-linear time complexity in the number of atoms by using any popular search structure, since we just need to retrieve the closest anchor for a specific patch, followed by a (fixed time cost) projection to the HR patch. ANR shares the time complexity (see Fig. 2), but requires much larger dictionaries of anchoring points for comparable performance, which makes it considerably slower as shown in our experiments. A+ is order(s) of magnitude faster than another successful efficient sparse coding approach, Zeyde et al. [11]. At the same time, A+ is 0.2 dB up to 0.7 dB better at any given dictionary size. With as few as 16 atoms A+ outperforms ANR and Zeyde et al. with dictionaries of 2048 atoms. This corresponds to an algorithmic speed up of 128 over ANR for the same quality level.

5 Conclusions

We proposed an enhanced highly efficient example-based super-resolution method, which we named Adjusted Anchored Neighborhood Regression, or shortly – A+. A+ succeeds in substantially surpassing the shortcomings of its predecessors such as ANR or SF. We proposed a different interpretation of the LR space, as a joint space of subspaces spanned by anchoring points and their closed neighborhood of prior samples. While the anchoring points are the unit l_2-norm atoms of a sparse dictionary, the characterizing neighborhood is formed by mined samples from the training samples. For each such atom and neighborhood a regression is learned offline and at test time this is applied to the correlated low resolution samples to super-resolve it. A+ is shown on standard benchmarks to improve 0.2 dB up to 0.7 dB in performance over state-of-the-art methods such as ANR or SF. At the same time it is indisputably the fastest method. It has the lowest time complexity and uses orders of magnitude less anchor points than ANR or SF for substantially better performance. As future work we plan to explore A+ for video processing and other real-time critical applications.

Acknowledgement. This work was partly supported by the ETH General Founding (OK) and the Flemish iMinds framework.

References

1. Timofte, R., De Smet, V., Van Gool, L.: Anchored neighborhood regression for fast example-based super resolution. In: ICCV, pp. 1920–1927 (2013)
2. Sun, J., Xu, Z., Shum, H.-Y.: Image super-resolution using gradient profile prior. In: CVPR, pp. 1–8 (2008)
3. Glasner, D., Bagon, S., Irani, M.: Super-resolution from a single image. In: ICCV, pp. 349–356 (2009)
4. Yang, J., Wright, J., Huang, T.S., Ma, Y.: Image super-resolution as sparse representation of raw image patches. In: CVPR, pp. 1–8 (2008)
5. Sun, J., Zhu, J., Tappen, M.F.: Context-constrained hallucination for image super-resolution. In: CVPR, pp. 231–238 (2010)
6. Michaeli, T., Irani, M.: Nonparametric blind super-resolution. In: ICCV, pp. 945–952 (2013)
7. Efrat, N., Glasner, D., Apartsin, A., Nadler, B., Levin, A.: Accurate blur models vs. image priors in single image super-resolution. In: ICCV, pp. 2832–2839 (2013)
8. Freeman, W.T., Pasztor, E.C., Carmichael, O.T.: Learning low-level vision. IJCV **40**(1), 25–47 (2000)
9. Chang, H., Yeung, D.-Y., Xiong, Y.: Super-resolution through neighbor embedding. In: CVPR, pp. 275–282 (2004)
10. Bevilacqua, M., Roumy, A., Guillemot, C., Alberi Morel, M.-L.: Low-complexity single-image super-resolution based on nonnegative neighbor embedding. In: BMVC, pp. 1–10 (2012)
11. Zeyde, R., Elad, M., Protter, M.: On single image scale-up using sparse-representations. In: Boissonnat, J.-D., Chenin, P., Cohen, A., Gout, C., Lyche, T., Mazure, M.-L., Schumaker, L. (eds.) Curves and Surfaces 2011. LNCS, vol. 6920, pp. 711–730. Springer, Heidelberg (2012)
12. Yang, C.-Y., Yang, M.-H.: Fast direct super-resolution by simple functions. In: ICCV, pp. 561–568 (2013)
13. Roweis, S., Lawrence, S.: Nonlinear dimensionality reduction by locally linear embedding. Science **290**, 2323–2326 (2000)
14. Timofte, R., Van Gool, L.: Adaptive and weighted collaborative representations for image classification. Pattern Recogn. Lett. **43**, 127–135 (2014)
15. Martin, D., Fowlkes, C., Tal, D., Malik, J.: A Database of human segmented natural images and its application to evaluating segmentation algorithms and measuring ecological statistics. In: ICCV, pp. 416–423 (2001)
16. Yang, J., Wright, J., Huang, T.S., Ma, Y.: Image super-resolution via sparse representation. IEEE Trans. Image Process. **19**(11), 2861–2873 (2010)

17. De Smet, V., Namboodiri, V.P., Van Gool, L.J.: Nonuniform image patch exemplars for low level vision. In: WACV, pp. 23–30 (2013)
18. Dong, C., Loy, C.C., He, K., Tang, X.: Learning a deep convolutional network for image super-resolution. In: Fleet, D., Pajdla, T., Schiele, B., Tuytelaars, T. (eds.) ECCV 2014, Part IV. LNCS, vol. 8692, pp. 184–199. Springer, Heidelberg (2014)

Multiple Ocular Diseases Classification with Graph Regularized Probabilistic Multi-label Learning

Xiangyu Chen[1]([⊠]), Yanwu Xu[1], Lixin Duan[1], Shuicheng Yan[2], Zhuo Zhang[1], Damon Wing Kee Wong[1], and Jiang Liu[1]

[1] Institute for Infocomm Research, Agency for Science,
Technology and Research, Singapore, Singapore
chenxy@i2r.a-star.edu.sg
[2] Department of Electrical and Computer Engineering,
National University of Singapore, Singapore, Singapore

Abstract. Glaucoma, Pathological Myopia (PM), and Age-related Macular Degeneration (AMD) are three leading ocular diseases in the world. In this paper, we proposed a multiple ocular diseases diagnosis approach for above three diseases, with Entropic Graph regularized Probabilistic Multi-label learning (EGPM). The proposed EGPM exploits the correlations among these three diseases, and simultaneously classifying them for a given fundus image. The EGPM scheme contains two concatenating parts: (1) efficient graph construction based on k-Nearest-Neighbor (k-NN) search; (2) entropic multi-label learning based on Kullback-Leibler divergence. In addition, to capture the characteristics of these three leading ocular diseases, we explore the extractions of various effective low-level features, including Global Features, Grid-based Features, and Bag of Visual Words. Extensive experiments are conducted to validate the proposed EGPM framework on *SiMES* dataset. The results of Area Under Curve (AUC) in multiple ocular diseases classification outperform the state-of-the-art algorithms.

1 Introduction

Vision is one of the most important senses which greatly influences an individuals quality of life. Studies have shown that many of the leading causes of vision impairment and blindness worldwide are irreversible and cannot be cured [1]. Glaucoma, Pathological Myopia (PM), and Age-related Macular Degeneration (AMD) are three leading ocular diseases. Simultaneously diagnosing Glaucoma, PM and AMD is one of the most challenging problems in medical imaging.

Glaucoma is a chronic eye disease that leads to vision loss, in which the optic nerve is progressively damaged. It is one of the common causes of blindness, and is predicted to affect around 80 million people by 2020 [1]. During the progression of glaucoma disease, the death of ganglion nerve cells often leads to changes in the appearance of the Optic Disc (OD) [2]. Glaucoma diagnosis is typically based on the medical history, intraocular pressure, and visual field loss tests together

© Springer International Publishing Switzerland 2015
D. Cremers et al. (Eds.): ACCV 2014, Part IV, LNCS 9006, pp. 127–142, 2015.
DOI: 10.1007/978-3-319-16817-3_9

with a manual assessment of the OD through ophthalmoscopy. Since the loss of vision in glaucoma eye is irreversible and permanent, early detection of this disease is a strong need.

Pathological Myopia (PM) is another leading cause of visual impairment and can lead to blindness in children if left undetected, which is primarily a genetic condition [3]. PM is a type of severe and progressive nearsightedness characterized by changes in the fundus of the eye, posterior staphyloma, and deficient corrected acuity [4]. It has been shown that PM related visual impairment affect the productivity and quality of life. It is essential to manage the progression of degenerative PM with early detection and treatment. Current detection of PM relies heavily on the manual screening and efforts of the clinicians, which is based on fundus image where retinal degeneration is observed in the form of Peripapillary Atrophy (PPA).

As the leading cause of vision loss, Age-related Macular Degeneration (AMD) is often associated to the presence of drusen [5]. AMD is a degenerative condition of aging which affects the area of the eye involved with central vision. AMD can be divided into Early AMD and Late AMD [6]. Early AMD is characterized by good vision and the presence of sparse drusen with risk of progression to late stage of AMD. Late AMD is distinguished by the loss of central vision caused by geographic atrophy, neovascularization or pigment epithelial detachment [12]. Hence it is important to detect Early AMD to halt its progress and prevent it from progressing to Late AMD.

With the advancement of retinal fundus imaging, several computer-aided diagnosis (CAD) methods and systems have been developed to automatically detect these three leading ocular diseases from retinal fundus image. However, current work mainly focus on detecting Glaucoma, PM, and AMD individually. Classifying these three leading diseases simultaneously is still an open research direction. There are some correlations among these three leading ocular diseases. In recent decades, the problem of low vision and blindness in elderly people became major and socially significant issue. The number of patients having age-related macular degeneration (AMD) in association with glaucoma grows all over the world [8], which attaches medical and social value to this multiple diseases diagnosis problem. Moreover, in recent study, myopic eyes are less likely to have AMD and diabetic retinopathy (DR) but more likely to have nuclear cataract and glaucoma [9].

Inspired by the correlations among Glaucoma, PM, and AMD, we develop an Entropic Graph regularized Probabilistic Multi-label learning (EGPM) method for harmoniously integrating the correlation information of these three diseases, and investigating the problem of learning to simultaneously diagnose them for a given fundus image. Different from previous algorithms that detect ocular disease independently, the proposed EGPM formulates the correlation information of different diseases of an image as a unit label confidence vector, which imposes inter-label constraints and manipulates labels interactively. It then utilizes the probabilistic Kullback-Leibler divergence and Shannon Entropy for problem formulation. Since a patient may have two or three ocular diseases at the same time, multiple ocular diseases detection is more oriented to real world diagnosis scenario.

2   Related Work

Multi-label learning is a hot and promising research direction in computer vision. In the past, there are several approaches proposed to exploit the multiple labels learning problem. For example, the work in [15] introduced a unified Correlative Multi-Label (CML) framework for classifying labels and modeling correlations between them. Chen et al. [19] solved the multi-label learning problem by utilizing a sylvester equation. However, in medical imaging analysis, multiple ocular diseases detection is still an open problem. In this paper, the proposed scheme exploits the medical problem of simultaneously diagnosing multiple ocular diseases based on entropic graph regularized probabilistic multi-label learning.

In the previous work [10], a graph-based semi-supervised learning (SSL) method was proposed for phone classification task. Unlike previous approaches, this method modeled the multi-class label confidence vector as a probabilistic distribution, and utilized the Kullback-Leibler (KL) divergence to gauge the pairwise discrepancy. The underlying philosophy is that such soft regularization term will be less vulnerable to noisy annotation or outliers. Here we adopt the same distance measure, yet in a different scenario (i.e. multiple ocular disease detection in medical imaging analysis), thus demanding new solution. In the setting of multi-label annotation in multimedia, the work in [20] proposed the Kullback-Leibler divergence based multi-label propagation, which encoded the label information of an image as a label vector and imposes inter-label constraints and manipulates labels interactively. In this paper, based on Kullback-Leibler Divergence and Shannon entropy, we propose a graph regularized probabilistic multi-label learning framework for harmoniously integrating the correlation information of different diseases, and investigating the problem of learning to simultaneously diagnose these three leading ocular diseases.

3   Feature Extraction

Detecting Glaucoma, PM and AMD is one of the most challenging problems in medical image analysis. In order to effectively capture the characteristics of these three leading ocular diseases, we explore the extractions of various popular features adopted in medical imaging and computer vision in this section. We extract three types of low-level features: Global Features, Grid-based Features, and Bag of Visual Words.

3.1   Global Features

Color Histogram: In computer version, color histogram is an effective representation of the distribution of colors in an image, where it represents the number of pixels that have colors in each of a fixed list of color ranges. The color histogram can be built for any kind of color space such as RGB. In this paper, we use the LAB color space [14], where it is a color-opponent space with L for lightness and A and B for color opponents. Different from RGB and other

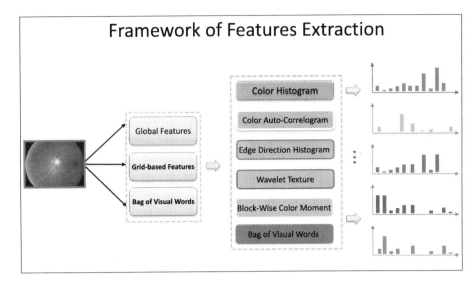

Fig. 1. Framework of features extraction. A set of effective and popularly used global and local features for each fundus image are extracted. Global Features: color histogram, color auto-correlogram, edge direction histogram, and wavelet texture; Grid-based Features: block-wise color moments are extracted; Local Features: bags of visual words.

color spaces, LAB is designed to approximate human vision, which aspires to perceptual uniformity. And the L component closely matches human perception of lightness. Here, we quantize each component of LAB color space uniformly into four bins. The color histogram for each component is calculated as:

$$L(i) = \frac{Z_i}{N}, i = 1, 2, ..., k, \qquad (1)$$

where Z_i is the number of pixels with value i, N is the total number of pixels in the image, and k is the size of the quantized bins (Fig. 1).

Color Auto-Correlogram: The color histogram describes the global color distribution of a image as mentioned above. However, it does not contain any spatial information and is therefore liable to false positives. In this paper, we compute color auto-correlogram for each fundus image, which characterize the color distributions and the spatial correlation of pairs of colors together. For color auto-correlogram, the first two dimensions are the colors of any pixel pair, and the third dimension is their spatial distance. Let I represent the entire set of image pixels and $I_c(i)$ represent the subset of pixels with color $c(i)$, then the color auto-correlogram can be computed as [16]:

$$r_{i,j}^{(t)} = P_{r_{p_1 \in I_{c_i}, p_2 \in I}} [p_2 \in I_{c(j)} \,\|\, |p_1 - p_2| = d], \qquad (2)$$

where $|p_1 - p_2|$ is the distance between pixels p_1 and p_2, and $i, j \in \{1, 2, ..., k\}$, $d \in 1, 2, ..., l$. Since color auto-correlogram only capture the spatial correlation between identical colors, the dimension is reduced from $O(N^2 d)$ to $O(Nd)$.

Edge Direction Histogram: Edge is an important feature to represent the content of the fundus images. Edge direction histogram builds a histogram with the direction of the gradients of the edges. Here, we employ the edge direction histogram as introduced in [17], which comprises a total of 73 bins (the first 72 bins are the count of edges with directions quantized at five degrees interval, and the last bin is the count of number of pixels that do not contribute to an edge). Canny filter is utilized to detect edge points, and Sobel operator is employed to compute the direction by the gradient of each edge point. The entries in histogram are normalized as follows [17]:

$$
E_i = \begin{cases} \frac{E(i)}{H_e}, & \text{if } i \in [0, ..., 71] \\ \frac{E(i)}{H}, & \text{if } i = 72 \end{cases} \tag{3}
$$

where $E(i)$ is the count of bin i in the edge direction histogram; H_e is the total number of edge points detected in the sub-block of an fundus image; and H is the total number of pixels in the sub-block.

Wavelet Texture: Textures are one of the basic features in visual content analysis, which are replications, symmetries and combinations of various basic patterns with some random variation. Texture analysis is important in many applications of image analysis such as classification, detection or segmentation. For texture analysis, we adopt the wavelet transformation, which involves filtering and sub-sampling. During the process of wavelet transformation, the fundus image is decomposed into four frequency sub-bands, LL, LH, HL, and HH (L and H stand for low frequency and high frequency respectively). There are two types of wavelet transform: Pyramid-structured Wavelet Transform (PWT) and Tree-structured Wavelet Transform (TWT). The PWT recursively decomposes the LL band. On the other hand, the TWT decomposes other bands such as LH, HL or HH. Wavelet transformation decomposes a signal with a family of basis functions. These basis functions $v_{ij}(x)$ are computed from a mother wavelet $v(x)$ [22] i.e.,

$$
v_{ij}(x) = 2^{-\frac{i}{2}} v(2^{-i}x - j), \tag{4}
$$

where i and j are the dilation and translation parameters.

The next step for wavelet transformation after the decomposition is feature vector construction. Mean and standard deviation of the energy distribution of each sub-band at each level are utilized to construct the feature vectors. For PWT, a feature vector with the dimension of $24 = 3 \times 4 \times 2$ will be obtained for the three-level decomposition. For TWT, the feature vector will be computed depend on how the sub-bands at each level are decomposed. After sequentially decomposing the LL, LH, and HL bands, a fixed decomposition tree can be obtained. And finally, a feature vector with the dimension of $104 = 52 \times 2$ will be obtained [22].

3.2   Grid-Based Features

Block-wise Color Moments: Color moments provide a measurement for color similarity between images. The basis of color moments lays in the assumption that:

the distribution of color in an image can be considered as a probability distribution. Color moments include three central moments: mean, standard deviation, and skewness. These three color moments have been validated to be efficient and effective in representing the color distributions of images. These three moments are defined as [7]:

$$\theta_i = \frac{1}{N} \sum_{j=1}^{N} b_{ij}. \tag{5}$$

$$\kappa_i = \left(\frac{1}{N} \sum_{j=1}^{N} (b_{ij} - \theta_i)^2\right)^{1/2}. \tag{6}$$

$$\delta_i = \left(\frac{1}{N} \sum_{j=1}^{N} (b_{ij} - \theta_i)^3\right)^{1/3}. \tag{7}$$

where b_{ij} is the value of the i-th color component of the image pixel j, and N is the total number of pixels in the image.

In these three color moments, mean can be understood as the average color value in the image. The standard deviation can be considered as the square root of the variance of the distribution. The skewness is a measure of the degree of asymmetry in the distribution. In this paper, we extract the block-wise color moments over 55 fixed grid partitions of the fundus image, which results in a block-wise color moments.

3.3 Bag of Visual Words

The bag of visual words model approach in computer vision, also known as bag-of-words model [23], is a simplifying representation used in natural language processing and information retrieval by treating local image features as words. In natural language processing, a bag-of-words is a sparse vector of occurrence counts of words; that is, a sparse histogram over the vocabulary. In computer vision, a bag-of-words is a sparse vector of occurrence counts of a vocabulary of local image features (codebook), which is a location-independent global feature; however, the properties of local features, such as intensity, rotation, scale and affine invariants can also be preserved. In this paper, the generation of bag of words comprises three steps:

- First, perform Gaussian filters on the gray scale version of the fundus images for detecting a set of key-points and scales respectively.
- Then, calculate the Scale Invariant Feature Transform (SIFT) over the local region defined by the key-point and scale.
- Finally, conduct the vector quantization on SIFT region descriptors for building the visual vocabulary by exploiting the k-means clustering. In this paper, we set $k = 500$.

4   Graph Regularized Probabilistic Multi-label Learning

The proposed entropic multi-label learning framework includes two concatenating parts: (1) k-Nearest-Neighbor (k-NN) Search based Graph Construction; (2) Entropic Multi-label Learning based on Kullback-Leibler Divergence.

4.1   Graph Construction

In this paper, we adopt the same representation and distance measure as in [10, 20], yet in a different scenario (i.e. multiple ocular diseases diagnosis in medical imaging analysis), thus demanding new solution. For graph construction, we utilize the an directed weighted graph $\mathcal{G} =< V,\ E >$. V is the node set and E is the edge set. Let V_l and V_u be the sets of labeled and unlabeled vertices respectively. $\mathcal{G}$ is equivalent to a weight matrix $\mathbf{W} = \{w_{ij}\} \in \mathbb{R}^{m \times m}$. To efficiently handle the data, the constructed graph is enforced to be sparse: the weight between two nodes w_{ij} is nonzero only when $j \in \mathcal{N}_i$. $\mathcal{N}_i$ stands for the local neighborhood of the i-th image. There are two main steps for graph construction: (1) Neighborhood Selection; and (2) Edge Weight Computation.

Neighborhood Selection. For the issue of neighborhood selection, there are two conventional strategies in previous work: ϵ-ball neighborhood and k-nearest-neighbor based neighborhood.

For ϵ-ball neighborhood selection, for a given image node x_i, any image x_j that satisfies $d(x_i,\ x_j) \leq \epsilon$ will be considered as the neighborhood of the node x_i, resulting in nonzero w_{ij}. Here $d(x_i,\ x_j)$ is a distance measure and ϵ is pre-specified threshold. The obtained weight matrix of the constructed graph is symmetric. However, for some images beyond a distance from the others, there is probably no edge connecting to other images.

For k-nearest-neighbor based neighborhood selection, for a given image node x_i, w_{ij} is nonzero only if the image x_j is among the k-nearest neighbors to the i-th image. Graphs constructed in this way may ensure a constant vertex degree and avoid over-dense sub-graphs and isolated vertices. Hence, we employ k-nearest-neighbor based neighborhood for graph construction in this paper.

Edge Weight Computation. For edge weight computation, the selection of inter-sample similarity is the core problem for graph-based multi-label learning. Basically, the message transmitted from the neighboring image nodes with higher weights will be much stronger than the others. The more similar an image is to another image, the stronger the interaction exists between them. There are two traditional ways to computing the edge weight: unweighted k-NN similarity and exponentially weighted similarity.

For unweighted k-NN similarity, if x_j is among the k-NN of x_i, then the similarity w_{ij} between x_i and x_j is 1; otherwise w_{ij} is 0. For undirected graph, the weight matrix is symmetric with $w_{ij} = w_{ji}$. For exponentially weighted similarity, given all chosen k-NN neighbors, their weights can be obtained as below:

$$w_{ij} = \exp\left(-\frac{d(x_i, x_j)}{\sigma^2}\right),\tag{8}$$

where $d(x_i, x_j)$ is the distance measure and σ is a free parameter to control the decay rate.

In this paper, we utilized an efficient weight computation method–*weighted linear neighborhood similarity* [18]. It is assumed that the image x_i can be linearly reconstructed from its k-NN. The weights are computed via solving the following optimization problem:

$$\min_{w_{ij}} \| x_i - \sum_{j \in \mathcal{N}_i} w_{ij} x_j \|^2 . \tag{9}$$

As introduced in [18], we adopt the constraints $w_{ij} \geq 0$ and $\sum_j w_{ij} = 1$. The kind of constraints could help exploit the correlations of the three ocular diseases.

4.2 Entropic Multi-label Learning Based on Kullback-Leibler Divergence

In this section, we let $M = \{M_l, M_u\}$ be the entire fundus images data set of multiple ocular diseases. $M_l = \{x_i, r_i\}_{i=1}^l$ is the set of labeled fundus images. $M_u = \{x_i\}_{i=l+1}^{l+u}$ is the set of unlabeled images. Here, x_i is the feature vector of the i-th fundus image and r_i is a multi-label vector of this fundus image. For r_i, its entry is set to be 1 if it is assigned with the corresponding label of ocular disease, otherwise its entry is 0. For graph regularized multi-label learning, the labels of M_u will be learned from that of M_l. As introduced in [10], in the measurable space $(Y, \mathcal{Y})$, the probability measure p_i is defined for each x_i of the fundus image. $Y \subset \mathbb{N}$ is the space of classifier outputs. $\mathcal{Y}$ stands for the σ-field of measurable subsets of Y. For binary classification, the value of $|Y|$ is 2. For multi-label classification, $|Y| > 2$. In this paper, we deal with the multiple ocular diseases classification and set $|Y| = 3$.

In the problem formulation, p_i and r_i are for the i-th fundus image, both of which are subject to the multinomial distributions. We let $p_i(y)$ be the probability that x_i belongs to class y, and utilize $\{r_j, j \in V_l\}$ to encode the supervision information of the labeled images of ocular diseases. When r_j is assigned a unique disease label, it becomes the so-called "one-hot" vector, where only the corresponding entry is 1, the rest is 0. When r_j is associated with multiple labels, it will be represented to be a probabilistic distribution with multiple non-zero entries. The following objective function for multi-label learning is based on the concept of Kullback-Leibler divergence [10] defined on two distributions:

$$B_1(p) = \sum_{l=1}^l K_L\left(r_i \| p_i\right) + \mu \sum_{i=1}^m K_L\left(p_i \| \sum_{j \in N(i)} w_{ij} p_j\right), \tag{10}$$

where $K_L(r_i \| p_i) = \sum_y r_i(y) \log \frac{r_i(y)}{p_i(y)}$, which stands for the KL divergence between r_i and p_i.

In this formulation, the first term of $B_1(p)$ will trigger a heavy penalty if the estimated value p_i deviates from the pre-specified r_i. The second term stems from the assumption that p_i can be linearly reconstructed from the estimations of its neighbors. And it will penalize the inconsistency between the p_i and its neighborhood estimation. μ is a free parameter to balance these two terms. The optimal solution of $B_1(p)$ can be obtained by $p^* = \arg_p \min B_1(p)$.

For solving the multiple ocular diseases classification, we employ a modified version of B_1 in Eq. (10) by introducing a new group of variables $\{q_i\}$ and Shannon entropy $H(q_i)$, which is shown as below:

$$B_2(p, q) = \sum_{l=1}^{l} K_L(r_i \parallel q_i) + \mu \sum_{i=1}^{m} K_L(p_i \parallel \sum_{j \in \mathcal{N}(i)} w_{ij} q_j)$$

$$+\eta \sum_{i=1}^{m} K_L(p_i \parallel q_i) + \xi \sum_{i=1}^{m} H(q_i). \tag{11}$$

where the third measure q_i is an approximated version of p_i, which is introduced to decouple the original term $\mu \sum_{i=1}^{m} K_L\big(p_i \parallel \sum_{j \in N(i)} w_{ij} p_j\big)$ in $B_1(p)$. To enforce consistency between them, the third term $\sum_{i=1}^{m} K_L(p_i \parallel q_i)$ is incorporated. Here $H(q) = \sum_y q(y) log q(y)$. The Eq. (11) could be solved by utilizing the similar method in [10].

5 Experiments

In this paper, in order to evaluate the performance of our proposed multiple diseases diagnosis method–Graph Regularized Probabilistic Multi-label Learning (EGPM), we perform extensive experiments on the Singapore Malay Eye Study (SiMES) database [13] for simultaneously detecting the three leading ocular diseases: Glaucoma, Pathological Myopia (PM), and age-related macular degeneration (AMD). As described in Sect. 3, we extract three different types of low-level features for conducting experiments and study the performance of the proposed EGPM with a total of four settings: (1) global features; (2) grid-based features; (3) bag of words; (4) global features + grid-based features + bag of words. The notation + indicates a combination of four types of features in the corresponding setting. We provide quantitative study on SiMES, with an emphasis on the comparison with six state-of-the-art related methods.

Table 1. The Baseline Algorithms.

Name	Methods
KNN	k-Nearest Neighbors [25]
SVM	Support Vector Machine [24]
LNP	Linear Neighborhood Propagation [18]
SPM	State-of-the-art algorithm for PM Detection [4]
SAMD	State-of-the-art algorithm for AMD Detection [21]
SGL	State-of-the-art algorithm for Glaucoma Detection [2]

5.1   Dataset

In this paper, we conduct the experiments on SiMES dataset. The Singapore Malay Eye Study (SiMES) is a population-based study, which examined a cross-sectional and age stratified sample of 3,280 randomly selected Malays aged from 40 to 80 years old living in Singapore. For each subject in this database, personal demographic/clinical data, a retinal fundus image, and a blood sample (used for genotyping) were collected during the clinic visit, which thus gives us three informatics domains containing completely different types of data [11].

In this dataset, the detection of Glaucoma, AMD, and PM have been made by clinicians. The detection of different diseases made by clinicians during the visit are used as the gold standard to evaluate the classification performance of all the methods in the experiments. We choose a subset of SiMES for experiments, which contains 2,258 subjects. In this subset dataset, there are 100 with glaucoma, 122 with AMD, and 58 with PM. For each disease, the distribution of the subjects who contracted the disease in the selected dataset is representative of the disease prevalence in the population.

5.2   Low-Level Features

As detailed in Sect. 3, in order to capture the characteristics of these three leading ocular diseases, we extract a set of effective and popularly used global and local features for each image. For global features, four types of features are extracted: 64-dimensional color histogram [14], 144-dimensional color auto-correlogram [16], 73-dimensional edge direction histogram [17], and 128-dimensional wavelet texture [22]. For grid-based features, 225-dimensional block-wise color moments are extracted [7]. For local features, 500-dimensional bags of visual words [23] are generated.

5.3   Evaluation Criteria

We utilize the area under the curve (AUC) of receiver operation characteristic curve (ROC) to evaluate the performance of multiple ocular diseases diagnosis. The ROC is plotted as a curve which shows the tradeoff between sensitivity TPR (true positive rate) and specificity TNR (true negative rate), which can be defined as

$$TPR = \frac{TP}{TP + FN}, \ TNR = \frac{TN}{TN + FP}, \tag{12}$$

where TP and TN are the number of true positives and true negatives, respectively, and FP and FN are the number of false positives and false negatives, respectively.

5.4   Baselines and Experimental Setup

In the experiments, we compare our proposed Entropic Graph regularized Probabilistic Multi-label learning (EGPM) with six baseline methods (as shown in

Table 2. The AUCs of different algorithms for simultaneously detecting the three lead-ing ocular diseases (i.e., Glaucoma, PM and AMD) on SiMES dataset. The combined visual features (global features + grid-based features + bag of words) are utilized in the experiment. The results of AUC marked in boldface are significantly better than others.

Methods	Glaucoma	Pathological Myopia	AMD
KNN	74.2%	86.5%	72.9%
SVM	76.7%	89.1%	75.0%
LNP	78.8%	90.1%	76.6%
SGL	81.0%	-	-
SPM	-	91.0%	-
SAMD	-	-	77.8%
Our proposed	**84.2 %**	**93.8 %**	**80.4%**

Table 1): Support Vector Machine (SVM) [24], k-Nearest Neighbors (KNN) [25], Linear Neighborhood Propagation (LNP) [18], SPM [4], SAMD [21], and SGL [2]. Amongst them, SVM is originally developed to solve binary-class or multi-class classification problem. Here we use its multi-class version by adopting the one-vs-one method. LNP is the state-of-the-art algorithms for semi-supervised learning. It bases on a linear construction criterion to calculate the edge weights of the graph, and disseminates the supervision information by a local propagation and updating process. SPM is the state-of-the-art algorithm for PM detection, which is a sparse learning based framework to recognize PM in retinal fundus images. SAMD is the state-of-the-art algorithm for AMD detection, which is an auto-matic framework for the detection of drusen images for AMD assessment. SGL is the state-of-the-art algorithm for Glaucoma detection, which is a reconstruction-based learning technique for glaucoma screening. Since SPM, SAMD and SGL are the individual ocular disease detection algorithms, we only give the AUCs of PM, AMD and Glaucoma for SPM, SAMD and SGL in Table 2, respectively.

For KNN, SVM, and LNP, we implement them under the aforementioned three settings using different feature types as well as their combinations. For each setting, all the methods for the automatic detections of the three leading ocular diseases (i.e., glaucoma, AMD and PM) are evaluated on SiMES dataset. All the experiments are implemented with Matlab and tested on a four core 3.4 GHz PC with 32 GB RAM.

5.5   Experiment Results Analysis

In the experiments, we systematically compare our proposed EGPM with six baselines (SVM, KNN, LNP, SPM, SAMD, and SGL) on SiMES. Below are the parameters and the adopted values for each method:

– For SVM algorithm, we adopt the RBF kernel. For its two parameters γ and C, we set $\gamma = 0.5$ and $C = 1$ in experiments after fine tuning.

Table 3. The AUCs of different algorithms under three setting of features on SiMES dataset for Glaucoma diagnosis. The results of AUC marked in boldface are significantly better than others.

Methods	KNN	SVM	LNP	Our proposed
Global features	71.2%	73.5%	75.2%	79.5%
Grid based features	69.1%	71.2%	73.0%	77.4%
Bag of words	68.4%	70.9%	72.6%	76.2%
Combined features	**74.2 %**	**76.7%**	**78.8 %**	**84.2%**

Table 4. The AUCs of different algorithms under three setting of features on SiMES dataset for AMD diagnosis. The results of AUC marked in boldface are significantly better than others.

Methods	KNN	SVM	LNP	Our proposed
Global features	70.2%	72.5%	73.9%	77.2%
Grid based features	69.3%	71.8%	72.5%	77.8%
Bag of words	68.1%	70.3%	71.6%	74.4%
Combined features	**72.9 %**	**75.0%**	**76.6 %**	**80.4%**

– For KNN, there is only one parameter k for tuning, which stands for the number of nearest neighbors and is trivially set as 500.
– For EGPM, we set the two parameters as $\mu = 9$, $\eta = 4$, and $\xi = 0.01$.
– For SGL, SPM, and SAMD, we use the similar setting as in their papers.

The AUCs of the seven methods for detecting the three leading ocular diseases (i.e., Glaucoma, PM, and AMD) on SiMES dataset are illustrated in Table 2. The combined visual features (global features + grid-based features +bag of words) are utilized in this experiment. For SGL, SPM and SAMD, we adopt the similar setting in their papers. Our proposed algorithm EGPM outperforms the other baseline algorithms significantly. For example, EGPM has an improvement 9.8% over SVM, 13.5% over KNN, 6.9% over LNP for detecting Glaucoma. For PM, EGPM has an improvement 5.3% over SVM, 8.4% over KNN, and 4.1% over LNP. For AMD, EGPM has an improvement 7.2% over

Table 5. The AUCs of different algorithms under three setting of features on SiMES dataset for PM diagnosis. The results of AUC marked in boldface are significantly better than others.

Methods	KNN	SVM	LNP	Our proposed
Global features	81.5%	84.1%	85.6%	88.4%
Grid based features	79.3%	82.3%	83.7%	86.3%
Bag of words	83.8%	86.5%	87.9%	90.3%
Combined features	**86.5 %**	**89.1%**	**90.1 %**	**93.8%**

SVM, 10.3 % over KNN, and 5.0 % over LNP. Comparing with the state-of-the-art algorithms of individual disease detection, the proposed EGPM outperforms SGL, SPM, and SAMD by achieving the AUC 84.2 %, 93.8 %, 80.4 %, respectively. The improvement is supposed to stem from the fact that our proposed algorithm encodes the disease label information of each image as a unit confidence vector, which imposes extra inter-label constraints. In contrast, other methods consider each disease label independently.

The comparison results of the detecting performance under four feature setting are listed in Tables 3, 4, and 5. Since the state-of-the-art algorithms (SGL, SPM, SAMD) of the individual ocular disease detection are based on their own

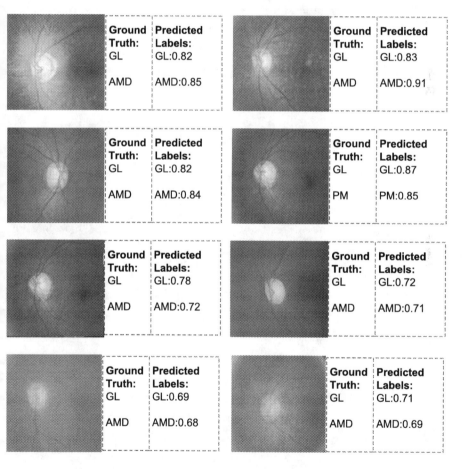

Fig. 2. Sample results diagnosed by our proposed EGPM algorithm. The order is from left top to right bottom. Each fundus image is attached the ground truth diagnosed by clinicians and the predicted labels with probabilities by EGPM. GL, AMD, and PM stand for Glaucoma, Age-related Macular Degeneration, and Pathological Myopia, respectively.

special visual features and retinal structures, the AUC results are not given in Tables 3, 4, and 5. From Table 3, we are able to observe that, for glaucoma detection, our proposed algorithm EGPM outperforms the three baseline algorithms based on the combined features. The AUC of the receiver operating characteristic curve in glaucoma detection is 84.2%. The similar results are shown in Tables 4 and 5 for AMD and PM detection respectively. For AMD detection, our proposed EGPM algorithm achieves 80.4%. For PM detection, the AUC of EGPM is 93.8%.

Recall that the proposed algorithm is a graph based probabilistic multi-label learning algorithm, wherein $p_i(y)$ expresses the probability for the i-th image to be associated with the y-th label, as detailed in Sect. 3.2. Figure 2 gives eight sample results by our proposed EGPM algorithm. For each fundus image, we attach the ground truth diagnosed by clinicians and the predicted labels with probabilities by EGPM. In the real world, the number of patients usually have AMD in association with glaucoma [8]. PM eyes are less likely to have AMD, but more likely to have glaucoma [9]. Hence, in our experimental results, Glaucoma and AMD are usually detected at the same time, as well as Glaucoma and PM (as shown in the fourth sample in Fig. 2). As shown in the fourth row of Fig. 2, even the quality of the fundus images is not good, our proposed EGPM still detects the glaucoma and AMD diseases. This validates the robustness and stability of the proposed method.

6   Conclusion

The proposed EGPM integrates the correlation information of Glaucoma, PM and AMD, and exploits the problem of learning to simultaneously classify these three ocular diseases. Two concatenating parts are included in EGPM: (1) k-Nearest-Neighbor (k-NN) search based graph construction; (2) Kullback-Leibler divergence based entropic multi-label learning. In addition, in order to capture the characteristics of Glaucoma, PM and AMD, the extractions of various effective low-level features are explored, including Global Features, Grid-based Features, and Bag of Visual Words.

References

1. Quigley, H.A., Broman, A.T.: The number of people with glaucoma worldwide in 2010 and 2020. Br. J. Ophthalmol. **90**(3), 262–267 (2006)
2. Xu, Y., Lin, S., Wong, D.W.K., Liu, J., Xu, D.: Efficient reconstruction-based optic cup localization for glaucoma screening. In: Mori, K., Sakuma, I., Sato, Y., Barillot, C., Navab, N. (eds.) MICCAI 2013, Part III. LNCS, vol. 8151, pp. 445–452. Springer, Heidelberg (2013)
3. Young, T.L., Ronan, S.M., Alvear, A.B., Wildenberg, S.C., Oetting, W.S., Atwood, L.D., Wilkin, D.J., King, R.A.: A second locus for familial high myopia maps to chromosome 12q. Am. J. Hum. Genet. **63**(5), 1419–1424 (1998)

4. Xu, Y., Liu, J., Zhang, Z., Tan, N.M., Wong, D.W.K., Saw, S.M., Wong, T.Y.: Learn to recognize pathological myopia in fundus images using bag-of-feature and sparse learning approach. In: International Symposium on Biomedical Imaging, pp. 888–891 (2013)
5. Bressler, N.M., Bressler, S.B., Fine, S.L.: Age-related macular degeneration. Surv. Ophthalmol. **32**(6), 375–413 (1988)
6. De Jong, P.T.: Age-related macular degeneration. N. Engl. J. Med. **355**(14), 1474–1484 (2006)
7. Stricker, M., Orengo, M.: Similarity of color images. In: SPIE Storage and Retrieval for Image and Video Databases III (1995)
8. Avetisov, S.E., Erichev, V.P., Budzinskaia, M.V., Karpilova, M.A., Gurova, I.V., Shchegoleva, I.V., Chikun, E.A.: Age-related macular degeneration and glaucoma: intraocular pressure monitoring after intravitreal injections. Vestn. Oftalmol. **128**(6), 3–5 (2012)
9. Pan, C.W., Cheung, C.Y., Aung, T., Cheung, C.M., Zheng, Y.F., Wu, R.Y., Mitchell, P., Lavanya, R., Baskaran, M., Wang, J.J., Wong, T.Y., Saw, S.M.: Differential associations of myopia with major age-related eye diseases: the Singapore Indian Eye Study. Ophthalmol **20**(2), 284–291 (2013)
10. Subramanya, A., Bilmes, J.: Entropic graph regularization in non-parametric semi-supervised classification. In: NIPS (2009)
11. Foong, A.W.P., Saw, S.M., Loo, J.L., Shen, S., Loon, S.C., Rosman, M., Aung, T., Tan, D.T.H., Tai, E.S., Wong, T.Y.: Rationale and methodology for a population-based study of eye diseases in Malay people: the Singapore Malay eye study (SiMES). Ophthalmic Epidemiol. **14**(1), 25–35 (2007)
12. Cheng, J., Wong, D.W.K., Cheng, X., Liu, J., Tan, N.M., Bhargava, M., Cheung, C.M.G., Wong, T.Y.: Early age-related macular degeneration detection by focal biologically inspired feature. In: ICIP (2012)
13. Shen, S.Y., Wong, T.Y., Foster, P.J., Loo, J.L., Rosman, M., Loon, S.C., Wong, W.L., Saw, S.M., Aung, T.: The prevalence and types of glaucoma in malay people: the singapore malay eye study. Invest. Ophthalmol. Vis. Sci. **49**(9), 3846–3851 (2008)
14. Shapiro, L.G., Stockman, G.C.: Computer Vision. Prentice Hall, Englewood Cliffs (2003)
15. Qi, G., Hua, X., Rui, Y., Tang, J., Mei, T., Zhang, H.: Correlative multi-label video annotation. In: ACM Multimedia (2007)
16. Huang, J., Kumar, S., Mitra, M., Zhu, W.-J., Zabih, R.: Image indexing using color correlogram. In: IEEE Conference on Computer Vision and Pattern Recognition (1997)
17. Park, D.K., Jeon, Y.S., Won, C.S.: Efficient use of local edge histogram descriptor. In: ACM Multimedia (2000)
18. Wang, F., Zhang, C.: Label propagation through linear neighborhoods. In: ICML (2006)
19. Chen, G., Song, Y., Wang, F., Zhang, C.: Semi-supervised multi-label learning by solving a sylvester equation. In: SIAM International Conference on Data Mining (2008)
20. Chen, X., Mu, Y., Yan, S., Chua, T.-S.: Efficient large-scale image annotation by probabilistic collaborative multi-label propagation. In: ACM Multimedia (2010)
21. Wong, D.W.K., Liu, J., Cheng, X., Zhang, J., Yin, F., Bhargava, M., Cheung, C.M.G., Wong, T.Y.: THALIA - An automatic hierarchical analysis system to detect drusen lesion images for amd assessment. In: ISBI, pp. 884–887 (2013)

22. Manjunath, B.S., Ma, W.-Y.: Texture features for browsing and retrieval of image data. IEEE Trans. Pattern Anal. Mach. Intell. **18**(8), 837–842 (1996)
23. Lowe, D.: Distinctive image features from scale-invariant keypoints. Int J. Comput. Vis. **2**(60), 91–110 (2004)
24. Collobert, R., Sinz, F.H., Weston, J., Bottou, L.: Large scale transductive svms. J. Mach. Learn. Res. **7**, 1687–1712 (2006)
25. Duda, R., Stork, D., Hart, P.: Pattern Classification. Wiley, New York (2000)

Deeply Learning Deformable Facial Action Parts Model for Dynamic Expression Analysis

Mengyi Liu[1,2], Shaoxin Li[1,2], Shiguang Shan[1(✉)],
Ruiping Wang[1], and Xilin Chen[1,3]

[1] Key Laboratory of Intelligent Information Processing of Chinese Academy of
Sciences (CAS), Institute of Computing Technology, CAS, Beijing 100190, China
{sgshan,wangruiping,xlchen}@ict.ac.cn
[2] University of Chinese Academy of Sciences (UCAS), Beijing 100049, China
[3] Department of Computer Science and Engineering, University of Oulu,
Oulu, Finland
{mengyi.liu,shaoxin.li}@vipl.ict.ac.cn

Abstract. Expressions are facial activities invoked by sets of muscle
motions, which would give rise to large variations in appearance mainly
around facial parts. Therefore, for visual-based expression analysis, localizing the action parts and encoding them effectively become two essential
but challenging problems. To take them into account jointly for expression analysis, in this paper, we propose to adapt 3D Convolutional Neural
Networks (3D CNN) with deformable action parts constraints. Specifically, we incorporate a deformable parts learning component into the
3D CNN framework, which can detect specific facial action parts under
the structured spatial constraints, and obtain the discriminative part-
based representation simultaneously. The proposed method is evaluated
on two posed expression datasets, CK+, MMI, and a spontaneous dataset
FERA. We show that, besides achieving state-of-the-art expression recognition accuracy, our method also enjoys the intuitive appeal that the part
detection map can desirably encode the mid-level semantics of different
facial action parts.

1 Introduction

Facial expression analysis plays an important role in many computer vision applications, such as human-computer interaction and movie making. Many works
have been done in the literature [1,2], but it remains unsolved. One of the key
problems is how to represent different facial expressions. In the past decade, all
kinds of local features have been exploited for facial expression analysis. However,
making use of these hand-crafted local features might be essentially not good
(if not wrong), considering that these features are also successfully exploited by
face-based identity recognition methods. In principle, features for expression and
identity recognition should be somehow exclusive.

To step out the trap, instead of manually designing local features, data-driven
representation learning or deep learning is becoming popular more recently,

© Springer International Publishing Switzerland 2015
D. Cremers et al. (Eds.): ACCV 2014, Part IV, LNCS 9006, pp. 143–157, 2015.
DOI: 10.1007/978-3-319-16817-3_10

which emphasizes to hierarchically learn features that can be optimal to specific vision task. Among them, Convolutional Neural Network (CNN) [3] is one of the most successful ones for still image classification. Later on, it is further extended to 3D CNN [4] in order to deal with video-based action recognition problem. Our initial thought is applying CNN or 3D CNN directly to expression analysis, but we soon find it is even not better than hand-crafted features, e.g. HOG 3D [5] or LBP-TOP [6].

So, we realize that deep learning methods like CNN also need to be adapted to some new problems by incorporating the priors in the specific domain. In the case of expression analysis, studies in psychology have shown that expressions are invoked by a number of small muscles located around certain facial parts, e.g. eyes, nose, and mouth. These facial parts contain the most descriptive information for representing expressions. This observation brings us to the same spirit of the Deformable Part Model (DPM) [7], a state-of-the-art method in object detection. In DPM, an object is modeled by multiple parts in a deformable configuration and a bank of part filters can be simultaneously learned in a discriminative manner. The difference in our case is that the parts here are action parts, which dynamically change with the episode evolution of the expression.

With above ideas in mind, in this paper, we make an attempt to adapt 3D CNN for jointly localizing the action parts and learning part-based representations for expression analysis, by imposing the strong spatial structural constraints of the dynamic action parts. Fortunately, we found that the CNN framework has offered flexible structures to address the above problem: (1) CNNs have explicitly considered the spatial locality especially for 2D images or 3D videos, which can generate the underlying feature maps similar to HOG features used in DPM; (2) CNNs apply multiple trainable filters in each layer, which can be naturally incorporated with the deformation operations of part filters. Thus it is intuitive to embed such a deformation layer into the CNNs framework for learning these part locations as well as their representations.

To implement the above main ideas, i.e., achieve joint action part localization and part-based representation learning under CNN framework, we employ 3D CNN [4] as the basic model for its ability of motion encoding in multiple contiguous frames. Specifically, to adapt it for our goal, a bank of 3D facial part filters are designed and embedded in the middle layer of the networks (referring to Fig. 1), and the deformable action parts models are trained discriminatively under the supervision provided by class labels in the last layer. The deep networks increase the interactions among different learning components, thus we can obtain a globally optimized model.

2   Related Works

Many existing works on dynamic expression recognition attempt to encode the motion occurring in certain facial parts. One category of the methods is based on local spatio-temporal descriptors, e.g. LBP-TOP [6] and HOG3D [5]. The features extracted in local facial cuboid have possessed the property of repeatability, which makes it robust to the intra-class variation and face deformation.

However, such rigid cuboids can only capture low-level information that lacks of semantic meanings, and they can hardly represent the complex variations over those mid-level facial action parts. Another category of the methods attempt to encode the motion of facial action parts using a certain number of facial landmarks. For example, in [8,9], Active Appearance Model [10] and Constrained Local Model [11] are used to encode shape and texture variations respectively. However, it is difficult to achieve accurate landmarks (or action parts) detection under expression variations due to the large non-rigid deformation. In addition, all the methods mentioned above treat the feature learning separately without considering the final objective of classification, thus making the learned feature and model lacking of specificity and discriminative power.

Owing to the ability of organizing several functional components as cascaded layers into a unified network, the deep model is especially suitable for integrating the action parts detection, feature construction within the classifier learning procedure. For video-based classification tasks, 3D CNN [4] is shown to be one of the state-of-the-art models in action recognition field which considers the motion information encoded in multiple contiguous frames. However, except for the additional temporal convolutional operations, there is no structure designed specifically for locating or encoding semantic action parts, which makes it unsatisfactory for direct using in expression recognition task. Considering the structured property of human face, a DPM inspired deformable facial part model can also be learned for dynamic expression analysis. Meanwhile, [12] proposed to embed a deformation handling layer into the traditional 2D CNN for robust pedestrian detection. However, without consideration of temporal variations, this method cannot be directly applied to deal with video-based classification tasks.

To cope with the limitations in current works, in this paper we make two improvements: (1) We extend the traditional 2D deformable part model to 3D, which models dynamic motion in more complex videos rather than static appearance in simple still images. (2) We transform the binary detection model into multi-class classification model, and even continuous prediction model due to the regression capability of neural networks. Such adaptation enables us to accomplish expression intensity estimation and discrete expression recognition simultaneously.

3   Method

3.1   Overview

As mentioned above, our method is an adapted 3D CNN, which jointly takes into account two goals: localizing the facial action parts and learning part-based representations. Overall, our deep architecture is shown in Fig. 1. As can be seen, there are seven successive layers in our deep network:

Input video segments are n contiguous frames extracted from a certain expression video. The face in each frame is detected and normalized to the size of 64×64 pixels.

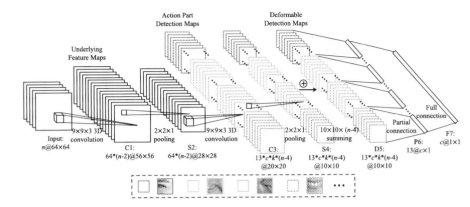

Fig. 1. An overview of the proposed deep architecture. The input n-frame video data is convolved with 64 **generic** 3D filters, and then mean-pooled to generate the underlying feature maps. Then the feature maps are convolved by $13 * c * k$ **specific** part filters to obtain the facial action part detection maps (where 13 is the number of manually defined facial parts, c is the number of classes, and k is the number of filters for one certain part in each class. The different colors represent the filter maps corresponding different parts). After the deformation maps weighting, the summed maps are processed by part-wise discriminative training to obtain the part-based estimation scores. Finally a full connection layer is used to predict the class label. **Best viewed in color** (Color figure online).

Underlying feature maps are obtained by convolving the input data using 64 spatio-temporal filters with the size of $9 \times 9 \times 3$. For translation invariance and dimension reduction, the filtered maps are then mean-pooled within non-overlapping $2 \times 2 \times 1$ spatial local region.

Action part detection maps are obtained by convolving the pooled underlying feature maps using a bank of class-specific 3D part filters. There are k filters for one certain part in each class to handle various manners of different people posing the same expression. Each detection map can be also regarded as response values of the whole face to a certain part filter. It is expected that the actual position of a detected action part arouses the largest response of the corresponding filter.

Deformable detection maps are obtained by summing up the part detection map and several deformation maps with learned weights. The deformation maps provide spatial constraints for detection maps according to the priors of facial configuration, which can fine-tune the detection scores and lead to a more reasonable result.

The partial connection layer concatenated to the deformable detection maps performs a part-wise discriminative learning for the part filters. As illustrated in Fig. 1, the different colors represent the detection maps corresponding to different facial action parts (We define 13 parts in this work). Totally 13 full connection structures are constructed for each part respectively for learning class-specific filters and outputs the part-based estimation scores. Finally we use a full connection layer to predict the expression label. The whole model is optimized globally with back-propagation.

3.2 3D Convolution

In 2D CNNs, convolutions are applied on 2D images or feature maps to encode only spatial information. When processing video data, it is desirable to consider the motion variation in temporal dimension, i.e. multiple contiguous image frames. In [4], the 3D convolution is achieved by convolving the 3D kernels/filters on the cube constructed by image frames. Generally, we use the central symmetric g_{ijm} with respect to f_{ijm} to give an element-level formulation:

$$V_{ij}^{xyz} = \sigma(\sum_{m}\sum_{p=0}^{P_i-1}\sum_{q=0}^{Q_i-1}\sum_{r=0}^{R_i-1} V_{(i-1)m}^{(x+p)(y+q)(z+r)} \cdot g_{ijm}^{pqr} + b_{ij}), \tag{1}$$

where V_{ij}^{xyz} is the value at position (x, y, z) on the j-th feature map in the i-th layer. P_i, Q_i, R_i are the sizes of the 3D filters (R_i is for temporal dimension, and g_{ijm}^{pqr} is the (p, q, r)-th value of the filter connected to the m-th feature map in the $(i-1)$-th layer). The function $\sigma(x) = max(0, x)$ is the nonlinear operation used in our model, named Rectified Linear Units (ReLU) [13]. Such non-saturating nonlinearity can significantly reduce the training time compared with those saturating functions, e.g. *sigmoid* and *tanh* [14]. Extending the $*$ operation from 2D to 3D, we also have a simplified version:

$$V_{ij} = \sigma(\sum_{m} V_{(i-1)m} * f_{ijm} + b_{ij}) \tag{2}$$

3.3 Deformable Facial Action Parts Model

Taking the same spirit of the Deformable Part Model (DPM) [7], in our task, the model of a face with N parts (we set $N = 13$ in this work, see Fig. 2) can be defined as a set of part models $(P_1, P_2, \ldots, P_N)$, where $P_l = (F_l, v_l, s_l, d_l)$.

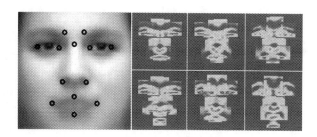

Fig. 2. The anchor positions of facial action parts (left) and illustration of the learned action parts filters for different expressions (right). For easy of visualization, we demonstrate the middle frame of the 3D filters. **Best viewed in color** (Color figure online).

Different from the original DPM, here $F_l = \{f_{[l,\theta]}|\theta = 1, 2, \ldots, c * k\}$ is a set of class-specific filters for detecting the l-th action parts of each expression respectively. v_l is a vector specifying the "anchor" positions for part l in the video, s_l is the size of the part detecting box, here the size is fixed by our 3D part filters in $C3$ layer, i.e. $9 \times 9 \times 3$. d_l is a weights vector of deformation maps specifying coefficients of a quadratic function defining deformation costs for possible placements of the part relative to the anchor.

Given the feature maps of a sample (i.e. the $S2$ layer), the l-th action part detection maps (i.e. the $C3$ layer) are obtained by convolving with a bank of part filters F_{3l} for response values. After the mean-pooling, the detection maps are summed with a set of weighted deformation maps to compute the deformable detection maps (i.e. the $D5$ layer). Note that here we process the operation for each 3D detection map separately corresponding to each single filter $f_{3[l,\theta]}$ in F_l. Formally, the scores on the map filtered by $f_{3[l,\theta]}$ in $D5$ layer is

$$D_{5[l,\theta]} = S_{4[l,\theta]} - d_l \cdot \phi_d(dx_l, dy_l, dz_l) + b,$$

$$S_{4[l,\theta]} = pool(C_{3[l,\theta]}), \tag{3}$$

$$C_{3[l,\theta]} = \sigma(\sum_m (S_{2m} * f_{3[l,\theta]m}) + b_{3[l,\theta]})),$$

where $[l, \theta]$ is the global index for the θ-th filter of the l-th part.

$$(dx_l, dy_l, dz_l) = (x_l, y_l, z_l) - v_l \tag{4}$$

gives the displacement of the l-th part relative to its anchor position, and

$$\phi_d(dx, dy, dz) = (dx, dy, dz, dx^2, dy^2, dz^2) \tag{5}$$

are deformation maps. Figure 3 shows an illustration of the deformable facial action part model. In general, the deformation cost is an arbitrary separable quadratic function of the displacements [7].

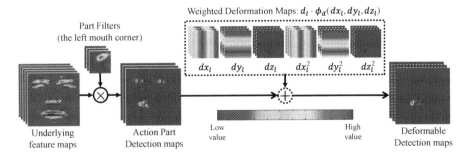

Fig. 3. An illustration of the deformable facial action part model. The part filters of left mouth corner may induce large response on the similar appearance position, e.g. eye corner. The spatial constraints provided by the deformation maps can effectively refine the detection maps. **Best viewed in color** (Color figure online).

In [12], only the maximum values of each deformable detection map are treated as the part scores for further prediction. However, in our multi-class recognition task, more diversified patterns are needed for describing each category particularly, rather than only tell "there is or not" in detection task. Therefore, the whole maps are retained for providing more information about the part filtered responses. Similar to [7,12], we conduct part-wise discriminative learning by partial connection to layer $P6$. Specifically, full connection structure are constructed for the maps of each part respectively and all the parameters in the part models (F_l, v_l, s_l, d_l) are optimized during the back-propagation.

4 Model Learning

4.1 Parameter Initialization

Training our deep model is a difficult task due to the millions of parameters. Therefore, we first initialize some important parameters and then update them all in the globally fine-tuning as in [15]. In this work, all the 3D convolution filters and the last two layers connection weights are chosen to be initialized.

Initialization of the filters. There are two kinds of filters in our model, i.e. the generic filters $\{f_{1m}\}$ and the specific part filters $\{f_{3[l,\theta]}\}$. Inspired by the work [16], we apply K-means clustering to learn centroids from the former feature maps and take them as the convolution filters. Specifically, we first learn 64 3D centroids from the input video, i.e. $\{f_{1m}\}$. Then we can obtain the $C1$ layer as

$$C_{1m} = \sigma(V_{input} * f_{1m} + b_{1m}). \tag{6}$$

The part filters $\{f_{3[l,\theta]}\}$ are learned from the pooled $S2$ layer. In the training set, we take the automatically detected $N = 13$ landmarks (as shown in Fig. 2, the initial anchor points are detected by SDM [17]) as the anchor positions of action parts, and sample the $9 \times 9 \times 3$ 3D cuboids around the anchors. The cuboids coming from the same position and same expression class are grouped up to learn k centroids, which are served as the class-specific part filters for layer $C3$. Totally there are $N * c * k$ filters in $\{f_{3[l,\theta]}\}$.

Initialization of the connection weights. After deformation handling layer $D5$, all the values of the same part, denoted as $D_{5[l,\cdot]}$, are fully connected to a subset of units in $P6$ layer, namely P_{6l}. We use W_{6l} to represent the connection weights corresponding to the l-th part, then

$$P_{6l} = \sigma(W_{6l}^T \, span(D_{5[l,\cdot]})). \tag{7}$$

where $span(\cdot)$ defines the operation of vectorization. Then the $P6$ is fully connected to $F7$:

$$F_7 = W_7^T P_{6[\cdot]}, \tag{8}$$

where $P_{6[\cdot]}$ represents the concatenated N part-based estimation scores, i.e. P_{6l}, in $P6$ layer. For initialization, we can directly use a linear transform for approximation. Therefore, the W_{6l} can be learned by a linear regression.

$$W_{6l} = Y^T span(D_{5[l,\cdot]})(span(D_{5[l,\cdot]})^T span(D_{5[l,\cdot]}) + \lambda I)^{-1} \tag{9}$$

where Y is the ground truth label matrix. Similarly, the W_7 can be learned as

$$W_7 = Y^T P_{6[\cdot]}(P_{6[\cdot]}^T P_{6[\cdot]} + \lambda I)^{-1} \tag{10}$$

4.2 Parameter Update

We update all the parameters after initialization by minimizing the loss function of square error

$$L(\mathcal{F}, \mathcal{D}, \mathcal{W}) = \frac{1}{2}||F_7 - Y||^2 = \frac{1}{2}e^2, \tag{11}$$

where $e = F_7 - Y$ is the error vector. $\mathcal{F} = \{F_1, \ldots, F_N\}$ and $\mathcal{D} = \{d_1, \ldots, d_N\}$ are part filters and weights vectors of deformation maps. $\mathcal{W} = \{\{W_{61}, \ldots, W_{6N}\}, W_7\}$ are connection matrices. The gradients of W_7 and P_{6l} can be computed by

$$\frac{\partial L}{\partial W_7} = P_{6[\cdot]}e^T, \tag{12}$$

$$\frac{\partial L}{\partial P_{6l}} = \frac{\partial L}{\partial P_{6[\cdot]}} \circ Mask_l = W_7\, e \circ Mask_l = \delta_{6l}, \tag{13}$$

where "$\circ$" represents element-wise multiplication and $Mask_1$ is a 0-1 vector to retain the connections only for the l-th part. For easy to express, we denote the gradient of P_{6l} as δ_{6l}. Then the gradients of W_{6l} and $D_{5[l,\cdot]}$ are

$$\frac{\partial L}{\partial W_{6l}} = span(D_{5[l,\cdot]})\delta_{6l}^T \circ I(P_{6l} > 0), \tag{14}$$

$$\frac{\partial L}{\partial D_{5[l,\cdot]}} = W_{6l}\delta_{6l} \circ I(P_{6l} > 0), \tag{15}$$

where $I(\cdot)$ is an index function to compute the derivative of ReLU. Given the gradient of $D_{5[l,\cdot]}$, we can obtain the the gradient of $D_{5[l,\theta]}$ at the same time by a simple reshape operation. The weights of deformation maps d_l can be updated according to its gradient

$$\frac{\partial L}{\partial d_l[t]} = \sum_\theta \frac{\partial L}{\partial D_{5[l,\theta]}} \circ \phi_d[t], \tag{16}$$

where $d_l[t]$ is the t-th component of the weights vector d_l and $\phi_d[t]$ is the t-th component of the deformation maps. Note that the $\partial L/\partial D_{5[l,\theta]}$ and $\phi_d[t]$ are both 3D feature maps. According to Eq. (3), we also have

$$\frac{\partial L}{\partial S_{4[l,\theta]}} = \frac{\partial L}{\partial D_{5[l,\theta]}} = \delta_{4[l,\theta]}, \tag{17}$$

then the gradient of $f_{3[l,\theta]}$ can be calculated as

$$\frac{\partial L}{\partial f_{3[l,\theta]}} = \delta_{4[l,\theta]} \frac{\partial S_{4[l,\theta]}}{\partial C_{3[l,\theta]}} \frac{\partial C_{3[l,\theta]}}{\partial f_{3[l,\theta]}}$$

$$= \sum_m S_{2m} * (up(\delta_{4[l,\theta]}) \circ I(C_{3[l,\theta]} > 0)). \tag{18}$$

where $up(\cdot)$ is the up-sampling using the same definition in [18].
The gradient of the first convolutional layer f_{1m} can be calculated with the chain rule in the same way as $f_{3[l,\theta]}$. When obtain all the gradient, we can update the parameters using the stochastic gradient descent as in [15]. Take W_7 for example, the update rule of of W_7 in the k-th iteration is

$$\Delta^{k+1} = \alpha \cdot \Delta^k - \beta \cdot \epsilon \cdot W_7^k - \epsilon \cdot \frac{\partial L}{\partial W_7^k}, \tag{19}$$

$$W_7^{k+1} = \Delta^{k+1} + W_7^k, \tag{20}$$

where Δ is the momentum variable [19], ϵ is the learning rate and α, β are tunable parameters. In the training process, the learning rate is set as a fixed value 0.01.

5   Experiments

We evaluate our model on two posed expression datasets, CK+ [8], MMI [20], and a spontaneous dataset FERA [21] in four aspects: (1) visualization of the deformable part detection maps; (2) the loss of training/test sets before and after parameter updating; (3) qualitative results of expression intensity prediction; (4) quantitative results of average expression recognition rate and overall classification accuracy.

5.1   Data

CK+ database contains 593 videos of 123 different subjects, which is an extended version of CK database [22]. All of the image sequences vary in duration from 10 to 60 frames and start from the neutral face to the peak expression. Among these videos, 327 sequences from 118 subjects are annotated with the seven basic emotions (i.e. Anger (An), Contempt (Co), Disgust (Di), Fear (Fe), Happy (Ha), Sadness (Sa), and Surprise (Su)) according to FACS [23].

MMI database includes 30 subjects of both sexes and ages from 19 to 62. In the database, 213 image sequences have been labeled with 6 basic expressions, in which 205 are with frontal face. Different from CK+, the sequences in MMI cover the complete expression process from the onset apex, and to offset. In general, MMI is considered to be more challenging for the subjects usually wear some accessories (e.g. glasses, mustaches), and there are also large inter-personal variations when performing the same expression. The number of samples for each expression in CK+ and MMI are illustrated in Table 1.

FERA database is a fraction of the GEMEP corpus [24] that has been put together to meet the criteria for a challenge on facial AUs and emotion recognition. As the labels on test set are unreleased, we only use the training set for evaluation (Table 2). The training set includes 7 subjects, and 155 sequences have been labeled with 5 expression categories: Anger (An), Fear (Fe), Joy (Jo),

Table 1. The number of samples for each expression in CK+ and MMI database.

Expression	An	Co	Di	Fe	Ha	Sa	Su
CK+	45	18	59	25	69	28	83
MMI	31	–	32	28	42	32	40

Table 2. The number of samples for each expression in FERA database.

Expression	An	Fe	Jo	Sa	Re
FERA	32	31	30	31	31

Sadness (Sa), and Relief (Re). FERA is more challenging than CK+ and MMI because the expressions are spontaneous in natural environment.

We adopt the strictly person-independent protocols on both two databases for evaluation. In detail, experiments are performed based on 15-fold cross validation in CK+ and 20-fold cross validation in MMI, exactly the same as that in [25] for fair comparison. For FERA, as the labels on test set are unreleased, we adopt leave-one-subject-out cross-validation on the training set.

5.2   Evaluation of the Model

The deep model requires equal size of image cube, i.e. n frames as shown in Fig. 1. Given a T-frame video, we can pick up $T - n + 1$ cubes as the input data. For training samples, according to the expression varying manner in a sequence, we assign soft label values to the $T - n + 1$ training sample, i.e. video segments, using a gaussian function. For test samples, there is no need to know the ground truth of expression frames. After obtaining the $T - n + 1$ predict label vector, an aggregation strategy proposed in [26] is employed to generate the final recognition result of the whole video.

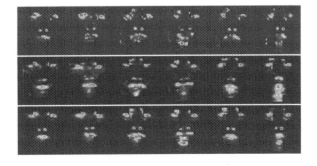

Fig. 4. Part detection maps of different part filters for different expressions. (We show the responses of all parts in one image by averaging the detection maps in the middle frame). **Best viewed in color** (Color figure online).

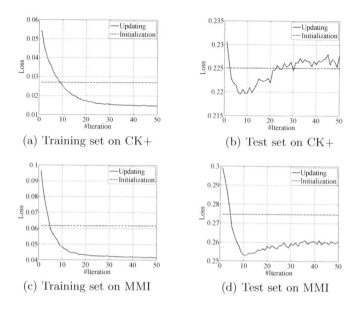

(a) Training set on CK+

(b) Test set on CK+

(c) Training set on MMI

(d) Test set on MMI

Fig. 5. The loss of training and test sets on CK+ and MMI database.

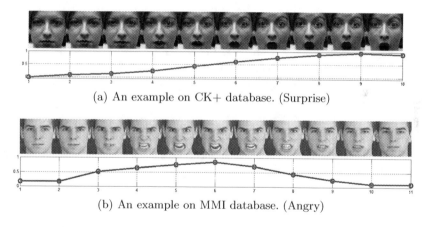

(a) An example on CK+ database. (Surprise)

(b) An example on MMI database. (Angry)

Fig. 6. The expression intensity prediction results for two test sequences. The predicted scores are all for a video segments. For easy to visualization, we demonstrate the middle frame of each video segment to show the temporal variations of the expression.

After training the deep model, the part based representation can be obtained in $D5$ layer, i.e. the deformable detection maps. Each map is composed of the response values of a certain part filter, which depict various appearance patterns of different expressions. In Fig. 4, we provide a visualization of some selected deformable part detection maps learned by our model.

Moreover, to evaluate the learning ability of our deep model, we demonstrate the loss (defined in Eq. 11) of training/test set before and after parameter updating in Fig. 5. As for validation purpose only, we conduct such experiments on one fold of CK+ and MMI respectively. In each figure, the blue curve is the loss of model using the initialized parameters for comparison. The red curve is the loss during the parameter updating, which shows a consistently decreasing trend on the training sets of both databases. However, it is easy to witness overfitting at a small number of iterations on the test sets, especially on CK+.

Our model can also provide the expression intensity prediction due to the regression ability of the neural networks. As presented in Sect. 5.1, a T-frame test sequence can generate $T - n + 1$ sub-segments for equal length inputs. Thus we can obtain $T - n + 1$ predict values for describing the changing of intensity during the whole expression process. We show some typical results of the intensity prediction along with the image/video data in Fig. 6.

5.3   Comparisons with Related Works

We compare our method, denoted by 3DCNN-DAP (Deformable Action Parts), with other related works under the same protocols adopted in [25]. Both average recognition rate and overall classification accuracy are measured. The results are listed in Tables 3 and 4 for CK+, Tables 5 and 6 for MMI, Tables 7 and 8 for FERA.

Specifically, to evaluate the most relevant work, the 3D CNN [4] fairly, we also conduct a similar parameter initialization using the same number of filters in each convolutional layer and a linear regression in the last full connection layer. The significant improvement shows that our deformable action part learning component has great advantages on task-specific feature representation.

Table 3. The average expression recognition rates on CK+ database.

Method	An	Co	Di	Fe	Ha	Sa	Su	Average
CLM [9]	70.1	52.4	92.5	72.1	94.2	45.9	93.6	74.4
AAM [8]	75.0	**84.4**	94.7	65.2	**100**	68.0	96.0	83.3
HMM [25]	–	–	–	–	–	–	–	83.5
ITBN [25]	**91.1**	78.6	94.0	83.3	89.8	76.0	91.3	86.3
HOG3D [5]	84.4	77.8	94.9	68.0	**100**	75.0	**98.8**	85.6
LBP-TOP [6]	82.2	77.8	91.5	72.0	98.6	57.1	97.6	82.4
3DCNN [4]	77.8	61.1	**96.6**	60.0	95.7	57.1	97.6	78.0
3DCNN-DAP	**91.1**	66.7	**96.6**	80.0	98.6	**85.7**	96.4	**87.9**

Table 4. The overall classification accuracy on CK+ database.

Method	CLM	AAM	ITBN	HOG3D	LBP-TOP	3DCNN	**3DCNN-DAP**
Accuracy	82.3	88.3	88.8	90.8	88.1	85.9	**92.4**

Table 5. The average expression recognition rates on MMI database.

Method	An	Di	Fe	Ha	Sa	Su	Average
HMM [25]	–	–	–	–	–	–	51.5
ITBN [25]	46.9	54.8	**57.1**	71.4	**65.6**	**62.5**	59.7
HOG3D [5]	61.3	53.1	39.3	78.6	43.8	55.0	55.2
LBP-TOP [6]	58.1	56.3	53.6	78.6	46.9	50.0	57.2
3DCNN [4]	58.1	21.9	25.0	83.3	53.1	**62.5**	50.7
3DCNN-DAP	**64.5**	**62.5**	50.0	**85.7**	53.1	57.5	**62.2**

Table 6. The overall classification accuracy on MMI database.

Method	ITBN	HOG3D	LBP-TOP	3DCNN	**3DCNN-DAP**
Accuracy	60.5	56.6	58.1	53.2	**63.4**

Table 7. The average expression recognition rates on FERA database.

Method	An	Fe	Jo	Sa	Re	Average
HOG3D [5]	43.8	33.3	74.2	54.8	48.4	50.9
LBP-TOP [6]	59.4	40.0	35.5	61.3	61.2	51.5
3DCNN [4]	34.4	26.7	64.5	51.6	54.8	46.4
3DCNN-DAP	50.0	58.1	73.3	51.6	48.4	**56.3**

Table 8. The overall classification accuracy on FERA database.

Method	HOG3D	LBP-TOP	3DCNN	**3DCNN-DAP**
Accuracy	51.0	51.6	46.5	**56.1**

6   Conclusions

In this paper, by borrowing the spirits of Deformable Part Models, we adapt 3D CNN to deeply learn the deformable facial action part model for dynamic expression analysis. Specifically, we incorporate a deformable parts learning component into the 3D CNN framework to detect special facial action parts under the structured spatial constraints, and obtain the deformable part detection maps to serve as the part-based representation for expression recognition. Such a deep model makes it possible to jointly localize the facial action parts and learn part-based representation. Impressive results beating the state-of-the-art are achieved on two challenging datasets.

To put it in another perspective, we have actually extended the deformable static part models to deformable dynamic part models under the CNN framework, which might also be validated by video-based event or behavior analysis.

In the future work, we will also try to consider more complex patterns of the action parts, e.g., of different sizes and shapes, or even with different time durations, to generate more flexible description of the facial expressions.

Acknowledgement. The work is partially supported by Natural Science Foundation of China under contracts nos. 61379083, 61272321, 61272319, and the FiDiPro program of Tekes.

References

1. Pantic, M., Rothkrantz, L.: Automatic analysis of facial expressions: the state of the art. IEEE T PAMI **22**, 1424–1445 (2000)
2. Zeng, Z., Pantic, M., Roisman, G., Huang, T.: A survey of affect recognition methods: audio, visual, and spontaneous expressions. IEEE T PAMI **31**, 39–58 (2009)
3. LeCun, Y., Bottou, L., Bengio, Y., Haffner, P.: Gradient-based learning applied to document recognition. Proc. IEEE **86**, 2278–2324 (1998)
4. Ji, S., Xu, W., Yang, M., Yu, K.: 3D convolutional neural networks for human action recognition. IEEE T PAMI **35**, 221–231 (2013)
5. Klaser, A., Marszalek, M.: A spatio-temporal descriptor based on 3D-gradients. In: BMVC (2008)
6. Zhao, G., Pietikainen, M.: Dynamic texture recognition using local binary patterns with an application to facial expressions. IEEE T PAMI **29**, 915–928 (2007)
7. Felzenszwalb, P., Girshick, R., McAllester, D., Ramanan, D.: Object detection with discriminatively trained part-based models. IEEE T PAMI **32**, 1627–1645 (2010)
8. Lucey, P., Cohn, J., Kanade, T., Saragih, J., Ambadar, Z., Matthews, I.: The extended cohn-kanade dataset (ck+): a complete dataset for action unit and emotion-specified expression. In: CVPRW (2010)
9. Chew, S., Lucey, P., Lucey, S., Saragih, J., Cohn, J., et al.: Person-independent facial expression detection using constrained local models. In: FG (2011)
10. Cootes, T., Edwards, G., Taylor, C., et al.: Active appearance models. IEEE T PAMI **23**, 681–685 (2001)
11. Cristinacce, D., Cootes, T.F.: Feature detection and tracking with constrained local models. In: BMVC (2006)
12. Ouyang, W., Wang, X.: Joint deep learning for pedestrian detection. In: ICCV (2013)
13. Nair, V., Hinton, G.: Rectified linear units improve restricted boltzmann machines. In: ICML (2010)
14. Krizhevsky, A., Sutskever, I., Hinton, G.: Imagenet classification with deep convolutional neural networks. In: NIPS (2012)
15. Zhu, Z., Luo, P., Wang, X., Tang, X.: Deep learning identity preserving face space. In: ICCV (2013)
16. Coates, A., Ng, A., Lee, H.: An analysis of single-layer networks in unsupervised feature learning. In: ICAIS (2011)
17. Xiong, X., De la Torre, F.: Supervised descent method and its applications to face alignment. In: CVPR (2013)
18. Bouvrie, J.: Notes on convolutional neural networks (2006)
19. Qian, N.: On the momentum term in gradient descent learning algorithms. Neural Netw. **12**, 145–151 (1999)

20. Valstar, M., Pantic, M.: Induced disgust, happiness and surprise: an addition to the MMI facial expression database. In: LRECW (2010)
21. Valstar, M.F., Mehu, M., Jiang, B., Pantic, M., Scherer, K.: Meta-analysis of the first facial expression recognition challenge. IEEE TSMCB **42**, 966–979 (2012)
22. Kanade, T., Cohn, J., Tian, Y.: Comprehensive database for facial expression analysis. In: FG (2000)
23. Ekman, P., Friesen, W.: Facial Action Coding System: A Technique for the Measurement of Facial Movement. Consulting Psychologists Press, Palo Alto (1978)
24. Bänziger, T., Scherer, K.R.: Introducing the geneva multimodal emotion portrayal (GEMEP) corpus. In: Scherer, K.R., Bänziger, T., Roesch, E.B. (eds.) Blueprint for Affective Computing: A Sourcebook, pp. 271–294. Oxford university Press, Oxford (2010)
25. Wang, Z., Wang, S., Ji, Q.: Capturing complex spatio-temporal relations among facial muscles for facial expression recognition. In: CVPR (2013)
26. Kanou, S., Pal, C., Bouthillier, X., Froumenty, P., Gülçehre, Ç., Memisevic, R., Vincent, P., Courville, A., Bengio, Y., Ferrari, R., et al.: Combining modality specific deep neural networks for emotion recognition in video. In: ICMI (2013)

A Novel Context-Aware Topic Model for Category Discovery in Natural Scenes

Zehuan Yuan and Tong Lu$^{(\boxtimes)}$

National Key Lab for Novel Software Technology, Nanjing University,
Nanjing, China
lutong@nju.edu.cn

Abstract. Automatic category discovery from images is a challenging problem in computer vision community especially from natural scene images due to the great variability in them. This paper proposes a novel context-aware topic model for category discovery in complex natural scenes. The proposed model constructs a generative probabilistic procedure from three-level features consisting of patch, region and the entire image by introducing latent topic variables to every patch and every region. Additionally, a new kind of scene context prior, namely, the spatial preference of categories, is also modeled using only a few parameters to reduce the ambiguity of categories in scene images. By regarding "topics" as "categories", category discovery is thus converted to the inference of the proposed probabilistic model, which will further be addressed under a Gibbs-EM framework effectively. Experimental results on two benchmark datasets comprising MSRC-v2 and SIFT Flow show its effectiveness and the advantages comparing with other methods.

1 Introduction

Unsupervised visual category discovery has been a research hot spot in computer vision community in the past decades due to its potential uses in automated visual content summarization, scene structure mining and automatic image labeling. Its ultimate target is to recognize visually similar categories and segment out their various instances by directly mining an unlabeled image set. Indeed, many efforts [1–14] have been made to achieve this goal. Roughly, for visual category discovery, most of them use either probabilistic graphical models or any clustering method to group image patterns such as patches and regions that have similar appearance and simultaneously co-occur in images. Although these methods obtain good results in particular datasets like MSRC-v2 [15], they still face a lot of challenges especially for complex natural scene images which more likely have much variability in their appearances.

Topic model (e.g., Latent Dirichlet Allocation (LDA) [16]) is a kind of generative probabilistic graphical model. These models are popular in unsupervised category discovery due to the strength of *Bag of Words* representation for an image when regarding topics as categories. As known, topic models are appearance-based and ignore any extra priors like the spatial compactness of objects. Unfortunately, the main challenges of category discovery for the images captured from

© Springer International Publishing Switzerland 2015
D. Cremers et al. (Eds.): ACCV 2014, Part IV, LNCS 9006, pp. 158–171, 2015.
DOI: 10.1007/978-3-319-16817-3_11

one natural scene generally include diversified shotting environments and complex image configurations due to occlusion, viewpoint variations and so on. Thus on one hand, scene context priors like the spatial preference of any category or category concurrence are necessary to be included to mitigate negative effects of photometry like weak illumination, shade or reflectance, and the large intra-class variability. For example, [17] introduces a context-aware topic model (CA-TM) to facilitate category discovery in natural scenes by including the spatial preference of each category. However, the learning of the prior of spatial preferences is separated from category discovery itself in their model. On the other hand, the features of different levels theoretically need to be integrated to extend a single level representation (sparse patches) in the traditional topic model since sparse patches are essentially insufficient to discriminate different topics. For example, besides image patches, [3] first introduces region features to reduce the ambiguity and enforce the spatial coherence of topic assignments.

In this paper, after integrating the image-level GIST feature [18] into category discovery, we bring forward a novel context-aware topic model named NCA-TM, which not only makes full use of multi-level representation of images from small patches to the entire image, but also succeeds in integrating the spatial preference of categories based on the conclusion that the GIST feature of an image can predict the location and the scale of instances of any category effectively [19]. Note that we model the prior explicitly in our graphical model by a few parameters instead of learning many global maps via complex steps as in [17]. NCA-TM assigns every region or patch a latent topic label and then derive each observation (e.g., features of patches, regions and images). In this way, category discovery is converted to the inference of NCA-TM and Gibbs-EM [20] is adopted to address it.

Our main contributions of this paper include:

1. We put forward a novel context-aware topic model by integrating multi-level image features, and
2. Spatial preference of categories is characterized in a more flexible way for assisting category discovery from complex natural scene images. The experimental results on two benchmark datasets consisting of MSRC-v2 and SIFT Flow [21] show the effectiveness of the proposed model.

The rest of the paper is organized as follows. Section 2 discusses the related work. In Sect. 3 we give our multi-level image representation. Section 4 shows the details of the proposed generative model for category discovery, and its inference is discussed in Sect. 5. Experimental results and discussions are given in Sect. 6, and finally Sect. 7 concludes the method.

2 Related Work

Currently, many techniques have been exploited in unsupervised category discovery. Roughly, these methods can be categorized into two classes: generative probabilistic models and clustering-based methods. The former searches for repeated patterns from a large number of unlabeled images using the variants of topic models [1–8], while the latter groups features or image regions with similar appearance through clustering methods [9–13]. Tuytelaars et al. [14] gives a systematic introduction and comparative study to the earlier methods.

Generative Probabilistic Model. Most generative methods are extensions to a topic model. Among these methods, the most typical one is Latent Dirichlet Allocation (LDA) [1], which regards image segments as documents and categories in images as topics for object discovery. Since the traditional LDA ignores the spatial compactness of words in images, [2,3,7] extend it by including spatial compactness priors. Besides, [6] uses extra information of correspondences between features to improve the results. Recently, [5] adds the mutual correlation between topics and scene spatial context to facilitate visual modeling. However, scene context priors have to be learned in advance in their methods.

Clustering-Based Methods. These methods are different from each other mainly on the strategies they considered to construct the similarity measurement between features or regions. For example, [11] uses link analysis on an appearance-similarity network between features and then constructs a structure-similarity matrix between features. As a result, the problem is reduced to spectral clustering to classify features belonging to the same object into the same group. Recently, [12] puts forward object-graphs to model regions, in which the regions of similar appearance and surrounding context are clustered together to form a object. They extend it to make the system automatic by searching for easy objects first and then hard objects gradually [13]. However, these methods are relatively limited to the ability to either image segmentation or features integration of different levels to compare regions. More details can be found in [14].

Additionally, there are methods [22–24] that unify category discovery and other applications simultaneously. For example, [17] considers scene labels to category discovery in order to perform scene classification. Rubinstein et al. [25] integrates unsupervised object discovery and image-cosegmentation under an MRF framework to co-segment co-occurring foreground objects. However, it only segments out instances of a single foreground object. Besides, [26] models unsupervised object class discovery under an multi-instance learning framework based on saliency detection. However, they only search for object classes rather than any categories in our model. Although [27] models any categories, they focus more on co-segmentation rather than constructing appearance model of each category explicitly.

3   Image Description

In our method, we represent each natural scene image I_d through three levels (See Fig. 1), namely, patch, region and image level features. Specifically, on the first level, we sample image patches P_d over the image densely and describe their appearances using SIFT. Then visual word w_{dp} is adopted to approximate the

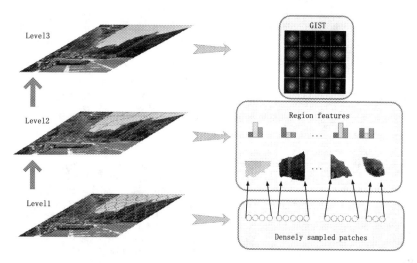

Fig. 1. Three-level image representation for an image. The first level are the features of dense image patches. The middle level corresponds to regions features and the top level has only one GIST feature of this image.

appearance of p_d by assigning it to the nearest word in the visual vocabulary pre-obtained by vector quantization of all the patch features. Simultaneously, we oversegment I_d into plenty of regions R_d to form the second level with each region r_d corresponding to a homogeneous area. Alike, we assign r_d with a visual word v_{dr} from an off-line region appearance codebook according to its feature. In addition, l_{dr} is used to represent the location of r_d corresponding to its center. There is only one image-level GIST g_d feature on the third level. To further remove redundancy, we perform PCA on traditional GIST features. Note that as the level goes up, the features pay more attention to entirety and by the contrary, more details are included into the features at the bottom level. The goal to construct the multi-level representation is to model the spatial compactness of each topic and its consistency to the spatial preference of categories in the scene.

4   The Proposed Generative Model

After the three-level representation of any image is generated, we further construct a generative probabilistic model (NCA-TM) to derive these observations. Like LDA, we regard each scene image as a document and categories in images as "topics". Topic proportions of images are represented by θ and for an image I_d, we need firstly sample its topic proportion $\theta_d \sim \mathrm{Dir}(\alpha)$ which governs the likelihood of each topic appearing in I_d. Thus topic labels of patches and regions are generated based on θ_d and finally all the observations of its three-level representation. To make all the parameters and the variables clear for understanding, we list all the notations in Table 1. The overall generative process is summarized in Table 2.

Table 1. Important notations in our model

Notations	Descriptions
$d = \{1, \cdots, |I|\}$	the index of all images I
$dr = \{1, \cdots, |R_d|\}$	the index of regions in R_d
$dp = \{1, \cdots, |P_d|\}$	the index of patches in P_d
$dt = \{1, \cdots, T\}$	the index of topics in t_d
$v_{dr} = \{1, \cdots, V\}$	the visual word of dr
$w_{dp} = \{1, \cdots, W\}$	the visual word of dp
$F_d = \mu_{dt}, s_{dt} | \forall dt \in t_d$	all attributes in d
μ_{dt}	the center of the topic t in d
s_{dt}	the scale of the topic t in d
l_{dr}	the region center of dr
g_d	the GIST features reduced by PCA
Latent variables	Description
$t_{dr} = \{1, \cdots, T\}$	the topic label of dr
$t_{dp} = \{1, \cdots, T\}$	the topic label of dp
$\theta_d \in [0, 1]^T$	the topic proportion of d
$\Psi \in \mathbf{R}^{T \times |V|}, \Phi \in \mathbf{R}^{T \times |W|}$	the probability of each word in each topic
Parameters	Description
Ω	the parameters of $P(g_d | F_d)$
Hyperparameters	Descriptions
α, β, γ	control the prior of $P(\theta|\alpha), P(\Phi|\beta)$ and $P(\Psi|\gamma)$ respectively

Table 2. The generative process of our generative model

(1) For each topic t, sample $\Phi_t \sim \mathrm{Dir}(\beta)$ and $\Psi_t \sim \mathrm{Dir}(\gamma)$,

(2) For each image I_d, sample its topic proportion $\theta_d \sim \mathrm{Dir}(\alpha)$ firstly,

(3) For each region $R_r \in I_d$, sample $t_{dr} \sim \mathrm{Multi}(\theta_d)$ and then sample $v_{dr} \sim \mathrm{Multi}(\Psi_{t_{dr}})$,

(4) For each patch $P_p \in R_r$, sample its visual word $w_{dp} \sim \mathrm{Multi}(\Phi_{t_{dr}})$,

(5) Given all sampled t_d, sample $g_d \sim P(g_d | F_d(t_d, l_d))$.

Generating the First Two-Level Features. Visual words of patches and regions can be treated as words in topic models. In another word, each visual word is derived from one unique latent topic and thus they are conditionally independent. However, since any region in the second level manifests a consistent appearance within it, we enforce the patches in one region to share the same topic as the region similar to [3]. Note that the proportion of different words in any topic is particular and stable, we model them as Φ and Ψ for patch words and region words, respectively. For each topic t, Φ_t is generated from a prior Dirichlet distribution $\Phi_t \sim Dir(\beta)$. Likewise, $\Psi_t \sim Dir(\gamma)$. Thus given a region r, we first select its topic t_{dr} via a multinomial distribution $t_{dr} \sim \mathrm{Multi}(\theta_d)$. Then its visual word v_r is sampled from $v_r \sim \mathrm{Multi}(\Phi_{t_{dr}})$. Simultaneously, the visual words of all the image patches in r are drawn from $\mathrm{Multi}(\Psi_{t_{dr}})$ one by one. Since we do not know any location priors of each topic and thus we assume $P(l_{dr}|t_{dr})$ is uniform.

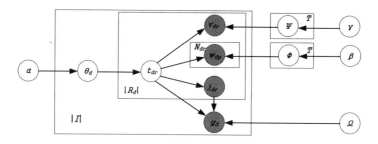

Fig. 2. The proposed graphical model.

Generating the Third-Level Features. As a kind of image level feature, GIST is representative for image characteristics such as the occurrence, location and scale of a single topic and spatial layout among topics. Note that these abstract attributes of topics in one image is also fixed after topic labels are sampled for all regions on the second layer. Thereby, we define $P(g_d | l_d, t_d) \equiv P(g_d | F_d)$ for any image I_d. F_d is a series of attribute functions $\{f^c(T_d, R_d, P_d), c = 1, \cdots, |F|\}$ where T_d is a collection of all t_{dr}. In order to simplify the modeling, we use only independent attributes for each topic: location μ and scale s. When we concatenate the two attributes of all topics together, $F_d = \{\mu_{dt}, s_{dt} | \forall t \in T_d\}$. Thus we sample g_d from $P(g_d | F_d)$. If we assume $P(F_d)$ is uniform, $P(g_d | F_d) \propto P(F_d, g_d)$. Assume that μ and s are conditionally independent, the generative process can be defined by

$$P(g_d | F_d) \propto P(F_d, g_d) = \prod_{t \in t_d} P(\mu_{dt}, g_d) P(s_{dt}, g_d) \tag{1}$$

We adopt the simple generalized linear model to formulate $P(s, g)$ and $P(\mu, g)$ rather than more complex mixtures of Gaussians in [19]:

$$P(\mu_{dt}, g_d) = G(\mu_{dt}; b_t^0 + \boldsymbol{b_t}^T g_d, \sigma 1_t^2) \tag{2}$$

$$P(s_{dt}, g_d) = G(s_{dt}; q_t^0 + \boldsymbol{q_t}^T g_d, \sigma 2_t^2) \tag{3}$$

where $\Omega = \{b_t^0, q_t^0, \sigma 1_t^2, \sigma 2_t^2, \boldsymbol{b_t}, \boldsymbol{q_t} | \forall t \in T\}$ are model parameters to learn.

Overall, the graphical model of our context-aware generative model is shown in Fig. 2. Given corresponding parameters, the joint distribution of all the variables can be obtained by

$$P(\boldsymbol{w}, \boldsymbol{v}, \boldsymbol{l}, \boldsymbol{g}, \boldsymbol{t}) = \int_\theta \int_{\Phi, \Psi} \prod_k P(\Psi_k | \gamma) P(\Phi_k | \beta) \prod_d^{|I|} P(\theta_d | \alpha) \prod_r^{|R|} P(t_{dr} | \theta_d) P(v_{dr} | \Psi_{t_{dr}})$$

$$P(l_{dr} | t_{dr}) \prod_{p \in r} P(w_{dp} | \Phi_{t_{dr}}) P(g_d | F(\boldsymbol{t_d}, \boldsymbol{l_d})) d\theta d\Psi d\Phi \tag{4}$$

5   Model Learning and Inference

The goal of category discovery corresponds to the inference of the graphical model, namely, maximizing the posterior distribution of latent variables given all observations $P(t|w, l, g, v; \Omega, \alpha, \beta, \gamma)$. Different from the traditional topic model, we also need to estimate the parameters Ω during the inference. Thereby, we adopt a Gibbs EM algorithm [20] to the model inference and parameter learning. The main difference between our method and the typical EM is that Gibbs EM uses Gibbs sampling to estimate the posterior distribution in the E-step. Likewise, the E-step and M-step are interleaved and process iteratively into convergence.

E-step: In the E-step, by integrating out θ, Φ and Ψ, t_{dr} can be sampled from a Gibbs sampling procedure. The distribution of t_{dr} conditioned on t_{-dr} is

$$P(t_{dr} = k|t_{-dr}, w, v, l, g; \Omega, \alpha, \beta, \gamma) \propto (n_{d,(\cdot)}^{k,-dr} + \alpha_k) \frac{n_{(\cdot),v_{dr}}^{k,-dr} + \beta_v}{\sum_{c=1}^{V} n_{(\cdot),c}^{k,-dr} + \beta_c}$$

$$\prod_{w_{dp}, p \in R_{dr}}^{W} \frac{A_{m_{w_{dp},k}^{(\cdot)} + \gamma w_{dp} - 1}^{m_{w_{dp},(\cdot)}^{dr}}}{A_{m_{(\cdot),k}^{(\cdot)} + \gamma - 1}^{m_{(\cdot),(\cdot)}^{dr}}} P(g_d|t_d, l_d; \Omega)$$

$$(5)$$

where $m_{w,k}^r$ denotes the number of patches in the region r with the visual word w and the topic label k. $n_{d,v}^{k,-r}$ represents the number of regions in the image d with the visual word v and their topic labels equal to k except the region r. If any dimension is not limited to some specific value, we use to $(\cdot)$ to replace it. A is the P-permutation operator.

M-step: In the M-step, we need to estimate Ω based on sampled t in the E-step. Firstly, for each topic t appearing in any image I_d, μ_{dt} are calculated following $\mu_{dt} = \frac{1}{N_{dt}} \sum_{t_{dr}=t} l_{dr}$ and alike, $s_{dt} = \frac{1}{N_{dt}} \sum_{t_{dr}=t} (l_{dr} - \mu_{dt})^2$. N_{dt} is the number of regions in I_d with their topic labels equal to t. As [19] validated, GIST feature is not sensitive to horizontal locations of topics. Thus we only calculate the two attributes along the vertical direction. When all u_{dt} and s_{dt} are calculated, the corresponding parameters Ω can be obtained by

$$B = (U^T U) U^T G \qquad Q = (S^T S) S^T G$$
$$\Sigma 1 = (U - GB^T)^T (U - GB^T)$$
$$\Sigma 2 = (S - GQ^T)^T (S - GQ^T)$$

$$(6)$$

where U and S are two $|D| \times T$ matrices with each element corresponding to u_{dt} and s_{dt}, respectively. G is a matrix with each row corresponding to g_d. $B, Q, \Sigma 1$ and $\Sigma 2$ are model parameters with each row representing $b, q, \sigma 1$ and $\sigma 2^2$ of each t, respectively. Experimental results show the simple generalized linear model also functions well to model the spatial preference of categories.

Simultaneously, after the Gibbs EM framework are converged, we can also get the characteristic visual word distributions Ψ and Φ. Since Ψ and Φ are conditionally independent on the samples of t, the evaluation of Ψ and Φ are not correlated. Thus they can be estimated as in the traditional LDA

$$\Phi_k^w = \frac{m_{w,k}^{(\cdot)} + \beta}{m_{(\cdot),k}^{(\cdot)} + W\beta} \quad \Psi_k^v = \frac{n_{(\cdot),v}^{k,(\cdot)} + \gamma}{n_{(\cdot),(\cdot)}^{k,(\cdot)} + V\gamma} \tag{7}$$

6 Experiments

6.1 Datasets

We evaluated our methods on two datasets: MSRC-v2 and SIFT Flow. MSRC-v2 dataset has altogether 21-categories (591 images). The SIFT Flow dataset includes images from 8 natural scene classes with 2688 images (256×256) and 33 categories in all the images totally. SIFT Flow is selected following two considerations: (1) all the images are captured in natural scenes with relatively stable context in each scene, and (2) all the images have pixel-level ground-truth labels. Note that all the images in MSRC-v2 are also resized into 256×256.

6.2 Experimental Settings

In order to generate three-level representation for an image, we first sample 12×12 patches densely in the image with step 3 pixels and then extract their SIFT features. These features are then vector quantized to form a codebook of size 500 using K-means. SLIC [28] is used to generate homogeneous regions for each image with the initial region-size 30 and then for each region, we extract its texture feature with 40 dimensions using the same filter bank as [12] and its 3-dimension color. Likewise, a region color codebook of size 20 and a texture codebook of size 200 are obtained by clustering all region color features and texture features, respectively. Additionally, for the third level GIST feature, we apply PCA to reduce the typical GIST feature of 512 dimensions to 64 to prevent overfitting of our selected generalized linear model. As to hyperparameters, we set $\alpha = 50/T, \beta = 200/W$ and $\gamma = 200/V$.

6.3 Evaluation Metrics

As [12] also states, it is difficult to ensure what each topic corresponds to. In another word, it may represent either an semantic category or a part of any category such as the window of any building. Thus without semantic information, it is difficult to evaluate it in the same way as image segmentation or labeling with supervised assistance, especially for the practical case that we don't know the topic number in advance. Thereby, we adopt the *purity* score to measure the coherence of topic assignments to pixels. Note that a higher *purity* score indicates that topic assignments are more consistent with ground-truth labels.

6.4   Evaluation and Results

Without smoothing topic assignments, several example raw results for MSRC-v2 and SIFT Flow are shown in Figs. 3 and 4, respectively. We find that most of the categories in the images are distinguished from each other despite some noise, which can be removed in any practical application. Note that windows are labelled as a different topic from that of buildings since there indeed exists semantic gap. Since the best topic number is not known to us and thus we report *purity* scores with different topic numbers. We find in Fig. 5 that for the two datasets, as the topic number arise, the performance become better and get the best performance within the interval $[1, 1.5] \times N$ where N is the ground-truth category number. Besides, it is not beneficial to our model that the topic number is too large.

In order to validate the effectiveness of modeling GIST and its implying scene context in NCA-TM, we conduct comparative study with our modified version (a), and the spatial LDA method [2] (b) on MSRC-v2 and SIFT Flow. In (a), we delete the variable g and related edges. Essentially, (a) is unsupervised spatial-LTM [3] because $P(l|z)$ is uniform in our model. Spatial LDA (b) only adds the prior that the patches of the same topic should be close and no any scene context prior is included. From Fig. 5, we can see our modeling of GIST has two different impacts for MSRC-v2 and SIFT Flow. Our model is inferior compared to (a) and (b) in MSRC-v2 and gets the best performance in SIFT Flow by the contrary. It is observed that for most of images in MSRC-v2, instances of the foreground categories are likely to locate in the center. Thus there are less stable context reflected by GIST since GIST indicates locations and scales of categories by the environment around them [19]. However, the images in SIFT Flow are from natural scenes with stable scene context (See Fig. 4 for image examples). Thereby, including GIST in the dataset like MSRC-v2 to category discovery has little improvement or even inferior performance. According to the comparison, we conclude that our modeling of GIST in NCA-TM is effective and necessary for natural scenes.

Simultaneously, we further compare the method (c) in [17] to show our modeling of GIST is more flexible and effective than their global location maps. Note that the method is intended to scene classification and it is an extension of DISC-LDA [24] to include global contexts and semantic labels. Thus we only simplify it by replacing DISC-LDA by spatial-LTM and the modeling of their global context does not change. The comparative results are shown in Fig. 5 and we find in SIFT Flow, our performance is superior to (c) obviously. The results further validate the intuition that GIST is effective and flexible to model scene contexts and category discovery in natural scenes can benefit from our model.

The modeling of the category spatial preference prior into category discovery is indeed explored earlier. However, our model moves forward by considering them as specific cases of our NCA-TM. Thereby, the proposed model is essentially a more generalized framework:

1. If we remove GIST features, namely the node of g and the related nodes of parameters in the graphical model, the model will be reduced to [7] where

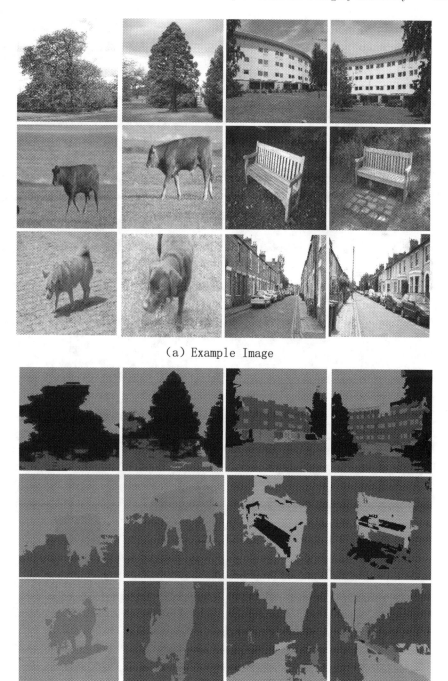

(a) Example Image

(b) category discovery results

Fig. 3. Example category results of MSRC-v2. Different colors in category discovery results represent different topics (Color figure online).

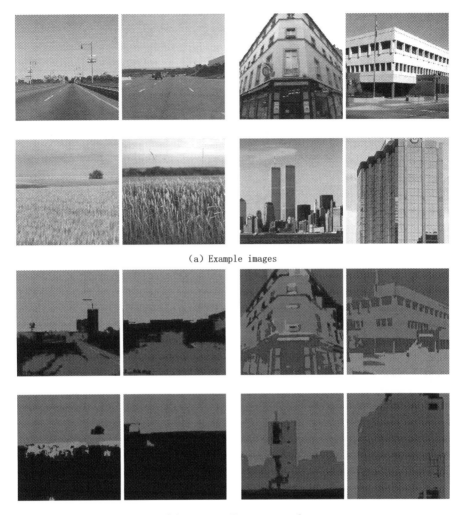

(a) Example images

(b) Category discovery results

Fig. 4. Category results of 4 scenes in SIFT Flow with two examples for each scene. Different from the experiments on MSRC-v2, we perform NCA-TM on 8 scenes respectively rather than all scene images together. Different colors also represent different topics. However, colors of different scene examples are independent (Color figure online).

they use Gaussian to model $P(l_d|t_d)$ rather than our uniform assumption. Thereby, their model can only enforce the same topic to the patches that are spatially compact.

2. If we replace GIST features with many global location maps of topics, namely cutting the image-related relation between t_d and g_d, the model will be similar to [17] for scene recognition. As known, global location map of categories is unstable and does not make use of valuable image-specific information.

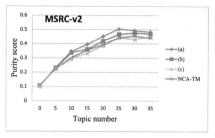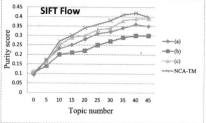

Fig. 5. Purity scores of MSRC-v2 and SIFT-Flow at different topic numbers.

Therefore, our model is a generalization to the existing models to use scene context prior and the spatial preference of categories for category discovery in natural scene images. Experimental results show our model outperforms these models especially in natural scene images.

To conclude, our model succeeds in modeling the scene context prior, the spatial preference of categories, and integrate multi-level features in a flexible and effective way and it is better for category discovery in natural scene images.

7 Conclusion

In this paper, we propose a novel context-aware topic model to make use of multi-level features and scene context priors to facilitate category discovery in natural scenes by a flexible and effective way. The model constructs a generative probabilistic procedure for all the three-level features by regarding "topics" as "categories". Category discovery corresponds to the inference of the model, which is addressed under the Gibss-EM framework. Experimental results show its effectiveness and the advantage in natural scenes. For future work, we will focus on modeling more complex and accessible scene contexts into category discovery in natural scenes.

Acknowledgement. The work described in this paper was supported by the Natural Science Foundation of China under Grant No. 61272218 and No. 61321491, the 973 Program of China under Grant No. 2010CB327903, and the Program for New Century Excellent Talents under NCET-11-0232.

References

1. Russell, B.C., Freeman, W.T., Efros, A.A., Sivic, J., Zisserman, A.: Using multiple segmentations to discover objects and their extent in image collections. In: CVPR, vol. 2, pp. 1605–1614 (2006)
2. Wang, X., Grimson, E.: Spatial latent dirichlet allocation. In: NIPS (2007)
3. Cao, L., Li, F.F.: Spatially coherent latent topic model for concurrent segmentation and classification of objects and scenes. In: ICCV, pp. 1–8 (2007)

4. Zhao, B., Fei-Fei, L., Xing, E.P.: Image segmentation with topic random field. In: Daniilidis, K., Maragos, P., Paragios, N. (eds.) ECCV 2010, Part V. LNCS, vol. 6315, pp. 785–798. Springer, Heidelberg (2010)

5. Lin, D., Xiao, J.: Characterizing layouts of outdoor scenes using spatial topic processes. In: ICCV, pp. 841–848 (2013)

6. Liu, D., Chen, T.: Unsupervised image categorization and object localization using topic models and correspondences between images. In: ICCV, pp. 1–7 (2007)

7. Liu, D., Chen, T.: Semantic-shift for unsupervised object detection. In: CVPR (2006)

8. Fergus, R., Li, F.F., Perona, P., Zisserman, A.: Learning object categories from internet image searches. Proc. IEEE **98**, 1453–1466 (2010)

9. Lee, Y.J., Grauman, K.: Shape discovery from unlabeled image collections. In: CVPR, pp. 2254–2261 (2009)

10. Lee, Y.J., Grauman, K.: Foreground focus: unsupervised learning from partially matching images. Int. J. Comput. Vis. **85**, 143–166 (2009)

11. Kim, G., Faloutsos, C., Hebert, M.: Unsupervised modeling of object categories using link analysis techniques. In: CVPR (2008)

12. Lee, Y.J., Grauman, K.: Object-graphs for context-aware visual category discovery. IEEE Trans. Pattern Anal. Mach. Intell. **34**, 346–358 (2012)

13. Lee, Y.J., Grauman, K.: Learning the easy things first: self-paced visual category discovery. In: CVPR, pp. 1721–1728 (2011)

14. Tuytelaars, T., Lampert, C.H., Blaschko, M.B., Buntine, W.L.: Unsupervised object discovery: a comparison. Int. J. Comput. Vis. **88**, 284–302 (2010)

15. Shotton, J., Winn, J.M., Rother, C., Criminisi, A.: Textonboost for image understanding: multi-class object recognition and segmentation by jointly modeling texture, layout, and context. Int. J. Comput. Vis. **81**, 2–23 (2009)

16. Blei, D.M., Ng, A.Y., Jordan, M.I.: Latent dirichlet allocation. J. Mach. Learn. Res. **3**, 993–1022 (2003)

17. Niu, Z., Hua, G., Gao, X., Tian, Q.: Context aware topic model for scene recognition. In: CVPR, pp. 2743–2750 (2012)

18. Oliva, A., Torralba, A.: Modeling the shape of the scene: a holistic representation of the spatial envelope. Int. J. Comput. Vis. **42**, 145–175 (2001)

19. Torralba, A.: Contextual priming for object detection. Int. J. Comput. Vis. **53**, 169–191 (2003)

20. Andrieu, C., de Freitas, N., Doucet, A., Jordan, M.I.: An introduction to mcmc for machine learning. Mach. Learn. **50**, 5–43 (2003)

21. Tighe, J., Lazebnik, S.: Superparsing - scalable nonparametric image parsing with superpixels. Int. J. Comput. Vis. **101**, 329–349 (2013)

22. Su, H., Sun, M., Li, F.F., Savarese, S.: Learning a dense multi-view representation for detection, viewpoint classification and synthesis of object categories. In: ICCV, pp. 213–220 (2009)

23. Li, L.J., Socher, R., Li, F.F.: Towards total scene understanding: classification, annotation and segmentation in an automatic framework. In: CVPR, pp. 2036–2043 (2009)

24. Niu, Z., Hua, G., Gao, X., Tian, Q.: Spatial-disclda for visual recognition. In: CVPR, pp. 1769–1776 (2011)

25. Rubinstein, M., Joulin, A., Kopf, J., Liu, C.: Unsupervised joint object discovery and segmentation in internet images. In: CVPR, pp. 1939–1946 (2013)

26. Zhu, J.Y., Wu, J., Wei, Y., Chang, E.I.C., Tu, Z.: Unsupervised object class discovery via saliency-guided multiple class learning. In: CVPR, pp. 3218–3225 (2012)

27. Yuan, Z., Lu, T., Shivakumara, P.: A novel topic-level random walk framework for scene image co-segmentation. In: Fleet, D., Pajdla, T., Schiele, B., Tuytelaars, T. (eds.) ECCV 2014, Part I. LNCS, vol. 8689, pp. 695–709. Springer, Heidelberg (2014)
28. Achanta, R., Shaji, A., Smith, K., Lucchi, A., Fua, P., Süsstrunk, S.: Slic superpixels compared to state-of-the-art superpixel methods. IEEE Trans. Pattern Anal. Mach. Intell. **34**, 2274–2282 (2012)

Robust Sharpness Metrics Using Reorganized DCT Coefficients for Auto-Focus Application

Zheng Zhang[(✉)], Yu Liu, Xin Tan, and Maojun Zhang

College of Information System and Management, National University of Defense Technology, Changsha 410073, Hunan, People's Republic of China
zhangzheng.ntu@gmail.com

Abstract. We present two new metrics for measuring sharpness of an image. Both methods exploit a reorganized Discrete Cosine Transform (DCT) representation and analyze the reorganized coefficients to use the most useful components for sharpness measuring. Our first metric utilizes optimal high and middle frequency coefficients for relative sharpness evaluation. It is well suitable for focus measure as it is super sensitive to the best-focus position and could predict stable and accurate focus values for various subjects and scenes with different lighting and noise conditions. Experiments demonstrate that it has high discrimination power even for high noisy and low-contrast images. The second metric constructs energy maps for each scale of reorganized DCT coefficients, and determines absolute sharpness/blurriness using the local maxima energy information. Compared with most existing no-reference sharpness/blurriness metrics, this metric is very efficient in sharpness measurement for images with different contents, and can be used in real-time auto-focus application. Experiments show that it correlates well with perceived sharpness.

1 Introduction

The perceptions of sharpness and blurriness are closely related to the details and clarity of an image. Most often they are used as antonyms since sharpness is inversely proportional to blurriness. For sharpness or blurriness measurement, subjective method that relies on human observations is accurate but has limited use for imaging applications. By contrast, objective metric which automatically assesses the degree of sharpness/blurriness is important for many applications of image processing and computer vision. One important application of sharpness measurement is for contrast-based auto-focus. In contrast-based auto-focus, a measure of focus is detected from each image acquired at different lens positions, and is used for adjusting the camera lens to locate the in-focus position by finding the maximum focus measure. Focus measure is normally defined in terms of sharpness, which is computed by a sharpness metric. Because the maximum focus measure corresponds to the best focused position, the sharpness metric largely determines focusing accuracy. Other important applications of sharpness measurement include image quality assessment, image enhancement and restoration, for all of which the sharpness evaluation may play critical roles in the design and optimization of the relevant algorithms.

© Springer International Publishing Switzerland 2015
D. Cremers et al. (Eds.): ACCV 2014, Part IV, LNCS 9006, pp. 172–187, 2015.
DOI: 10.1007/978-3-319-16817-3_12

The accurate evaluation of image sharpness is a difficult problem because sharpness is affected by many factors such as the image content, illumination, noise and spatial activity [1,2]. Our motivation of developing new sharpness metrics is twofold. Firstly, we are interested in accurate and robust relative sharpness measures. A relative sharpness metric is designed to predict sharpness of images that have the same content but may fail for different images. It is often used as a focus measure for auto-focus systems where the relative largest sharpness point determines the best-focus position. For actual autofocusing, the subjects being focused vary across scenes, being static or dynamic, having strong or poor contrast, with different illumination conditions that may cause serious noisy distortion and poor image quality. Although various relative sharpness metrics for focus measurement have been proposed [3–10], seldom methods are reported to be suitable for autofocusing in different scenes under severe illumination conditions. We are motivated to design a new relative sharpness metric that is robust to noise, illuminations, scene movements and low-contrast image contents. Secondly, we are also interested in evaluating an absolute value of sharpness for an given image. An absolute sharpness measure means its evaluation is not relative to a reference image, *i.e.*, it is a no-reference sharpness measure. It can discriminate the degree of sharpness among images that have different contents. Existing no-reference sharpness metrics are oriented to estimate extra parameters [1,2,11–13], and tend to have high computation complexity. These methods may produce accurate estimations but may not be suitable for situations where limited computation resource is available and real-time performance is needed. For our purpose, we desire a simple and efficient absolute sharpness metric which would be used combined with the relative sharpness metric for efficient autofocusing.

In this work, we first propose a robust DCT-based relative sharpness metric, where we exploit reorganized DCT coefficients to select the most suitable components that have high effect on sharpness measure. A nice property of our metric is that it has high discrimination power even for high noisy and low-contrast images.It is very suitable for focus measure as it is super sensitive to the best-focus position and could predict stable and accurate focus values for various subjects and scenes with different lighting and noise conditions. We also present an efficient DCT-based absolute sharpness metric. This metric exploits the same framework of the reorganized DCT representation. It correlates well with perceived sharpness and is efficient in sharpness measurement for images with different contents. We demonstrate the performance of our metrics by comparing them against several most commonly used metrics both on public Gaussian blur images of the LIVE dataset [14] and the captured out-of-focus sequences.

2   Related Work

Many sharpness metrics are developed mainly for the application of auto-focus, where these metrics are used to give a relative evaluation of sharpness for measuring focus. Because an auto-focus system generally requires real-time performance for various scenes under different illumination conditions, these relative sharpness metrics are required to be robust and efficient. Existing spatial-domain relative sharpness metrics [3,4,15] often determine sharpness by exploiting edge, gray scale, histogram or correlation information, while frequency-domain methods [6–9,16,17] first transform image to a frequency domain using the fast Fourier transform (FFT) [18], DCT [6–9] or discrete wavelet transform (DWT) [16,17], and then compute sharpness with the high or middle frequency components of the transformed data. Generally, spatial-domain sharpness measures are relative computational efficiency, but mostly sensitive to noise [19,20]. This would cause many local maxima in focus curve especially for scenes under low illumination conditions, making it difficult for autofocusing to find the best focused position. Frequency-domain methods usually require more computational cost as they need an extra frequency transform step. Because they calculate sharpness based on selecting of desired high or middle frequency coefficients, they are relatively insensitive to noise [5,20].

Besides these relative sharpness metrics, there are also many no-reference metrics that are designed for absolute sharpness evaluation. In theory, an absolute sharpness metric can give an absolute evaluation of image sharpness regardless of the image contents. One typical way is to exploit the information of edges [21–23]. The method of [21] first detects edges of an image and then evaluate the blurriness based on the edge widths. The work [22] presents two blurriness metrics that are based on an analysis of the edges and adjacent regions in an image. In [23], the authors present the notion of just noticeable blur (JNB) and integrate it into a probability summation model. The work [24] improves the method of [12] by incorporating a visual attention model. Similarly, [23] also uses the concept of JNB and combines it with the cumulative probability of detecting blur at an edge. There are also spatial algorithms that do not rely on measuring the spread of edges. For example, the method of [25] utilizes eigenvalues of an image to evaluate sharpness.

Various frequency methods are also proposed for absolute sharpness/ blurriness estimation. The work [26] computes sharpness using the average 2D kurtosis of the 8×8 DCT blocks. The work [11] presents a blurriness metric that is based on histogram computation of non-zero DCT coefficients. The method [27] uses Harr wavelet transform for sharpness analysis. In [28], a sharpness metric that uses both frequency contents and spatial features in one framework in order to avoid the pitfalls of alternative methods. The work [2] also utilizes both spectral and spatial features of an image, where the magnitude spectrum and the total spatial variation is measured for sharpness evaluation.

3   The Proposed Relative Sharpness Metric

We propose a relative sharpness metric that is designed for sharpness evaluation of images having similar scenes. This metric is suitable for auto-focus application where the primary requirement is to evaluate the relative sharpnesses of a sequence images of the same scene being focused. Our method is in the DCT domain. Compared with other transform algorithms such as FFT or DWT, DCT has an important advantage is that DCT can be computed efficiently by using optimized DCT-specific platforms [29, 30] and fast computation algorithms [31]. Another advantage is many video encoding algorithms are based on block-based DCT data [32, 33]. This allows us to exploit the already available DCT coefficients and may reach sharpness metrics of high efficiency.

3.1   A Reorganized DCT Representation

DCT is an algorithm that transforms image data of spatial-domain into frequency-domain. Let $f(x, y)$ denotes the spatial pixel value at (x, y) of an image with size $M \times N$, $F(i, j)$ denotes the corresponding DCT frequency components, the mapping between $f(x, y)$ and $F(i, j)$ is:

$$F(i, j) = \sum_{(x, y)} f(x, y) C_{ij}(x, y; M, N) \tag{1}$$

where C_{ij} are orthogonal 2D basis functions, defined as

$$C_{ij} = c_i(x; M) c_j(y; N) \tag{2}$$

where

$$c_\varphi(z; A) = \alpha(\varphi; A) cos(\frac{\pi \varphi (2z + 1)}{2A}) \tag{3}$$

$$\alpha(\varphi; A) = \begin{cases} \frac{1}{\sqrt{A}} & \text{if } \varphi = 0; \\ \sqrt{\frac{2}{A}} & \text{otherwise.} \end{cases} \tag{4}$$

For sharpness measure, we are interested in using 8×8 DCT which carries the transform on 8×8 pixel blocks. Several efficient algorithms and hardware implementation solutions exist for this block based DCT [6]. The operation of 8×8 DCT would result in a series of 64 coefficients $\{F(i, j) | i = 0, 1, \cdots, 7, j = 0, 1, \cdots, 7\}$, where $F(0, 0)$ is the DC coefficient, and the others are AC coefficients. Each of these coefficients represents a particular spatial frequency.

A typical image is consisted of a set of smooth regions delimited by edge discontinuities. After applied block-based DCT operation, the image energy of smooth regions is compacted into the DC coefficientstogether with a few high-frequency AC coefficients, while the energy of edges is compacted into a small number of high-frequency AC coefficients [33, 34]. This energy compaction property of DCT allows us to select a set of high-frequency components that are related to the edges in spatial domain for measuring sharpness. We exploit a reorganization strategy of DCT coefficients [32, 34] for finding the most suitable components that have high effect on focus measure. In this reorganization, each 8×8 block is taken as a three scale tree of coefficients with 10 subbands decomposition, as shown in Fig. 1(a). After that, the coefficients of the same subbands for all blocks are grouped together and put onto their corresponding positions (Fig. 1(b)). Figure 1(c) shows an example of the reorganization representation of one image. It is seen that this form of reorganization of block-based DCT

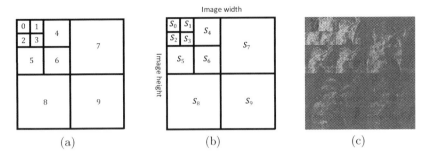

Fig. 1. Reorganization strategy of DCT coefficients. (a) Each 8×8 block is taken as three-scale tree with ten-subband decomposition; (b) The reorganization representation for an image where coefficients of the same subbands for all 8×8 blocks are grouped together and put onto their corresponding positions; (c) reorganization result of Lena image;

Table 1. Energy ratios of each coefficient to the total four coefficients in each subband of Lena image. Each ratio is computed using energy of the corresponding coefficients collected from all blocks.

Subband 4	$F(0,2)$	$F(0,3)$	$F(1,2)$	$F(1,3)$
	0.5348	0.1576	0.2070	0.1006
Subband 5	$F(2,0)$	$F(2,1)$	$F(3,0)$	$F(3,1)$
	0.4706	0.3001	0.1159	0.1159
Subband 6	$F(2,2)$	$F(2,3)$	$F(3,2)$	$F(3,3)$
	0.4806	0.2355	0.1674	0.1165

coefficients has structural similar characteristics to the three-scale multiresolution decomposition of discrete wavelet transform [35]. For example, the DCT subbands S_7, S_8 and S_9 correspond to the level-1 HL, LH and HH subbands of DWT separately.

3.2   The Metric

Our sharpness measures exploit the structural similarities between the subbands of multi-scale DWT and the reorganized subbands of block-based DCT. For three-level DWT data, low frequency components increase with the level of subbands, where the subbands of level-1 and level-2 are dominated by high and middle frequency coefficients. Since the subbands $\{S_i | i = 7, 8, 9\}$ and $\{S_i | i = 4, 5, 6\}$ of reorganized DCT correspond to the level-1 and level-2 subbands of DWT respectively, it is reasonable to calculate the sharpness using the components in these DCT subbands regions.

To select the optimum coefficient components that have high discrimination power, we analyze and compare the different effects of using middle and high frequencies on measuring sharpness. According to the structural similarities

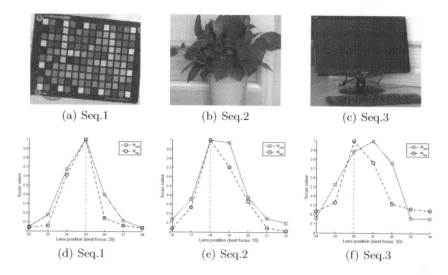

Fig. 2. Comparison of middle-frequency and high-frequency based sharpness measure. Above: best-focus images of three sequences taken with different subjects; Below: sharpness or focus values of few neighbor positions around the best focused position are shown.

between reorganized DCT and DWT coefficients, we select middle frequencies from subbands (4, 5, 6) and high frequencies from subbands (7, 8, 9) for each 8×8 DCT block. Taking signal power of all coefficients in the corresponding subbands to measure sharpness is one possible way, but it would certainly need high computational cost. Since the histograms of corresponding coefficients collected from all blocks shows that the signal energy is usually concentrated in the lower frequency bands [36], we use the coefficients centralized in upper left corner of each subband. Table 1 gives the energy ratios of each coefficient to all coefficients in the corresponding subbands of Lena image. These ratios are computed using all block data. It is seen that about half of the energy associated with subbands 4, 5 and 6 is taken up by the corresponding upper left coefficients. Hence, we choose the three upper left corner coefficients for the case of middle frequency based metric, i.e., $F(0,2)$ of subband 4, $F(2,0)$ of subband 5 and $F(2,2)$ of subband 6. We define the middle-frequency sharpness metric of single block as follows:

$$M_{mid} = |F(0,2)|^2 + |F(2,0)|^2 + |F(2,2)|^2 \tag{5}$$

The high frequency based metric is defined in a similar way. In the three scale tree decomposition (Fig. 1(a)), each coefficient of subbands 4, 5, and 6 is associated with four children in subbands 7, 8 and 9 respectively. For instance, coefficients $F(0,4)$, $F(0,5)$, $F(1,4)$ and $F(1,5)$ are the four children of the parent coefficient $F(0,2)$. It can be found that much of the energy of subbands 7, 8, and 9 is also concentrated in the corresponding four children. We define the high

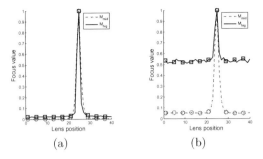

(a)   (b)

Fig. 3. Sharpness measures on the synthetic noisy image sequence. (a–b) the focus curves on Seq.1 without (a) and with white Gaussian noise (b); Note that each point of the focus curves is normalized by the corresponding maximum sharpness.

frequency metric as follows:

$$M_{hig} = \sum_{i=0}^{1}\sum_{j=4}^{5}|F(i,j)|^2 + \sum_{i=4}^{5}\sum_{j=0}^{1}|F(i,j)|^2 + \sum_{i=4}^{5}\sum_{j=4}^{5}|F(i,j)|^2 \qquad (6)$$

Figure 2 gives the focus curves of the two measures on three sequences. The average sharpness of all blocks are taken into account for focus evaluation. It is seen that both measures have a peak at the best focused position, but M_{hig} gives sharper focus curves. For Seq.3 only M_{hig} gives sharpest value at the correct focus position. These figures indicate that M_{hig} is more sensitive to best focused position. Figure 3 plots focus curves of the two measures for the images with and without noise added, where the synthetic noisy image is generated by adding Gaussian noise with standard deviation 20 to Seq.1. We can see that though both measures produce maxima values at the best focused position, M_{mid} shows more robust performance as its focus curve is less effected by noise, while M_{hig} has smaller dynamic sharpness range around the peak. We may conclude that using high frequencies for focus measuring, *e.g.*, M_{hig}, would have higher discrimination power as they are more sensitive to the best-focus position, but may be effected by noise. On the contrast, the middle frequency based measures like M_{mid} shows very strong robustness of anti-noise but may lack of discriminativity in ambiguous cases. Our proposed relative sharpness metric M_{reodct} combines both middle and high frequencies in a linear form defined as follows:

$$M_{reodct} = \lambda M_{mid} + M_{hig}^* \qquad (7)$$

where λ is a factor that balances the effect of both measures M_{mid} and M_{hig}^*. M_{hig}^* is a variant of M_{hig} and is defined as:

$$\begin{aligned} M_{hig}^* = &|F(0,4)|^2 + |F(0,5)|^2 + |F(1,4)|^2 \\ &+ |F(4,0)|^2 + |F(4,1)|^2 + |F(5,0)|^2 \\ &+ |F(4,4)|^2 + |F(4,5)|^2 + |F(5,4)|^2 \end{aligned} \qquad (8)$$

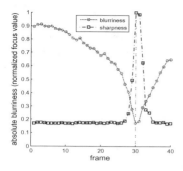

Fig. 4. Blurriness and focus value curves of one sample sequence.

where three coefficient components, *i.e.*, $F(1,5)$, $F(5,1)$ and $F(5,5)$ are removed from the part of M_{hig}. We find this in addition to being less computation consuming but almost reduces no performance of the measure.

3.3   Sharpness Detection Ability (SDA) Measure

A good sharpness measure should decrease with an increasing blurring. Higher measure difference between the consecutive values indicates stronger discrimination ability. Let M_t denotes the normalized focus measure of image frame t, σ_t is the corresponding Gaussian blur standard deviation. Give measures on frames $t = 1, \cdots, T$, we define a new metric named Sharpness Detection Ability measure (SDA) to quantify the sharpness functions. SDA is defined as a psychometric function [37] which can be modeled as follows:

$$SDA = \frac{1}{T} \sum_{t=1}^{T} 1 - exp\left(- \left| \frac{M_{t+1} - M_t}{\sigma_{t+1} - \sigma_t} \right|^{\frac{1}{\sigma_{t+1}}} \right) \tag{9}$$

SDA is designed to produce higher value on larger sharpness differences with smaller blur deviation between consecutive images. This means it is a good indicator of sensitivity to best focus. Additionally, if the consecutive sharpness measure differences change inverse proportionally with the corresponding deviation differences, the metric would produce larger value which indicates better sharpness discrimination power.

4   The Proposed Absolute Sharpness Metric

4.1   Our Motivation

One problem of the initialization stage in autofocusing is to set the size of focusing-step properly. A smaller focusing-step size should be used when the starting image is sharper, and a larger step should be used when the image is blurred. This requires to know the absolute sharpness or blurriness of the starting image.

Another problem is to decide which direction to move the focus motor. Searching in a wrong direction would causes slow focusing which is a bad visual experience. Since the arbitrary starting position may be severely blurred or very close to best-focus position, it is difficult to successfully judge the direction efficiently for all cases.

Figure 4 shows blurriness (i.e., the absolute sharpness) and focus value curves for one focusing sequence. It is seen that the absolute sharpness curve monotonously decreases with the increase of focus value, showing high discriminative power in distinguishing blurriness even in the area where the focus value curve is very flat. This motivates us to exploit both absolute sharpness and focus value (i.e., the relative sharpness) for solving the aforementioned problems. Using the relative sharpness measures of autofocusing to decide the absolute blurriness of image would meet problems. This is because that they are highly dependent on image content, and they provide relative sharpness values that are meaningful only for an entire focusing sequence captured at the same scene. Most existing absolute sharpness/blurriness estimation algorithms [11,12,27] are proposed for image quality assessment. They are not suitable for our task due to their high computational complexity.

4.2   The Algorithm

This algorithm is inspired by the work [27] that uses Harr wavelet transform (HWT) for blur detection. In this work, image edges are classified into four types: Dirac-Structure, Astep-Structure, Gstep-Structure, and Roof-Structure. When blur happens both Dirac-Structure and Astep-Structure edges will disappear, and Gstep-Structure as well as Roof-Structure tend to lose their sharpness. The algorithm performs edge detection by finding the local maxima on three-scale HWT of the image, and counts the numbers of each edge type according to a set of rules. As a result, the blur degree is calculated using the ratio of the number of Roof-Structure and Gstep-Structure edges that lost their sharpness to the total number of Roof-Structure and Gstep-Structure edges.

The above blur detection method works effectively for out-of-focus or linear motion blur. However, the use of HWT that consumes much extra computational resources would not be suitable for the auto-focus application where the main processing is in the DCT domain. Moreover, we find that the algorithm is fairly sensitive to noise. In our method, blur estimation is performed in the DCT domain where we exploit the reorganized DCT representation described in Sect. 3.1. An energy map for each level i of the three-level ($i = 1, 2, 3$) DCT coefficients is firstly constructed as follows:

$$E_i(k, l) = \sqrt{\left(S_{i1}(k, l)\right)^2 + \left(S_{i2}(k, l)\right)^2} \qquad (10)$$

where $\{S_{ij} | j = 1, 2, 3\}$ with $S_{ij} = S_{(3-i) \times 3 + j}$ denote the subbands associated with the level i decomposition in the reorganized DCT representation, as illustrated in Fig. 1(b). In Eq. 10, the coefficients of subbands S_3, S_6, S_9 are neglected

---

Algorithm 1. Absolute sharpness or blurriness estimation using the reorganized block DCT

---

(1). Compute 8×8 DCT of the image of interest, construct energy maps E_i using Eq. 10 for each scale of DCT coefficients in the reorganized representation.

(2). Find the local maxima of each block for every energy map to obtain three edge maps EM_i.

(3). Set $N_{rg} \leftarrow 0$, $N_{blur} \leftarrow 0$; **for** *every point* (k, l) **do**

> **if** $EM_1(k, l) \geq T_1 || EM_2(k, l) \geq T_1 || EM_3(k, l) \geq T_1$ **then**
>> **if** $EM_1(k, l) \leq EM_2(k, l) \leq EM_3(k, l) ||$
>> $EM_2(k, l) \geq EM_1(k, l) \&\& EM_2(k, l) \geq EM_3(k, l)$ **then**
>>> $N_{rg} \leftarrow N_{rg} + 1$;
>>> **if** $EM_2(k, l) \leq T_2$ **then**
>>>> $N_{blur} \leftarrow N_{blur} + 1$;

(4). Compute blurriness $B = \frac{N_{blur}}{N_{rg}}$.

---

for energy calculation. This is because that these subbands consist of relative higher frequency components, of which the energy is more easily affected by noise. After that, three edge maps $\{EM_i | i = 1, 2, 3\}$ of the same size are extracted by finding the local maxima of every block in each energy map. The block size of E_i is $2^{a-i} \times 2^{a-i}$, where a is usually set to 3 or 4.

Considering that the energy of DCT coefficient tends to centralize in upper left corner of each subband, we can construct E_1 by only using the upper left coefficients of each block. For instance, $\{F_{i,j} | i = 4, 5; j = 0, 1;\}$ and $\{F_{i,j} | i = 0, 1; j = 4, 5;\}$ of each 8×8 block are used to construct E_1 for the case when $a = 3$. Accordingly the maxima energy of the 4 coefficients of each block are then taken as the local maxima for building edge map EM_1. This would significantly increase the computational efficiency.

Two threshold parameters $T_i(i = 1, 2)$ $(T_2 \geq T_1)$ are used in our algorithm. T_1 is used for detecting edge points, and T_2 is for judging edge points that lose sharpness. For any Gstep-Structure or Roof-Structure edge point (k, l), our algorithm decides whether this point is blurred by: $EM_2(k, l) < T_2$. Since the edge map EM_1 is based on high frequency coefficients, it is more sensitive to noise. By contrast, the use of edge map EM_2 for finding blurred points leads to strong anti-noise ability. The presented method is summarized in Algorithm 1.

5   Experiments

We first evaluate our proposed relative sharpness metric on public available dataset. A total of five spatial-domain measures and four DCT-based measures are compared with the proposed metric M_{reodct}. The spatial-domain measures include the Tenengrad or Sobe function M_{sob}, the Squared gradient M_{sqg}, the sum of differences across rows and columns M_{smd}, the sum of Laplacians M_{sml}, and the energy of Laplacians M_{eol}. Definitions of these measures are

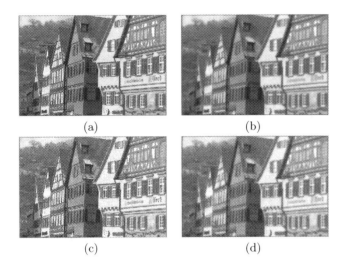

Fig. 5. Above row: two sample Gaussian blur images of the same scene from the LIVE dataset [14], (a) blur deviation $\sigma = 0$, (b) $\sigma = 2.624972$; Below row: white noise is added to the corresponding images (c–d), with noise deviation $\sigma_{noise} = 30$.

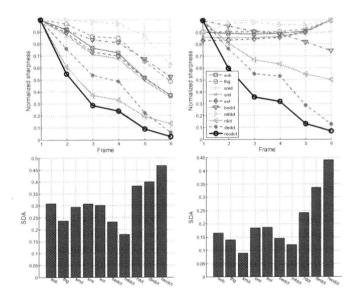

Fig. 6. Above row: sharpness measures on "building" sequence without (a) and with noise (b); Below row: the corresponding SDA evaluations.

not given here as they can be explicitly found in several related works [3,7,9]. The four DCT-based methods include the Bayes spectral entropy based measure M_{bsedct} [6], the middle frequency component based measure M_{mfdct} [7], the ratio of AC and DC energy based measure M_{rdct} [8], and the block direction

Table 2. SDA accuracy between different sharpness measures on LIVE Gaussian blur sequences with sythetic noises.

Measure	$\sigma_{noise} = 30$					
	M_{sob}	M_{sml}	M_{eol}	M_{bedct}	M_{dirdct}	M_{reodct}
Coinsinfountain	0.1018	0.0920	0.0911	0.2169	0.3484	**0.3640**
Ocean	0.1018	0.0920	0.0911	0.2169	0.3484	**0.3640**
Statue	0.1516	0.1455	0.1455	0.2023	**0.3437**	0.3213
Dancers	0.1976	0.2099	0.2077	0.3134	0.3619	**0.4145**
Paintedhouse	0.1599	0.1562	0.1562	0.1956	0.3819	**0.4001**
Stream	0.1174	0.1160	0.1105	0.3160	0.3158	**0.4674**
Bikes	0.2223	0.2435	0.2409	0.3177	0.3569	**0.4316**
Flowersoih35	0.1972	0.1910	0.1859	0.3064	0.3224	**0.4516**
Parrots	0.1592	0.1655	0.1656	0.2688	**0.3532**	0.3511
Studentsculpture	0.1157	0.1257	0.1282	0.2705	0.3694	**0.4520**
Building2	0.0862	0.0795	0.0702	0.3263	0.3916	**0.4919**
Plane	0.2178	0.2216	0.2222	0.3145	0.3430	**0.4040**
Woman	0.1287	0.1351	0.1297	0.2369	0.3641	**0.3648**
House	0.2271	0.2233	0.2214	0.2169	0.3960	**0.4116**
Rapids	0.1550	0.1563	0.1523	0.3385	0.3688	**0.4469**
Womanhat	0.0772	0.0752	0.0749	0.1456	0.2879	**0.3047**
Caps	0.2155	0.2171	0.2177	0.2011	0.3405	**0.3568**
Lighthouse	0.1903	0.1797	0.1770	0.2853	0.4055	**0.4604**
Sailing1	0.1464	0.1476	0.1449	0.2716	0.3987	**0.4691**
Carnivaldolls	0.1046	0.0987	0.0968	0.2339	0.3366	**0.3626**
Lighthouse2	0.0875	0.1044	0.1075	0.2426	0.3367	**0.3884**
Sailing2	0.1556	0.1618	0.1643	0.1867	0.3989	**0.4111**
Cemetry	0.1126	0.1312	0.1339	0.3070	0.3644	**0.4476**
Manfishing	0.1815	0.1707	0.1610	0.2140	0.3324	**0.3967**
Sailing3	0.1267	0.1261	0.1253	0.1415	0.2561	**0.2681**
Churchandcapitol	0.1674	0.1884	0.1956	0.3430	0.4112	**0.4512**
Monarch	0.3166	0.3136	0.3166	0.3642	0.3881	**0.4181**
Sailing4	0.2495	0.2413	0.2374	0.3545	0.4010	**0.4598**

information based measure M_{dirdct} [9]. The public available dataset LIVE [14] is used for the comparison experiments. LIVE provides 145 Gaussian blur images which are created from 29 input images. Figure 5 shows example Gaussian blur images of LIVE.

Figure 6(a) plots the sharpness evaluation results on one blur image sequence named "buildings" of LIVE (Fig. 6). Figure 6(c) gives the corresponding evaluations of SDA. The DCT based sharpness measures like M_{rdct}, M_{dirdct} and the

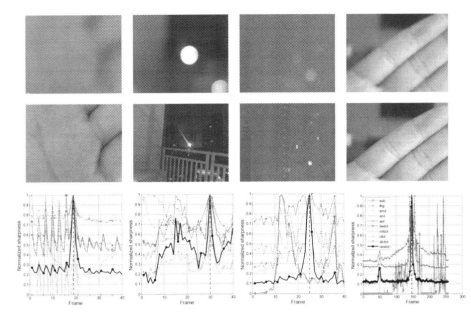

Fig. 7. From left to right: sharpness measuring on example sequences of scenes with low contrast ("Hand"), strong lighting ("LightBeam"), high noise ("NightBuilding") and moving objects ("MovingFingers").

proposed one show relative better performance than all spatial-domain functions. To test noise sensitivity of the proposed measure, white Gaussian noise of standard deviation σ_{noise} is added to the blur images, and the 10 sharpness measures are tested again. Figure 6(b) and (d) gives the results on the noised "buildings" sequence. We can see all measures except of M_{reodct} and M_{dirdct} are seriously affected by noise. Table 2 gives SDA evaluations of the 6 measures including M_{sob}, M_{sml}, M_{eol}, M_{rdct}, M_{dirdct} and M_{reodct} on the 29 LIVE Gaussian image sequences with synthetic noise. It is found that M_{reodct} shows very robust performance and outperforms other measures both in accuracy and robustness.

The proposed sharpness measure is also tested on four real focusing sequences, which are labeled as "Hand", "LightBeam", "NightBuilding" and "MovingFingers". As shown in Fig. 7, the Hand sequence is poor in contrast, the LightBeam has strong lighting distortions, the NightBuilding is captured at low illumination, and the MovingFingers is a sequence of moving subject. For all evaluation, the center window of size $\frac{1}{3}w \times \frac{1}{3}h$ (w and h denote the image width and height separately) is taken as the area for sharpness calculation. For the Hand sequence, we can see from the focus curves that only M_{reodct} gives largest sharpness dynamic range and correct position of best focus. In sequence LightBeam, the factors such as halo edges and illumination changes would largely affect the sharpness measure. Multiple peaks and many fluctuations may exist, as seen from the focus curves. The results show that the proposed measure M_{reodct} is

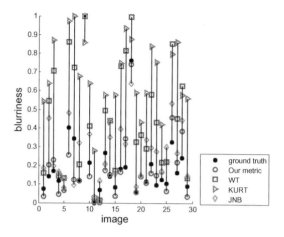

Fig. 8. Blur estimation for sample Gaussian blurred images of LIVE dataset, of which the blurred image set is obtained by filtering 29 input images with different content using Gaussian kernel of different standard deviation σ. For all images, our algorithm uses $T_1 = 5$, $T_2 = 10$, while other algorithms use the optimal parameters as suggested. The normalized σ is taken as the ground truth of blurriness.

able to give the correct maximum measure for this complex case. For sequence NightBuilding which is polluted by noise due to the low illumination, M_{reodct} shows the best performance of anti-noise. It also produces stable and reliable estimations when the subject is moving, as can be seen from the result of the sequence MovingFingers.

We have tested the proposed no-reference metric of absolute sharpness on the Gaussian blur sequence of the public LIVE dataset. From the given 145 Gaussian blur images, we select 29 blurred images that have different blur σ and image contents. Three commonly used metrics are chosen for performance comparison: the wavelet transform method (WT) [27], the kurtosis method (KURT) [26], and the just noticeable blur method (JNB) [12]. The parameters of each algorithm are set according to the optimal suggestions described in the relevant work. Figure 8 gives the result of the four metrics for judging blurred points. It is seen that our metric outperforms other methods both in robustness and accuracy.

6 Conclusion

In this work, we propose two sharpness metrics by exploiting a reorganized DCT representation. The first metric selects the most suitable components that have high effect on sharpness measuring. This metric has high discrimination power even for high noisy and low-contrast images. We have used it for auto-focus application where it shows super sensitive to the best-focus position and could predict stable sharpness measures for various subjects and scenes with different lighting and noise conditions. We also present an efficient DCT-based absolute sharpness metric. This metric exploits the same framework of the reorganized DCT representation. It correlates well with perceived sharpness and is efficient in sharpness measurement for images with different contents. We demonstrate the performance of our metrics by comparing them against several most commonly used metrics both on public and the captured out-of-focus sequences.

References

1. Ciancio, A., da Costa, A.L.N.T., da Silva, E.A.B.: No-reference blur assessment of digital pictures based on multifeature classifiers. IEEE Trans. Image Process. **20**, 64–75 (2011)
2. Vu, C.T., Phan, T.D., Chandler, D.M.: S3: a spectral and spatial measure of local perceived sharpness in natural images. IEEE Trans. Image Process. **21**, 934–945 (2011)
3. Santos, A., Solorzano, C.O.D., Vaquero, J.J., Pena, J.M., Malpica, N., Pozo, F.D.: Evaluation of autofocus functions in molecular cytogenetic analysis. J. Microsc. **188**, 264–272 (1997)
4. Yousefi, S., Rahman, M., Kehtarnavaz, N.: A new auto-focus sharpness function for digital and smart-phone cameras. IEEE Trans. Consum. Electron. **57**, 1003–1009 (2011)
5. Choi, J., Kang, H., Lee, C.M., Kang, M.G.: Noise insensitive focus value operator for digital imaging systems. IEEE Trans. Consum. Electron. **56**, 312–316 (2010)
6. Kristan, M., Pers, J., Perse, M., Kovacic, S.: A bayes-spectral-entropy-based measure of camera focus using a discrete cosine transform. Pattern Recogn. Lett. **27**, 1431–1439 (2006)
7. Lee, S.Y., Kumar, Y., Cho, J.M., Lee, S.W., Kim, S.W.: Enhanced autofocus algorithm using robust focus measure and fuzzy reasoning. IEEE Trans. Circ. Syst. Video Technol. **18**, 1237–1246 (2008)
8. Shen, C.H., Chen, H.H.: Robust focus measure for low-contrast images. In: IEEE International Conference on Consumer Electronics (2006)
9. Jeon, J., Lee, J., Paik, J.: Robust focus measure for unsupervised auto-focusing based on optimum discrete cosine transform coefficients. IEEE Trans. Consum. Electron. **57**, 1–5 (2011)
10. Lee, M.E., Chen, C.F., Lin, T.N., Chen, C.N.: The application of discrete cosine transform combined with the nonlinear regression routine on optical auto-focusing. In: IEEE International Conference on Consumer Electronics (2009)
11. Marichal, X., Ma, W.Y., Zhang, H.: Blur determination in the compressed domain using dct information. In: IEEE International Conference on Image Processing (1999)
12. Ferzli, R., Karam, L.J.: A no-reference objective image sharpness metric based on the notion of just noticeable blur. IEEE Trans. Image Process. **18**, 717–728 (2009)
13. Shen, J., Li, Q., Erlebacher, G.: Hybrid no-reference natural image quality assessment of noisy, blurry, jpeg2000, and jpeg images. IEEE Trans. Image Process. **20**, 2089–2098 (2011)
14. Sheikh, H.R., Wang, Z., Cormack, L., Bovik, A.C.: Live image qaulity assessment database release 2. http://live.ece.utexas.edu/research/quality
15. Zhang, Y., Zhang, Y., Wen, C.: A new focus measure method using moments. Image Vis. Comput. **18**, 959–965 (2000)

16. Kautsky, J., Flusser, J., Zitova, B., Simberova, S.: A new wavelet-based measure of image focus. Pattern Recogn. Lett. **23**, 1785–1794 (2002)
17. Yang, G., Nelson, B.J.: Wavelet-based autofocusing and unsupervised segmentation of microscopic images. In: IEEE International Conference on Intelligent Robots and Systems (2003)
18. Horn, B.K.P.: Focusing. Technical report, Massachusetts Institute of Technology (1968)
19. Choi, K.S., Lee, J.S., Ko, S.J.: New autofocusing technique using the frequency selective weighted median filter for video cameras. IEEE Trans. Consum. Electron. **45**, 820–827 (1999)
20. Chen, C.Y., Hwang, R.C., Chen, Y.-J.: A passive auto-focus camera control system. Appl. Soft Comput. **10**, 296–303 (2010)
21. Marziliano, P., Dufaux, F., Winkler, S., Ebrahimi, T.: A no-reference perceptual blur metric. In: IEEE International Conference on Image Processing (2002)
22. Marziliano, P., Dufaux, F., Winkler, S., Ebrahimi, T.: Perceptual blur and ringing metrics application to jpeg2000. Sig. Process. Image Commun. **19**, 163–172 (2004)
23. Narvekar, N.D., Karam, L.J.: A no-reference image blur metric based on the cumulative probability of blur detection. IEEE Trans. Image Process. **20**, 2678–2683 (2011)
24. Sadaka, N.G., Karam, L.J., Ferzli, R., Abousleman, G.P.: A no-reference perceptual image sharpness metric based on saliency-weighted foveal pooling. In: IEEE International Conference on Image Processing (2008)
25. Wee, C.Y., Paramesran, R.: Image sharpness measure using eigenvalues. In: 9th International Conference on Signal Processing (2008)
26. Caviedes, J., Oberti, F.: A new sharpness metric based on local kurtosis, edge and energy information. Sig. Process. Image Commun. **19**, 147–161 (2004)
27. Tong, H., Li, M., Zhang, H., Zhang, C.: Blur detection for digital images using wavelet transform. In: IEEE International Conference on Multimedia and Expo (2004)
28. Shaked, D., Tastl, I.: Sharpness measure: towards automatic image enhancement. In: IEEE International Conference on Image Processing (2005)
29. Balam, S., Schonfeld, D.: Associative processors for video coding applications. IEEE Trans. Circuits Syst. Video Technol. **16**, 241–250 (2006)
30. Huan, J., Parris, M., Lee, J., DeMara, R.F.: Scalable fpga-based architecture for dct computation using dynamic partial reconfiguration. ACM Trans. Embed. Comput. Syst. **9**, 1–18 (2009)
31. Cho, N.I., Lee, S.U.: Fast algorithm and implementation of 2d discrete cosine transform. IEEE Trans. Circ. Syst. **38**, 297–305 (1991)
32. Xiong, Z., Guleryuz, O., Orchard, M.T.: A dct-based embedded image coder. Signal Process. Lett. **3**, 289–290 (1996)
33. Ma, L., Li, S., Zhang, F., Ngan, K.N.: Reduced-reference image quality assessment using reorganized dct-based image representation. IEEE Trans. Multimedia **13**, 824–829 (2011)
34. Zhao, D., Gao, W., Chan, Y.K.: Morphological representation of dct coefficients for image compression. IEEE Trans. Circuits Syst. Video Technol. **12**, 819–823 (2002)
35. Mallat, S.: A theory for multiresolution signal decomposition: the wavelet representation. IEEE Trans. Pattern Anal. Mach. Intell. **11**, 674–693 (1989)
36. Lam, E.Y., Goodman, J.W.: A mathematical analysis of the dct coefficient distributions for images. IEEE Trans. Image Process. **9**, 1661–1666 (2000)
37. Robson, J.G., Graham, N.: Probability summation and regional variation in contrast sensitivity across the visual field. Vision. Res. **21**, 409–418 (1981)

DisLocation: Scalable Descriptor Distinctiveness for Location Recognition

Relja Arandjelović[(✉)] and Andrew Zisserman

Department of Engineering Science, University of Oxford, Oxford, UK
relja@robots.ox.ac.uk

Abstract. The objective of this paper is to improve large scale visual object retrieval for visual place recognition. Geo-localization based on a visual query is made difficult by plenty of non-distinctive features which commonly occur in imagery of urban environments, such as generic modern windows, doors, cars, trees, etc. The focus of this work is to adapt standard Hamming Embedding retrieval system to account for varying descriptor distinctiveness. To this end, we propose a novel method for efficiently estimating distinctiveness of all database descriptors, based on estimating local descriptor density everywhere in the descriptor space. In contrast to all competing methods, the (unsupervised) training time for our method (DisLoc) is linear in the number database descriptors and takes only a 100 s on a single CPU core for a 1 million image database. Furthermore, the added memory requirements are negligible (1 %).

The method is evaluated on standard publicly available large-scale place recognition benchmarks containing street-view imagery of Pittsburgh and San Francisco. DisLoc is shown to outperform all baselines, while setting the new state-of-the-art on both benchmarks. The method is compatible with spatial reranking, which further improves recognition results.

Finally, we also demonstrate that 7 % of the least distinctive features can be removed, therefore reducing storage requirements and improving retrieval speed, without any loss in place recognition accuracy.

1 Introduction

We consider the problem of visual place recognition, where the goal is to build a system which can geographically localize a query image, and do so in near real-time. Such a system is useful for geotagging personal photos [1], mobile augmented reality [2], robot localization [3], or to aid automatic 3D reconstruction [4].

A common approach is to cast place recognition as a visual object retrieval problem: the query image is used to visually search a large database of geo-tagged images [5], and highly ranked images are returned to the user as location suggestions [6–8]. Visual retrieval is usually conducted by extracting local descriptors, such as SIFT [9], quantizing them into visual words [10], and representing images as bag-of-visual-words (BoW) histograms. The BoW histograms are sparse because large visual vocabularies are commonly used [10,11]. Retrieval

© Springer International Publishing Switzerland 2015
D. Cremers et al. (Eds.): ACCV 2014, Part IV, LNCS 9006, pp. 188–204, 2015.
DOI: 10.1007/978-3-319-16817-3_13

is then performed by computing distances between sparse BoW histograms, which can be done efficiently by using an inverted index [10]. Many works have further improved on this core system by using larger vocabularies [11,12], soft-assignment [13,14], more accurate descriptor matching [15], enforcing geometric consistency [10,11,15], or learning better descriptors [16,17]. Further improvements of retrieval systems specifically targeted at location recognition have been made, namely removal of confusing features [6], training of per-location classifiers [18,19], and better handling of repetitive structures commonly found on façades of modern buildings [8].

In this work we focus on improving localization performance by exploiting distinctiveness of local descriptors – distinctive features should carry more weight than non-distinctive features. Automatically determining which features are distinctive or not should be quite helpful in location recognition, especially in urban environments where many features look alike (e.g. descriptors extracted from corners of generic modern office windows are all very similar). A traditional method for weighting features based on their distinctiveness is the inverse document frequency (idf) weighting [10] which down-weights frequently occurring visual words. However, this method operates purely on the visual word level, while recent retrieval methods imply that a finer-level descriptor matching is required for better retrieval accuracy [15,20–25]. Therefore, we investigate descriptor distinctiveness on a sub-visual-word level for which we extend the Hamming Embedding (HE) approach [15,20] (reviewed in Sect. 2).

Our method, DisLoc (Sect. 3), uses local density of descriptor space as a measure of descriptor distinctiveness, i.e. descriptors which are in a densely populated region of the descriptor space are deemed to be less distinctive (Fig. 1). This approach is in line with the idf weighting [10] where frequent visual words are deemed to be less distinctive, but, unlike idf, our method estimates descriptor density on a finer level than visual words. Similar motivation is used in the second nearest neighbour test [9] where descriptor matches are rejected if the nearest descriptor to the query descriptor is not significantly closer than the second nearest. This test tends to be overly aggressive as two database descriptors can naturally be very similar due to depicting the same object; in this case the second nearest neighbour test would reject perfectly good matches. In contrast, our method is much softer in nature because matches are weighted based on the local density of descriptor space, which is estimated robustly such that a few repeated descriptors do not affect density estimates much.

1.1 Related Work

Distinctiveness has been investigated in a supervised setting where [6] remove confusing features based on their geographical distribution. In [26], only repeatable visual words for a particular scene are kept. Classifiers can be learnt to automatically estimate visual word importance for every location [18,19]. However, all four methods suffer from two major problems: (1) much like idf weighting, they are limited to operate on the visual word level; and (2) they are not scalable enough. The four methods are impractical on a large scale as they require

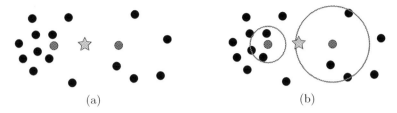

(a)   (b)

Fig. 1. Descriptor distinctiveness. Full circles represent database descriptors in the descriptor space. The red and green full circles are the closest database descriptors to the query (cyan star) and are equidistant from it. (a) The baseline Hamming Embedding method treats the green and red descriptors equally due to their equal distance from the query. (b) The red and green circles depict the local neighbourhood (radius is equal to the distance to the third nearest neighbour) for the red and green descriptors, respectively. DisLoc weights the green feature more because the relative distance to the query with respect to the neighbourhood radius is smaller for the green than for the red descriptor, implying that green is a better match (Color figure online).

querying with each image in the database: [6] does this to discover confusing features, [18] for selecting negatives with hard-negative mining, while [19,26] need it for constructing the image graph [27]. Even though this processing is only performed offline, it is still impractical as the computational complexity is quadratic in the number of database features. For a database with millions of images (such as the San Francisco landmarks dataset [7] used in this work), which contains billions of local descriptors, it is unreasonable to use a method with quadratic computational cost. For example, using each image from the San Francisco dataset (1M images, Sect. 4.1) to query the dataset using the baseline retrieval method (Hamming Embedding, Sect. 4.2) with fast spatial verification [11] (required for all four methods), takes 2.2 days on a single core (estimated from a random sample of 10k images). The quadratic nature of the approaches means that for a 10 M database one would need a cluster with 100 computers to work for 2.2 days. In contrast, we propose a method which is *linear* in the number of database features, which takes only 100 CPU seconds (Sect. 3.1) to compute for the 1 M image San Francisco dataset. Furthermore, unlike [6,18], our method is completely unsupervised.

Measures of local descriptor density have been used to improve retrieval, but were commonly applied at the image descriptor level [28–30] (e.g. density of BoW histograms is investigated) rather than at the level of local patch descriptors (e.g. SIFT); applying these methods directly onto patch descriptors is impossible as it would require a prohibitive amount of extra RAM. Furthermore, all three methods are also quadratic in nature and therefore not scalable enough. Finally, [21] exploit descriptor-space density on the patch descriptor level, but their method suffers from two problems: (1) it is, again, quadratic in nature; and (2) requires storing an extra floating point value per descriptor. For the example of the San Francisco dataset from which we extract 0.8 billion features, assuming single-precision floats (i.e. 4 bytes), [21] would require an extra 3.3 GB of RAM, which is a 31 % increase over the baseline and our method. In contrast, our DisLoc method is scalable as the necessary offline preprocessing is linear in the number of database features, and only a fixed (i.e. does not increase with database size) and negligible amount of extra memory is required (103 MB in total).

2 Hamming Embedding for Object Retrieval

In this section we provide a short overview of the Hamming Embedding [15] method for large scale object retrieval, which has been shown to outperform BoW-based methods [15,20,23,24]. We will use it as our baseline (Sect. 4.2) and, in Sect. 3, extend it to incorporate our descriptor distinctiveness weighting.

We follow the notation and framework of Tolias et al. [24] which encapsulates many popular retrieval methods, including bag-of-words (BoW) [10], Hamming Embedding (HE) [15], burstiness normalization [20] and VLAD [31]. An image is described by a set $\mathcal{X} = \{x_1, \ldots, x_n\}$ of n local descriptors. The k-means vector quantizer q maps a descriptor x_i into a visual word ID $q(x_i)$, such that $q(x_i) \in \mathcal{C}$, where $\mathcal{C} = \{c_1, \ldots, c_k\}$ is the visual vocabulary of size k. Finally, $\mathcal{X}_c$ is a subset of descriptors in $\mathcal{X}$ assigned to the visual word c, i.e. $\mathcal{X}_c = \{x \in \mathcal{X} : q(x) = c\}$. The similarity K between two image representations $\mathcal{X}$ and $\mathcal{Y}$ is defined as:

$$K(\mathcal{X}, \mathcal{Y}) = \gamma(\mathcal{X})\gamma(\mathcal{Y}) \sum_{c \in \mathcal{C}} w_c M(\mathcal{X}_c, \mathcal{Y}_c) \tag{1}$$

where $\gamma(.)$ is a normalization factor, w_c is a constant which depends on visual word c, and M is a similarity defined between two sets of descriptors assigned to the same visual word. For the case of BoW and HE, w_c is typically chosen to be the square of the inverse document frequency (idf). The normalization factor is usually defined such that the self-similarity of an image is $K(\mathcal{X}, \mathcal{X}) = 1$. For Hamming Embedding retrieval [15,20], a B-dimensional binary signature is stored for every database descriptor, in order to provide more accurate descriptor matching; the signature is constructed in a LSH-like [32] manner (for more details see [15]). The similarity function M takes the following form for the special case of Hamming Embedding [15] with burstiness normalization [20] (assuming $\mathcal{X}$ and $\mathcal{Y}$ are representations of the query and database images, respectively):

$$M(\mathcal{X}_c, \mathcal{Y}_c) = \sum_{x \in \mathcal{X}_c} |\mathcal{Y}_c(x)|^{-1/2} \sum_{y \in \mathcal{Y}_c} f(h(b_x, b_y)) \tag{2}$$

where b_x and b_y are binary signatures of local descriptors x and y, h is the Hamming distance, f is a weighting function which associates weights for all possible values of the Hamming distance, and $|\mathcal{Y}_c(x)|$ is the number of elements in the set $\mathcal{Y}_c(x)$ of database descriptors that match with x:

$$\mathcal{Y}_c(x) = \{y \in \mathcal{Y}_c : f(h(b_x, b_y)) \neq 0\} \tag{3}$$

Finally, the weighting function f is defined as the truncated non-normalized Gaussian [20]:

$$f(h) = \begin{cases} e^{-h^2/\sigma^2} & , \ h \leq 1.5\sigma \\ 0 & , \ otherwise \end{cases} \tag{4}$$

where the Gaussian bandwidth parameter σ is typically chosen to be one quarter of the number of bits B used for the binary signatures [20,33] (e.g. a common setting is $B = 64$ and $\sigma = 16$).

Discussion. Here we explain, in less formal terms, the intuition behind mathematical definitions presented in this section (which were adapted from [24]). Equation (1) simply decomposes the image similarity across different visual words, which enables efficient computation of the similarity between the query and all database images by employing an inverted index. It also accounts for inverse document frequency weighting (w_c), and normalizes the scores in order to not bias the similarity towards images with a large number of descriptors (e.g. for the BoW case, Eq. (1) reduces to cosine similarity between tf-idf weighted BoW vectors). The binary signatures b_x and b_y help perform precise matching between the two descriptors by rejecting some false matches that a pure BoW system would accept, at a cost of increased storage (to store the signatures) and processing (to compute Hamming distances) requirements. This is done by thresholding the Hamming distance in Eq. (4), where descriptor matches whose Hamming distances are larger than 1.5σ are discarded, while others are given increasing weights for decreasing distances. For comparison, a BoW system would simply correspond to $f(h) = 1$ for all h. Finally, the visual burstiness effect is countered by the burstiness normalization [20] in Eq. (2).

3   Scalable Descriptor Distinctiveness

This section proposes a method for determining descriptor distinctiveness and incorporating it into the standard retrieval framework presented in the previous section. Apart from improving retrieval performance, there are two main requirements: (1) the method must not have quadratic computational complexity in order to be scalable to databases containing millions of images, and (2) storage requirements should not increase drastically, i.e. no additional information should be kept on a per-descriptor basis but only a fixed amount (i.e. not dependant on the database size) of additional RAM can be justified. Both of these requirements distinguish our work from previous works, a review of which is given in Sect. 1.1.

The key idea of our method is to estimate the local density of the descriptor space around each database descriptor, and weight descriptors depending on their distinctiveness which is inverse to the local density; we call it Local Distinctiveness (DisLoc). Figure 1 illustrates this point: given two database features (red and green) equally distant from the query (star), it is clear that the green one is more likely to be a correct match than the red one. This is because the red descriptor is surrounded by many other descriptors (i.e. descriptor density is large, distinctiveness is small) and is therefore not distinctive, and, for example, the second nearest neighbour test of [9] would reject the match. On the other hand, the green descriptor is quite distinctive as there is a small concentration of other descriptors around it, so it might be a correct match for the query.

The Hamming Embedding retrieval system (reviewed in Sect. 2), would add the same weight, $f(h)$ (Eq. (4)), to the images from which the red and green features came from, because h is the same for both of them. We therefore modify the weighting function to adjust the Gaussian bandwidth based on descriptor distinctiveness, i.e. we propose to make σ (Eq. (4)) a function of the database descriptor. Increasing σ allows for larger Hamming distances to be tolerated when deciding if two descriptors match, while reducing it increases the selectivity; Fig. 1b illustrates this. More formally, we modify the definition of M and f (Eqs. (2) and (4), respectively) to incorporate σ being a function of the local descriptor, i.e. its visual word c and binary signature b (recall that $\mathcal{X}$ and $\mathcal{Y}$ are the representations of the query and database images, respectively):

$$M(\mathcal{X}_c, \mathcal{Y}_c) = \sum_{x \in \mathcal{X}_c} |\mathcal{Y}_c(x)|^{-1/2} \sum_{y \in \mathcal{Y}_c} f(h(b_x, b_y), c, b_y) \qquad (5)$$

$$f(h, c, b_y) = \begin{cases} e^{-h^2/\sigma(c, b_y)^2} & , \ h \leq 1.5\sigma(c, b_y) \\ 0 & , \ otherwise \end{cases} \qquad (6)$$

3.1   Scalable Estimation of $\sigma(c, b)$

The key remaining problem is how to robustly estimate $\sigma(c, b)$ for all database descriptors, and obey our two design goals: do not incur quadratic computational cost, nor store extra information on a per-descriptor basis (e.g. one could be tempted to store $\sigma(c, b)$ for every descriptor) thus requiring much more RAM which is usually the limiting factor for any large scale retrieval system.

We propose to precompute and store $\sigma(c, b)$ for all possible values of the visual word c and binary signature b. However, this is impractical – there are 2^B possible B-dimensional binary signatures, and for reasonably – sized signatures (e.g. typically $B = 64$) there are too many combinations to compute and store. Therefore, we propose a small approximation – the B-dimensional binary signature b is divided into m blocks where each of the blocks is $l = \frac{B}{m}$ dimensional, so that b is a concatenation of $b^{(1)}, b^{(2)}, \ldots, b^{(m)}$. The blocks represent subspaces of the full descriptor space and we assume, akin to Product Quantization [34], that the subspaces are relatively independent of each other, i.e. if a descriptor is distinctive, it is also likely that it is distinctive in many of the m subspaces. Then, $\sigma(c, b)$ is approximated as the sum of σ's in the individual subspaces: $\sigma(c, b) = \sum_{i=1}^{m} \sigma_i(c, b^{(i)})$. Splitting the large B-dimensional binary vector into several parts makes our problem manageable due to dealing with smaller dimensional binary signatures – for each visual word c, instead of storing a table of $\sigma(c, b)$ values which has 2^B entries, we store m tables $\sigma_i(c, b^{(i)})$ with $2^l = 2^{B/m}$ values each. For a typical setting where $B = 64$, $m = 8$ and therefore $l = 64/8 = 8$ bits, the number of stored and computed elements decreases from $2^{64} = 1.8 \times 10^{19}$ to $8 \times 2^8 = 2048$.

The problem now becomes: for all visual words c and all signature blocks (i.e. subspaces) s, compute and store $\sigma_s(c, b^{(s)})$ for all values of $b^{(s)}$. As discussed earlier, we propose to make $\sigma_s(c, b^{(s)})$ proportional to the binary signature distinctiveness, which is inversely proportional to the local descriptor density, and therefore proportional to the local neighbourhood size. The local neighbourhood for a given signature can be estimated as the minimal hypersphere which contains its p neighbours, the radius of this hypersphere is equal to the distance to the p-th nearest neighbour. This strategy is illustrated in Fig. 1b ($p = 3$), where the local neighbourhood is automatically estimated – the red descriptor's neighbourhood is smaller (i.e. descriptor density is larger, so it is less distinctive) than the green one's. Other measures of local neighbourhood size exist as well, such as a softer approach of [35], but we found the overall place recognition performance of our method to be robust to various neighbourhood size definitions.

We simply make $\sigma_s(c, b^{(s)})$ equal to the local neighbourhood radius, i.e. the Hamming distance to the p-th nearest neighbour of signature $b^{(s)}$ in visual word c. The p parameter is set automatically as the average number of neighbours across all database descriptors (in the same visual word c and subspace s) which are closer than the default value of σ_{def}/m, where σ_{def} is defined as the value from Sect. 2, i.e. $\sigma_{def} = B/4$ [20,33]. In other words, if all descriptors are uniformly distributed in the descriptor space, the estimated $\sigma(c, b)$ would be identical for all b and equal to the default σ_{def} of the baseline Hamming Embedding method (Sect. 2).

Implementation Details: $\sigma_s(c, b^{(s)})$ Computation. It is simple and fast to compute the distance to the p-th nearest neighbour for all possible values of $b^{(s)}$ (remember that $b^{(s)}$ is l-dimensional, and l is small, with $l = 8$ there are only 256 different values of $b^{(s)}$). For this purpose we define a lookup table $t_s(c, b^{(s)})$ which stores the number of descriptors quantized to visual word c which have the binary signature $b^{(s)}$ in subspace s. This table can be populated with a single pass through the inverted index (i.e. the computational complexity is by definition $O(n)$, where n is the number of descriptors in the database). To compute the distance to the p-th nearest neighbour for a particular value $b_i^{(s)}$, one can simply use a brute force approach: go through the list of binary signatures $b_j^{(s)}$ in the non-decreasing order of hamming distance $h(b_i^{(s)}, b_j^{(s)})$ and accumulate $t_s(c, b_j^{(s)})$ along the way. The traversal is terminated once the accumulated number reaches p, signifying that $h(b_i^{(s)}, b_j^{(s)})$ is the distance of the p-th nearest neighbour.

Implementation Details: Normalization. We make sure that on average $\sigma(c, b)$ is the same as the default σ_{def} so that no bias is introduced, such as consistently under/overestimating $\sigma(c, b)$ which by coincidence might work better for a particular benchmark. We therefore normalize $\sigma(c, b)$ by subtracting the mean over all $\mathcal{X}_c$ and adding σ_{def}. Therefore, the final estimate of $\sigma(c, b)$ is computed as $\sigma_{final}(c, b) = v_c + \sigma(c, b) = v_c + \sum_{i=1}^{m} \sigma_i(c, b^{(i)})$, where $v_c = \sigma_{def} - mean_{x \in \mathcal{X}_c}(\sigma(c, b_x))$; it is clear that this ensures that $mean_{x \in \mathcal{X}_c}(\sigma_{final}(c, b_x)) = \sigma_{def}$. In order to be able to conduct the normalization at run-time, a single extra floating point number, v_c, needs to be stored for every visual word c.

Computational Speed. As mentioned earlier, the table $t_s(c, b_i^{(s)})$ can be populated with a single pass over all database descriptors, which is $O(n)$, where n is their count. The brute force search for the p-th nearest neighbour distance is $O(2^l \times 2^l) = O(2^{2l})$ so this part of the algorithm is independent of the database size as l is a constant.

On a single core (i5 3.30 GHz), the entire computation takes only 100 s for the San Francisco dataset (Sect. 4.1) which contains 1 M images and 0.8 billion local features. Furthermore, even though there is no real need for speeding it up as 100 s for a one off preprocessing task is very efficient, the algorithm is easily parallelizable as the computations are performed completely independently for all visual words c and subspaces s.

Storage Requirements. For every visual word c, at runtime one needs to have access to v_c (a single precision floating point number, 4 bytes) and m (typically equal to 8) lookup tables $\sigma_s(c, b^{(s)})$, which contain 2^l (typically equal to $2^8 = 256$) values. The $\sigma_s(c, b^{(s)})$ values can only take integer numbers from 0 to l as they are the only possible Hamming distances for l-length binary signatures. However, for our parameter settings we observe that all obtained values are between 1 and 4, therefore only 2 bits are needed to encode them. The total number of bits for storing all necessary information, for visual vocabulary size k, is therefore: $k \times (32 + 2 \times m \times 2^l)$, which for our parameter settings $k = 200k$, $m = 8$, $l = 8$ equals 103 MB. Note that no information is stored on a per-feature basis, i.e. for any size dataset, comprising of potentially millions of images, one only requires 103 MB of extra storage, which is negligible. On the other hand, the method of [21] requires storing a floating point number for every database feature, which for 0.8 billion features of the San Francisco dataset (Sect. 4.1) would require extra 3.3 GB of RAM. This is a 31 % increase in baseline's storage needs; in contrast, our method increases storage requirements by less than 1 %.

3.2   Removal of Unhelpful Features

Up to this point we have shown how to compute distinctiveness of every descriptor in the database – larger $\sigma(c, b)$ corresponds to larger distinctiveness. We note that very non-distinctive features are not useful for retrieval or place recognition, as (1) they don't convey much information, and (2) it is unlikely that query features will match to them as the adapted Gaussian bandwidth $\sigma(c, b)$ is quite tight. Therefore, we propose to investigate removing non-distinctive descriptors, namely, to remove all descriptors from the database whose $\sigma(c, b)$ is below a certain threshold. Experimental results (Sect. 4.3) indeed show that 7 % of features can be removed safely without any degradation in place recognition performance, while 24 % of features can be removed in exchange for a small reduction in recognition performance. The removal of features directly translates to reduced storage and RAM requirements, as well as place recognition speedup.

4   Experimental Setup and Recognition Results

4.1   Datasets and Evaluation Procedure

Location recognition performance is evaluated on two standard large scale datasets containing street-view images of Pittsburgh [8] and San Francisco [7].

Pittsburgh [8]. The dataset contains 254 k perspective images generated from 10.6 k Google Street View panoramas of Pittsburgh downloaded from the internet. There are 24 k query images generated from 1 k panoramas taken from an independent dataset, Google Pittsburgh Research Dataset, which has been created at a different time. We follow the evaluation protocol of [8] where ground truth is generated automatically by using the provided GPS coordinates; a database image is deemed as a positive if it is within 25 m from the query image. It should be noted that a perfect location recognition score is unachievable as some queries (1.2 %) do not have any positives (as all database images are further away than 25 m), some positives are not within 25 m due to GPS inaccuracies ([8] reports GPS accuracy to be between 7 and 15 m), and the construction of the ground truth does not take into account occlusions which can occur due to large camera displacements.

San Francisco Landmarks [7]. The dataset contains 1.06 million perspective images generated from 150 k panoramas of San Francisco, while the query set contains 803 images taken at different times using mobile phones. Ground truth is provided in terms of building IDs which appear in the query and database images; as in [7,8], positives for a particular query are all database images which contain a query building.

There are two versions of the ground truth provided by the database authors – the original April 2011 version used by [7,8], and an updated April 2014 version which contains fixes but has not been used in a paper yet due to its recency. Unless otherwise stated, we report results on the latest ground truth version (April 2014), while when comparing to previous methods [7,8] we use the same version as them (the first version from April 2011) in order to be fair.

Finally, it should be noted that there are still some problems with the ground truth – 6.5 % queries do not contain any positives making the maximal obtainable location recognition score to be 93.5 %. Furthermore, we have encountered a few more ground truth errors, such as cases where the side of the building imaged in a query is not visible in any of the database images of the same building.

Evaluation Measure. Localization performance is evaluated in the same way for the two datasets, as defined by their respective authors [7,8], as recall at N retrievals. Namely, a query is deemed to be correctly localized if at least one positive image is retrieved within the top N positions. We use two types of graphs to visualize the performance: (1) *recall@N*: recall as a function of the number of top N retrievals; and (2) *rank-gain@N*: relative decrease in the number of required top retrievals such that the recall is the same as the baseline method at N retrievals. An example of a *rank-gain@N* curve is Fig. 2d, where our method,

DisLoc, achieves 33.3 % at $N = 30$, which means that 33.3 % less retrievals were needed for DisLoc to achieve the same recall as the baseline achieves at $N = 30$ (i.e. DisLoc only needs to return 20 images).

4.2   Baseline

We have implemented a baseline retrieval system based on the Hamming Embedding [15] with burstiness normalization [20], details of which are discussed in Sect. 2. We extract upright RootSIFT [36] descriptors from Hessian-Affine interest points [37], and quantize them into 200 k visual words. To alleviate quantization errors, multiple assignment [13] to five nearest visual words is performed, but in order not to increase memory requirements this is done on query features only, as in [14]. A 64-bit Hamming Embedding (HE) [15] signature is stored together with each feature in order to improve feature matching precision. The visual vocabulary and Hamming Embedding parameters are all trained on a random subsample of features from the respective datasets.

As shown in Fig. 4, our baseline (HE) already sets the state of the art on both datasets, and by a large margin. For example, on the Pittsburgh benchmark at $N = 10$ the baseline gets 77.3 % while the best previous result (Adaptive weights [8]) achieves 61.5 %. The superior performance of the baseline can be explained by the fact that Hamming Embedding with burstiness normalization has been shown to outperform bag-of-words methods due to increased feature matching precision [15, 20, 23, 33].

4.3   Results

Unless otherwise stated, none of the following experiments performs spatial reranking [11] as our aim is to improve the performance of the core retrieval system. Spatial reranking or any other postprocessing technique [29, 33, 38, 39] can be applied on top of our method, and we show results for spatial reranking later in Sect. 4.4.

Note that the Pittsburgh benchmark contains many more query images than San Francisco (24 k compared to 803), which explains why the Pittsburgh performance graphs are smoother and differences between methods are easier to see (large number of query images implies performance differences are statistically significant).

Figure 2 shows the performance of our DisLoc method compared to the Hamming Embedding baseline. DisLoc clearly outperforms the baseline on both benchmarks and at all sizes of retrieved lists. For example, for the San Francisco dataset DisLoc achieves a rank-gain of 37.5 % at $N = 80$, namely DisLoc only needs to retrieve 50 images in order to achieve the same recall (87.2 %) as the baseline obtains with 80 retrievals. This directly corresponds to a more user-friendly system as a much shorter list of suggestions has to be shown to a user in order to achieve the same success rate. Rank-gain is consistently larger than 20 % for all N on both benchmarks.

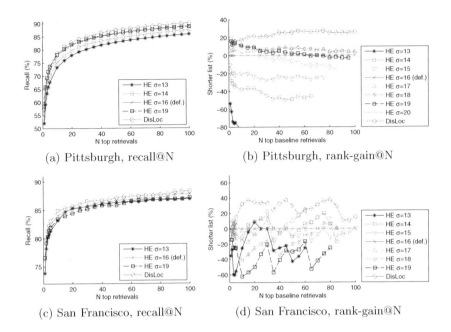

(a) Pittsburgh, recall@N

(b) Pittsburgh, rank-gain@N

(c) San Francisco, recall@N

(d) San Francisco, rank-gain@N

Fig. 2. Localization performance evaluation. DisLoc always outperforms the baseline by a large margin. It also outperforms various settings of the baseline's σ parameter.

We also investigate if the baseline's performance can be improved by tweaking the σ parameter; Fig. 2 also shows the results of these experiments. The default parameter value σ = 16 [20,33] indeed performs the best with the performance being relatively stable in the range between 14 and 18. DisLoc outperforms all baselines regardless of the tweaked σ, further proving its superiority.

Figure 3 shows some qualitative examples of place recognition, where Dis-Loc outperforms the baseline due to successful estimation of distinctive vs non-distinctive features.

Comparison with State of the Art. As noted in Sect. 4.2, our Hamming Embedding baseline already advances the new state of the art on both benchmarks (Fig. 4). Since DisLoc consistently outperforms this baseline, it sets the new state of the art for both datasets. The best competitor is the Adaptive weights method [8] which discovers repetitive structures in an image and uses them to perform a more natural soft assignment of local descriptors. The paper [8] also tests several baselines (included in Fig. 4) such as Fisher Vectors (FV), tf-idf, etc. DisLoc consistently beats all existing methods, for example, on the Pittsburgh dataset at N = 10 DisLoc achieves 78.7 % while the best competitor, Adaptive weights [8], gets 61.5 %. Furthermore, the recall at N = 50 when the performance of all methods starts to saturate is also much larger – 87.4 % compared to 73 %. DisLoc with only top 3 retrievals achieves a better recall than Adaptive weights at 25 and 50 retrievals for the Pittsburgh and San Francisco benchmarks, respectively.

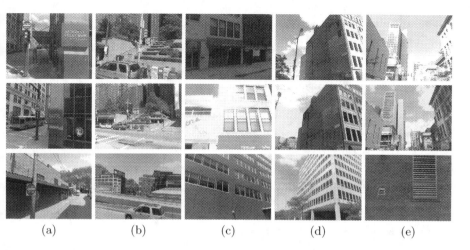

(a)   (b)   (c)   (d)   (e)

Fig. 3. Qualitative examples from the Pittsburgh benchmark. Each column shows one example, the query image is shown in the top row, and the first results returned by DisLoc and the baseline are shown in the middle and bottom rows, respectively. The baseline is often confused by non-distinctive features coming from traffic signs (a), cars (b), windows (c–d), and various repetitive structures (e). DisLoc often successfully overcomes these problems.

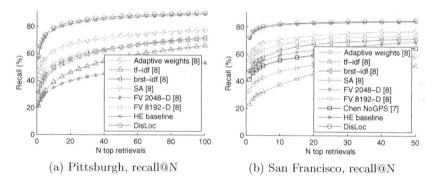

(a) Pittsburgh, recall@N   (b) San Francisco, recall@N

Fig. 4. Comparison with state of the art. The two graphs are taken from [8] and amended with our Hamming Embedding baseline and the DisLoc method. For the San Francisco dataset and this figure only, we use the April 2011 version of the ground truth for fair comparison with [7,8], as explained in Sect. 4.1.

Removal of Unhelpful Features. Figure 5 shows the effects of removing non-distinctive features, i.e. all features whose σ is estimated to be below a threshold are removed. It can be seen that removing 7 % of features doesn't change the localization performance, while quite good performance is maintained after removing 24 % of the features. Removing 50 % of features makes the system work worse than the baseline for $N < 55$. Therefore, without compromising localization quality one can save 7 % of storage/RAM while simultaneously increasing

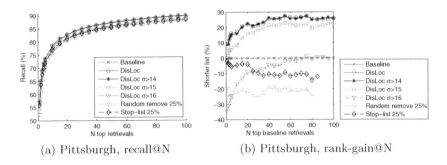

(a) Pittsburgh, recall@N   (b) Pittsburgh, rank-gain@N

Fig. 5. Removal of unhelpful features. Keeping only features for which DisLoc assigns σ larger than 14, 15 and 16 reduces storage/RAM requirements by 7 %, 24 % and 50 %. Random removal or stop-word removal of 25 % of features combined with the baseline method works much worse than the DisLoc competitors.

localization speed (as the posting lists get shorter due to a smaller number of features). With a small decrease in localization performance, a 24 % saving in storage is obtainable. We have observed similar trends on the San Francisco benchmark as well.

We compare the DisLoc-based feature removal method with two additional baselines which don't use automatic distinctiveness estimation: (1) random removal: discards 25 % of the features randomly (i.e. no selection criterion is used); and (2) stop-list [10]: removes 25 % of the features by discarding the most frequent visual words. Both strategies perform poorly (Fig. 5) compared to the DisLoc alternative – with the same number of removed features (25 %) DisLoc outperforms the two baselines with a large margin. Even with 50 % of the features removed, the DisLoc method significantly outperforms random removal for $N > 4$, as well as stop-list for $N > 25$.

4.4   Pushing the Localization Performance Further

In this section we evaluate using postprocessing methods to further increase place recognition performance.

Spatial Reranking. We use the standard fast spatial reranking method of [11] where the top 200 images are checked for spatial consistency with the query, using an affine transformation with verticality constraint. As expected, the method increases precision (Fig. 6) reflected in the increased recall at small N. For the San Francisco benchmark, DisLoc without spatial reranking beats the baseline with spatial reranking. Our method, DisLoc, continues to outperform the baseline method after spatial reranking on both benchmarks.

Unique Landmark Suggestions. In real-world location recognition, retrieval results should be processed to improve user experience. Namely, it would be frustrating for a user if a place recognition system provides the same wrong

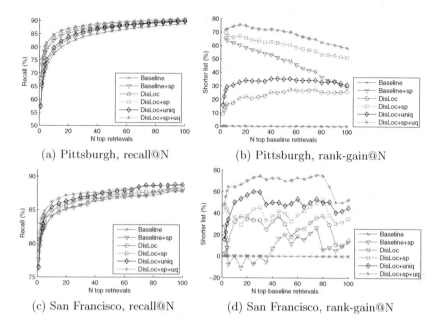

(a) Pittsburgh, recall@N (b) Pittsburgh, rank-gain@N

(c) San Francisco, recall@N (d) San Francisco, rank-gain@N

Fig. 6. Postprocessing performance evaluation. The "+sp" suffix signifies that spatial reranking is performed (on top 200 images), the "+uniq" suffix signifies that unique landmark suggestions are returned to the user. DisLoc continues to outperform the baseline after spatial reranking. For the San Francisco benchmark, DisLoc without spatial reranking outperforms the baseline with spatial reranking. Returning unique landmarks further improves the place recognition performance.

answer multiple times. Simple diversification of results alleviates this problem and prevents the user from being buried with false retrievals.

For the San Francisco dataset where building IDs are known for every database image, one can simply avoid returning the same building ID more than once, i.e. only the first instance of a building ID is kept. For the Pittsburgh dataset there is no building ID meta data available, but GPS coordinates of all database images are known. We therefore tessellate Pittsburgh into 25-by-25 m squares and only return the top ranked images from each square. For datasets which do not contain any meta information, a vision-based diversification approach can be used, such as [19,40,41].

As expected, the proposed diversification approach further improves location recognition performance (Fig. 6).

5 Conclusions

DisLoc has been shown to consistently outperform the baseline Hamming Embedding system on standard place recognition benchmarks: Pittsburgh and San Francisco landmarks, containing street-view images of those cities. Furthermore, DisLoc sets the state-of-the-art for both benchmarks by a large margin.

Standard post-processing methods such as spatial reranking and result diversification have been shown to be compatible with DisLoc, and to further improve its performance. Furthermore, non-distinctive local descriptors can be discarded from the inverted index, therefore lowering memory requirements by 7%–24% and speeding up the system.

Acknowledgement. We thank A. Torri and D. Chen for sharing their datasets, and are grateful for financial support from ERC grant VisRec no. 228180 and a Royal Society Wolfson Research Merit Award.

References

1. Quack, T., Leibe, B., Van Gool, L.: World-scale mining of objects and events from community photo collections. In: Proceedings of the CIVR (2008)
2. Chen, D.M., Tsai, S.S., Vedantham, R., Grzeszczuk, R., Girod, B.: Streaming mobile augmented reality on mobile phones. In: International Symposium on Mixed and Augmented Reality, ISMAR (2009)
3. Cummins, M., Newman, P.: FAB-MAP: probabilistic localization and mapping in the space of appearance. Int. J. Rob. Res. **27**, 647–665 (2008)
4. Agarwal, S., Snavely, N., Simon, I., Seitz, S.M., Szeliski, R.: Building Rome in a day. In: Proceedings of the ICCV (2009)
5. Schindler, G., Brown, M., Szeliski, R.: City-scale location recognition. In: Proceedings of the CVPR (2007)
6. Knopp, J., Sivic, J., Pajdla, T.: Avoiding confusing features in place recognition. In: Daniilidis, K., Maragos, P., Paragios, N. (eds.) ECCV 2010, Part I. LNCS, vol. 6311, pp. 748–761. Springer, Heidelberg (2010)
7. Chen, D.M., Baatz, G., Koeser, K., Tsai, S.S., Vedantham, R., Pylvanainen, T., Roimela, K., Chen, X., Bach, J., Pollefeys, M., Girod, B., Grzeszczuk, R.: City-scale landmark identification on mobile devices. In: Proceedings of the CVPR (2011)
8. Torii, A., Sivic, J., Pajdla, T., Okutomi, M.: Visual place recognition with repetitive structures. In: Proceedings of the CVPR (2013)
9. Lowe, D.: Distinctive image features from scale-invariant keypoints. IJCV **60**, 91–110 (2004)
10. Sivic, J., Zisserman, A.: Video Google: a text retrieval approach to object matching in videos. In: Proceedings of the ICCV, vol. 2, pp. 1470–1477 (2003)
11. Philbin, J., Chum, O., Isard, M., Sivic, J., Zisserman, A.: Object retrieval with large vocabularies and fast spatial matching. In: Proceedings of the CVPR (2007)
12. Nister, D., Stewenius, H.: Scalable recognition with a vocabulary tree. In: Proceedings of the CVPR, pp. 2161–2168 (2006)
13. Philbin, J., Chum, O., Isard, M., Sivic, J., Zisserman, A.: Lost in quantization: improving particular object retrieval in large scale image databases. In: Proceedings of the CVPR (2008)
14. Jégou, H., Douze, M., Schmid, C.: Improving bag-of-features for large scale image search. IJCV **87**, 316–336 (2010)
15. Jegou, H., Douze, M., Schmid, C.: Hamming embedding and weak geometric consistency for large scale image search. In: Forsyth, D., Torr, P., Zisserman, A. (eds.) ECCV 2008, Part I. LNCS, vol. 5302, pp. 304–317. Springer, Heidelberg (2008)

16. Philbin, J., Isard, M., Sivic, J., Zisserman, A.: Descriptor learning for efficient retrieval. In: Daniilidis, K., Maragos, P., Paragios, N. (eds.) ECCV 2010, Part III. LNCS, vol. 6313, pp. 677–691. Springer, Heidelberg (2010)
17. Simonyan, K., Vedaldi, A., Zisserman, A.: Learning local feature descriptors using convex optimisation. IEEE PAMI **36**, 1573–1585 (2014)
18. Gronat, P., Obozinski, G., Sivic, J., Pajdla, T.: Learning and calibrating per-location classifiers for visual place recognition. In: Proceedings of the CVPR (2013)
19. Cao, S., Snavely, N.: Graph-based discriminative learning for location recognition. In: Proceedings of the CVPR (2013)
20. Jégou, H., Douze, M., Schmid, C.: On the burstiness of visual elements. In: Proceedings of the CVPR (2009)
21. Jégou, H., Douze, M., Schmid, C.: Exploiting descriptor distances for precise image search. Technical report, INRIA (2011)
22. Aly, M., Munich, M., Perona, P.: CompactKdt: compact signatures for accurate large scale object recognition. In: IEEE Workshop on Applications of Computer Vision (2012)
23. Sattler, T., Weyand, T., Leibe, B., Kobbelt, L.: Image retrieval for image-based localization revisited. In: Proceedings of the BMVC (2012)
24. Tolias, G., Avrithis, Y., Jégou, H.: To aggregate or not to aggregate: selective match kernels for image search. In: Proceedings of the ICCV (2013)
25. Qin, D., Wengert, C., Van Gool, L.: Query adaptive similarity for large scale object retrieval. In: Proceedings of the CVPR (2013)
26. Turcot, T., Lowe, D.G.: Better matching with fewer features: the selection of useful features in large database recognition problems. In: ICCV Workshop on Emergent Issues in Large Amounts of Visual Data (WS-LAVD) (2009)
27. Philbin, J., Zisserman, A.: Object mining using a matching graph on very large image collections. In: Proceedings of the ICVGIP (2008)
28. Jégou, H., Harzallah, H., Schmid, C.: A contextual dissimilarity measure for accurate and efficient image search. In: Proceedings of the CVPR (2007)
29. Qin, D., Gammeter, S., Bossard, L., Quack, T., Van Gool, L.: Hello neighbor: accurate object retrieval with k-reciprocal nearest neighbors. In: Proceedings of the CVPR (2011)
30. Delvinioti, A., Jégou, H., Amsaleg, L., Houle, M.E.: Image retrieval with reciprocal and shared nearest neighbors. In: VISAPP - International Conference on Computer Vision Theory and Applications (2014)
31. Jégou, H., Douze, M., Schmid, C., Pérez, P.: Aggregating local descriptors into a compact image representation. In: Proceedings of the CVPR (2010)
32. Andoni, A., Indyk, P.: Near-optimal hashing algorithms for approximate nearest neighbor in high dimensions. Comm. ACM **51**, 117–122 (2008)
33. Tolias, G., Jégou, H.: Visual query expansion with or without geometry: refining local descriptors by feature aggregation. Pattern Recogn. **47**, 3466–3476 (2014)
34. Jégou, H., Douze, M., Schmid, C.: Product quantization for nearest neighbor search. IEEE PAMI **33**, 117–128 (2011)
35. Van der Maaten, L., Hinton, G.: Visualizing data using t-SNE. J. Mach. Learn. Res. **9**, 2579–2605 (2008)
36. Arandjelović, R., Zisserman, A.: Three things everyone should know to improve object retrieval. In: Proceedings of the CVPR (2012)
37. Mikolajczyk, K., Schmid, C.: Scale & affine invariant interest point detectors. IJCV **1**, 63–86 (2004)

38. Chum, O., Philbin, J., Sivic, J., Isard, M., Zisserman, A.: Total recall: automatic query expansion with a generative feature model for object retrieval. In: Proceedings of the ICCV (2007)
39. Chum, O., Mikulik, A., Perd'och, M., Matas, J.: Total recall II: query expansion revisited. In: Proceedings of the CVPR (2011)
40. Kennedy, L., Naaman, M.: Generating diverse and representative image search results for landmarks. In: Proceedings of the World Wide Web (2008)
41. van Leuken, R.H., Garcia, L., Olivares, X., van Zwol, R.: Visual diversification of image search results. In: Proceedings of the World Wide Web (2009)

Discriminative Collaborative Representation for Classification

Yang Wu[1](✉), Wei Li[2], Masayuki Mukunoki[1], Michihiko Minoh[1],
and Shihong Lao[3]

[1] Academic Center for Computing and Media Studies,
Kyoto University, Kyoto 606-8501, Japan
yangwu@mm.media.kyoto-u.ac.jp,
{mukunoki,minoh}@media.kyoto-u.ac.jp
[2] Institute of Scientific and Industrial Research, Osaka University,
Ibaraki-shi 567-0047, Japan
seuliwei@126.com
[3] OMRON Social Solutions Co., LTD, Kyoto 619-0283, Japan
lao_shihong@oss.omron.co.jp

Abstract. The recently proposed l_2-norm based collaborative representation for classification (CRC) model has shown inspiring performance on face recognition after the success of its predecessor — the l_1-norm based sparse representation for classification (SRC) model. Though CRC is much faster than SRC as it has a closed-form solution, it may have the same weakness as SRC, i.e., relying on a "good" (properly controlled) training dataset for serving as its dictionary. Such a weakness limits the usage of CRC in real applications because the quality requirement is not easy to verify in practice. Inspired by the encouraging progress on dictionary learning for sparse representation, which can much alleviate this problem, we propose the discriminative collaborative representation (DCR) model. It has a novel classification model well fitting its discriminative learning model. As a result, DCR has the same advantage of being efficient as CRC, while at the same time showing even stronger discriminative power than existing dictionary learning methods. Extensive experiments on nine widely used benchmark datasets for both controlled and uncontrolled classification tasks demonstrate its consistent effectiveness and efficiency.

1 Introduction

Sparse representation based classification (SRC) [1] has recently attracted a lot of attention due to its simplicity and striking performance on some visual classification tasks especially face recognition. While most followers have focused on exploring new applications or designing new dictionary learning models to

Electronic supplementary material The online version of this chapter (doi:10. 1007/978-3-319-16817-3_14) contains supplementary material, which is available to authorized users.

D. Cremers et al. (Eds.): ACCV 2014, Part IV, LNCS 9006, pp. 205–221, 2015.
DOI: 10.1007/978-3-319-16817-3_14

further improve its performance on those exemplary recognition tasks, there are also a few papers on exposing the intrinsic reasons for its effectiveness or even expressing different opinions. Among these voices, there is a distinctive argument: it is the collaborative representation of the test sample using all the training samples that truly results in SRC's success but not its l_1-norm based sparsity [2]. To prove that, a new model named collaborative representation based classification (CRC) has been proposed which uses the l_2-norm based regularization to replace the l_1-norm based sparsity term. Primary experiments on face recognition have shown that CRC performs no worse than SRC. However, considering that SRC requires a controlled training set with sufficient samples per class for ensuring a good performance [3], it is likely that CRC may need similar pre-conditions since both of them directly use the training data as the reconstruction dictionary.

To alleviate the dependence on the quality of training data, great efforts have been put into dictionary learning (DL) models [4–6] for enhancing SRC. They generally aim at learning a dictionary and/or classification model for better exploring the discriminative ability of the training data. Existing DL approaches are very diverse in model design and optimization, resulting in different performances and speeds. As far as we are aware, these approaches are all proposed for sparse representation, and the l_0-norm or l_1-norm based sparsity usually leads to a high computational cost. Since the efficient l_2-norm based collaborative representation has already shown some of its discriminative power, it is interesting and valuable to see whether DL can also be explored to further improve its performance while at the same time keep being efficient. This study is planned for presenting the first attempt in this direction.

More concretely, we propose a novel dictionary learning model called discriminative collaborative representation (DCR), which has stronger discriminative power than state-of-the-art DL models while at the same time utilizes the efficient l_2-norm to regularize the representation coefficients. In addition to that, a novel classification model directly derived from the learning model is adopted. We will show that DCR learns faster and performs better than its competitors on various classification tasks.

2   Related Work

Dictionary learning has recently become an active research topic. Though it has been used for many applications, we are focusing on classification tasks.

As its name shows, dictionary learning approaches usually directly target at learning a discriminative dictionary. A representative work is the meta-face learning approach [7] which learns class-specific sub-dictionaries independently. Later on, the DLSI model [8] was proposed to improve the discrimination ability of the sub-dictionaries and also explore their shared common bases via exploring the incoherence between the sub-dictionaries. Very recently, a new model called DL-COPAR [6] develops DLSI's idea on exploring the common bases of sub-dictionaries [8] by explicitly separating the particularity (class-specific sub-dictionaries) and commonality (a common sub-dictionary) in dictionary learning.

There are also some other approaches working in the direction of learning a discriminative classification model using the sparse representation coefficients. Representative approaches include supervised dictionary learning [9] using the logistic regression model, discriminative K-SVD (D-KSVD) [10] with a linear regression model, and the label consistent K-SVD (LC-KSVD) model [4] which adds one more linear regression term to D-KSVD to further enhance the label consistency within each class.

Taking into account the effectiveness of both directions, the work of Fisher discrimination dictionary learning (FDDL) [5] explicitly combines discriminative dictionary learning and coefficients based classification model learning, and uses both of them in its two classification models as well.

The proposed DCR, however, integrates the key ideas behind all these three groups and uses l_2-norm regularization terms for efficiency while pursuing effectiveness and comprehensiveness. Moreover, DCR has a novel classification model which coincides well with its learning model. The model optimization with closed-form solutions for alternating steps and the comprehensiveness of experiments in this paper are also different from those in the literature.

It's worth noticing that the work of Discriminative k-metrics [11] extends q-flats to metrics and introduces discrimination, resulting in a similar formula with part of DCR. However, its collaborative representation (CR) exists only in within-class metrics, while DCR is an inter-class CR model. The work on structured sparsity [12] also has a CR-like model, but it embeds GMM/MAP-EM for representation and uses PCA to generate dictionary and regularize coefficients, which are much unlike DCR.

3 Discriminative Collaborative Representation

3.1 Sparse/Collaborative Representation

Given a training dataset $X = [X_1, \ldots, X_L] \in \mathbb{R}^{d \times n}$, where n denotes the total number of samples, d denotes their feature dimension, L is the number of classes, and $X_i, \forall i \in \{1, \ldots, L\}$ denotes the n_i samples belonging to class i. Both sparse representation and collaborative representation seeks a linear combination of all the training samples X to best reconstruct an arbitrary test sample $y \in \mathbb{R}^d$. And such a reconstruction is regularized by some norm of the reconstruction coefficients to make the solution unique. It can be modeled by the following optimization problem:

$$\hat{\alpha} = \arg\min_{\alpha} \|y - X\alpha\|_2^2 + \lambda_1 \|\alpha\|_p, \tag{1}$$

where λ_1 is a trade-off parameter for balancing the reconstruction error and the squared norm of α. In general, the l_p-norm can be any feasible norm. Since l_0-norm leads to a combinatorial optimization problem which is hard to be solved efficiently, SRC chooses the l_1-norm which to some extent ensures the sparsity of α, coinciding with the belief that the sparse coefficients have great discriminative ability. Differently, CRC takes the l_2-norm (actually the squared l_2-norm is used for easier optimization) which cannot make α sparse any more, but it leads to an efficient closed-form solution with good classification performance [2] as well.

3.2 Dictionary Learning for DCR

Reconstruction using the training data itself makes the performance of SRC and CRC largely depend on the properties of the training data X. To alleviate such a dependance, there is a research direction of learning a better dictionary D from X to replace it for the reconstruction. Inspired by the existing dictionary learning (DL) approaches, we design our dictionary learning model for DCR as:

$$\langle D^*, W^*, T^*, A^* \rangle = \arg \min_{D, W, T, A} \left\{ r\left(X, D, A\right) + \lambda \left(\|A\|_F^2 + \|D\|_F^2 \right) + \gamma f\left(W, T, A\right) \right\}, \quad (2)$$

where $D \in \mathbb{R}^{d \times K}$ with K items is the learned dictionary from X (usually $K \leq n$); $A \in \mathbb{R}^{K \times n}$ denotes the reconstruction coefficients over D for all the n training samples; W and T denote the learned parameters of the discriminative model $f(W, T, A)$ for classification with A; $r(X, D, A)$ is the discriminative reconstruction model defined over D (called the discriminative fidelity in [5]); $\|\cdot\|_F$ denotes the Frobenius norm which is a generalization of l_2-norm from dealing with vectors to operating on matrices. λ and γ are two unavoidable trade-off parameters, for which the discussion will be given in Sect. 4.

Most of the existing DL models can be covered by the above general model if we replace the Frobenius norm with a sum of l_0-norms or l_1-norms (except some models do not have the $f(W, T, A)$ term). The differences of them mainly consist in their detailed design of $r(X, D, A)$, $f(W, T, A)$ and the regularization of D, which largely influences the performance and speed of the model. Different from existing models, we propose to use the following formula for $r(X, D, A)$ in our model:

$$r\left(X, D, A\right) = \|X - DA\|_F^2 + \sum_{i=1}^{L} \left\| X_i - D_i A_i^i - D_0 A_i^0 \right\|_F^2 + \sum_{i=1}^{L} \sum_{j=1, j \neq i}^{L} \left\| D_i A_j^i \right\|_F^2. \quad (3)$$

In this formula, $D = [D_0, D_1, \ldots, D_L]$ denotes the dictionary to be learned, where D_0 is a common sub-dictionary shared by all the classes while D_i with $i \in \{1, \ldots, L\}$ stands for a class-specific sub-dictionary. Accordingly, A_j^i denotes the coefficients corresponding to the sub-dictionary D_i for those samples from X_j (i.e. the columns of A_j^i correspond to class j). When the physical meanings are concerned, the first term is the *global reconstruction error* (ensuring that the whole dictionary D can well represent X); the second term is the *class-specific reconstruction error* (forcing D_i together with D_0 to be able to well represent X_i); and the third term is the *confusion factor* (restricting D_i's ability on reconstructing samples from any other classes rather than i). Please note that the first term and the second term are not the same. The second term doesn't count $D_j, \forall j \neq i$. Putting them together is to force D discriminative.

For $f(W, T, A)$, we use the same discriminative model as the one for LC-KSVD [4] (more precisely the LC-KSVD2 model in the original paper)[1]:

$$f(W, T, A) = 4 \|Q - TA\|_F^2 + \|H - WA\|_F^2,   \tag{4}$$

where $H = [\mathbf{h}_1, ..., \mathbf{h}_n] \in \mathbb{R}^{L \times n}$ are label vectors for X with $\mathbf{h}_i = [0, \ldots, 0, 1, 0, \ldots, 0]^T \in \mathbb{R}^L$ indicating which class $\mathbf{x}_i$ is belonging to, and $Q = [\mathbf{q}_1, ..., \mathbf{q}_n] \in \mathbb{R}^{K \times n}$ are ideal sparse codes for X with $\mathbf{q}_i = [0, \ldots, 0, 1, \ldots, 1, 0, \ldots, 0]^T \in \mathbb{R}^K$ in which only the items corresponding to D_k is 1 when $\mathbf{x}_i$ is belonging to class k. In fact, given the structure of D, Q can be directly derived from H. The discriminative model aims at learning a linear mapping T which can map the coefficients A to the desired Q, while at the same time learning a linear regression model W which can transfer A to its corresponding label vectors. Therefore, W can be viewed as the model parameters of a linear classifier, while T acts like a parter of W which has greater modeling ability (with more parameters) than it. Such a design has been proved to be very effective in LC-KSVD, and it is more efficient than the Fisher discriminant based discriminative model in FDDL.

3.3   Optimization

Like other DL models, the optimization can only be done by alteratively optimize model parameters (D, T, and W) and coefficients A until convergence.

Initialization D and A. We simply utilize principle component analysis (PCA) to initialize D_0 and $D_i, \forall i \in \{1, \ldots, L\}$ with X and X_i, respectively. However, it is also possible to initialize D with random numbers, which will only cost a few more optimization iterations.

Unfortunately, there is no plausible way to initialize T and W without knowing A, while initializing A also needs some existing T and W. Therefore, we choose to discard $f(W, T, A)$ at first, so that A can be initialized based only on an initial D. More concretely, A can be computed in a class-by-class way thanks to the decomposition ability of the Frobenius norm. In another word, for each $i \in \{1, \ldots, L\}$, A_i can be initialized independently as follows.

$$A_i^* = \arg\min_{A_i} \left\{ \|X_i - DA_i\|_F^2 + \left\|X_i - DS_{0i}S_{0i}^T A_i\right\|_F^2 + \left\|DS_{\backslash 0i}S_{\backslash 0i}^T A_i\right\|_F^2 + \lambda \|A_i\|_F^2 \right\},   \tag{5}$$

where

$$S_i = \begin{bmatrix} O_{\sum_{m=1}^{i-1} K_m \times K_i} \\ I_{K_i \times K_i} \\ O_{\sum_{m=i+1}^{L} K_m \times K_i} \end{bmatrix}, \forall i \in \{0, 1, \ldots, L\},   \tag{6}$$

$$S_{0i} = [S_0, S_i],$$
$$S_{\backslash 0i} = [S_1, \cdots, S_{i-1}, S_{i+1}, \cdots, S_L],$$

---

[1] We follow LC-KSVD on balancing the two parts with a factor of 4 for simplicity, though a better factor may exist.

with $K_i, i \in \{0, 1, \ldots, L\}$ denoting the dictionary size of D_i. Here S_{0i} is a matrix for selecting D_0 and D_i, while $S_{\backslash 0i}$ is for discarding D_0 and D_i. O and I denote the zero matrix and the identity matrix, respectively. The optimization problem of Eq. 5 can be rewritten into a simpler form

$$A_i^* = \arg\min_{A_i} \left\{ \|R_i - Z_i A_i\|_F^2 + \lambda \|A_i\|_F^2 \right\}, \tag{7}$$

where

$$R_i = \begin{bmatrix} X_i \\ X_i \\ O_{d \times n_i} \end{bmatrix}, Z_i = \begin{bmatrix} D \\ D S_{0i} S_{0i}^T \\ D S_{\backslash 0i} S_{\backslash 0i}^T \end{bmatrix}. \tag{8}$$

Therefore, A_i has a computationally very efficient closed-form solution just like the CRC model:

$$A_i^* = \left(Z_i^T Z_i + \lambda \cdot I \right)^{-1} Z_i^T R_i. \tag{9}$$

Optimizing D, T, and W When Given A. Once A is given, the term $\lambda \|A\|_F^2$ becomes a constant, however, D is still impossible to be optimized as a whole because the objective function in Eq. 2 has two terms which are functions of sub-dictionaries $D_i, i \in \{0, 1, \ldots, L\}$ but not the overall dictionary D. Therefore, we optimize D_is one-by-one, assuming the others are fixed.

First, for each **class-specific sub-dictionary** $D_i, i \in \{1, \ldots, L\}$, suppose all $D_j, j \in \{0, \ldots, L\}, j \neq i$ are fixed, we can reform the objective function for optimizing D_i as

$$D_i^* = \arg\min_{D_i} \left\{ \|U_i - D_i V_i\|_F^2 + \lambda \|D_i\|_F^2 \right\}, \tag{10}$$

where

$$U_i = \left[X - D_{\backslash i} A^{\backslash i}, (X_i - D_0 A_i^0), O_{d \times (n - n_i)} \right], \quad V_i = \left[A^i, A_i^i, A_{\backslash i}^i \right]. \tag{11}$$

In Eq. 11, $D_{\backslash i}$ denotes all the $D_j, j \in \{0, \ldots, L\}, j \neq i$ together and $A^{\backslash i}$ denotes their corresponding coefficients (i.e. without A^i). Conceptually, "$\backslash i$" means without class i. $O_{d \times (n - n_i)}$ denotes a $d \times (n - n_i)$ dimensional zero matrix, where $n_i, i \in \{1, \ldots, L\}$ is the number of samples in class i and $n = \sum_{i=1}^{L} n_i$. Equation 10 has a closed-form solution

$$D_i^* = U_i V_i^T \left(V_i V_i^T + \lambda \cdot I \right)^{-1}. \tag{12}$$

Then, for the **common sub-dictionary** D_0, when $D_i, i \in \{1, \ldots, L\}$ are all given, the optimizing objective function for D_0 can also be reformed as

$$D_0^* = \arg\min_{D_0} \left\{ \|U_0 - D_0 V_0\|_F^2 + \lambda \|D_0\|_F^2 \right\}, \tag{13}$$

where

$$U_0 = \left[X - D_{\backslash 0} A^{\backslash 0}, (X - D_{\backslash 0} \hat{A}^{\backslash 0}) \right], \quad V_0 = \left[A^0, A^0 \right], \tag{14}$$

with

$$\hat{A}^{\backslash 0} = \begin{bmatrix} A_1^1 & 0 & \cdots & 0 \\ 0 & A_2^2 & \cdots & 0 \\ \vdots & \vdots & \ddots & \vdots \\ 0 & 0 & \cdots & A_L^L \end{bmatrix}. \tag{15}$$

Similarly, Eq. 13 has a closed-form solution

$$D_0^* = U_0 V_0^T \left(V_0 V_0^T + \lambda \cdot I \right)^{-1}. \tag{16}$$

After getting A and D, optimizing T becomes solving a simple linear regression problem:

$$T^* = \arg\min_T \|Q - TA\|_F^2, \tag{17}$$

whose solution is $T^* = QA^T(AA^T)^{-1}$. Similarly, W also has a closed-form solution $W^* = HA^T(AA^T)^{-1}$.

Note that optimizing D_i depends on a given $D_{\backslash i}$, therefore, once D_i is updated, it should be used to update each $D_j, j \neq i$ in $D_{\backslash i}$. This is a chicken-and-egg problem, so a straightforward solution is updating all the D_is iteratively until they are converged (i.e. getting very small changes). However, since we are iterating between optimizing A and updating D, T, and W, a converged D will soon been changed once A is recomputed. Therefore, in our implementation, we ignored the iteration in D's optimization, and found that it still worked very well for our experiments.

Optimizing A When Given D, T, and W. Similar to initializing A, when D, T, and W are given, optimizing A is equivalent to optimizing A_i for each $i \in \{1, \ldots, L\}$ independently as follows.

$$A_i^* = \arg\min_{A_i} \left\{ \begin{array}{l} \|X_i - DA_i\|_F^2 + \|X_i - DS_{0i}S_{0i}^T A_i\|_F^2 + \|DS_{\backslash 0i}S_{\backslash 0i}^T A_i\|_F^2 \\ +\lambda \|A_i\|_F^2 + \gamma \left(4 \|Q_i - TA_i\|_F^2 + \|H_i - WA_i\|_F^2 \right) \end{array} \right\}, \tag{18}$$

which is very much like Eq. 5 except the last two additional terms, and it can be rewritten into Eq. 7 as well, leading to the same solution as Eq. 9. The differences are the values of R_i and Z_i, which now contain two extra terms about T and W as follows.

$$R_i = \begin{bmatrix} X_i \\ X_i \\ O_{d \times n_i} \\ 2\sqrt{\gamma}Q_i \\ \sqrt{\gamma}H_i \end{bmatrix}, Z_i = \begin{bmatrix} D \\ DS_{0i}S_{0i}^T \\ DS_{\backslash 0i}S_{\backslash 0i}^T \\ 2\sqrt{\gamma}T \\ \sqrt{\gamma}W \end{bmatrix}. \tag{19}$$

3.4   Classification Model

After learning D, T, and W from training samples, we can use them for classifying an input test sample $\mathbf{y}$, or a set of test samples Y for set-based classification.

Both tasks will be verified in our experiments. For simplicity, we use Y to stand for both cases, i.e., Y can be a feature vector for single sample or a matrix whose columns are individual samples belonging to the same set.

Unlike the classification models in the existing approaches, our classification model for DCR directly coincides with its dictionary learning model. For each candidate class $i \in \{1, \ldots, L\}$, suppose Y belongs to class i, then we can compute A_i according to:

$$A_i^* = \arg\min_{A_i} \left\{ \begin{array}{c} \|Y - DA_i\|_F^2 + \|Y - DS_{0i}S_{0i}^T A_i\|_F^2 + \|DS_{\backslash 0i}S_{\backslash 0i}^T A_i\|_F^2 \\ + \lambda \|A_i\|_F^2 + \gamma \left(4 \|Q_i - TA_i\|_F^2 + \|H_i - WA_i\|_F^2\right) \end{array} \right\}, \quad (20)$$

whose solution has exactly the same form as the one for Eq. 18. The only change needs to make is replacing X_i with Y. Therefore, we get a collaborative representation error $E_i(Y)$ for class i:

$$E_i(Y) = \|Y - DA_i^*\|_F^2 + \|Y - DS_{0i}S_{0i}^T A_i^*\|_F^2 + \|DS_{\backslash 0i}S_{\backslash 0i}^T A_i^*\|_F^2$$
$$+ \lambda \|A_i^*\|_F^2 + \gamma \left(4 \|Q_i - TA_i^*\|_F^2 + \|H_i - WA_i^*\|_F^2\right). \quad (21)$$

Then Y is classified by

$$C(Y) = \arg\min_i E_i(Y). \quad (22)$$

We do have tried other existing classification models like the linear projection model for LC-KSVD and found that they are not as good as the proposed classification model, which fits the learning model better and looks more reasonable. Detailed comparison is omitted in this paper due to the space limits.

3.5   Convergence and Computational Complexity

We present the computational complexity for each component/operation of our dictionary learning model and the classification model in Table 1. Since the components of our models only contain simple matrix operations, these complexity functions can be easily verified by checking the corresponding equations. Note that we have used the assumption $L \ll K$, which is generally true, for simplifying some of them when it is necessary. It has been proved that alternating optimization (AO) globally converges for iteration sequences initialized at arbitrary points and it is locally, q-linearly (faster than linearly) convergent to any local minimizer that satisfies some mild assumptions [13], so the AO algorithms can usually converge very quickly. In our case, DCR always converges within 3 to 8 iterations in all the experiments to be presented.[2] Therefore, the subtotal complexity listed in the training stage, which covers the initialization and a single iteration, can also stand for the complexity of the whole alternative optimization process. It can be seen that DCR scales less than linearly with d, L, and n, but nearly proportionally to K^3. Therefore, when the dictionary size is fixed/predetermined, it scales well with the dimensionality of the data and the

---

[2] Please refer to the supplementary material for more discussions and experimental results.

Table 1. Computational complexity of DCR. d, K, L, and n refer to the feature dimensionality, the size of the dictionary, the number of classes and the number of samples, respectively.

Training (Dictionary Learning)	
Operation	**Complexity**
Initializing A	$\mathcal{O}\left(dK^2L + K^3L + dKn\right)$
Optimizing D	$\mathcal{O}\left(dKLn + n\sum_{i=0}^{L} K_i^2 + \sum_{i=0}^{L} K_i^3\right)$
• Computing U_i	$\mathcal{O}\left(dn\sum_{j\neq i} K_j + dK_0 n_i\right)$
• Computing D_i^*	$\mathcal{O}\left(dK_i n + n\sum_{i=1}^{L} K_i^2 + \sum_{i=1}^{L} K_i^3\right)$
• Computing $U_0 \& D_0^*$	$\mathcal{O}\left(dK_0 n + nK_0^2 + K_0^3\right)$
Optimizing T	$\mathcal{O}\left(K^2 n + K^3\right)$
Optimizing W	$\mathcal{O}\left(KLn + K^2 n + K^3 +\right)$
Optimizing A	$\mathcal{O}\left((d + K + L)K(KL + n)\right)$
• Computing $Z_i \& A_i^*$	$\mathcal{O}\left((d + K + L)K(K + n_i)\right)$
Sub-total	$\mathcal{O}\left((K + n)dKL + K^3L + K^2 n\right)$

Testing (Classifying) each sample	
Operation	**Complexity**
Optimizing A	$\mathcal{O}\left((d + K + L)KL\right)$
Computing $E_i(Y), \forall i$	$\mathcal{O}\left((d + K + L)KL\right)$
Classification	$\mathcal{O}(L)$
Sub-total	$\mathcal{O}\left((d + K + L)KL\right)$

number of samples. In the testing stage, classifying a single sample has a reasonable complexity. Note that it is benefited from the fact that $\left(Z_i^T Z_i + \lambda \cdot I\right)^{-1} Z_i^T$ can be pre-computed using the learned model. As it will be shown in the next section, DCR has a significantly more efficient learning model than other related dictionary learning methods, while its classification model is comparable to the best of them in efficiency.

4   Experiments on Real-World Applications

We try DCR on solving various real-world classification problems including face recognition in controlled laboratory environments, uncontrolled person re-identification in a real airport surveillance scenario, texture classification with great scale, viewpoint, and illumination changes, and fine-grained object categorization for differentiating leaf species and food subcategories. For each of these four types of classification problems, we choose two different and representative benchmark datasets for evaluating the performance of DCR, comparing with CRC, SRC, and other related dictionary learning models including FDDL, LC-KSVD, and DL-COPAR. We used the version of SRC embedded in the FDDL code, and implemented CRC by ourselves. Codes for all the other methods were got from their authors. State-of-the-art results on specific datasets from other unrelated methods are also listed for reference. Whenever applicable, we conduct 10 times random training and test data sampling for result averaging.

For a clear overview and comparison of all the experiments and their corresponding results, we briefly introduce each classification problem and the concrete tasks, whilst having the dataset statistics listed together with the classification performance in uniform tables. Representative samples images are given to those less well-known datasets for a better understanding. To be brief and clear, the analysis and discussion of the results is stated in a separate subsection after the individual subsections.

4.1 Experimental Settings

The same features and sub-dictionary sizes (for DL models only) have been used for all these models to ensure a relatively fair comparison. Though it is possible that different models may favor different dictionary size settings, it is unaffordable to perform a brute-force best setting search for each of them on every dataset due to its high computational cost. Concretely, we had the sub-dictionary sizes (K_0 and $K_i, i \in \{1, \ldots, L\}$) chosen as follows: $K_0 = 5$ and $K_i = 15$ for the Extended Yale B dataset; $K_0 = 3$ and $K_i = 6$ for the AR dataset; $K_0 = 10$ and $K_i = 23$ for the iLIDS-MA dataset; $K_0 = 4$ and $K_i = 8$ for the iLIDS-AA dataset; $K_0 = 2$ and $K_i = 10$ for the KTH-TIPS dataset; $K_0 = 5$ and $K_i = 15$ for the CUReT dataset; $K_0 = 3$ and $K_i = 10$ for the Swedish Leaf dataset; and $K_0 = 3$ and $K_i = 6$ for the PFID Food dataset. For the comparisons with the ScatNet features on texture classification datasets, we have $K_0 = 2$ and K_i equal to the number of training samples per class for every setting. For all our experiments, we used the same trade-off parameters for DCR: $\lambda = 1.0 \times 10^{-4}$ and $\gamma = 2.5 \times 10^{-7}$. For the other methods, we had the following setting for their trade-off parameters (fixed as well): $\lambda = 1.0 \times 10^{-4}$ for SRC and CRC; $\lambda_1 = 1.0 \times 10^{-4}$, $\lambda_2 = 5.0 \times 10^{-3}$, $\gamma = 0.001$ and $w = 0.05$ for FDDL; $\alpha = 1.0 \times 10^{-6}$, and $\beta = 2.5 \times 10^{-7}$ for LC-KSVD. These parameters were chosen by extensive but not brute-force testing for making the results as good as possible for all the methods, while at the same time made to be consistent across them. It's worth mentioning that DCR's performance is stable w.r.t. a large range of λ (from 10^{-8} to 10^{-2}) and γ (from 0 to 10^{-4}). Details on how the performances change with these parameters are omitted due to the space limit. The other parameters (if exist) for the methods compared with were kept as they are in their original codes.

4.2 Experiment Details

Controlled Face Recognition. Face recognition, more specifically, controlled face recognition in laboratory environments, has been tested on by almost every sparse/collaborative representation based model. We follow such a tradition and choose two widely-used benchmark datasets for our experiments: the Extended Yale B [14] dataset and the AR [15] dataset. The former one contains illumination and facial expression variations, while the later covers one more variation – disguises changes. The AR dataset used here is the one mentioned in [1] and [5], which is a subset of the original dataset. We use the same 504-dimensional feature representation (generated by random matrix projection) as the one adopted in

Table 2. The benchmark datasets used for face recognition, their statistics, and the average recognition accuracy for each compared method. The best results are in bold, while those worth mentioning are marked in italic.

Dataset	Statistics				Performance of Methods (%)					
	Samples	Classes	Training samples (per Class)	Test samples (per Class)	SRC	CRC	FDDL	LC-KSVD	DL-COPAR	DCR
	(NS)	(NC)	(NTrS(/NC))	(NTsS(/NC))	[1]	[2]	[5]	[4]	[6]	
Ext. Yale B	2414	38	half ($\sim$ 32)	half ($\sim$ 32)	95.1	*97.6*	96.8	94.4	92.8	**98.2**
AR	1400	100	700 (7)	700 (7)	89.8	*91.9*	91.7	67.7	69.4	**93.4**

[4] for Extended Yale B dataset, and the 300-dimensional Eigenfaces for AR dataset. The statistics of the experimental data and the final recognition rates are presented in Table 2.

Uncontrolled Person Re-identification. Person re-identification is a problem of identifying people again when they travel across non-overlapping cameras or reappear in the view of the same camera after disappearing for some time. Though any possible cues can be used for solving it, body appearance is mostly concerned. Since almost all the benchmark datasets were built from data captured in real scenarios without specific environmental settings, it is a good uncontrolled recognition problem which is much unlike the above face recognition problem.

In this paper, we work on the two newly built datasets "iLIDS-MA" and "iLIDS-AA" [16] collected from the i-LIDS video surveillance data captured at an airport. This data was originally released by the Home Office of UK. Both of them contain multiple images for each human individual captured by two non-overlapping cameras (camera 1 and camera 3 in their original setting), and there are large viewpoint changes. The iLIDS-MA dataset has 40 persons with exactly 46 manually cropped images per camera for each person, while the iLIDS-AA dataset contains as many as 100 individuals with totally 10754 images (each individual has 21 to 243 images) collected by an automatic tracking algorithm (thus localization errors and unequal class sizes may exist). For result averaging, we random sample certain amount of images per person (23 for iLIDS-MA, and up to 46 for iLIDS-AA) from each camera for training and test, respectively. Some randomly chosen samples are shown in Fig. 1. We use the same 400-dimensional color and texture histograms based features as adopted in [17] for all the methods. Following [18], we perform multiple-shot re-identification (i.e., set-based classification). Therefore, the set-based classification model of DCR is used, while the simple minimum point-wise distance between two sets is adopted for other methods except CSA [18]. Since personal re-identification is commonly treated as a ranking problem and we expect to see the correct match in the top-ranked few candidates, we report the cumulative recognition rate at rank top 10 % instead of the rank-1 recognition accuracy. The results are shown in Table 3.

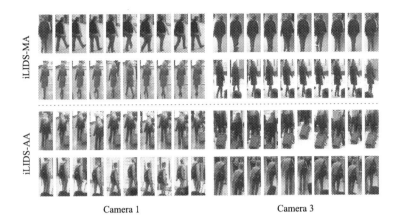

Camera 1   Camera 3

Fig. 1. Some randomly chosen image examples of iLIDS-MA and iLIDS-AA datasets.

Table 3. The benchmark datasets used for person re-identification, their statistics, and the average recognition rates (at rank 10 %) of compared methods. The best results are in bold, while those worth mentioning are marked in italic.

Dataset	Statistics				Performance of methods (%)						
	NS	NC	NTrS(/NC)	NTsS(/NC)	CSA [18]	SRC	CRC	FDDL	LC-KSVD	DL-COPAR	DCR
iLIDS-MA	3680	40	920 (23)	920 (23)	80.5	77.0	72.3	82.3	82.3	**85.3**	*83.3*
iLIDS-AA	≤9200	100	≤4600 (≤46)	≤4600 (≤46)	51.5	*77.9*	64.2	70.0	73.7	*66.6*	**80.3**

Texture Classification. Unlike other classification tasks, texture classification is useful for verifying the effectiveness of a classification model on working with the texture cue only. Two representative benchmark datasets: KTH-TIPS with 10 classes and CUReT with 61 classes, are chosen for our experiments because they both have enough samples for each class (satisfying SRC's one precondition). However, these two datasets share the same difficulty of having great within-class variations including illumination, viewpoint and scale changes. We use the PRI-CoLBP$_0$ feature proposed in [19] as the raw feature representation which is designed to be somewhat robust to these variations. By doing so, it is more meaningful to compare our results with the state-of-the-art shown in [19], which was generated by Kernel SVM (KSVM) with a χ^2 kernel. The experimental results are listed in Table 4.

Fine-Grained Object Categorization. Fine-grained object categorization concerns the classification of sub-categories, thus it lies in the continuum between basic level categorization and identification of individuals. Though it has not been as popular as those two extremes, recently its importance has been rediscovered by the community. We experiment on two specific tasks: identifying leaf species in the popular Swedish leaf dataset, and classifying fast food subcategories in the subset of 61 food classes from the Pittsburgh Food Image

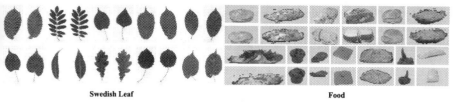

Swedish Leaf   Food

Fig. 2. Some representative samples from the Swedish leaf dataset and the Pittsburgh Food Image Dataset, respectively.

Table 4. The benchmark datasets used for texture classification, their statistics, and the average recognition accuracy for each compared method. The best results are in bold, while those worth mentioning are marked in italic.

Dataset	NS	NC	Statistics					Performance of Methods (%)							
			NTrS (/NC)	NTsS (/NC)	Zhang et al.[20]	Caputo et al.[21]	KSVM [19]	SVM	SRC	CRC	FDDL	LC-KSVD	DL-COPAR	DCR
KTH-TIPS	810	10	400 (40)	410 (41)	96.1	94.8	98.3	86.1	95.7	*97.1*	69.9	88.5	*58.5*	**98.7**
CUReT	5612	61	2806 (46)	2806 (46)	95.3	98.5	98.6	82.9	82.4	*93.3*	4.9	93.0	*10.3*	**98.9**

Dataset (PFID) [23]. These two tasks covers the problem of using mainly shape cue and the one which is rich of color, texture and shape information. The PFID dataset is more challenging due to the large within-class variations and possibly different data distributions in the training and test subsets. More concretely, there are 3 different instances in the same food sub-category, which were bought from different chain stores on different days, and each instance has six images taken from different viewpoints. In our experiment, two instances are randomly chosen for training while the other is left for testing, so we had 3 trials for result averaging. Representative samples from these two datasets are shown in Fig. 2, and the categorization accuracies can be found in Table 5.

4.3   Result Analysis and Discussion

All the results shown above clearly demonstrate the effectiveness and robustness of DCR. On seven of the eight datasets, DCR performs the best, exceeding all related models and those methods which represent the state-of-the-art. For only iLIDS-MA dataset, its performance is slightly lower than DL-COPAR, but still

Table 5. The benchmark datasets used for fine-grained object categorization, their statistics, and the average recognition accuracy for each compared method. The best results are in bold, while those worth mentioning are marked in italic.

Dataset	NS	NC	Statistics				Performance of Methods (%)							
			NTrS (/NC)	NTsS (/NC)	Spatial PACT [22]	Yang et al. [23]	SVM	SRC	CRC	FDDL	LC-KSVD	DL-COPAR	DCR
Swedish Leaf	1125	15	375 (25)	750 (50)	97.9	N/A	95.0	95.8	*99.1*	92.2	99.0	*43.7*	**99.2**
Food	1098	61	732 (12)	366 (6)	N/A	28.2	18.4	31.1	*34.9*	17.5	22.0	*16.7*	**37.3**

Table 6. The benchmark datasets used for texture classification, their statistics, and the average recognition accuracy for each compared method. The best results are in bold, while those worth mentioning are marked in italic.

Dataset	Statistics				Performance of Methods (%)					
	NS	NC	NTrS (/NC)	NTsS (/NC)	KSVM [19]	SRC	CRC	LC-KSVD	ScatNet [24]	DCR DCR
KTH-TIPS_5	810	10	50 (5)	760 (76)	64.4	19.9	35.7	56.6	70.4	**75.0**
KTH-TIPS_20	810	10	200 (20)	610 (61)	83.3	22.5	50.3	60.4	*94.39*	**94.41**
KTH-TIPS_40	810	10	400 (40)	410 (41)	88.6	24.7	54.1	73.6	*97.7*	**97.8**
UIUC_5	1000	25	125 (5)	815 (35)	33.6	21.3	30.0	47.5	49.5	**57.6**
UIUC_10	1000	25	250 (10)	750 (30)	30.2	24.0	34.8	52.0	60.8	**71.4**
UIUC_20	1000	25	500 (20)	500 (20)	28.5	27.6	41.8	61.6	74.6	**78.4**

higher than all the others. The high scores on texture datasets and the leaf dataset are mainly because the adopted PRI-CoLBP$_0$ features themselves are already very effective (see KSVM's or SVM's performance) and there are plenty of samples per class. Though we have tried our best to use the original codes from the authors for the existing methods (like SRC), there may be slight differences between the results reported in the literature and the ones shown here, which may be due to the usage of different features, different data caused by random sampling, and possibly slightly different parameter settings. Note that FDDL and DL-COPAR seem to significantly over-fit the training data on the last four datasets, which is even worse than using SRC itself.

Though we've already shown some state-of-the-art results from unrelated methods, there are definitely uncovered ones, especially when different features are used. In order to show the superiority of proposed classifier DCR, we take texture classification as an example to show how it performs comparing with those strongest competitors using the same newly proposed feature ScatNet [24]. We use the latest code of ScatNet from its authors, and have the method proposed in [24] (ScatNet with a linear SVM classifier) included for comparison as well (simply denoted by "ScatNet"). Since the KTH-TIPS dataset is enhanced from CUReT, we use another dataset UIUC instead of CUReT for the comparison, and set different sample sizes (number of samples per class) to show how this factor influence the performances. The results presented in Table 6 demonstrate that DCR consistently performs better than that of ScatNet and other methods which are most competitive in former experiments, especially in the small sample size cases.

In general, there are two important conclusions which could be easily derived from the details of the results.

1. *DCR learns a good dictionary for collaborative representation.* In all the experiments, dictionary learning in DCR consistently and greatly improves the performance of collaborative representation (compared with CRC).
2. *DCR appears less over-fitting and more effective than other dictionary learning models in our experiments*, which is very significant, especially on those datasets with few samples per class (such as AR, Food, KTH-TIPS_5, UIUC_5,

Table 7. Computational cost comparison with all the related methods on all concerned classification tasks. The best results are in bold, and the best results for dictionary learning based methods are underlined.

Dataset	Training Time (ms/sample)						Test Time (ms/sample)					
	SRC	CRC	FDDL	LC-KSVD	DL-COPAR	DCR	SRC	CRC	FDDL	LC-KSVD	DL-COPAR	DCR
Extended Yale B	0	0	2386	116.6	1274	<u>57.6</u>	3093	16.9	1257	**<u>0.56</u>**	18.9	9.7
iLIDS-AA	0	0	134715	6059	539.4	<u>124.2</u>	8420	**9.8**	10349	21.1	48.7	<u>16.6</u>
KTH-TIPS	0	0	1138	265.2	3154	<u>25.0</u>	2830	**0.18**	2371	<u>4.4</u>	6.9	8.8
Swedish Leaf	0	0	1753	<u>219.6</u>	1806	346.1	4149	**0.77**	3470	<u>3.2</u>	9.2	7.8

and UIUC_10) and large within-class variations (such as iLIDS-AA, KTH-TIPS, CUReT and Food).

4.4   Computational Cost

We choose a representative dataset for each problem to compare the actual training/test time for all the adopted sparse/collaborative representation based models. The results are averaged over the 10 trials if applicable, and we report them in the "per sample" manner to eliminate the influence of dataset size. All the methods compared are implemented in Matlab and ran on a 2.67 GHz machine with 20 GB memory (more than actually needed). The results listed in Table 7 show that the learning model of DCR is generally more efficient than those of other dictionary learning methods (especially its analogues FDDL and DL-COPAR). Though LC-KSVD is very fast in the testing stage as it needs only a linear projection, the test time of DCR is comparable to that of LC-KSVD. This is unlike FDDL which needs expensive optimization even at the test stage. We can verify the correctness of the theoretical complexity (shown in Table 1) by comparing it with the actual computational time. Take "Extended Yale B" as an example, the theoretical complexity for training is $\mathcal{O}(2.72 \times 10^{10})$ while the actual training time is about 6.8 times of 2.72×10^{10}, showing that they match each other very well.

5   Conclusions

We have proposed a novel dictionary learning model DCR for classification, which to the best of our knowledge is the first one for the l_2-norm based collaborative representation. Extensive experimental results on 9 benchmark datasets for 4 types of tasks have shown that DCR is more effective and less over-fitting than the state-of-the-art. Its performance is also superior to the latest results from some unrelated methods. Moreover, DCR learns its dictionary faster than the other related dictionary learning models due to the closed-form solutions for each sub-problem in the alternative optimization. Future work includes a comparison of the concerned models on how their performances change when the trade-off parameters ar e tuned, which may reveal new interesting findings on the effectiveness of each component and the models' sensitivity to these parameters.

Acknowledgement. This work was supported by "R&D Program for Implementation of Anti-Crime and Anti-Terrorism Technologies for a Safe and Secure Society", Funds for integrated promotion of social system reform and research and development of the Ministry of Education, Culture, Sports, Science and Technology, the Japanese Government.

References

1. Wright, J., Yang, A., Ganesh, A., Sastry, S., Ma, Y.: Robust face recognition via sparse representation. IEEE TPAMI **31**, 210–227 (2009)
2. Zhang, L., Yang, M., Feng, X.: Sparse representation or collaborative representation: which helps face recognition? In: ICCV (2011)
3. Wright, J., Ma, Y., Mairal, J., Spairo, G., Huang, T., Yan, S.: Sparse representation for computer vision and pattern recognition. Proc. IEEE **98**, 1031–1044 (2010)
4. Jiang, Z., Lin, Z., Davis, L.: Learning a discriminative dictionary for sparse coding via label consistent K-SVD. In: CVPR, pp. 1697–1704 (2011)
5. Yang, M., Zhang, L., Feng, X., Zhang, D.: Fisher discrimination dictionary learning for sparse representation. In: ICCV, pp. 543–550 (2011)
6. Kong, S., Wang, D.: A dictionary learning approach for classification: separating the particularity and the commonality. In: Fitzgibbon, A., Lazebnik, S., Perona, P., Sato, Y., Schmid, C. (eds.) ECCV 2012, Part I. LNCS, vol. 7572, pp. 186–199. Springer, Heidelberg (2012)
7. Yang, M., Zhang, L., Yang, J., Zhang, D.: Metaface learning for sparse representation based face recognition. In: ICIP, pp. 1601–1604 (2010)
8. Ramirez, I., Sprechmann, P., Sapiro, G.: Classification and clustering via dictionary learning with structured incoherence and shared features. In: CVPR, pp. 3501–3508 (2010)
9. Mairal, J., Bach, F., Ponce, J., Sapiro, G., Zisserman, A.: Supervised dictionary learning. In: NIPS, pp. 1033–1040 (2009)
10. Zhang, Q., Li, B.: Discriminative K-SVD for dictionary learning in face recognition. In: CVPR, pp. 2691–2698 (2010)
11. Szlam, A., Sapiro, G.: Discriminative k-metrics. In: Proceedings of the 26th Annual International Conference on Machine Learning, ICML 2009, pp. 1009–1016. ACM, New York (2009)
12. Yu, G., Sapiro, G., Mallat, S.: Solving inverse problems with piecewise linear estimators: from gaussian mixture models to structured sparsity. IEEE Trans. Image Process. **21**, 2481–2499 (2012)
13. Bezdek, J.C., Hathaway, R.J.: Convergence of alternating optimization. Neural, Parallel Sci. Comput. **11**, 351–368 (2003)
14. Georghiades, A., Belhumeur, P., Kriegman, D.: From few to many: illumination cone models for face recognition under variable lighting and pose. IEEE TPAMI **23**, 643–660 (2001)
15. Martinez, A., Benavente, R.: The ar face database. CVC Technical report 24 (1998)
16. Bak, S., Corvee, E., Bremond, F., Thonnat, M.: Boosted human re-identification using riemannian manifolds. Image Vis. Comput. **30**, 443–452 (2012)

17. Wu, Y., Minoh, M., Mukunoki, M., Lao, S.: Robust object recognition via third-party collaborative representation. In: ICPR (2012)
18. Wu, Y., Minoh, M., Mukunoki, M., Li, W., Lao, S.: Collaborative sparse approximation for multiple-shot across-camera person re-identification. In: AVSS, pp. 209–214 (2012)
19. Qi, X., Xiao, R., Guo, J., Zhang, L.: Pairwise rotation invariant co-occurrence local binary pattern. In: Fitzgibbon, A., Lazebnik, S., Perona, P., Sato, Y., Schmid, C. (eds.) ECCV 2012, Part VI. LNCS, vol. 7577, pp. 158–171. Springer, Heidelberg (2012)
20. Zhang, J., Marszalek, M., Lazebnik, S., Schmid, C.: Local features and kernels for classification of texture and object categories: a comprehensive study. IJCV **73**, 213–238 (2007)
21. Caputo, B., Hayman, E., Fritz, M., Eklundh, J.O.: Classifying materials in the real world. Image Vis. Comput. **28**, 150–163 (2010)
22. Wu, J., Rehg, J.: Centrist: a visual descriptor for scene categorization. IEEE TPAMI **33**, 1489–1501 (2011)
23. Yang, S., Chen, M., Pomerleau, D., Sukthankar, R.: Food recognition using statistics of pairwise local features. In: CVPR, pp. 2249–2256 (2010)
24. Bruna, J., Mallat, S.: Invariant scattering convolution networks. IEEE Trans. Pattern Anal. Mach. Intell. **35**, 1872–1886 (2013)

Thread-Safe: Towards Recognizing Human Actions Across Shot Boundaries

Minh Hoai[1,2]([✉]) and Andrew Zisserman[1]

[1] Visual Geometry Group, Department of Engineering Science,
University of Oxford, Oxford OX1 3PJ, UK
[2] Department of Computer Science, Stony Brook University,
Stony Brook, NY 11794, USA
minhhoai@cs.stonybrook.edu

Abstract. We study the task of recognizing human actions in video whilst paying attention to the shot and thread editing structure. Most existing action recognition algorithms ignore this structure, but it is generally present in edited TV and film material.

To this end, we make the following contributions: first, we introduce a new dataset of human actions to study the occurrence/reoccurrence of patterns of human actions in edited TV material; second, we propose composing a video into threads of related shots, removing some of the discontinuities due to shot boundaries; and third, we show the benefits of utilizing video threads in recognizing human actions. The experiments demonstrate that human action retrieval accuracy can be improved using threads.

1 Introduction

Humans are the primary focus of many TV shows, and consequently recognizing their actions is important for automated semantic analysis of TV material. This importance is well recognized, and several datasets (e.g., [1–4]) and many approaches have been proposed (e.g., [1,2,4–7]). Existing approaches, however, ignore the structure and discontinuities in edited material. For examples, many algorithms track object patches or compute motion cues across shot boundaries, which are irrelevant to the actual content of an action.

In this paper, we propose to embrace the editing structure when recognizing human actions. We reverse the editing and decompose a video into *threads* [8]. Each thread is an ordered sequence of shots, filming the same scene by the same camera. Recall that a scene is typically filmed by multiple cameras at multiple angles, and a video is composed by cutting and joining video clips from multiple cameras. These video clips are referred to as shots and the transitions between them are shot boundaries.

Figure 1 shows a typical video sequence and illustrates the importance of considering threads when recognizing human actions. This video sequence depicts a scene of an affectionate kiss. It consists of several shots, which can be connected

© Springer International Publishing Switzerland 2015
D. Cremers et al. (Eds.): ACCV 2014, Part IV, LNCS 9006, pp. 222–237, 2015.
DOI: 10.1007/978-3-319-16817-3_15

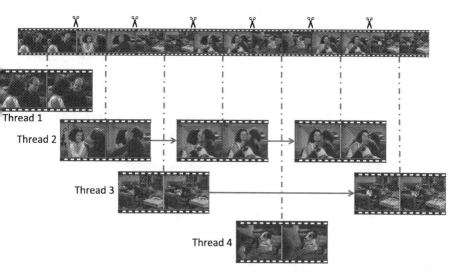

Fig. 1. A typical scene with shots and threads. This video sequence of an affectionate kiss consists of several interleaving threads. Thread 1 sets the context for the kiss, while Threads 2 and 3 portray the kiss at different angles. Thread 4 shows a dog being amused by the affection between two people. This thread shows a part of the scene, but it is completely irrelevant to the kissing action.

to form several interleaving threads. Apart from removing abrupt discontinuities due to shot boundaries, threads can be used to separate parts of the video sequence that are irrelevant to the action of interest.

Video threads and shot grouping have been considered before, but primarily for scene segmentation. Zhai & Shah [9] proposed an MCMC algorithm for clustering shots into scenes. Yeung et al. [10] constructed shot connectivity graph and used hierarchical clustering for scene segmentation. Kender & Yeo [11] detected scene boundaries by measuring coherence between shots and taking the local minima. Chasanis et al. [12] used sequence alignment and shot threading for scene detection. Cour et al. [8] proposed a weakly supervised algorithm that uses screenplays and close captions to parse a movie into a hierarchy of scenes, threads, and shots. Lehane et al. [13,14] considered repeating shots with still cameras and used Finite State Machines to detect dialogues. Pickup & Zisserman [15] used threads to spot visual continuity errors in movies. Tapaswi et al. [16] utilized threads for visualizing character interactions. All of these works, however, do not study human actions and the benefits of video threading in recognition.

Unfortunately, no existing datasets for human actions, including [2–4,17–19], can be used to study the editing structure and the benefits of using threads for recognition, as they lack annotation and contextual surround (video sequences before and after the actions). Therefore, we introduce here a new dataset of human actions. Our dataset contains more than 4000 video samples, divided into shots with annotated occurrences of human actions. The data is extracted from a large collection of TV series with different types of genres. This dataset is the first of its kind, and this is a contribution of our paper.

2   Dataset

We introduce a large dataset of video threads with annotated occurrences of human actions. The dataset consists of video samples for 13 popular actions, extracted from 15 different TV series. The video samples are divided into shots, and Amazon Mechanical Turk (MTurk) is used to verify the occurrence of human actions in the shots. This dataset can be used to study the occurrence/reoccurrence patterns of human actions in edited TV material and the benefits of using video threads to recognize human actions. These tasks can not be performed with existing human action datasets [2–4,17–19]. The dataset is available at http://www.robots.ox.ac.uk/~vgg/data/threadsafe.

2.1   Data Collection with Script Mining

The data is extracted from a large collection of edited TV material. This collection consists of 15 different TV series, each with two entire seasons. The TV series are: Frasier, Married With Children, Millennium, Friends, Andromeda, Gilmore Girls, Smallville, Farscape, Seinfeld, Scrubs, Lost, The Big Bang Theory, Star Trek TNG, Desperate Housewives, and Roswell. These TV series cover a wide range of genres, from family and friends to crime investigation and science fiction. There are 658 different episodes. The duration of each episode ranges from 20 to 60 min.

To obtain rough locations of human actions, we use video-aligned scripts [20]. Scripts are text documents that contain dialogs and scene descriptions. Scripts are generally available for popular TV shows. All TV series considered in our dataset have scripts, which are publicly available on the Internet. Scripts, however, do not provide time synchronization with the video. Following [20], we resolve this issue by synchronizing script dialogs with subtitles. Subtitles are already synchronized with videos through timestamps, and they can be easily downloaded from the Internet or copied from DVDs. Using dynamic time warping, we match script text with subtitles and transfer the time information from subtitles to scripts.

From the scene descriptions in video-aligned scripts, we collect video samples for 13 actions: answer phone, drive car, eat, fight, get out car, shake hand, hug, kiss, run, sit down, sit up, stand up, and high five. These actions frequently occur in TV shows. They are the superset of the actions considered in Hollywood2 [2] and TVHI [4] datasets, two benchmarks for human action recognition.

To collect video samples from scene descriptions, we build a text search engine. For a particular action, we first identify a set of relevant keywords and phrases. For example, the keywords and phrases for *Shakehand* are: "shake-hand", "handshake", "shake * * hand", and "hand * * shake". Here, the "*" is a wild card, and it can be matched to any word. The search engine also supports

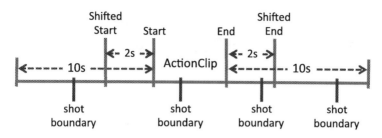

Fig. 2. Video intervals for annotation. We ask MTurk workers to annotate the extended video sequence of an action clip. The video sequence is divided into non-overlapping intervals based on shot boundaries and the start and end markings of the action clip. The shot boundaries depicted here are just for illustrative purpose; their actual locations vary.

word stemming, so "shake" is equivalent to "shakes" and "shaking". With wildcard and stemming support, searching for "shake * * hand" will return all the following sentences if they are in the scene descriptions: (1) they shake hands; (2) he shakes her hand; and (3) Leonard, shaking Penny's hand, smiled excitedly. We refer the video samples obtained using this way as ActionClips (ACs).

2.2 Annotation Verification and Refinement

We use MTurk to verify and refine the annotation for the ACs that were automatically obtained using aligned scripts. We also collect annotation for the video sequences that immediately precede or follow the action clips. For each AC, we first extend it by 10 s at both ends of the clip, as illustrated in Fig. 2. This extended sequence will be referred to as a Ten second Extended Action Clip (TEAC). We divide the TEAC into non-overlapping intervals based on: (1) shot boundaries; (2) the start and the end of the AC; and (3) the shifted start time (2 s earlier) and the shifted end time (2 s later) of the AC. This division procedure is illustrated in Fig. 2. Each obtained interval is a video shot or a part of a video shot. Hereafter, we will refer to these intervals simply as shots for brevity. We ask three MTurk workers to identify the shots that visually contain the action of interest.

2.3 Dataset Statistics and Consistency of Annotation

Table 1 displays dataset statistics and the consistency of annotation. The second and third columns show the number of clips and the number of shots for each of the 13 actions. Altogether, there are around 5000 video samples with 64000 shots. Each *shot* is labeled by three MTurk workers, and the last three columns of Table 1 shows the percentage of shots where all three MTurk workers agree. The overall percentage of agreement is 86.3 %, and 9.1 % of the shots is unanimously marked as containing the action of interest. The percentage of shots containing the action of interest varies from action to action. This is because human actions

Table 1. Dataset statistics and annotation consistency. Each shot is annotated by three MTurk workers. The last three columns show the percentage of shots that receive the same annotation from all MTurk workers. The percentage of unanimous decision is 86.3 %.

Action	#clips	#shots	%shots with agreed annotation		
			No	Yes	No/Yes
AnswerPhone	237	2768	62.8 %	25.6 %	88.4 %
DriveCar	171	2419	82.8 %	4.5 %	87.3 %
Eat	307	3539	64.1 %	11.0 %	75.1 %
Fight	383	6268	68.4 %	9.7 %	78.1 %
GetOutCar	159	2246	87.5 %	4.5 %	92.0 %
Shakehand	181	2090	78.0 %	7.8 %	85.8 %
Hug	431	4831	70.6 %	17.4 %	88.0 %
Kiss	774	8550	75.4 %	12.0 %	87.4 %
Run	1441	20758	80.4 %	6.6 %	87.0 %
SitDown	459	4921	83.0 %	6.2 %	89.2 %
SitUp	133	1608	84.5 %	3.0 %	87.5 %
StandUp	274	3421	87.9 %	4.3 %	92.2 %
Highfive	53	571	87.6 %	5.4 %	93.0 %
Total	5003	63990	77.2 %	9.1 %	86.3 %

are different and they are portrayed differently in edited TV material. For example, a video sample for AnswerPhone tends to alternate between two threads of two people talking on the phone for an extended period of time. This is why the percentage of AnswerPhone shots in an AnswerPhone sample is relatively high (25.6 %). Meanwhile, the action SitUp or StandUp are usually shown briefly. This explains the low percentages of SitUp and StandUp shots.

2.4   Temporal Extent of Actions

Where does an action occur? To answer this question, we report the percentage of times ACs and their surrounding video sequences contain the action of interest. Refer to Fig. 3 and consider an ActionClip (AC). Let PreAC and PostAC be the video sequences obtained by extending the action clip to the previous or next shot boundaries. PreAC2 and PostAC2 are the extension before PreAC and after PostAC, respectively. The occurrence percentage of the actions in these video parts are reported in Table 2. Here, a video sequence is believed to contain an action of interest if it contains a shot that is marked to contain the action by at least two MTurk workers.

As can be seen in Table 2, the action samples obtained using video-aligned scripts are useful, but noisy. On the one hand, the occurrence percentage for an action inside ACs is high, 52.3 %. On the other hand, this action-occurrence

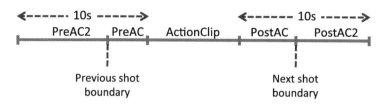

Fig. 3. Video sequences surrounding an action clip. Given an ActionClip (AC), PreAC and PostAC are obtained by extending the AC to the closest shot boundaries. PreAC2 and PostAC2 are continual extensions of PreAC and PostAC.

percentage is far from 100 %. Furthermore, consider the occurrence percentage for all combined temporal locations (last column of Table 2). The mean value is 71.3 %, which is essentially the percentage of times a verbally-described action is visually seen. This reflects the nature of scene descriptions in video scripts: many of them are based on inference instead of visualization. For example, an out-of-frame handshake between two people can still be inferred based on other cues such as audio or the greeting scenario.

The AC is the best location to extract an action sample because its action-occurrence percentage is significantly higher than those of other temporal locations. However, AC does not usually contain the entire action as the action percentage for PreAC and PostAC are also significant. Thus, perhaps the AC should be extended to capture the action in its entirety. We propose to consider Extended Action Clip (EAC), obtained by extending the AC to the previous and next shot boundaries, but clipping the extension at 2s. This 2s clipping is to avoid a situation where the previous or next shot boundaries are far away. Table 3 shows the action-occurrence percentage for EAC and its preceding and following video sequences. Notably, the action-occurrence percentage for PostEAC is significantly higher than PreEAC. This suggests that the beginning of an action is more precisely aligned with a scene description than the end of the action.

3   Video Threads

A video sequence is decomposed into interleaving threads. Each thread is an ordered sequence of video shots filmed from the same camera for the same scene. This section describes a shot boundary detection algorithm and the algorithm for joining shots into threads.

3.1   Shot Boundary Detection

Shot boundary detection is a very well studied area [21–23]. Our algorithm is based on several principles suggested in [21,22] such as temporal discontinuity and adaptive threshold, but it uses more recent visual features namely HOG [24] and SIFT [25]. Based on HOG, the algorithm produces a set of candidate shot boundaries by thresholding the difference between pairs of consecutive frames.

Table 2. Occurrence percentage for human actions at different temporal locations. AC is the video sample automatically obtained by video-aligned script. PreAC, PreAC2, PostAC, and PostAC2 are video sequences before or after AC, as depicted in Fig. 3.

	PreAC2	PreAC	AC	PostAC	PostAC2	Anywhere
AnswerPhone	13.9%	17.3%	73.8%	67.5%	54.9%	89.9%
DriveCar	5.8%	4.1%	43.9%	13.5%	16.4%	53.8%
Eat	13.0%	13.0%	55.0%	42.3%	42.0%	81.4%
Fight	16.2%	11.2%	34.5%	10.2%	20.4%	44.4%
GetOutCar	3.1%	7.5%	54.7%	21.4%	9.4%	69.2%
Shakehand	6.1%	18.2%	49.2%	23.2%	11.0%	70.2%
Hug	11.4%	22.0%	68.4%	40.6%	27.6%	87.9%
Kiss	9.3%	21.7%	70.9%	21.2%	13.4%	86.6%
Run	13.3%	12.5%	44.2%	18.5%	20.2%	61.0%
SitDown	3.9%	11.3%	51.4%	23.7%	10.9%	81.0%
SitUp	5.3%	6.8%	41.4%	13.5%	6.8%	58.6%
StandUp	9.5%	15.0%	50.7%	13.5%	11.3%	75.5%
Highfive	9.4%	24.5%	41.5%	5.7%	7.5%	67.9%
Mean	9.2%	14.3%	52.3%	24.2%	19.4%	71.3%

Subsequently, SIFT matching is used to remove false candidates. Evaluated on the TVHI dataset [4], this shot boundary detection algorithm has no false positive and 1 false negative. The details of HOG proposal and SIFT verification are given below.

Shot Boundary Proposal Using HOG. For each video frame of a video sequence, our algorithm first normalizes the frame to 128×96 pixels and computes the HOG feature vector with cell size of 8. Let $\mathbf{h}_i$ be the HOG feature vector for frame i, and let d_i be the HOG-difference between frame i and its previous frame: $d_i = ||\mathbf{h}_i - \mathbf{h}_{i-1}||_1$. Centering at i, consider the values of HOG-difference in a temporal window around i (i.e., $\{d_{i-5}, \cdots, d_{i+5}\}$), and let m_i and s_i be the mean and standard deviation respectively. We first discard all frames i such that $d_i < threshold$, where $threshold$ is set to be the 98.5 percentile of all HOG-difference values. We further remove all frames where the HOG difference is not significantly higher than the mean value of the HOG differences in the supporting window. Specifically, we remove frame i from the list of shot boundary candidates if $d_i < m_i + 1.5s_i$. This procedure can be performed in real time because: (i) HOG feature extraction is fast, and (ii) the mean and standard deviation for a sliding window can be computed using convolution.

False Positive Removal with SIFT Matching. The set of candidate boundaries returned by the above procedure can still contain false positives due to fast

Table 3. Action-occurrence percentage for extended action clip. EAC: obtained by extending the AC to the previous and next shot boundaries, but clipping the extension at 2s. PreEAC: the video sequence right before EAC. PostEAC: the video sequence right after EAC.

	PreEAC	EAC	PostEAC
AnswerPhone	15.6 %	82.7 %	71.3 %
DriveCar	6.4 %	45.0 %	19.9 %
Eat	16.9 %	64.5 %	59.0 %
Fight	17.2 %	36.3 %	21.1 %
GetOutCar	5.0 %	60.4 %	17.6 %
Shakehand	8.3 %	61.3 %	17.1 %
Hug	16.2 %	77.3 %	40.4 %
Kiss	13.2 %	78.6 %	20.4 %
Run	15.1 %	50.7 %	24.4 %
SitDown	6.8 %	67.3 %	18.5 %
SitUp	6.8 %	49.6 %	12.8 %
StandUp	10.6 %	65.0 %	15.0 %
Highfive	11.3 %	64.2 %	7.5 %
Mean	11.5 %	61.8 %	26.5 %

motion. We address this problem using SIFT matching [25]. Two video frames are considered to be in the same shot if there are at least 40 geometrically valid matches (the horizontal and vertical distance between two matched descriptors must be smaller than a quarter of the frame width and height respectively). SIFT matching is much slower than HOG computation. Fortunately, we only need to perform SIFT matching for a small set of shot boundary candidates.

3.2 Joining Video Shots into Threads

Given an ordered sequence of video shots $s_1, \cdots, s_k$, we link shots into threads as follows. First, we construct an undirected connectivity graph where each node represents a shot. Two nodes i and j are connected if $0 < i - j < 10$ and the first frame of shot i can be matched with the last frame of shot j (using SIFT matching [25]). We then find all connected components of the graph. Each connected component defines a video thread of shots. The complexity for building the graph and for finding the connected components is $O(k)$, i.e., linear in the number of shots.

Table 4 shows some summary statistics of threads and shots in TEACs. Some actions such as Fight and Run contain more threads than other actions. Compared Columns (A) and (B), it can be seen that not all threads contain an action of interest. In fact, the proportion of threads that contain an action can be small (e.g., GetOutCar and SitDown). This suggests the importance of considering

Table 4. Mean numbers of threads and shots in TEACs. Column A: mean number of threads. B: mean number of threads containing the action of interest. C: mean number of shots in threads without the action. D: mean number of shots in threads with the action. E: percentage of shots that contain the action in the threads that contain the action.

	Mean #threads		Mean #shots		E
	A	B	C	D	
AnswerPhone	5.24	2.07	1.34	1.65	89.9 %
DriveCar	8.09	1.78	1.32	1.32	93.8 %
Eat	5.02	1.73	1.38	1.56	88.6 %
Fight	11.91	4.87	1.31	1.45	91.9 %
GetOutCar	7.39	1.21	1.36	1.43	85.0 %
Shakehand	4.90	1.24	1.41	1.80	73.4 %
Hug	5.08	1.75	1.28	1.71	80.6 %
Kiss	4.78	1.54	1.36	1.72	78.8 %
Run	8.67	2.13	1.28	1.38	88.4 %
SitDown	4.74	1.12	1.34	1.53	80.8 %
SitUp	5.64	1.17	1.34	1.66	76.4 %
StandUp	5.70	1.22	1.37	1.71	76.0 %
Highfive	4.56	1.25	1.30	1.89	66.4 %
Mean	6.29	1.77	1.34	1.60	82.3 %

threads for recognizing human actions. Compared Columns (C) and (D), on average, a thread that does not contain an action has fewer shots than a thread that does. For threads that contain an action, the percentages of shots containing the action are high, varying from 66.4 % to 93.8 % (last column of Table 4).

4   Experiments and Analysis

4.1   Experimental Setup

Training and Testing Data. We split video samples into the test and training subsets such that the two subsets do not share samples from the same TV series. We split the TV series into two separate subsets, aiming to have scene and genre diversity in both training and testing sets. In particular, the following TV series are used for training: Frasier, Married With Children, Millennium, Friends, Andromeda, Gilmore Girls, Smallville, and Farscape. In testing, to ensure the correctness of test data, a video sequence (or thread) is considered positive only if all three MTurk workers believe it contains the action. In training, to increase the amount of training data, a video sequence (or thread) is considered as a positive training sample if it is annotated to contain the action by at least two MTurk workers.

Trajectory Features. The feature representation is based on improved Dense-Trajectory Descriptors (DTDs) [6]. DTD extracts dense trajectories and encodes gradient and motion cues along trajectories. Each trajectory leads to four feature vectors: Trajectory, HOG, HOF, and MBH, which have dimensions of 30, 96, 108, and 192 respectively. We refer the reader to [6] for more details.

The procedure for extracting DTDs is the same as [6] with two subtle modifications: (i) videos are normalized to have the height of 360 pixels, and (ii) frames are extracted at 25 fps. These modifications are added to standardize the feature extraction procedure across videos and datasets. They do not significantly alter the performance of the action recognition system [26]f.

Fisher Vector Encoding. To encode features, we use Fisher vectors [27]. A Fisher vector encodes both first and second order statistics between the feature descriptors and a Gaussian Mixture Model (GMM). In [6], Fisher vector shows an improved performance over bag of features for action classification. Following [6,27], we first reduce the dimension of DTDs by a factor of two using Principal Component Analysis (PCA). We set the number of Gaussians to $k = 256$ and randomly sample a subset of 1,000,000 features from the training sets of TVHI and Hollywood2 to learn the GMM. There is one GMM for each feature type. A video sequence is represented by a $2dk$ dimensional Fisher vector for each descriptor type, where d is the descriptor dimension after performing PCA. As in [6,27], we apply power ($\alpha = 0.5$) and L_2 normalization to the Fisher vectors. We combine all descriptor types by concatenating their normalized Fisher vectors, leading to a single feature vector of $109,056$ dimensions.

Least-Squares SVM. For classification, we propose to use Least-Squares Support Vector Machines (LSSVM) [28]. LSSVM, also known as kernel Ridge regression [29], has been shown to perform equally well as SVM in many classification benchmarks [30]. LSSVM has a closed-form solution, which is a computational advantage over SVM. Furthermore, once the solution of LSSVM has been computed, the solution for a reduced training set obtaining by removing any training data point can found efficiently. This enables reusing training data for further calibration (e.g., used in [26,31,32]). This section reviews LSSVM and the leave-one-sample-out formula.

Given a set of n data points $\{\mathbf{x}_i | \mathbf{x}_i \in \Re^d\}_{i=1}^n$ and associated labels $\{y_i | y_i \in \{1, -1\}\}_{i=1}^n$, LSSVM optimizes the following:

$$\underset{\mathbf{w},b}{\text{minimize}} \ \lambda ||\mathbf{w}||^2 + \sum_{i=1}^n (\mathbf{w}^T \mathbf{x}_i + b - y_i)^2. \tag{1}$$

For high dimensional data ($d \gg n$), it is more efficient to obtain the solution for $(\mathbf{w}, b)$ via the representer theorem, which states that $\mathbf{w}$ can be expressed as a linear combination of training data, i.e., $\mathbf{w} = \sum_{i=1}^n \alpha_i \mathbf{x}_i$. Let $\mathbf{K}$ be the kernel matrix, $k_{ij} = \mathbf{x}_i^T \mathbf{x}_j$. The optimal coefficients $\{\alpha_i\}$ and the bias term b can be found using closed-form formula: $[\boldsymbol{\alpha}^T, b]^T = \mathbf{My}$. Where $\mathbf{M}$ and other auxiliary variables are defined as:

$$\mathbf{R} = \begin{bmatrix} \lambda\mathbf{K} & 0_n \\ 0_n^T & 0 \end{bmatrix}, \mathbf{Z} = \begin{bmatrix} \mathbf{K} \\ 1_n^T \end{bmatrix}, \mathbf{C} = \mathbf{R} + \mathbf{ZZ}^T, \mathbf{M} = \mathbf{C}^{-1}\mathbf{Z}, \mathbf{H} = \mathbf{Z}^T\mathbf{M}. \quad (2)$$

If $\mathbf{x}_i$ is removed from the training data, the optimal coefficients can be computed:

$$\begin{bmatrix} \boldsymbol{\alpha}_{(i)} \\ b_{(i)} \end{bmatrix} = \begin{bmatrix} \boldsymbol{\alpha} \\ b \end{bmatrix} + \left(\frac{[\boldsymbol{\alpha}^T \; b]\mathbf{z}_i - y_i}{1 - h_{ii}} \right) \mathbf{m}_i. \quad (3)$$

Here, $\mathbf{z}_i$ is the ith column vector of $\mathbf{Z}$ and h_{ii} is the ith element in the diagonal of $\mathbf{H}$. Note that $\mathbf{R}, \mathbf{Z}, \mathbf{C}, \mathbf{M}$, and $\mathbf{H}$ are independent of the label vector $\mathbf{y}$. Thus, training LSSVMs for multiple classes is efficient as these matrices need to be computed once. A more gentle derivation of the above formula is given in [33].

4.2   The Benefits of Knowing Relevant Video Threads

Not every thread of a video sequence is relevant for recognizing human actions, as we discussed earlier. This subsection shows the empirical benefits of knowing relevant threads.

Consider the task of classifying whether a video sequence contains an action of interest. We create training data for this experiment by combining EACs of all actions. For a particular action, the positive samples are EACs that are annotated to contain the action, and the negative samples are EACs for other actions. Recall that an EAC is believed to contain the action if it has a shot containing the action (agreed by at least two MTurk workers). Similarly, we create a test set by extracting EACs from testing TV series (which are disjoint from training TV series). However, for testing, we only use EACs that are unanimously agreed to contain the actions by all MTurk workers. This is to ensure the correctness of test data.

We consider several methods, with and without video threading. In all cases the task is to classify whether an EAC contains the action of interest in the test data. However, we change the *representation* of the EAC in both training and testing over the different methods as follows. If video threading is not used, a feature vector (using Fisher vector encoding of dense trajectories) is computed for the entire video sequence, ignoring the discontinuities due to shot boundaries. If video threading is used, an EAC is divided into several threads and a feature vector (using Fisher vector encoding) is computed for each thread independently. The feature vectors of all threads are then aggregated to be the feature vector for the EAC. The task considered in this subsection should not be confused with individual thread classification, which is investigated in the next subsection.

We measure performance using Average Precision (AP), which is an accepted standard for action recognition [2,4,34–38]. Table 5 compares the performance of using and not using threads. *Clip* is a popular approach [6,34,37], which treats an EAC as the whole and extract feature trajectories across shot boundaries.

Table 5. The benefits of discarding irrelevant threads in training and testing. This shows APs of several methods for classifying video clips. *Clip*: a video clip is treated as the whole, with dense trajectories computed across shot boundaries. *AllThreads*: a video clip is decomposed into threads and dense trajectories and a Fisher Vectors are computed for each thread separately; each clip is then represented by the mean of Fisher Vectors. *AllThreads+Clip*: combining AllThreads and Clip (by concatenating feature vectors). *RelevantThreads*: similar to AllThreads, but assuming we know which threads contain the actions so irrelevant threads can be discarded. These results indicate the importance of finding relevant threads.

Action	Ignore threads	Use threads		
	Clip	AllThreads	AllThreads+Clip	RelevantThreads
AnswerPhone	22.1	21.6	23.2	31.5
DriveCar	44.5	51.7	49.6	70.8
Eat	38.1	35.0	38.9	37.3
Fight	35.8	29.5	35.0	55.6
GetOutCar	21.9	26.0	24.5	41.5
Shakehand	20.9	18.9	21.2	30.6
Hug	41.2	39.3	40.6	44.2
Kiss	69.6	68.8	69.8	76.6
Run	87.7	88.3	88.8	94.9
SitDown	71.5	69.7	71.3	80.2
SitUp	16.1	14.5	13.7	12.1
StandUp	19.1	17.8	20.1	26.6
Highfive	13.2	11.9	12.2	9.3
Mean	38.6	37.9	39.1	47.0

AllThreads is the method that decomposes an EAC into threads and computes feature trajectories for each thread separately. Here, we join the shots of a thread together and compute dense trajectories normally, as explained in Subsect. 4.1. For an EAC with multiple threads, we average the feature vectors of all threads and perform L2-normalization. Notably, AllThreads is slightly worse than Clip. This suggests that the shot boundaries may provide some indicative cues toward recognizing human actions in edited material, even though they are not parts of an action. *AllThreads+Clip* is the method that combine both threads and the whole EAC, by concatenating feature vectors computed for both. *Relevant-Threads* is the method that only aggregates feature vectors for threads that contain the actions. This leads to huge AP improvement, suggesting the importance of identifying relevant threads.

4.3 Video Thread Classification

The previous subsection shows the benefits of knowing relevant threads. In this subsection, we consider the task of recognizing those threads, as opposed to classifying the whole action clip.

We create the training data for this experiment by combining positive threads of EACs of all actions. For a particular action, the positive samples are threads that are annotated to contain the action, and the negative samples are positive threads for other actions. In training, a thread is believed to contain the action if it has a shot containing the action (agreed by at least two MTurk workers). Similarly, we create a test set of positive threads of testing EACs. For testing, we only use threads that are unanimously agreed to contain the actions by all MTurk workers. Again, this is to ensure the correctness of test data.

Table 6 shows the performance for recognizing relevant action threads. *Clip* is the method in which training samples are the whole EACs without considering threads. As can be seen, Clip performs relatively poorly compared to

Table 6. Recognizing relevant threads of human actions. This table shows the APs for action recognition where the testing samples are video threads. *Clip*: training samples are EACs without using threads. *PT*: training samples are threads; positive samples are positive threads extracted inside the EACs. *PT+NITAP, PT+NITAN, PT+POTAP*: same as PT but with additional training samples. NITAP: use negative threads inside EACs as positive training samples. NITAN: use negative threads inside EACs as negative training samples. POTAP: use positive threads outside EACs as positive training samples.

Action	Clip	Training data are video threads			
		PT	Using additional training threads		
			PT+NITAP	PT+NITAN	PT+POTAP
AnswerPhone	25.4	27.9	20.2	28.4	23.2
DriveCar	54.7	63.5	52.8	60.5	67.5
Eat	31.0	33.4	23.3	31.4	34.5
Fight	28.9	46.3	44.5	43.0	48.7
GetOutCar	23.0	36.5	19.3	34.6	38.1
Shakehand	21.2	28.3	21.2	28.8	26.3
Hug	38.7	43.5	41.6	39.7	44.4
Kiss	72.0	75.2	64.7	74.2	76.2
Run	92.4	93.7	85.8	93.4	94.1
SitDown	77.7	77.8	63.9	77.1	79.0
SitUp	12.4	11.3	3.4	12.2	9.6
StandUp	22.4	24.3	11.4	22.5	25.0
Highfive	13.8	8.4	5.0	8.3	9.3
Mean	39.5	43.8	35.2	42.6	44.3

PT. PT is the method in which training samples are threads. *PT+NITAP*, *PT+NITAN*, *PT+POTAP*: are similar to PT, but with additional training samples. PT+NITAP is the method where negative threads inside EACs are mistakenly used as additional positive training samples. As can be seen, a mistake for identifying relevant threads is devastating. This reaffirms the importance for identifying relevant threads. PT+NITAN is the method where negative threads inside EACs are used as additional negative training samples. Surprisingly, this does not improve the performance. This is perhaps due to the importance of contextual cues: a thread might not portray an action, but still provides discriminative cue for recognizing the action. PT+POTAP is the method where additional positive training samples are positive threads extracted outside EACs (i.e., either PreEACs or PostEACs). PT+POTAP improves the performance of PT; this reemphasizes the importance of having more relevant threads in training data. However, the improvement is slim. This indicates the high degree of similarity between the additional and the original data. Recall that the positive threads outside an EAC may just be the continuation of the positive threads inside.

Several conclusions can be drawn from this experiment and the experiment in Subsect. 4.2. First, it is beneficial to consider threads. Second, it is important to identify the relevant threads. Third, it is perhaps not so beneficial to consider additional training threads from action clips (EACs or TEACs) where we already collect some positive training threads.

5 Summary

We have considered the task of recognizing human actions in TV material and discussed the problem of ignoring the discontinuity due to shot boundaries. Towards addressing the problem, we have introduced a large dataset with annotated occurrences of human actions in video shots. We used our dataset to study video threads and human actions, and our experiments confirmed the importance of considering and identifying relevant video threads in action recognition.

Acknowledgements. This work was supported by the EPSRC grant EP/I012001/1 and a Royal Society Wolfson Research Merit Award.

References

1. Laptev, I., Marszalek, M., Schmid, C., Rozenfeld, B.: Learning realistic human actions from movies. In: Proceedings of the IEEE Conference on Computer Vision and Pattern Recognition (2008)
2. Marszalek, M., Laptev, I., Schmid, C.: Actions in context. In: Proceedings of the IEEE Conference on Computer Vision and Pattern Recognition (2009)
3. Kuehne, H., Jhuang, H., Garrote, E., Poggio, T., Serre, T.: HMDB: a large video database for human motion recognition. In: Proceedings of the International Conference on Computer Vision (2011)

4. Patron-Perez, A., Marszalek, M., Reid, I., Zisserman, A.: Structured learning of human interactions in TV shows. IEEE Trans. Pattern Anal. Mach. Intell. **34**, 2441–2453 (2012)
5. Hoai, M., Lan, Z.Z., De la Torre, F.: Joint segmentation and classification of human actions in video. In: Proceedings of the IEEE Conference on Computer Vision and Pattern Recognition (2011)
6. Wang, H., Schmid, C.: Action recognition with improved trajectories. In: Proceedings of the International Conference on Computer Vision (2013)
7. Hoai, M., Zisserman, A.: Talking heads: detecting humans and recognizing their interactions. In: Proceedings of the IEEE Conference on Computer Vision and Pattern Recognition (2014)
8. Cour, T., Jordan, C., Miltsakaki, E., Taskar, B.: Movie/Script: alignment and parsing of video and text transcription. In: Forsyth, D., Torr, P., Zisserman, A. (eds.) ECCV 2008, Part IV. LNCS, vol. 5305, pp. 158–171. Springer, Heidelberg (2008)
9. Zhai, Y., Shah, M.: Video scene segmentation using markov chain monte carlo. IEEE Trans. Multimed. **8**, 686–697 (2006)
10. Yeung, M., Yeo, B.L., Liu, B.: Segmentation of video by clustering and graph analysis. Comput. Vis. Image Underst. **71**, 94–109 (1998)
11. Kender, J., Yeo, B.L.: Video scene segmentation via continuous video coherence. In: Proceedings of the IEEE Conference on Computer Vision and Pattern Recognition (1998)
12. Chasanis, V.T., Likas, A.C., Galatsanos, N.P.: Scene detection in videos using shot clustering and sequence alignment. IEEE Trans. Multimed. **11**, 89–100 (2009)
13. Lehane, B., O'Connor, N.E., Murphy, N.: Dialogue sequence detection in movies. In: Leow, W.-K., Lew, M., Chua, T.-S., Ma, W.-Y., Chaisorn, L., Bakker, E.M. (eds.) CIVR 2005. LNCS, vol. 3568, pp. 286–296. Springer, Heidelberg (2005)
14. Lehane, B., O'Connor, N.E., Smeaton, A.F., Lee, H.: A system for event-based film browsing. In: Göbel, S., Malkewitz, R., Iurgel, I. (eds.) TIDSE 2006. LNCS, vol. 4326, pp. 334–345. Springer, Heidelberg (2006)
15. Pickup, L., Zisserman, A.: Automatic retrieval of visual continuity errors in movies. In: ACM International Conference on Image and Video Retrieval (2009)
16. Tapaswi, M., Bauml, M., Stiefelhagen, R.: Storygraphs: visualizing character interactions as a timeline. In: Proceedings of the IEEE Conference on Computer Vision and Pattern Recognition (2014)
17. Schuldt, C., Laptev, I., Caputo, B.: Recognizing human actions: a local svm approach. In: Proceedings of the International Conference on Pattern Recognition (2004)
18. Gorelick, L., Blank, M., Shechtman, E., Irani, M., Basri, R.: Actions as space-time shapes. IEEE Trans. Pattern Anal. Mach. Intell. **29**, 2247–2253 (2007)
19. Reddy, K.K., Shah, M.: Recognizing 50 human action categories of web videos. Mach. Vis. Appl. **24**, 971–981 (2012)
20. Everingham, M., Sivic, J., Zisserman, A.: "hello! my name is ... Buffy" - automatic naming of characters in tv video. In: Proceedings of the British Machine Vision Conference (2006)
21. Boreczky, J.S., Rowe, L.A.: Comparison of video shot boundary detection techniques. J. Electron. Imaging **5**, 122–128 (1996)
22. Lienhart, R.: Comparison of automatic shot boundary detection algorithms. In: SPIE, vol. 3656 (1998)
23. Lienhart, R.: Reliable transition detection in videos: a survey and practitioner's guide. Int. J. Image Graph. **1**, 469–486 (2001)

24. Dalal, N., Triggs, B.: Histograms of oriented gradients for human detection. In: Proceedings of the IEEE Conference on Computer Vision and Pattern Recognition (2005)
25. Lowe, D.: Distinctive image features from scale-invariant keypoints. Int. J. Comput. Vis. **60**, 91–110 (2004)
26. Hoai, M., Zisserman, A.: Improving human action recognition using score distribution and ranking. In: Cremers, D., Reid, I., Saito, H., Yang, M.-H. (eds.) ACCV 2014. LNCS, vol. 9007, pp. 3–20. Springer, Heidelberg (2014)
27. Perronnin, F., Sánchez, J., Mensink, T.: Improving the fisher Kernel for large-scale image classification. In: Daniilidis, K., Maragos, P., Paragios, N. (eds.) ECCV 2010, Part IV. LNCS, vol. 6314, pp. 143–156. Springer, Heidelberg (2010)
28. Suykens, J.A.K., Vandewalle, J.: Least squares support vector machine classifiers. Neural Process. Lett. **9**, 293–300 (1999)
29. Saunders, C., Gammerman, A., Vovk, V.: Ridge regression learning algorithm in dual variables. In: Proceedings of the International Conference on Machine Learning (1998)
30. Suykens, J.A.K., Gestel, T.V., Brabanter, J.D., DeMoor, B., Vandewalle, J.: Least Squares Support Vector Machines. World Scientific, Singapore (2002)
31. Tommasi, T., Caputo, B.: The more you know, the less you learn: from knowledge transfer to one-shot learning of object categories. In: Proceedings of the British Machine Vision Conference (2009)
32. Hoai, M.: Regularized max pooling for image categorization. In: Proceedings of the British Machine Vision Conference (2014)
33. Cawley, G.C., Talbot, N.L.: Fast exact leave-one-out cross-validation of sparse least-squares support vector machines. Neural Netw. **17**, 1467–1475 (2004)
34. Vig, E., Dorr, M., Cox, D.: Space-variant descriptor sampling for action recognition based on saliency and eye movements. In: Fitzgibbon, A., Lazebnik, S., Perona, P., Sato, Y., Schmid, C. (eds.) ECCV 2012, Part VII. LNCS, vol. 7578, pp. 84–97. Springer, Heidelberg (2012)
35. Marin-Jimenez, M.J., Yeguas, E., de la Blanca, N.P.: Exploring STIP-based models for recognizing human interactions in TV videos. PRL **34**, 1819–1828 (2013)
36. Jiang, Y.-G., Dai, Q., Xue, X., Liu, W., Ngo, C.-W.: Trajectory-based modeling of human actions with motion reference points. In: Fitzgibbon, A., Lazebnik, S., Perona, P., Sato, Y., Schmid, C. (eds.) ECCV 2012, Part V. LNCS, vol. 7576, pp. 425–438. Springer, Heidelberg (2012)
37. Mathe, S., Sminchisescu, C.: Dynamic eye movement datasets and learnt saliency models for visual action recognition. In: Fitzgibbon, A., Lazebnik, S., Perona, P., Sato, Y., Schmid, C. (eds.) ECCV 2012, Part II. LNCS, vol. 7573, pp. 842–856. Springer, Heidelberg (2012)
38. Gaidon, A., Harchaoui, Z., Schmid, C.: Recognizing activities with cluster-trees of tracklets. In: Proceedings of the British Machine Vision Conference (2012)

Segmentation

Consistent Foreground Co-segmentation

Jiaming Guo[1], Loong-Fah Cheong[1], Robby T. Tan[3],
and Steven Zhiying Zhou[1,2]($\boxtimes$)

[1] Department of ECE, National University of Singapore, Singapore, Singapore
elezzy@nus.edu.sg
[2] National University of Singapore Research Institute, Suzhou, China
[3] SIM University, Singapore, Singapore

Abstract. When the foreground objects have variegated appearance
and/or manifest articulated motion, not to mention the momentary
occlusions by other unintended objects, a segmentation method based
on single video and a bottom-up approach is often insufficient for their
extraction. In this paper, we present a video co-segmentation method
to address the aforementioned challenges. Departing from the objectness attributes and motion coherence used by traditional figure-ground
separation methods, we place central importance in the role of "common
fate", that is, the different parts of the foreground should persist together
in all the videos. To accomplish this idea, we first extract seed superpixels by a motion-based figure/ground segmentation method. We then
formulate a set of linkage constraints between these superpixels based on
whether they exhibit the characteristics of common fate or not. An iterative constrained clustering algorithm is then proposed to trim away the
incorrect and accidental linkage relationships. The clustering algorithm
also performs automatic model selection to estimate the number of individual objects in the foreground (e.g. male and female birds in courtship),
while at the same time binding the parts of a variegated object together
in a unified whole. Finally, a multiclass labeling Markov randome field is
used to obtain a refined segmentation result. Our experimental results on
two datasets show that our method successfully addresses the challenges
in the extraction of complex foreground and outperforms the state-of-
the-art video segmentation and co-segmentation methods.

1 Introduction

Imagine how, starting with a lack of models for most categories of objects, a
developing young infant, say 7–8 month old, can come to acquire the faculty
of segmenting the world into objects. It is believed that young infants gradually perceive individual objects as unified, bounded, and persisting by repeated
observations from different perspectives and how objects interact with others [1].
However, the computational process underpinning this developmental process is
not well-explored. Imagine another (common) scenario where we are given multiple videos with the same tag, but no further information is provided; how
can we automatically augment the tag with more fine-grained information such

© Springer International Publishing Switzerland 2015
D. Cremers et al. (Eds.): ACCV 2014, Part IV, LNCS 9006, pp. 241–257, 2015.
DOI: 10.1007/978-3-319-16817-3_16

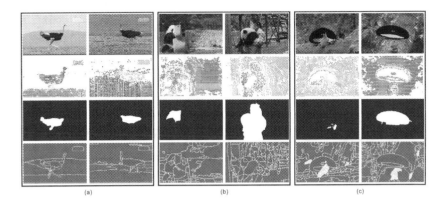

Fig. 1. Challenges of video foreground co-segmentation: variegated objects (such as the ostrich and the panda's variegated black and white appearance), objects hardly separable from the background (such as the inconspicuous female Bird of Paradise in (c)), and motion ambiguities caused by articulated motions of many animals, and extraneous objects moving together momentarily by chance (e.g. the green toy horse in (b)). **First row:** Original videos. **Second row:** Video segmentation results from [10]. **Third row:** The selected object proposals of [8]. **Fourth row:** Results of the proposed video foreground co-segmentation method (Color figure online).

as the segmentation of the tagged object [2]? These two scenarios provide the motivation for our work.

Our work is akin to the traditional figure-ground separation albeit in a multiple video setting. We prefer calling it foreground separation rather than figure-ground separation in such multiple video setting, as not necessarily all the figures in the individual videos are of interest — some figural objects are only present fleetingly and/or coincidentally. Despite some such subtle differences, our problem has many similarities with the traditional figure-ground separation works. Of course, figure-ground separation has been a longstanding important problem. Despite many attempts made over decades [3–9], the problem remains difficult or even ill-defined. In those methods based on a single image, classical mid-level visual cues to figure/ground assignment such as convexity and parallelism are used [3–6]. However, most proposed representations are still too local and bottom-up to handle the complex variability in natural images. They were usually demonstrated solely on line images, with a few exceptions [4,5].

The reason why figural assignment is hard is because it is not a purely bottom-up phenomenon [11]. Top-down cues such as familiar shape contours play a role [12], especially in natural scenes where many objects may not have convex shape or have holes. Moreover, the figure itself may contain multiple objects, which may be spatially separated with each other so that many of the figure-ground segmentation methods may fail to extract the whole figure due to their continuity assumption about the figure.

When we are viewing a dynamic scene, motion cue provides strong information about figural assignment. Despite the utility of motion cues, not many methods exploit motion for figure extraction. Recently, video segmentation methods [9,10,13] divide the video into motion layers, though the focus of these methods has been not so much on figure-ground separation. For simple scenes (e.g. near planar) or object motions (e.g. rigid), these approaches of course *also* yield figure and ground as two layers, but for more complex scenes and object motions, this simple strategy would fail. The natural world, unfortunately, abounds with such motions, such as the slithering motion of snake, the articulated motion of ostrich in Fig. 1(a), and indeed, almost all animal motions. The video segmentation approach is also plagued by the practical difficulties of obtaining accurate optical flow. Figure 1 illustrates two of these difficulties. In the third row of Fig. 1(a), the elongated head and neck of the ostrich are poorly delineated because of the well-known short-boundary bias of standard pairwise MRF model and the failure of the objectness measure [14,15] to cover the whole figure; in Fig. 1(c), the smaller female Bird of Paradise in the near ground fails to be separated from the background due to the paucity of textural details in the female bird.

From the above brief review of the figure-ground separation problem, we can make the following observations. The image-based methods are often plagued by over-segmentation, due to the variegated appearance of many objects and the non-convex shapes of many real-world objects. While the image-based methods can use motion cues to bind object segments together, they often over-rely on motion coherence which limits its applicability for natural motions. The use of motion cue also does not guarantee accurate figure outline due to the practical difficulty of estimating optical flow (See the second row of Fig. 1).

In our problem setting, the use of motion (or form for that matter) brings another complication: How to determine whether a group of segments (coherent in motion or form) are from the same object, but not from different objects moving together momentarily? One example is shown in Fig. 1(b) where a panda is playing with a toy horse. In other videos, there might be multiple moving objects. Some might be only momentarily present, but some might be interacting with one another on a prolonged basis, for instance, the two Birds of Paradise in courtship ritual in Fig. 1(c). In the former example, imagine we are trying to segment all the pandas in a group of videos bearing the tag "panda". Then, clearly we are not interested in the toy horse. In the latter example, there might be strong reasons to regard the multiple objects as a single foreground entity.

In solving our problem of video foreground separation, we need to handle the aforementioned difficulties faced by the image-based approach as well as those using dynamic cues. Our definition of foreground is much more generic than those used for figure-ground separation; we eschew assumptions used by the preceding approaches, such as those based on objectness and motion coherence. As we have at our disposal multiple video sequences, with the foreground of interest appearing in all of them, the foreground is simply an object that is recurring in all the videos, moving differently from the background but having certain permanence quality about it. Operationally, this permanence quality is checked by requiring the different parts of the foreground should persist together in all the videos. In other words, the goodness of the foreground is based upon

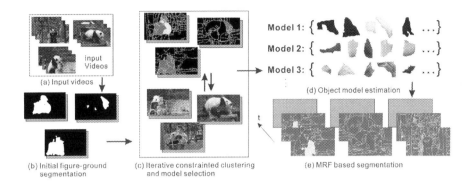

Fig. 2. Algorithm overview with steps (a) to (e).

"common fate", which we believe is a much more generic assumption than those used for figure-ground separation. By observing the appearance under different environment, we will be able to tease out the stable from the accidental, not getting entangled in possibly spurious correlations of features.

Figure 2 shows an overview of the proposed method. It first performs an initial motion based figure-ground segmentation within each video to get seed superpixels for foreground and background. We also generate initial pair-wise to-link and not-to-link constraints between these superpixels based on whether they manifest the characteristics of common fate or not. Using these seed superpixels and their pair-wise constraints, we propose an iterative constrained clustering algorithm, in which the grouping together of articulated or variegated objects is promoted by retaining and making use of the correct and common constraints, whereas the removal of spurious connections is cast as discovering and pruning of violated constraints. We also need to perform model selection in the constrained clustering step because we want to allow for multiple objects in the foreground. Finally, we perform multiple and multiclass labeling Markov random fields (MRFs) to obtain the final refined co-segmentation result.

We test our method on a newly created dataset, CFViSC as well as on the MOViSC dataset from [16]. The videos of CFViSC highlight the aforementioned video foreground segmentation challenges. Our experiments in Sect. 3 show that our method successfully addresses these challenges and outperforms the state-of-the-art video segmentation [8,10,13] and co-segmentation [16] methods in term of foreground segmentation accuracy.

1.1 Related Works

Video Segmentation: Video segmentation methods such as [10,13] make use of dense trajectories and the associated motion cues for grouping. Due to the lack of explicit notion of how the figure looks like, they simply assume that the figure is the content moving in the scene. Clearly, this is not fine-grained enough in many cases where some extraneous objects of no interest are also moving or momentarily interacting with the figure. Another limitation of these methods arises when there are objects with articulated motions. In this case, relying on the pair-wise motion distance is likely to result in over-segmentation.

Some other methods make use of dense optical flow between two frames for figure-ground segmentation [17,18]. They are also easily plagued by the practical difficulties of obtaining accurate optical flow. The work of [9] aims to address this issue by simultaneously estimating accurate flow and solving for a figure-ground segmentation that yields good flow estimates. While it is able to recover fine structures, it still faces the limitation of a two-layer segmentation and would suffer from the various ambiguity problems mentioned above.

Recently, several video segmentation methods built upon object proposals [14,15] are proposed to detect the primary object in videos [7,8]. When faced with the scenario in Fig. 1(b), they are still likely to suffer from the aforementioned issue as they are unable to determine whether there is an object with variegated appearance or there are multiple objects moving together. Other modes of failure include: the employed object proposal method may fail to generate adequately good proposals to correctly cover the whole figure. Even when there exist good object proposals, the segmentation algorithm may fail to identify them and select the bad ones. This is likely to happen especially when the object has non-compact shape. For instance, in Fig. 1(a), due to the variegated appearance and its articulated motion, the selected object proposals by [8] does not cover the neck and the feet of the ostrich (third row, Fig. 1(a)).

Co-segmentation: The problem of object co-segmentation is first addressed by [19] on an image pair. The usage of object proposals has also been introduced to co-segmentation [20,21]. They share with other object-based approaches the same limitation mentioned in the preceding paragraph.

There are other co-segmentation works that segment objects using videos [16,22]. The former [22] formulates subspace clustering for video co-segmentation which jointly utilizes appearance feature across multiple videos and motion features within each video to segment the foreground of interest. The assumption that the motion of each object forms a low-rank subspace makes this work incapable of handling objects with articulated motion. While it can treat multiple objects as foreground, it cannot provide further segmentation into the individual foreground objects. The latter [16] formulates a distant-dependent Chinese Restaurant Process across multiple videos based on motion cues and appearance cues, but the co-segmentation results are not organized into foreground and background explicitly. It also suffers from severe over-segmentation when dealing with complex scenes with a lot of clutter.

Table 1 compares our method with the previous video and image object co-segmentation methods. As explained above, our method can handle foreground with variegated appearance and non-compact shape, foreground comprising multiple objects (with the number of objects unknown), and finally, can remove extraneous or spurious objects momentarily present in the scene or interacting with the foreground. Note from Table 1 that [16,24] are also able to handle extraneous objects that are only present in some of the scenes. They termed this kind

Table 1. Comparison of our algorithm with previous video and image co-segmentation methods (top and bottom halves respectively). MS: whether an algorithm can perform model selection. MF: whether an algorithm is designed for multiple figure object segmentation. CM: whether an algorithm can deal with the content misalignment issues (see text for discussion). Hetero-FG: whether an algorithm can identify a heterogeneous object as a single object. Y and N represent yes and no respectively

Method	MS	MF	CM	Hetero-FG
Ours	Y	Y	Y	Y
ddCRP [16]	Y	Y	Y	N
ObMiC [21]	N	Y	N	Y
SC&QPBO [22]	N	N	N	Y
DC-M [23]	N	Y	N	N
MFC [24]	N	Y	Y	Y
OC [20]	N	N	N	Y

of images or videos as exhibiting content misalignment. One big difference is that they choose to retain these extraneous objects in the foreground. In principle, both these two and our methods utilize the information to discard or retain these extraneous objects, depending on the needs of the applications.

2   Proposed Method

Given a set of N videos $\mathcal{V} = \{V_1, V_2, ..., V_N\}$, we first run the motion-aware superpixel segmentation of [25] for each frame within each video, and then represent each video as a collection of superpixels, i.e., $\mathcal{S} = \{S_1, S_2, ..., S_N\}$, where S_i denotes the superpixel collection of V_i. Our video co-segmentation method presented in this section is based on these superpixels as input.

2.1   Discovering Seed Superpixels and Initial Pairwise Constraints

The objective in this step is to perform a rudimentary foreground-background segmentation in each video to obtain a set of seed superpixels and some initial pairwise constraints among these selected superpixels. In this rudimentary foreground-background segmentation, often only fragments of the foreground are selected, together with extraneous background or other undesirable objects. Thus, further processing of foreground-background separation will be needed.

To extract the seed superpixels, we adopt the latest technique in computing the motion saliency map [18] and the inside-outside map [26]. The motion saliency measure of [18] exploits the center-surround difference on optical flow field to separate the foreground. It is relatively robust to any complex intra-object motion differences that could arise from self-occlusion or articulated motion. For instance, it allows the head and neck of the ostrich in Fig. 1(a)

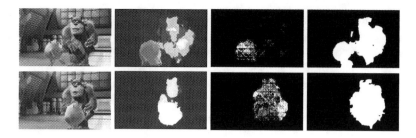

Fig. 3. First column: Two original frames. **Second column:** motion saliency measure. **Third column:** inside-outside measure, with intensity indicating degree of inside-ness. **Fourth column:** extracted patches by combining motion saliency and inside-outside measure.

to have different motion from the body, as long as the contrast with the background is large enough. The drawback is that it depends on sufficient motion contrast (see the missing arm in the second column, second row of Fig. 3), and could be sensitive to spurious motion contrast due to depth discontinuities in the background.

The inside-outside map of [26] is based on first detecting motion boundaries, and then based on these incomplete boundaries, computes the inside-outside map via a point-in-polygon rule. Specifically, any ray starting from a point inside the polygon (or any closed curve) should intersect the boundary of the polygon an odd number of times. According to our observation, this inside-outside measure significantly outperforms the motion saliency measure when the foreground has a small motion contrast against the background. However, it is erroneous when the foreground object possesses large intra-object motion differences, since in this case, the differences could raise too many edges in the interior of the foreground, violating the basic premise of the point-in-polygon rule.

Figure 3 shows both the motion saliency map and the inside-outside map of two frames of a video, where their aforementioned pros and cons are well-illustrated in the second and third columns. We found that the two measures can actually complement each other to resolve their drawbacks. Thus, we combine them to extract those seed superpixels s that are likely to cover the foreground region:

$$\mathcal{S}^{F} = \{s \mid \overline{sal}(s) > \alpha \ \text{ or } \ \overline{in}(s) > \beta \},\qquad(1)$$

where $\mathcal{S}^{F}$ denotes the collection of seed superpixels (F stands for figure); $\overline{sal}(\cdot)$ and $\overline{in}(\cdot)$ represent the average motion saliency and the inside points ratio of a superpixel respectively; α and β are the thresholds. The fourth column of Fig. 3 shows initial foreground-background separation results. Despite the relatively good result of the foreground-background segmentation for this example, there are plenty of other examples where the initial segmentation is inadequate, for instance, the panda shown in Fig. 2.

After the rudimentary foreground-background segmentation, our next aim is to generate the pair-wise constraints among the extracted seed superpixels of each input video. These constraints will eventually guide the formation of the correct foreground model in a constrained clustering setting. Denoting $\mathcal{S}_n^{\mathrm{F}}$ as the seed superpixels of video V_n, we want to build for $\mathcal{S}_n^{\mathrm{F}}$ a constraint matrix $\mathbf{Z}_n = \{Z_{ij}\}_{N_n \times N_n}$, $N_n = |\mathcal{S}_n^{\mathrm{F}}|$:

$$
Z_{ij} = \begin{cases} +1, & (s_i, s_j) \in \mathcal{M} \\ -1, & (s_i, s_j) \in \mathcal{C} \\ 0, & \text{otherwise.} \end{cases} \tag{2}
$$

where $\mathcal{M}$ denotes the set of to-link constraints, and $\mathcal{C}$ denotes the set of not-to-link constraints. The not-to-link constraints forbid two objects that are physically separated to be linked together and are computed based on the following simple spatial relationship: $(s_i, s_j) \in \mathcal{C}$ if there is no path (i.e. a sequence of nodes connected by edges) from s_i to s_j in an adjacency graph built for the seed superpixels of the current frame. To compute $\mathcal{M}$, we select a pair of superpixels (s_i, s_j) that are adjacent in a frame, and warp them to the next and previous 5 frames using the forward and the backward optical flow respectively. If the warped superpixels still remain close to each other, i.e., exhibiting common-fate, (s_i, s_j) are selected to be in $\mathcal{M}$; otherwise, no constraints are assigned to (s_i, s_j).

Since we rely only on the gestalt law of common fate to generate constraints, the graphs are robust to intra-object motion difference arising from self-occlusion or articulated motions. For instance, the different parts of the ostrich are linked together due to the fact they stay connected despite the articulated motions. Evidently, there would still be incorrect constraints, such as those to-link constraints that arise when there are different objects interacting with each other in a single video (e.g. the panda and the toy horse). This is where one needs to use multiple videos to tease out the stable aspect of the foreground appearance.

In order to estimate the background model, we also need to extract the seed superpixels that can represent the background. We used the simple boundary prior proposed by [27], namely, we select those superpixels that reside along the image boundary but do not belong to $\mathcal{S}^{\mathrm{F}}$, and denote the set as $\mathcal{S}^{\mathrm{B}}$.

2.2   Iterative Constrained Clustering and Model Selection

Given N input videos $\mathcal{V} = \{V_1, V_2, ..., V_N\}$, seed superpixels $\mathcal{S}^{\mathrm{F}} = \{\mathcal{S}_1^{\mathrm{F}}, \mathcal{S}_2^{\mathrm{F}}, \ldots, \mathcal{S}_N^{\mathrm{F}}\}$, constraint matrices $\mathcal{Z} = \{\mathbf{Z}_1, \mathbf{Z}_2, \ldots, \mathbf{Z}_N\}$ and an affinity matrix $\mathbf{W} \in \mathcal{R}^{M \times M}$ ($M = \sum_{n=1}^{N} |\mathcal{S}_n^{\mathrm{F}}|$), which describes the similarity between all seed superpixels, the objective in this subsection is to estimate the number of cluster K and divide the seed superpixels into K clusters, each of which models a foreground object.

To accomplish the objective, we rely on the to-link constraints to provide the necessary prior to bind the non-uniformly colored zones of say, a panda or a leopard together in one cluster. However, recall that some constraints in our $\mathbf{Z}_n$

Algorithm 1. Iterative Constrained Clustering and Model Selection

---

Input: $\mathbf{W}$, $\mathcal{Z} = \{\mathbf{Z}_1, \mathbf{Z}_2, \ldots, \mathbf{Z}_N\}$, T, CM
   $\mathbf{G}_0 = \mathrm{diag}(\mathbf{Z}_1, \mathbf{Z}_2, \ldots, \mathbf{Z}_N)$;
   for $t = 1 \rightarrow T$ **do**
      $\mathbf{G}_t = \mathbf{G}_{t-1}$;
      for $n = 1 \rightarrow N$ **do**
         Compute the matrix $\mathbf{G}_t^n$ by (3);
         Get the clustering result L_n by (4);
         Compute $R(\mathbf{Z}_n)$, the violated constraint ratio of $\mathbf{Z}_n$;
      end for
      if no violated constraints detected **then**
         $\mathbf{G}^* = \mathbf{G}_t$ and break;
      end if
      Select the constraint matrix $\mathbf{Z}_n$ with the largest $R(\mathbf{Z}_n)$;
      Update $\mathbf{Z}_n$ by (5) and update $\mathbf{G}_t$ accordingly;
   end for
   Get the model number K and the final clustering result L^* by clustering $\mathbf{W}$ s.t. $\mathbf{G}^*$;
   if CM $== 0$ **then**
      Remove the clusters that are not common;
      Adjust K and L^* accordingly;
   end if
   return K and L^*

---

may be incorrect due to the interaction between different objects or to the errors from the initial foreground-background segmentation. Thus, we need to prune these incorrect constraints to avoid incorrect binding or incorrect separation when clustering the superpixels.

Based on the assumption made in the last subsection, namely, those correct constraints must be stable and recur for all input videos while those incorrect ones should not recur in most videos, we propose an iterative constrained clustering algorithm to deal with the aforementioned issues. Our key idea is similar to the cross-validation procedure, where the incorrect constraints from one matrix $\mathbf{Z}_n$ are detected by finding the inconsistency between the clustering results and the remaining $(N-1)$ constraint matrices. The proposed algorithm is summarized in Algorithm 1.

For the sake of clarity, let's first assume we have two simple input videos. The first video contains a flapping flag with red and white stripes, and the second contains a flapping flag with red, white and blue stripes (in this case, by the end of the process, our extracted foreground must contain only white and red stripes, since they consistently appear in the two videos). In our algorithm, we extract superpixels from the areas of the flags, and create a similarity matrix $\mathbf{W}$ based on color appearance of these superpixels. We generate constraint matrices: $\mathbf{Z}_1$ and $\mathbf{Z}_2$, where $\mathbf{Z}_1$ will provide the links between the red and white superpixels, and $\mathbf{Z}_2$ will provide the links for the red, white and blue superpixels. Our idea here is that if we remove the links in $\mathbf{Z}_1$, and do the clustering on $\mathbf{W}$ subject to $\mathbf{Z}_2$, we end up with the blue stripes included in the foreground. However, if we remove the links in $\mathbf{Z}_2$, and do the clustering on $\mathbf{W}$ subject to $\mathbf{Z}_1$, the extracted foreground will comprise only the white and red stripes grouped together, because there is no link to the blue superpixels. For the latter case, there will be inconsistency between the clustering result and the constraints described by $\mathbf{Z}_2$, necessitating $\mathbf{Z}_2$ to be corrected or updated. Through this verification process, we can prune incorrect constraints and this forms the core of our algorithm.

For more detailed discussion of Algorithm 1, we start with combining all constraints $\mathcal{Z}$ into a matrix $\mathbf{G}_0$, such that $\mathbf{G}_0 = \mathrm{diag}(\mathbf{Z}_1, \mathbf{Z}_2, \ldots, \mathbf{Z}_N)$. In every iteration t, our goal is to select one $\mathbf{Z}_n$ that currently has the highest violated constraint ratio, and then to update it. To achieve this, in the second loop (the n-loop), we first remove each set of constraints one by one. We denote $\mathbf{G}_t^n$ the $\mathbf{G}_t$ with $\mathbf{Z}_n$ removed from the matrix:

$$\mathbf{G}_t^n(i,j) = \begin{cases} 0, & \text{if } (i,j) \in \Omega_n, \\ \mathbf{G}_t(i,j), & \text{otherwise.} \end{cases} \tag{3}$$

where Ω_n is a set of indices of $\mathbf{Z}_n$ that we want to remove.

Next, we perform the following constrained clustering:

$$\text{Cluster on } \mathbf{W}, \text{ s.t. } \mathbf{G}_t^n. \tag{4}$$

In each iteration n, we are interested only in the clustering results of the foreground superpixels, denoted as L_n. Since $\mathbf{Z}_n$ is excluded in this round, it has no effect on L_n. Subsequently, we can compare L_n to $\mathbf{Z}_n$ and record the violated constraints of $\mathbf{Z}_n$. If $\mathbf{Z}_n(i,j) = +1$ but $L_n(i) \neq L_n(j)$, or $\mathbf{Z}_n(i,j) = -1$ but $L_n(i) = L_n(j)$, then we increase the number of violation. The ratio of violated constraint of $\mathbf{Z}_n$, denoted as $R(\mathbf{Z}_n)$, is then computed as the number of violation over the number of all constraints.

Having processed the n-loop, we choose the constraint matrix that has the highest violated constraint ratio, and then update it as follows:

$$\mathbf{Z}_n(i,j) = \begin{cases} 0, & \text{if } \mathbf{Z}_n(i,j) \text{ violates } L_n, \\ \mathbf{Z}_n(i,j), & \text{otherwise.} \end{cases} \tag{5}$$

This will create new configurations of links that are more consistent, since those that are inconsistent with the others are pruned.

Figure 4 visualizes the constraint updating process by Algorithm 1. It can be seen that the incorrect constraints such as those to-link ones between the

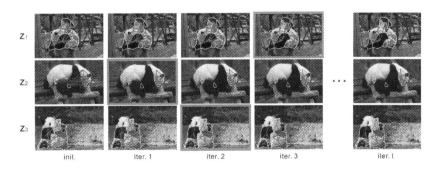

Fig. 4. The constraint updating process by Algorithm 1 on the panda sequences. The constraint graphs having the highest violated constraint ratio and thus selected for update in each iteration are bordered in orange (Color figure online).

panda and the toy horse or those not-to-link ones within the panda are success-fully removed iteratively, while the correct and common to-link constraints that connect the panda's white and black patches remain alive.

We stop the iteration when no more violation of constraint is found or the preset maximum iteration limit is reached. The cluster number K and the final clustering result L^* are obtained by running the constrained clustering algorithm based on the final overall constraint matrix $\mathbf{G}^*$. A final minor point is that, as discussed in Sect. 1, one can choose to discard or retain the extraneous objects extracted, depending on the needs. We use the parameter CM for this purpose. In our implementation, we set CM == 0 which means that the clusters that do not appear in all input videos should be removed. For some applications, if we want to allow some foreground objects to irregularly occur, then the flag CM is set to 1.

Implementation Details. We extract the normalized color histogram as the feature descriptors of superpixels as in [16,23] and compute the pair-wise affinity using the following formula:

$$\mathbf{W}(i,j) = \exp\left\{ -\frac{\|\chi^2(c_i, c_j)\|^2}{\sigma_c} \right\}, \tag{6}$$

where c_i denotes the color histogram and $\chi^2(\cdot, \cdot)$ represents the χ^2-distance between two histograms. To perform constrained clustering, we adopt the Ex-haustive and Efficient Constraint Propagation method (EECP) from [28] to incorporate the constraints into the affinity matrix. As EECP does not have an in-house step to perform model selection, we adopt the state-of-the-art SCAMS method from [29] to perform simultaneous clustering and model selection on the modified affinity matrix. Please refer to [28] and [29] for the details of the EECP and the SCAMS algorithms respectively.

2.3 MRF Based Object Segmentation

Assuming the seed superpixels have been clustered by Algorithm 1 into K groups for the foreground, $\mathcal{F} = \{\mathcal{F}_1, \mathcal{F}_2, \ldots, \mathcal{F}_K\}$, we now augment it with the back-ground seed superpixels $\mathcal{S}^{\mathrm{B}}$. We then learn a $K+1$ class SVM classifier that can infer an appropriate distance metric to distinguish the $K+1$ classes. This is done in an one-vs-all scheme by using one of $\mathcal{F}_k$ or $\mathcal{S}^{\mathrm{B}}$ as positive data and the others as negative data. Normalized color histograms are used as the feature descriptors in this step.

Having obtained the appropriate distance metrics for the foreground object models and the background model, we can use them to refine the segmentation results via a graph-cut method [30,31]. We define a graph over each video's superpixels with nodes representing superpixels and edges between two nodes corresponding to the cost of a cut between two superpixels. Then, we seek to minimize the following energy function for multi-class video segmentation:

$$E(\mathbf{f}) = \sum_{i \in \mathcal{S}} D_i(f_i) + \lambda \sum_{i,j \in \mathcal{N}} V_{i,j}(f_i, f_j) \tag{7}$$

where $\mathbf{f}$ is the label vector of the superpixel nodes with each element $f_i \in [1, K+1]$, and $\mathcal{N}$ defines the spatiotemporal neighborhood of the superpixels. The data term $D_i(f_i)$ penalizes the labeling of the superpixel x_i with f_i, which is described as $D_i(f_i) = 1 - P_{f_i}(x_i)$, where $P_{f_i}(x_i)$ is the estimated probability of assigning x_i with label f_i, calculated using the learnt one-vs-all SVM for f_i. The smoothness term $V_{i,j}(f_i, f_j)$ encourages the labeling to be spatiotemporally consistent, and is defined as:

$$V_{i,j}(f_i, f_j) = \begin{cases} e^{-(\omega_1 d_c + \bar{\omega}_1 d_f)}, & \text{if } f_i \neq f_j \text{ and } A_{ij}^s = 1, \\ e^{-(\omega_2 d_c + \bar{\omega}_2 d_o)}, & \text{if } f_i \neq f_j \text{ and } A_{ij}^t = 1, \\ 0, & \text{if } f_i = f_j. \end{cases} \tag{8}$$

where $A_{ij}^s = 1$ and $A_{ij}^t = 1$ indicate spatial adjacency and temporal adjacency respectively. The spatial adjacency is only based on the spatial relationship in a single frame, as we want to keep the MRF to a simple pairwise clique. To define temporal adjacency, we warp the superpixels forward and backward to the adjacent frames using optical flow, and then, those superpixels in the adjacent frames that overlap the warped area are selected as the temporal neighbors. The weights w_i and $\bar{w}_i$ ($w_i + \bar{w}_i = 1$) are used to trade off the influence of the color distance and the motion distance. We define the color distance $d_c(i, j)$ as the χ^2-distance between the color histograms of the superpixels, and the motion distance $d_f(i, j)$ between spatially adjacent superpixels as the Euclidean distance between the mean motions of the pixels in the superpixels. For temporally adjacent superpixels, their motion distance $d_o(i, j)$ is computed as the average area of two way after-motion overlap, which indicates how likely it is for x_i to move to x_j and vice versa.

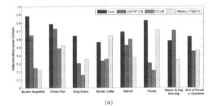 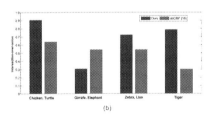

Fig. 5. Comparison of segmentation accuracies on (a) CFViCS and (b) MOViCS.

3 Experiments

We applied our method on two datasets and compared the results with those from the state-of-the-art video segmentation methods and video co-segmentation methods. To quantify the results, we employed the intersection-over-union (IOU) metric which is defined as $M(S, G) = \frac{S \cap G}{S \cup G}$, where S is the segmentation result and G is the ground truth. As the video segmentation methods do not link figure objects across videos, we computed their IOU metrics independently in each video and obtain the average as the final IOU figure, while for the video co-segmentation method, the IOU metric was computed jointly in all videos, with S restricted to the segments having the same label. For those videos whose foregrounds have multiple objects, we did not include for comparison those video segmentation methods that can only generate two-layer segmentation.

Exp. on the CFViCS Dataset: We built the Complex Foreground Video Co-Segmentation (CFViCS) dataset that comprises of 8 sets of videos selected to cover the challenges mentioned in Sect. 1. The ground truth of this dataset was manually annotated, and is depicted in the second rows of (a) through (h) of Fig. 6. The CM parameter in Algorithm 1 is set to 0 for this dataset.

Figure 5(a) depicts the IOU metrics on the CFViCS. It shows that our method achieved the best performance on most of the sequences, and in average

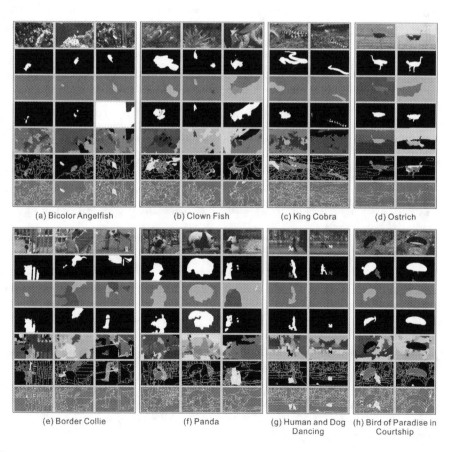

(a) Bicolor Angelfish   (b) Clown Fish   (c) King Cobra   (d) Ostrich

(e) Border Collie   (f) Panda   (g) Human and Dog Dancing   (h) Bird of Paradise in Courtship

Fig. 6. Segmentation results on the CFViCS dataset. In each example, from top to bottom: original video frames, ground truth, results of [10] post-processed by [13], results of [8], results of [16], results of our method after Algorithm 1, and our final results with MRF refinement. Best viewed in color (Color figure online).

outperformed the ddCRP [16] by 20 %, the VS [8] by 39 %, and the Moseg ([10] postprocessed by [13]) by 25 %.

The segmentation results on the CFViCS are shown in Fig. 6. The VS [8] performed poorly in nearly all the sequences in this dataset, and the chief reason was the difficulties in obtaining enough good object proposals when the foreground or background is complex. The video segmentation algorithm obtained by postprocessing [10] with [13] tended to have a good performance when the foreground undergoes rigid motions, as can be seen in the Clown Fish sequences (Fig. 6(b)) and the Border Collie sequences (Fig. 6(e)). However, its performance degraded severely when confronted with articulated motion and inaccurate optical flow estimates (Fig. 6(c) and (d)). In comparison, our method was able to resolve the ambiguity arising from articulated motion and rectify the errors caused by inaccurate optical flow.

The ddCRP method [16] does not organize the segmentation into foreground and background, which to some degree increases the difficulty in matching the foreground across videos. Even if it succeeds in matching, it is likely to oversegment those complex foreground objects with variegated appearance (Fig. 6(e) and (f)). In comparison, it can be seen from the sixth row of Fig. 6 that our iterative constrained clustering and model selection algorithm manages to group different parts of the heterogeneous foreground together.

Exp. on the MOViCS Dataset: We also tested our method on the Multi-Object Video Co-Segmentation (MOViCS) dataset from [16]. This dataset allows the foreground to comprise of objects irregularly occurring in the videos. Thus, for experimental comparison, we set the CM parameter in Algorithm 1 to 1.

The comparison between our method and the ddCRP of [16] on the MOViCS is shown in Figs. 5(b) and 7. Our method outperformed the ddCRP [16] in three out of four sets of videos, and by 17 % in average. Again, as can be seen in Fig. 7, the ddCRP [16] was likely to generate a severely over-segmented results on both the foreground and background, whereas our method was able to capture the foreground objects as unified entities.

The model selection results of our method on the CFViCS and the MOViCS are also shown in Table 2. It can be seen that our method obtained correct model selection results in half of the video sets. Even for those incorrect cases, the

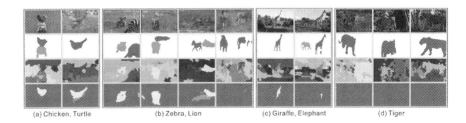

(a) Chicken, Turtle   (b) Zebra, Lion   (c) Giraffe, Elephant   (d) Tiger

Fig. 7. Segmentation results on the MOViCS dataset. In each example, from top to bottom: original video frames, ground truth, results of [16], and results of our method.

errors in the model selection were mainly due to some background patches being incorrectly extracted as foreground (see Figs. 6 and 7). Most of these patches were separated from the true foreground objects. Thus they could be easily removed by some user interaction if necessary.

Table 2. The true numbers of objects in the foreground (#GT) and the model selection results of our method (#MS).

Video set	#GT	#MS	Video set	#GT	#MS
CFViCS					
Bicolor Angelfish	1	2	Human and Dog Dancing	2	2
Border Collie	1	3	Ostrich	1	1
Clown Fish	1	2	Panda	1	1
King Cobra	1	1	Bird of Paradise in Courtship	2	2
MOViCS					
Chicken, Turtle	2	4	Giraffe, Elephant	2	2
Zebra, Lion	2	3	Tiger	1	2

4   Conclusions

We have presented a video co-segmentation framework for the separation of complex foreground and background. We first perform an initial figure/ground separation using motion cues to obtain seed superpixels and their pairwise constraints. An iterative constrained clustering algorithm is then put forth for model selection and estimation. Finally, a multiclass labeling MRF is used to obtain refined segmentation results. We have tested our method on the CFViCS and the MOViCS datasets; the experimental results demonstrate its success in addressing the challenges present in realistic foreground extraction.

Acknowledgement. This work was partially supported by the Singapore PSF grant 1321202075 and the grant from the National University of Singapore (Suzhou) Research Institute (R-2012-N-002).

References

1. Spelke, E.S.: Principles of object perception. Cogn. Sci. **14**, 29–56 (1990)
2. Wang, M., Ni, B., Hua, X.S., Chua, T.S.: Assistive tagging: a survey of multimedia tagging with human-computer joint exploration. ACM Comput. Surv. **44** (2012)
3. Fowlkes, C., Martin, D., Malik, J.: On measuring the ecological validity of local figure/ground cues. In: ECVP (2003)
4. Maire, M.: Simultaneous segmentation and figure/ground organization using angular embedding. In: Daniilidis, K., Maragos, P., Paragios, N. (eds.) ECCV 2010, Part II. LNCS, vol. 6312, pp. 450–464. Springer, Heidelberg (2010)

5. Ren, X., Fowlkes, C.C., Malik, J.: Figure/ground assignment in natural images. In: Leonardis, A., Bischof, H., Pinz, A. (eds.) ECCV 2006. LNCS, vol. 3952, pp. 614–627. Springer, Heidelberg (2006)

6. Stahl, J., Wang, S.: Convex grouping combining boundary and region information. In: ICCV (2005)

7. Lee, Y., Kim, J., Grauman, K.: Key-segments for video object segmentation. In: ICCV (2011)

8. Zhang, D., Javed, O., Shah, M.: Video object segmentation through spatially accurate and temporally dense extraction of primary object regions. In: CVPR (2013)

9. Sun, D., Wulff, J., Sudderth, E.B., Pfister, H., Black, M.J.: A fully-connected layered model of foreground and background flow. In: CVPR (2013)

10. Brox, T., Malik, J.: Object segmentation by long term analysis of point trajectories. In: Daniilidis, K., Maragos, P., Paragios, N. (eds.) ECCV 2010, Part V. LNCS, vol. 6315, pp. 282–295. Springer, Heidelberg (2010)

11. Peterson, M.A.: Low-level and high-level contributions to figure-ground organization. In: Wagemans, J. (ed.) Oxford Handbook of Perceptual Organization. Oxford University Press, Oxford (2014)

12. Peterson, M., Gibson, B.: Must figure-ground organization precede object recognition? an assumption in peril. Psychol. Sci. 5, 253–259 (1994)

13. Ochs, P., Brox, T.: Object segmentation in video: a hierarchical variational approach for turning point trajectories into dense regions. In: ICCV (2011)

14. Alexe, B., Deselaers, T., Ferrari, V.: What is an object? In: CVPR (2010)

15. Endres, I., Hoiem, D.: Category independent object proposals. In: Daniilidis, K., Maragos, P., Paragios, N. (eds.) ECCV 2010, Part V. LNCS, vol. 6315, pp. 575–588. Springer, Heidelberg (2010)

16. Chiu, W.C., Fritz, M.: Multi-class video co-segmentation with a generative multi-video model. In: CVPR (2013)

17. Criminisi, A., Cross, G., Blake, A., Kolmogorov, V.: Bilayer segmentation of live video. In: CVPR (2006)

18. Rahtu, E., Kannala, J., Salo, M., Heikkilä, J.: Segmenting salient objects from images and videos. In: Daniilidis, K., Maragos, P., Paragios, N. (eds.) ECCV 2010, Part V. LNCS, vol. 6315, pp. 366–379. Springer, Heidelberg (2010)

19. Rother, C., Kolmogorov, V., Minka, T., Blake, A.: Cosegmentation of image pairs by histogram matching incorporating a global constraint into MRFs. In: CVPR (2006)

20. Vicente, S., Rother, C., Kolmogorov, V.: Object cosegmentation. In: CVPR (2011)

21. Fu, H., Xu, D., Zhang, B., Lin, S.: Object-based multiple foreground video co-segmentation. In: CVPR (2014)

22. Wang, C., Guo, Y., Zhu, J., Wang, L., Wang, W.: Video object co-segmentation via subspace clustering and quadratic pseudo-boolean optimization in an MRF framework. IEEE Trans. Multimedia 23 (2014)

23. Joulin, A., Bach, F., Ponce, J.: Multi-class cosegmentation. In: CVPR (2012)

24. Kim, G., Xing, E.P.: On multiple foreground cosegmentation. In: CVPR (2012)

25. Galasso, F., Cipolla, R., Schiele, B.: Video segmentation with superpixels. In: Lee, K.M., Matsushita, Y., Rehg, J.M., Hu, Z. (eds.) ACCV 2012, Part I. LNCS, vol. 7724, pp. 760–774. Springer, Heidelberg (2013)

26. Papazoglou, A., Ferrari, V.: Fast object segmentation in unconstrained video. In: ICCV (2013)

27. Lempitsky, V., Kohli, P., Rother, C., Sharp, T.: Image segmentation with a bounding box prior. In: ICCV (2009)

28. Lu, Z., Ip, H.H.S.: Constrained spectral clustering via exhaustive and efficient constraint propagation. In: Daniilidis, K., Maragos, P., Paragios, N. (eds.) ECCV 2010, Part VI. LNCS, vol. 6316, pp. 1–14. Springer, Heidelberg (2010)
29. Li, Z., Cheong, L.F., Zhou, S.Z.: SCAMS: simultaneous clustering and model selection. In: CVPR (2014)
30. Boykov, Y., Veksler, O., Zabih, R.: Fast approximate energy minimization via graph cuts. TPAMI **23**, 1222–1239 (2001)
31. Cheng, H.T., Ahuja, N.: Exploiting nonlocal spatiotemporal structure for video segmentation. In: CVPR (2012)

On Multiple Image Group Cosegmentation

Fanman Meng[1], Jianfei Cai[2]([⊠]), and Hongliang Li[1]

[1] School of Electronic Engineering, University of Electronic Science
and Technology of China, Chengdu, Sichuan, China
[2] School of Computer Engineering,
Nanyang Technological University, Singapore, Singapore
asjfcai@ntu.edu.sg

Abstract. The existing cosegmentation methods use intra-group information to extract a common object from a single image group. Observing that in many practical scenarios there often exist multiple image groups with distinct characteristics but related to the same common object, in this paper we propose a multi-group image cosegmentation framework, which not only discoveries intra-group information within each image group, but also transfers the inter-group information among different groups so as to more accurate object priors. Particularly, we formulate the multi-group cosegmentation task as an energy minimization problem. Markov random field (MRF) segmentation model and dense correspondence model are used in the model design and the Expectation-Maximization algorithm (EM) is adapted to solve the optimization. The proposed framework is applied on three practical scenarios including image complexity based cosegmentation, multiple training group cosegmentation and multiple noise image group cosegmentation. Experimental results on four benchmark datasets show that the proposed multi-group image cosegmentation framework is able to discover more accurate object priors and significantly outperform state-of-the-art single-group image cosegmentation methods.

1 Introduction

Cosegmentation automatically extracts common objects from multiple images by forcing the segments to be consistent, which can be used in many applications, such as image classification [1], image retrieval [2] and object recognition [3]. Such a task is extremely challenging when dealing with large variations of common objects and the interferences of complex backgrounds. In the past several years, many cosegmentation methods have been proposed, which usually add foreground consistency constraint into traditional segmentation models to achieve the common object extraction, such as graphcut based cosegmentation [2,4–6], random walker based cosegmentation [7], active contours based cosegmentation [8], discriminative clustering based cosegmentation [9], and heat diffusion based cosegmentation [10].

Although these methods have been successfully used in some scenarios, they mainly focus on the cosegmentation of a single image group, where intra-group information is discovered to achieve the common object extraction. However,

© Springer International Publishing Switzerland 2015
D. Cremers et al. (Eds.): ACCV 2014, Part IV, LNCS 9006, pp. 258–272, 2015.
DOI: 10.1007/978-3-319-16817-3_17

in many other scenarios, multiple image groups with different characteristics but related to the same common object can be formed or already exist. For example, (1) for a given image group with large number of images, we can divide them into several subgroups such as low-complexity image group and complex image group. (2) Many training datasets for one general object often contain image groups of multiple classes, such as multiple types of "face" in face recognition and multiple kinds of "bird" species in image classification. (3) The Internet images of an object (e.g., a landmark) may be retrieved from several web engines such as Google and Flicker, which naturally results in the generation of several image groups with distinct characteristics according to the searching engines. The common existence of image groups naturally brings up the questions: *how to do cosegmentation when there exist multiple image groups with distinct characteristics? how to use the segmentation of one group to help another group?*

There are two straightforward solutions: one is to cosegment each image group independently; the other is to merge all the image groups into one and then use the existing cosegmentation technique to solve it. The problem with such straightforward methods is that they ignore the subtle prior information among image groups, which could be very helpful for cosegmentation as illustrated in the following examples.

– The in-between group information can provide more accurate object prior and make the model more robust to the background interferences. For example, in the top row of Fig. 1(a), *Shiny Cowbird* has very smooth texture (just black), which can be easily cosegmented within this group even with complex background. Then, its segmentation results can be used to help the cosegmentation of *Swainson Warbler* group that has complicated texture, as shown in the bottom row of Fig. 1(a).
– Multiple group cosegmentation can simplify the cosegmentation in terms of the object prior generation and computational cost. For example, based on some image complexity analysis, we can classify the image group into two subgroups: simple image group and complex image group, as shown in Fig. 1(b). The object prior can be easily and accurately generated from the simple image group rather than all images. In addition, since the size of the simple image group is smaller than the original one, it will also reduce the time cost of the cosegmentation significantly.
– Multiple group cosegmentation might be able to help on removing noise images. For example, the images of an object retrieved from Google and Flicker are likely to contain independent noise images. By comparing among different groups, we can easily filter out the noise images.

In this paper we propose a framework for multi-group image cosegmentation which utilises the in-between group information to improve the cosegmentation performance, and can be used in many applications, such as image classification, object detection and object recognition. Particularly, we formulate multi-group image cosegmentation as an energy minimization problem,

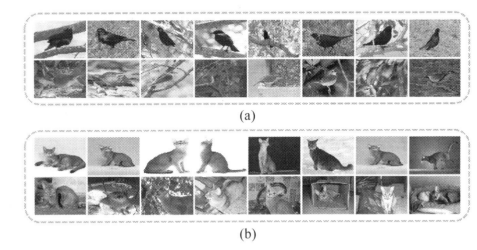

(a)

(b)

Fig. 1. Examples of the usefulness of inter-group information in cosegmentation. (a): two subspecies groups of bird (with smooth texture and complex texture, respectively). (b): simple background group and complex background group generated from a given image group.

where our overall energy function consists of three terms: traditional single image segmentation term that enforces foreground and background to be smooth and discriminatory, traditional single group term that enforces the consistency between image pairs from the same group, and a novel multiple group term that enforces the consistency between image pairs from different image groups through transferring structure information between image groups. We also introduce hidden variables in the energy function to select useful image pairs within a group and across the groups. The proposed model is finally minimized by the Expectation-Maximization algorithm (EM) algorithm with some adaptations and customizations. Furthermore, we apply our framework on three practical scenarios including image complexity based cosegmentation, multiple training group cosegmentation and multiple noise image group cosegmentation. Experimental results on four benchmark datasets show that our proposed multi-group segmentation significantly outperforms the existing methods in terms of both quantitative intersection-over-union (IOU) values and visual quality.

2   Related Work

The existing cosegmentation methods focus on segmenting common object from a group of images, which is usually designed by adding the foreground consistency constraint into traditional segmentation models, i.e.

$$E = \sum_i E^{image}(I_i) + \sum_{(i,j)} E^{global}(I_i, I_j) \tag{1}$$

where E^{image} is the traditional single image segmentation term (single term) to ensure the segment smoothness, and E^{global} is the multiple image term (global term), which is to make the segments consistent with each other. The cosegmentation is then achieved by minimizing (1). Since adding the global term usually makes the energy minimization of (1) difficult, it is critical to design appropriate single term and global term for easy optimization. In the existing methods, several efficient single and global terms have been designed. For example, markov random field segmentation [2,4–6], random walker segmentation [7], heat diffusion segmentation [11,12], and active contours segmentation have been used for E^{image}, while ℓ_1 norm [2], ℓ_2 norm [4] and reward measurement [5] have been proposed for E^{global} to trade off between accurate foreground similarity measurement and simple model minimization. In general, non-linear region similarity measurement is more accurate to measure the foreground consistency, but at cost of difficult energy minimization and local minimum solution. In contrast, linear region similarity measurement can result in simple model optimization, although it is not as accurate as the non-linear region similarity measurement.

Recently, more strategies have been introduced to evaluate the global term E^{global}, such as the region similarity evaluation by clustering output [9,13], random forest based objectness evaluation model [14], the matric rank for scale invariant objects [15], second order graph matching method [16], co-saliency model [17], graph transduction learning [18] and consistent functional maps [19]. Note that these methods are still based on the model in (1). In other words, they still focus on single image group cosegmentation, where the group level information has not been explored.

There are a few cosegmentation methods that involve multiple image groups, which partially motivated us. In particular, Kim et al. [20] proposed a web photo streams based cosegmentation, which tries to extract common objects from multiple web photo streams. Their method focuses on extracting multiple classes of objects from streams by skillfully incorporating the photo storylines, which can improve the classification accuracy via the iteration of segmentation and classification. However, the method is essentially similar to combining the photo streams into a single image group, which does not sufficiently use the group level information in the cosegmentation. Meng et al. [21] recently proposed a feature adaptive cosegmentation method, which tries to learn the feature model adaptive to each image group using simple and complicated image subgroups. Since it focuses on the feature learning, its cosegmentation is still within one group.

3 Proposed Framework for Multiple Image Group Cosegmentation

3.1 Problem Formulation

Denoting multiple image groups as $\mathbf{I}^i$, we aim at extracting the common objects ω_j^i from each given image I_j^i, where I_j^i refers to the j-th image in the i-th image group $\mathbf{I}^i$. Without lose of generalization, let's consider two image groups for simplicity:

$\mathbf{I}^0 = \{I_1^0, \cdots, I_{N_0}^0\}$ and $\mathbf{I}^1 = \{I_1^1, \cdots, I_{N_1}^1\}$, where N_i is the number of images in group i, $i \in \{0, 1\}$. Denoting $\mathbf{w}^0 = \{\omega_1^0, \cdots, \omega_{N_0}^0\}$ and $\mathbf{w}^1 = \{\omega_1^1, \cdots, \omega_{N_1}^1\}$ as the set of the common object regions ω_j^i, the goal becomes extract $\mathbf{w}^0$ and $\mathbf{w}^1$ from $\mathbf{I}^0$ and $\mathbf{I}^1$, respectively.

As illustrated in Fig. 2, our basic idea is to combine the single-image consistency, the single-group consistency and the multi-group consistency whenever it is necessary so as to achieve better common object extraction. We formulate the problem as an energy minimization problem with the overall energy function:

$$E = \sum_{i=0}^{1} \alpha_i E_I(\mathbf{w}^i) + \beta_i E_S(\mathbf{w}^i) + \gamma_i E_M(\mathbf{w}^i, \mathbf{w}^{1-i}), \qquad (2)$$

where E_I is the **single image segmentation term** that enforces foreground and background to be smooth and discriminatory, E_S is the **single group term** that enforces the consistency between image pairs from the same group, E_M is the **multiple group term** that enforces the consistency between image pairs from different image groups, and α_i, β_i and γ_i are tradeoff factors. In the following, we describe the three terms in detail.

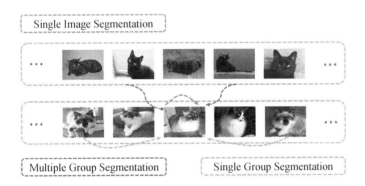

Fig. 2. Illustration of our main idea of combining single image segmentation, single group segmentation and multiple group segmentation.

Single group term $E_S(\mathbf{w}^i)$. Given a foreground set $\mathbf{w}^i$ with N_i foregrounds, $E_S(\mathbf{w}^i)$ is used to evaluate the consistencies between its elements. Particularly, in our model we evaluate the consistency by the sum of the similarities between each pair of images, i.e.

$$E_S(\mathbf{w}^i) = \sum_{(k,l),k \neq l} \mathbf{z}_{sg}(k,l) S(\omega_k^i, \omega_l^i) \qquad (3)$$

with the similarity function defined as

$$S(\omega_k^i, \omega_l^i) = \sum_{p \in \omega_k^i} -\log(P(p|F_{\omega_l^i})), \qquad (4)$$

where $P(p|F_{\omega_l^i})$ is the probability of pixel p belonging to the Gaussian Mixture Model (GMM) feature model $F_{\omega_l^i}$ of foreground ω_l^i, (k,l) represents foreground pair (ω_k^i, ω_l^i) in set $\mathbf{w}^i$, and $\mathbf{z}_{sg}(k,l)$ is a hidden binary variable to indicate whether ω_k^i and ω_l^i are paired or not with 1 for pairing and 0 for not pairing. Note that (4) is essentially the GMM similarity measurement that has been widely used in MRF models. There are also many other similarity measurements such as ℓ1-norm [2], ℓ2-norm [4], which could also be adopted here. The reason we choose the GMM similarity measurement is that it is a linear measurement, which leads to simple energy minimization. The introduce of $\mathbf{z}_{sg}(k,l)$ in (3) is to create useful image pairs for consistency enforcement and avoid bringing in bad image pairs that might deteriorate the performance. All these hidden variables together form a matrix $\mathbf{z}_{sg}$ with size $N_i \times N_i$.

Multiple group term $E_M(\mathbf{w}^i, \mathbf{w}^{1-i})$. The multiple group term transfers foreground information among the image groups. Here, we define it as

$$E_M(\mathbf{w}^i, \mathbf{w}^{1-i}) = \sum_{(k,l)} \mathbf{z}_{sm}(k,l) S_m(\omega_k^i, \omega_l^{1-i}), \tag{5}$$

where (k,l) represents a foreground pair of $(\omega_k^i, \omega_l^{1-i})$ from the two different foreground sets, $\mathbf{z}_{sm}(k,l)$ is the hidden binary variable to indicate whether ω_k^i and ω_l^{1-i} from different image groups are paired or not, similar to $\mathbf{z}_{sg}(k,l)$, and S_m is the similarity measurement between foreground pair $(\omega_k^i, \omega_l^{1-i})$. All $\mathbf{z}_{sm}(k,l)$ together form a matrix $\mathbf{z}_{sm}$ with size $N_i \times N_{1-i}$.

Different from the similarity measurement S defined in (4), for the image pair similarity at group level we often want to transfer structure information such as shape from one group (e.g. simple group) to the other (e.g. complex group). Thus, we define the group-level similarity measurement as

$$S_m(\omega_k^i, \omega_l^{1-i}) = \sum_{p \in \omega_k^i} \|f_k^i(p) - f_l^{1-i}(p + \mathbf{v}(p))\|_1, \tag{6}$$

where f_k^i and f_l^{1-i} are the features of image I_k^i and I_l^{1-i}, respectively, $p + \mathbf{v}(p)$ is a pixel in image I_l^{1-i} corresponding to pixel p in image I_k^i, and $\mathbf{v}(p)$ is the flow vector of pixel p. We use the SIFT flow method [22] to obtain the flow vector set $\mathbf{v}$. The feature f_k^i could be SIFT, color, or other features, depending on the applications.

Single image term $E_I(\mathbf{w}^i)$. Single image term is to ensure the smoothness of the segmentation and the distinction of the foreground and the background. Following common MRF segmentation model, $E_I(\mathbf{w}^i)$ is defined as

$$E_I(\mathbf{w}^i) = \sum_{k=1}^{N_i} S(\omega_k^i, \omega_k^i) + S(\bar{\omega}_k^i, \bar{\omega}_k^i) + V(\omega_k^i) \tag{7}$$

where S is the same as that in (4), $\bar{\omega}_k^i = \{p|p \in \Omega_k^i, p \notin \omega_k^i\}$ is the background, Ω_k^i is the pixel set of image I_k^i, and $V(\omega_k^i)$ is the smoothness term regularizing the segment mask ω_k^i. We select V as the pairwise term in the common MRF segmentation model [2]. The first two terms in (7) are essentially the data terms, respectively measuring how well foreground and background pixels match the foreground and background GMM feature models of the image itself.

3.2   Optimization Solution

We now present our solution to the optimization problem of (2). Considering there are hidden variables in (2), we adapt the EM to find the solution, which consists of two alternatively iterative steps: E-step and M-step. In the E-step, we update the hidden variables $\mathbf{z}_{sg}^i$ and $\mathbf{z}_{sm}^i$ based on the feature consistency of the segments, while in the M-step we refine the segments based on the updated hidden variables. In the following, we describe the two steps in detail.

E-step: Updating z. In the E-step, we update $\mathbf{z}$ by the K nearest-neighbor search. Given the segmentation results in the t-th iteration, we represent each segment by a feature such as color or SIFT. Then, for each segment ω, we calculate its K nearest neighbors denoted as $\mathbf{N}(\omega)$. For a segment pair (ω and ω_k), we set the corresponding hidden variable $z = 1$ if $\omega_k \in \mathbf{N}(\omega)$; otherwise, $z = 0$. In this way, we update $\mathbf{z}_{sg}$ and $\mathbf{z}_{sm}$ respectively when the images are in the same group or different groups.

The nearest neighbors are usually searched based on a certain distance metric such as Euclidean distance or Qi-square distance. We observe that these distances may not handle the region interferences very well. For example, in Fig. 3(a), the current foreground contains $A + B$, where A is the object region we want while B is the noise region. Directly using those common distance metrics might find the nearest neighbors that contain both A and B such as Fig. 3(b) and exclude the ideal neighbors such as Fig. 3(c). To avoid such cases, we define the region distance between two foregrounds as

$$D(\omega, \omega_k) = \frac{1}{|\omega_k|} \sum_{q \in \omega_k} \min_{p \in \omega} d(f(p), f(q)), \tag{8}$$

where $f(p)$ is the feature representation of pixel p and d is the Euclidean distance. In this way, the foreground in Fig. 3(c) will have a small distance to that in Fig. 3(a). To speed up the process, we compute the distance in (8) based on the segment (superpixel) obtained by the simple linear iterative clustering (SLIC) superpixel generation method [23] (with the pixel number 300).

M-step: Refining Cosegmentation. In the M-step, we fix $\mathbf{z}_{sg}$ and $\mathbf{z}_{sm}$, and want to refine $\mathbf{w}^0$ and $\mathbf{w}^1$ by minimizing (2). However, directly minimizing (2) is difficult since it involves two image groups and each image group contains multiple images. To make the problem trackable, we propose to solve each image segmentation separately by fixing the foregrounds of other images as constants. In this way, we divide the minimization problem into many sub-minimization

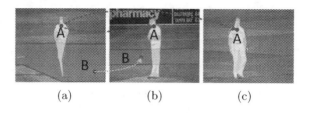

(a)   (b)   (c)

Fig. 3. An example of foreground distance measurement for K nearest-neighbor search.

problems. The energy function of each sub-minimization problem becomes

$$E_k^i = \alpha_i [S(\omega_k^i, \omega_k^i) + S(\bar{\omega}_k^i, \bar{\omega}_k^i) + V(\omega_k^i)]$$
$$+ \beta_i \sum_{l,l \neq k} \mathbf{z}_{sg}^i(k,l) S(\omega_k^i, \omega_l^i) + \gamma_i \sum_l \mathbf{z}_{sm}^i(k,l) S_m(\omega_k^i, \omega_l^{1-i}). \qquad (9)$$

Since the similarity measurements S and S_m are designed as linear measurement, the energy in (9) is submodular. Hence, (9) can be efficiently minimized by the classical graphcut algorithm [24]. By solving the sub-minimization problem in (9) one by one, we then update all ω_j^i.

Overall Algorithm. Algorithm 1 summarizes the proposed EM based solution. Note that the input includes two 2×2 matrices M_1 and M_2, which are used to specify the propagation relationship and the similarity features used so as to accommodate different application scenarios. Specifically, if we want to use the foreground information of the j-th group for the cosegmentation of the i-th group, we set $M_1(i,j) = 1$; otherwise, we set $M_1(i,j) = 0$. The diagonal elements $M_1(i,i)$ are always set to 1. M_2 is used to specify the features used in the propagation. In this research, we mainly consider color and SIFT features. We set $M_2(i,j)$ to 0 or 1 to respectively indicate color or SIFT feature used in the information transfer from group j to group i. Note that $M_2(i,i)$ specifies the transfer feature used within group i. Based on M_1 and M_2, we can easily design the transfer direction and the corresponding feature used in the transfer.

For the initialization, we set the initial region $\mathbf{w}_0^i, i = 1, 2$ as the rectangles with a fixed distance of $0.1 \times W$ (W is the image width) to the image boundary. $\mathbf{z}_{sg}^0$ is set as zero matrix with one on the diagonal, and $\mathbf{z}_{sm}^0$ is set as zero matrix. The M-step and E-step are run iteratively until the stop condition is met, i.e. reaching the maximum number of iterations N_{stop}. Typically, the EM algorithm converges in four iterations and thus we set $N_{stop} = 4$.

4   Experiments

In this section, we verify the proposed method via three cosegmentation applications: image complexity based group cosegmentation, multiple training group cosegmentation and multiple noise image group cosegmentation. We use four benchmark datasets, including ICoseg [25], Caltech-UCSD Birds 200 [26], Cat-Dog [27] and Noise Image dataset [28].

Algorithm 1. Proposed multiple group cosegmentation.

Input:
 Two image groups $\mathbf{I}^0$ and $\mathbf{I}^1$
 The relationship matrix M_1 and M_2.
Output:
 The common foreground region sets $\mathbf{w}^0$ and $\mathbf{w}^1$.
1: Setting iteration $t = 1$, the initial segments $\mathbf{w}_t^i, i = 0, 1$, $\mathbf{z}_{sg}^t$ and $\mathbf{z}_{sm}^t$;
2: **while** $t \leq N_{stop}$ **do**
3:    // M-step
4:    **for** each image I_j^i in $\mathbf{I}^i, i = 0, 1$ **do**
5:       Based on $\mathbf{w}_t^i, i = 0, 1$, $\mathbf{z}_{sg}^t$ and $\mathbf{z}_{sm}^t$, update ω_j^i for $\mathbf{w}_{t+1}^i$ by minimizing (9);
6:    **end for**
7:    // E-step
8:    Based on $\mathbf{w}_{t+1}^i, i = 0, 1$, update $\mathbf{z}_{sg}^{t+1}$ and $\mathbf{z}_{sm}^{t+1}$;
9:    $t = t + 1$;
10: **end while**
11: **return** $\mathbf{w}_{t+1}^i, i = 0, 1$;

4.1   Image Complexity Based Group Cosegmentation

Here, we consider the scenario of extracting a common object from a given single image group with large number of images, where some images are of simple background while others have complex background, which are difficult to segment. Following the image complexity analysis in [21], we can divide the given image group into simple image group and complex image group. For simple image group, we can easily extract the object out by using the single image group cosegmentation (setting γ_i in (2) to 0). Then, for the complex image group we perform the multiple image group cosegmetnation using our proposed framework, where the prior information generated from the simple image group is transferred to help the complex image group cosegmentation.

We test this scenario on the ICoseg dataset [25]. Color feature is selected for information transfer between the simple group and the complex group. Figure 4 shows some segmentation results of the images with complex backgrounds from the three classes *cheetah, elephant* and *panda2*. We can see that the proposed method can extract the common objects from interfered backgrounds, which is largely due to the accurate object prior provided by the simple group.

We next objectively evaluate the proposed method by IOU value, which is defined as the ration of the intersection area of the segment and the groundtruth to their union. We use the average value of the IOU results over all the classes of the ICoseg dataset to verify the performance. The average IOU values of the proposed method and the existing methods on ICoseg dataset are shown in the second column of Table 1, where we also compare the methods of our framework without and with the multiple group term, denoted as *ours+s* and *ours+m*, respectively. It can be seen that our proposed method with the multiple group term achieves the best performance with the highest IOU value of 0.7086 on the ICoseg dataset. Note that some image classes in ICoseg only contain

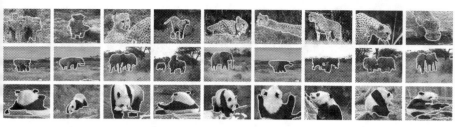

Fig. 4. The segmentation results of the proposed method on ICoseg dataset.

small number of images (smaller than ten), which is not suitable for simple and complex group division. Thus, for these small classes, only single image group cosegmentation of the proposed method is performed.

Table 1. The IOU values (Precision value for the Noise Image dataset) of the proposed method and the existing methods on Icoseg, Bird, Cat-Dog and Noise Image dataset.

Method	Icoseg	Bird	Cat	Noise
[9]	0.3947	0.2340	–	0.5270
[11]	0.3927	0.1806	0.4534	0.4695
[13]	0.4264	0.2384	–	0.6168
[28]	0.6763	0.2480	0.3950	0.5892
Ours+s	0.6514	0.3897	0.6235	–
Ours+m	0.7086	0.3957	0.6550	0.8627

Figure 5 further gives some visual comparison among different methods. We can see that the results of the single group based method often obtain large noise regions, such as the meadow in the *Liverpool* class (the first two columns). This is mainly because these noise regions repeatedly appear in the image group, which are then being considered as part of the foregrounds. Compared with other methods, our proposed group-level cosegmentation method can successfully remove those noise regions due to the nice prior extracted from the simple image group.

4.2 Multiple Training Group Cosegmentation

In this subsection, we consider the scenario of given a training collection of a general object such as bird or cat, where there already exists some groupings according to the type of the species. Some subspecies can be easily extracted according to a certain feature while segmenting the others is challenging due to the complicated texture of the object. For such dataset, we apply the single-group image cosegmentation (*ours+s*) using either color or SIFT feature on one

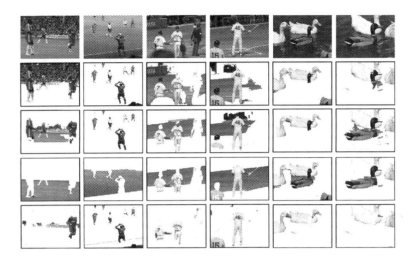

Fig. 5. From top to bottom: the original images, the segmentation results of [13,28], ours+s and ours+m methods.

selected group that can be easily segmented, and then apply our multi-group image cosegmentation (*ours+m*) on other groups using SIFT feature to transfer the object prior from the easy group to each of the other groups.

For this scenario, we test the proposed method on two classification datasets: Cat-Dog dataset and Caltech-UCSD Bird dataset. The Cat-Dog dataset contains 12 subspecies of cat with about 200 images per class, and we use all the classes. In Bird dataset, there are 200 species of bird with about 30 images per class. We select 13 continuous classes from number 026 (Bronzed Cowbird) to 038 (Great Crested Flycatcher) for verification. Considering some easy group has relatively large number of images, when applying the multi-group cosegmentation, the image matching between groups becomes very time-consuming. In order to reduce the computational cost, only a subset of the images with small number of images is used as the easy group to help cosegment other groups. Specifically, in the Cat-Dog dataset, Bombay cat group with 23 images is used as the easy group, and for UCB-Bird dataset, we select a subset of 029 American Crow with 18 images as the easy group.

Figures 6 and 7 show the segmentation results of some difficult groups in the Cat-Dog dataset and the Bird Dataset using our proposed method. Here, we give examples of the images with interfered backgrounds. We can see that the proposed method can locate the objects from these complicated backgrounds, such as the cat in the indoor scene.

The IOU values of ours method *Ours+m*, *Ours+s* and the existing methods on these two datasets are shown in the fourth and fifth columns in Table 1. Again, the proposed multi-group cosegmentation achieves the best performance. Meanwhile, we can see the significant improvement of cosegmentation is mainly caused by our single group version. The reason is that we use several new strategies to

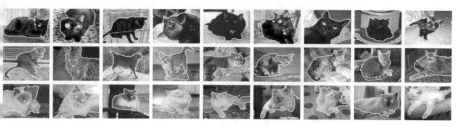

Fig. 6. The segmentation results of some difficult groups in Cat-Dog dataset using our proposed method.

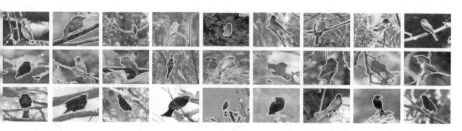

Fig. 7. The segmentation results of some difficult groups in Bird dataset using our proposed method.

improve the single image group cosegmentation performance, such as the dynamic re-neighboring across images, new neighbor selection method and simultaneously considering the segmentation on multiple image and single image. These strategies are able to result in the significant improvement of cosegmentation, especially when the dataset is challenging (such as Bird and Cat with the IOU values of 0.24 and 0.45, respectively). Meanwhile, it can also be seen that our multiple group version can further improve the IOU values over the single group version.

4.3   Noise Image Based Cosegmentation

In this experiment, we intend to demonstrate that our multi-group cosegmentation can help on removing noise or irrelevant images from a given internet image collection of a general object that for example could be the search results of multiple search engines, such as Google and Bing. We can divide the image collection into multiple groups according to its sources, i.e. where an image is coming from. By assuming the noise images are different from different sources, we can easily remove the noise images in one group by checking whether the noise images appear in another group or not. Such a noise removing method is much simpler than the one proposed in [28].

For demonstration purpose, we construct a noise dataset from the one in [28] to illustrate our idea. Specifically, we add different objects into a common object image set so as to form two different groups. For example, we respectively add a number of face and bird images into the car image set to form two different car groups. Note that for each group, we allow the repetition of the noise images, which cannot be handled by [28].

Some example results of the proposed method are shown in Fig. 8, where the top and bottom rows correspond to the results of the two different groups. We can see that the proposed method can delete the noise images successfully, as evident by no segmentation mask in those noise images. Since it is not meaningful to calculate IOU with empty segmentation mask, here we use the precision value as the evaluation metric, which is defined as the ratio of the number of correctly labelled pixels to the total number of pixels. The precision results of the proposed method are given in the last column of Table 1, which shows the significant improvement by using the proposed multiple group cosegmentation.

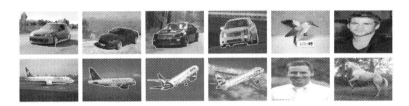

Fig. 8. The segmentation results of the proposed method on the Noise image dataset. Note that the noise images are identified in the cosegmentation since they have no segmentation masks.

5   Conclusion

In this paper, we have proposed a multi-group image cosegmentation framework, which is formulated as an energy minimization problem. The proposed energy model consists of three terms: the single image segmentation term, the single group term and the multiple group term, which, together with the hidden variables, can effectively ensure the right consistency to be enforced within an image, within a group and across different groups. The proposed model is minimized by the EM algorithm incorporated with the adopted K-nearest neighbor search and the graphcut algorithm. The experiments on three practical cosegmentation tasks and four benchmark image datasets have clearly demonstrated the usefulness and powerfulness of utilizing inter-group information.

Acknowledgement. This work was supported in part by the Major State Basic Research Development Program of China (973 Program 2015CB351804), NSFC (No. 61271289), the Singapore National Research Foundation under its IDM Futures Funding Initiative and administered by the Interactive & Digital Media Programme Office, Media Development Authority, the Ph.D. Programs Foundation of Ministry of Education of China (No. 20110185110002), and by The Program for Young Scholars Innovative Research Team of Sichuan Province, China (No. 2014TD0006).

References

1. Chai, Y., Rahtu, E., Lempitsky, V., Van Gool, L., Zisserman, A.: TriCoS: a tri-level class-discriminative co-segmentation method for image classification. In: Fitzgibbon, A., Lazebnik, S., Perona, P., Sato, Y., Schmid, C. (eds.) ECCV 2012, Part I. LNCS, vol. 7572, pp. 794–807. Springer, Heidelberg (2012)
2. Rother, C., Kolmogorov, V., Minka, T., Blake, A.: Cosegmentation of image pairs by histogram matching-incorporating a global constraint into MRFs. In: IEEE Conference on Computer Vision and Pattern Recognition, pp. 993–1000 (2006)
3. Zhu, H., Lu, J., Cai, J., Zheng, J., Thalmann, N.M.: Multiple foreground recognition and cosegmentation: an object-oriented CRF model with robust higher-order potentials. In: IEEE Winter Conference on Applications of Computer Vison (2014)
4. Mukherjee, L., Singh, V., Dyer, C.R.: Half-integrality based algorithms for cosegmentation of images. In: IEEE Conference on Computer Vision and Pattern Recognition, pp. 2028–2035 (2009)
5. Hochbaum, D.S., Singh, V.: An efficient algorithm for co-segmentation. In: International Conference on Computer Vision, pp. 269–276 (2009)
6. Vicente, S., Kolmogorov, V., Rother, C.: Cosegmentation revisited: models and optimization. In: Daniilidis, K., Maragos, P., Paragios, N. (eds.) ECCV 2010, Part II. LNCS, vol. 6312, pp. 465–479. Springer, Heidelberg (2010)
7. Collins, M., Xu, J., Grady, L., Singh, V.: Random walks based multi-image cosegmentation: quasiconvexity results and GPU-based solutions. In: IEEE Conference on Computer Vision and Pattern Recognition, pp. 1656–1663 (2012)
8. Meng, F., Li, H., Liu, G., Ngan, K.N.: Image cosegmentation by incorporating color reward strategy and active contour model. IEEE Trans. Cybern. **43**, 725–737 (2013)
9. Joulin, A., Bach, F., Ponce, J.: Discriminative clustering for image co-segmentation. In: IEEE Conference on Computer Vision and Pattern Recognition, pp. 1943–1950 (2010)
10. Chai, Y., Lempitsky, V., Zisserman, A.: BiCoS: a bi-level co-segmentation method for image classification. In: International Conference on Computer Vision, pp. 2579–2586 (2011)
11. Kim, G., Xing, E.P., Fei-Fei, L., Kanade, T.: Distributed cosegmentation via submodular optimization on anisotropic diffusion. In: International Conference on Computer Vision, pp. 169–176 (2011)
12. Kim, G., Xing, E.P.: On multiple foreground cosegmentation. In: IEEE Conference on Computer Vision and Pattern Recognition (2012)
13. Joulin, A., Bach, F., Ponce, J.: Multi-class cosegmentation. In: IEEE Conference on Computer Vision and Pattern Recognition, pp. 542–549 (2012)
14. Vicente, S., Rother, C., Kolmogorov, V.: Object cosegmentation. In: IEEE Conference on Computer Vision and Pattern Recognition, pp. 2217–2224 (2011)
15. Mukherjee, L., Singh, V., Peng, J.: Scale invariant cosegmentation for image groups. In: IEEE Conference on Computer Vision and Pattern Recognition, pp. 1881–1888 (2011)
16. Rubio, J., Serrat, J., López, A., Paragios, N.: Unsupervised co-segmentation through region matching. In: IEEE Conference on Computer Vision and Pattern Recognition, pp. 749–756 (2012)
17. Li, H., Ngan, K.N.: A co-saliency model of image pairs. IEEE Trans. Image Process. **20**, 3365–3375 (2011)

18. Ma, T., Latecki, L.J.: Graph transduction learning with connectivity constraints with application to multiple foreground cosegmentation. In: IEEE Conference on Computer Vision and Pattern Recognition (2013)

19. Wang, F., Huang, Q., Guibas, L.J.: Image co-segmentation via consistent functional maps. In: IEEE International Conference on Computer Vision (ICCV), pp. 849–856. IEEE (2013)

20. Xing, G.K.E.P.: Jointly aligning and segmenting multiple web photo streams for the inference of collective photo storylines. In: IEEE Conference on Computer Vision and Pattern Recognition (2013)

21. Meng, F., Li, H., Ngan, K.N., Zeng, L., Wu, Q.: Feature adaptive co-segmentation by complexity awareness. IEEE Trans. Image Process. **22**, 4809–4824 (2013)

22. Liu, C., Yuen, J., Torralba, A.: Sift flow: dense correspondence across scenes and its applications. IEEE Trans. Pattern Anal. Mach. Intell. **33**, 978–994 (2011)

23. Achanta, R., Shaji, A., Smith, K., Lucchi, A., Fua, P., Süstrunk, S.: Slic superpixels compared to state-of-the-art superpixel methods. IEEE Trans. Pattern Anal. Mach. Intell. **34**, 2274–2282 (2012)

24. Boykov, Y., Veksler, O., Zabih, R.: Fast approximate energy minimization via graph cuts. IEEE Trans. Pattern Anal. Mach. Intell. **23**, 1222–1239 (2001)

25. Batra, D., Kowdle, A., Parikh, D.: iCoseg: interactive co-segmentation with intelligent scribble guidance. In: IEEE Conference on Computer Vision and Pattern Recognition, pp. 3169–3176 (2010)

26. Welinder, P., Branson, S., Mita, T., Wah, C., Schroff, F., Belongie, S., Perona, P.: Caltech-UCSD Birds 200. Technical Report CNS-TR-2010-001, California Institute of Technology (2010)

27. Parkhi, O.M., Vedaldi, A., Zisserman, A., Jawahar, C.V.: Cats and dogs. In: IEEE Conference on Computer Vision and Pattern Recognition (2012)

28. Rubinstein, M., Joulin, A., Kopf, J., Liu, C.: Unsupervised joint object discovery and segmentation in internet images. In: IEEE Conference on Computer Vision and Pattern Recognition (2013)

Reconstructive Sparse Code Transfer for Contour Detection and Semantic Labeling

Michael Maire[1,2]([✉]), Stella X. Yu[3], and Pietro Perona[2]

[1] TTI Chicago, Chicago, USA
mmaire@ttic.edu
[2] California Institute of Technology, Pasadena, USA
perona@caltech.edu
[3] ICSI, University of California at Berkeley, Berkeley, USA
stellayu@berkeley.edu

Abstract. We frame the task of predicting a semantic labeling as a sparse reconstruction procedure that applies a target-specific learned transfer function to a generic deep sparse code representation of an image. This strategy partitions training into two distinct stages. First, in an unsupervised manner, we learn a set of dictionaries optimized for sparse coding of image patches. These generic dictionaries minimize error with respect to representing image appearance and are independent of any particular target task. We train a multilayer representation via recursive sparse dictionary learning on pooled codes output by earlier layers. Second, we encode all training images with the generic dictionaries and learn a transfer function that optimizes reconstruction of patches extracted from annotated ground-truth given the sparse codes of their corresponding image patches. At test time, we encode a novel image using the generic dictionaries and then reconstruct using the transfer function. The output reconstruction is a semantic labeling of the test image.

Applying this strategy to the task of contour detection, we demonstrate performance competitive with state-of-the-art systems. Unlike almost all prior work, our approach obviates the need for any form of hand-designed features or filters. Our model is entirely learned from image and ground-truth patches, with only patch sizes, dictionary sizes and sparsity levels, and depth of the network as chosen parameters. To illustrate the general applicability of our approach, we also show initial results on the task of semantic part labeling of human faces.

The effectiveness of our data-driven approach opens new avenues for research on deep sparse representations. Our classifiers utilize this representation in a novel manner. Rather than acting on nodes in the deepest layer, they attach to nodes along a slice through multiple layers of the network in order to make predictions about local patches. Our flexible combination of a generatively learned sparse representation with discriminatively trained transfer classifiers extends the notion of sparse reconstruction to encompass arbitrary semantic labeling tasks.

© Springer International Publishing Switzerland 2015
D. Cremers et al. (Eds.): ACCV 2014, Part IV, LNCS 9006, pp. 273–287, 2015.
DOI: 10.1007/978-3-319-16817-3_18

1   Introduction

A multitude of recent work establishes the power of learning hierarchical representations for visual recognition tasks. Noteworthy examples include deep autoencoders [1], deep convolutional networks [2,3], deconvolutional networks [4], hierarchical sparse coding [5], and multipath sparse coding [6]. Though modeling choices and learning techniques vary, these architectures share the overall strategy of concatenating coding (or convolution) operations followed by pooling operations in a repeating series of layers. Typically, the representation at the topmost layer (or pooled codes from multiple layers [6]) serves as an input feature vector for an auxiliary classifier, such as a support vector machine (SVM), tasked with assigning a category label to the image.

Our work is motivated by exploration of the information content of the representation constructed by the rest of the network. While the topmost or pooled features robustly encode object category, what semantics can be extracted from the spatially distributed activations in the earlier network layers? Previous work attacks this question through development of tools for visualizing and probing network behavior [7]. We provide a direct result: a multilayer slice above a particular spatial location contains sufficient information for semantic labeling of a local patch. Combining predicted labels across overlapping patches yields a semantic segmentation of the entire image.

In the case of contour detection (regarded as a binary labeling problem), we show that a single layer sparse representation (albeit over multiple image scales and patch sizes) suffices to recover most edges, while a second layer adds the ability to differentiate (and suppress) texture edges. This suggests that contour detection (and its dual problem, image segmentation [8]) emerge implicitly as byproducts of deep representations.

Moreover, our reconstruction algorithm is not specific to contours. It is a recipe for transforming a generic sparse representation into a task-specific semantic labeling. We are able to reuse the same multilayer network structure for contours in order to train a system for semantic segmentation of human faces.

We make these claims in the specific context of the multipath sparse coding architecture of Bo *et al.* [6]. We learn sparse codes for different patch resolutions on image input, and, for deeper layers, on pooled and subsampled sparse representations of earlier layers. However, instead of a final step that pools codes into a single feature vector for the entire image, we use the distributed encoding in the setting of sparse reconstruction. This encoding associates a high-dimensional sparse feature vector with each pixel. For the traditional image denoising reconstruction task, convolving these vectors with the patch dictionary from the encoding stage and averaging overlapping areas yields a denoised version of the original image [9].

Our strategy is to instead swap in an entirely different dictionary for use in reconstruction. Here we generalize the notion of "dictionary" to include any function which takes a sparse feature vector as input and outputs predicted labels for a patch. Throughout the paper, these transfer dictionaries take the form of a set of logistic regression functions: one function for predicting the label of each

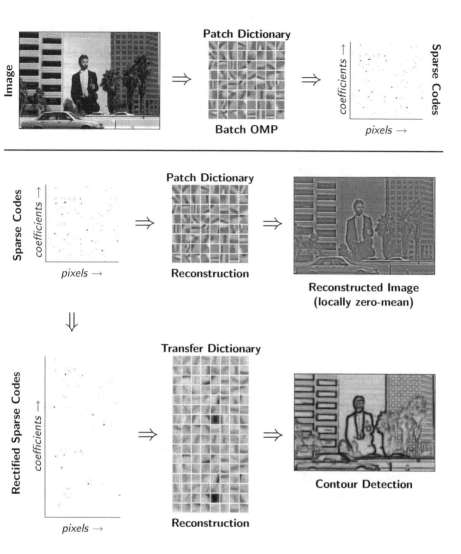

Fig. 1. Reconstructive sparse code transfer. *Top:* Applying batch orthogonal matching pursuit (BOMP) [10,11] against a learned appearance dictionary determines a sparse code for each patch in the image. We subtract means of patch RGB channels prior to encoding. *Bottom:* Convolving the sparse code representation with the same dictionary reconstructs a locally zero-mean version of the input image. Alternatively, rectifying the representation and applying a transfer function (learned for contour detection) reconstructs an edge map. For illustrative purposes, we show a small single-layer dictionary (64 11 × 11 patches) and simple transfer functions (logistic classifiers) whose coefficients are rendered as a corresponding dictionary. Our deeper representations (Fig. 2) are much higher-dimensional and yield better performing, but not easily visualized, transfer functions.

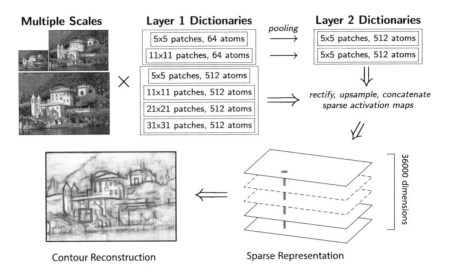

Fig. 2. Multipath sparse coding and reconstruction network. We resize an image to 6 different scales (3 shown) and encode each using dictionaries learned for different patch sizes and atom counts. Encoding sparsity is 2 and 4 nonzero coefficients for 64 and 512 atom dictionaries, respectively. The output representation of the smaller dictionaries is pooled, subsampled, and fed to a second sparse coding layer. We then rectify all sparse activation maps, upsample them to the original grid size, and concatenate to form a 36000-dimensional sparse representation for each pixel on the image grid. A set of logistic classifiers then transform the sparse vector associated with each pixel (red vertical slice) into a predicted labeling of the surrounding patch (red box) (Color figure online).

pixel in the output patch. For a simplified toy example, Fig. 1 illustrates the reconstruction obtained with such a dictionary learned for the contour detection task. Figure 2 diagrams the much larger multipath sparse coding network that our actual system uses to generate high-dimensional sparse representations. The structural similarity to the multipath network of Bo *et al.* [6] is by design. They tap part of such a network for object recognition; we tap a different part of the network for semantic segmentation. This suggests that it may be possible to use an underlying shared representation for both tasks.

In addition to being an implicit aspect of deep representations used for object recognition, our approach to contour detection is entirely free of reliance on hand-crafted features. As Sect. 2 reviews, this characteristic is unique amongst competing contour detection algorithms. Sections 3, 4, and 5 describe the technical details behind our two-stage approach of sparse coding and reconstructive transfer. Section 6 visualizes and benchmarks results for our primary application of contour detection on the Berkeley segmentation dataset (BSDS) [12]. We also show results for a secondary application of semantic part labeling on the Labeled Faces in the Wild (LFW) dataset [13,14]. Section 7 concludes.

2   Related Work

Contour detection has long been a major research focus in computer vision. Arbeláez et al. [8] catalogue a vast set of historical and modern algorithms. Three different approaches [8,15,16] appear competitive for state-of-the-art accuracy. Arbeláez et al. [8] derive pairwise pixel affinities from local color and texture gradients [17] and apply spectral clustering [18] followed by morphological operations to obtain a global boundary map.

Ren and Bo [15] adopt the same pipeline, but use gradients of sparse codes instead of the color and texture gradients developed by Martin et al. [17]. Note that this is completely different from the manner in which we propose to use sparse coding for contour detection. In [15], sparse codes from a dictionary of small 5×5 patches serve as replacement for the textons [19] used in previous work [8,17]. Borrowing the hand-designed filtering scheme of [17], half-discs at multiple orientations act as regions over which codes are pooled into feature vectors and then classified using an SVM. In contrast, we use a range of patch resolutions, from 5×5 to 31×31, without hand-designed gradient operations, in a reconstructive setting through application of a learned transfer dictionary. Our sparse codes assume a role different than that of serving as glorified textons.

Dollár and Zitnick [16] learn a random decision forest on feature channels consisting of image color, gradient magnitude at multiple orientations, and pairwise patch differences. They cluster ground-truth edge patches by similarity and train the random forest to predict structured output. The emphasis on describing local edge structure in both [16] and previous work [20,21] matches our intuition. However, sparse coding offers a more flexible methodology for achieving this goal. Unlike [16], we learn directly from image data (not predefined features), in an unsupervised manner, a generic (not contour-specific) representation, which can then be ported to many tasks via a second stage of supervised transfer learning.

Mairal et al. [22] use sparse models as the foundation for developing an edge detector. However, they focus on discriminative dictionary training and per-pixel labeling using a linear classifier on feature vectors derived from error residuals during sparse coding of patches. This scheme does not benefit from the spatial averaging of overlapping predictions that occurs in structured output paradigms such as [16] and our proposed algorithm. It also does not incorporate deeper layers of coding, an aspect we find to be crucial for capturing texture characteristics in the sparse representation.

Yang et al. [23] study the problem of learning dictionaries for coupled feature spaces with image super-resolution as an application. We share their motivation of utilizing sparse coding in a transfer learning context. As the following sections detail, we differ in our choice of a modular training procedure split into distinct unsupervised (generic) and supervised (transfer) phases. We are unique in targeting contour detection and face part labeling as applications.

3   Sparse Representation

Given image I consisting of c channels ($c = 3$ for an RGB color image) defined over a 2-dimension grid, our sparse coding problem is to represent each $m \times m \times c$

patch $x \in I$ as a sparse linear combination z of elements from a dictionary $D = [d_0, d_1, \ldots, d_{L-1}] \in \Re^{(m \cdot m \cdot c) \times L}$. From a collection of patches $X = [x_0, x_1, \ldots]$ randomly sampled from a set of training images, we learn the corresponding sparse representations $Z = [z_0, z_1, \ldots]$ as well as the dictionary D using the MI-KSVD algorithm proposed by Bo $et~al.$ [6]. MI-KSVD finds an approximate solution to the following optimization problem:

$$\underset{D,~Z}{\operatorname{argmin}} \left[||X - DZ||_F^2 + \lambda \sum_{i=0}^{L-1} \sum_{j=0, j \neq i}^{L-1} |d_i^T d_j| \right] \tag{1}$$

$$s.t.~\forall i,~||d_i||_2 = 1 \text{ and } \forall n,~||z_n||_0 \leq K$$

where $|| \cdot ||_F$ denotes Frobenius norm and K is the desired sparsity level. MI-KSVD adapts KSVD [24] by balancing reconstruction error with mutual incoherence of the dictionary. This unsupervised training stage is blind to any task-specific uses of the sparse representation.

Once the dictionary is fixed, the desired encoding $z \in \Re^L$ of a novel patch $x \in \Re^{m \cdot m \cdot c}$ is:

$$\underset{z}{\operatorname{argmin}} ||x - Dz||^2 \quad s.t.~||z||_0 \leq K \tag{2}$$

Obtaining the exact optimal z is NP-hard, but the orthogonal matching pursuit (OMP) algorithm [10] is a greedy iterative routine that works well in practice. Over each of K rounds, it selects the dictionary atom (codeword) best correlated with the residual after orthogonal projection onto the span of previously selected codewords. Batch orthogonal matching pursuit [11] precomputes correlations between codewords to significantly speed the process of coding many signals against the same dictionary. We extract the $m \times m$ patch surrounding each pixel in an image and encode all patches using batch orthogonal matching pursuit.

4   Dictionary Transfer

Coding an image I as described in the previous section produces a sparse matrix $Z \in \Re^{L \times N}$, where N is the number of pixels in the image and each column of Z has at most K nonzeros. Reshaping each of the L rows of Z into a 2-dimensional grid matching the image size, convolving with the corresponding codeword from D, and summing the results approximately reconstructs the original image. Figure 1 (middle) shows an example with the caveat that we drop patch means from the sparse representation and hence also from the reconstruction. Equivalently, one can view D as defining a function that maps a sparse vector $z \in \Re^L$ associated with a pixel to a predicted patch $P \in \Re^{m \times m \times c}$ which is superimposed on the surrounding image grid and added to overlapping predictions.

We want to replace D with a function $F(z)$ such that applying this procedure with $F(\cdot)$ produces overlapping patch predictions that, when averaged, reconstruct signal $\widehat{G}$ which closely approximates some desired ground-truth labeling G. G lives on the same 2-dimensional grid as I, but may differ in number of channels. For contour detection, G is a single-channel binary image indicating presence or absence of an edge at each pixel. For semantic labeling, G may have as many channels as categories with each channel serving as an indicator function for category presence at every location.

We regard choice of $F(\cdot)$ as a transfer learning problem given examples of sparse representations and corresponding ground-truth, $\{(Z_0, G_0), (Z_1, G_1), \ldots\}$. To further simplify the problem, we consider only patch-wise correspondence. Viewing Z and G as living on the image grid, we sample a collection of patches $\{g_0, g_1, \ldots\}$ from $\{G_0, G_1, \ldots\}$ along with the length L sparse coefficient vectors located at the center of each sampled patch, $\{z_0, z_1, \ldots\}$. We rectify each of these sparse vectors and append a constant term:

$$\hat{z}_i = \begin{bmatrix} \max(z_i^T, 0), & \max(-z_i^T, 0), & 1 \end{bmatrix}^T \tag{3}$$

Our patch-level transfer learning problem is now to find $F(\cdot)$ such that:

$$F(\hat{z}_i) \approx g_i \quad \forall i \tag{4}$$

where $\hat{z}_i \in \Re^{2L+1}$ is a vector of sparse coefficients and $g_i \in \Re^{m \times m \times h}$ is a target ground-truth patch. Here, h denotes the number of channels in the ground-truth (and its predicted reconstruction).

While one could still choose any method for modeling $F(\cdot)$, we make an extremely simple and efficient choice, with the expectation that the sparse representation will be rich enough that simple transfer functions will work well. Specifically, we split $F(\cdot)$ into a set $[f_0, f_1, ..., f_{(m^2 h - 1)}]$ of independently trained predictors $f(\cdot)$, one for each of the $m^2 h$ elements of the output patch. Our transfer learning problem is now:

$$f_j(\hat{z}_i) \approx g_i[j] \quad \forall i, j \tag{5}$$

As all experiments in this paper deal with ground-truth in the form of binary indicator vectors, we set each $f_j(\cdot)$ to be a logistic classifier and train its coefficients using L2-regularized logistic regression.

Predicting $m \times m$ patches means that each element of the output reconstruction is an average of outputs from m^2 different $f_j(\cdot)$ classifiers. Moreover, one would expect (and we observe in practice) the accuracy of the classifiers to be spatially varying. Predicted labels of pixels more distant from the patch center are less reliable than those nearby. To correct for this, we weight predicted patches with a Gaussian kernel when spatially averaging them during reconstruction.

Additionally, we would like the computation time for prediction to grow more slowly than $O(m^2)$ as patch size increases. Because predictions originating from similar spatial locations are likely to be correlated and a Gaussian kernel gives distant neighbors small weight, we construct an adaptive kernel $\mathcal{W}$, which approximates the Gaussian, taking fewer samples with increasing distance, but upweighting them to compensate for decreased sample density. Specifically:

$$\mathcal{W}(x, y; \sigma) = \begin{cases} \mathcal{G}(x, y; \sigma)/\rho(x, y) & \text{if } (x, y) \in \mathcal{S} \\ 0 & \text{otherwise} \end{cases} \tag{6}$$

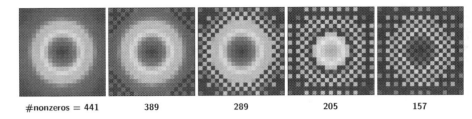

<table>
<tr><td>#nonzeros = 441</td><td>389</td><td>289</td><td>205</td><td>157</td></tr>
</table>

Fig. 3. Subsampled patch averaging kernels. Instead of uniformly averaging over-lapping patch predictions during reconstruction, we weight them with a Gaussian kernel to model their spatially varying reliability. As a classifier evaluation can be skipped if its prediction will receive zero weight within the averaging procedure, we adaptively sparsify the kernel to achieve a runtime speedup. Using the aggressively subsampled *(rightmost)* kernel is 3x faster than using the non-subsampled *(leftmost)* version, and offers equivalent accuracy. We also save the expense of training unused classifiers.

where $\mathcal{G}$ is a 2D Gaussian, $\mathcal{S}$ is a set of sample points, and $\rho(x, y)$ measures the local density of sample points. Figure 3 provides an illustration of $\mathcal{W}$ for fixed σ and sampling patterns which repeatedly halve density at various radii.

We report all experimental results using the adaptively sampled approximate Gaussian kernel during reconstruction. We found it to perform equivalently to the full Gaussian kernel and better than uniform patch weighting. The adaptive weight kernel not only reduces runtime, but also reduces training time as we neither run nor train the $f_j(\cdot)$ classifiers that the kernel assigns zero weight.

5   Multipath Network

Sections 3 and 4 describe our system for reconstructive sparse code transfer in the context of a single generatively learned patch dictionary D and the result-ing sparse representation. In practice, we must offer the system a richer view of the input than can be obtained from coding against a single dictionary. To accomplish this, we borrow the multipath sparse coding framework of Bo *et al.* [6] which combines two strategies for building richer representations.

First, the image is rescaled and all scales are coded against multiple dictio-naries for patches of varying size. Second, the output sparse representation is pooled, subsampled, and then treated as a new input signal for another layer of sparse coding. Figure 2 describes the network architecture we have chosen in order to implement this strategy. We use rectification followed by hybrid average-max pooling (the average of nonzero coefficients) between layers 1 and 2. For 5×5 patches, we pool over 3×3 windows and subsample by a factor of 2, while for 11×11 patches, we pool over 5×5 windows and subsample by a factor of 4.

We concatenate all representations generated by the 512-atom dictionaries, rectify, and upsample them so that they live on the original image grid. This results in a 36000-dimensional sparse vector representation for each image pixel. Despite the high dimensionality, there are only a few hundred nonzero entries per pixel, so total computational work is quite reasonable.

The dictionary transfer stage described in Sect. 4 now operates on these high-dimensional concatenated sparse vectors ($L = 36000$) instead of the output of a single dictionary. Training is more expensive, but classification and reconstruction is still cheap. The cost of evaluating the logistic classifiers scales with the number of nonzero coefficients in the sparse representations rather than the dimensionality. As a speedup for training, we drop a different random 50 % of the representation for each of the logistic classifiers.

6   Experiments

We apply multipath reconstructive sparse code transfer to two pixel labeling tasks: contour detection on the Berkeley segmentation dataset (BSDS) [12], and semantic labeling of human faces (into skin, hair, and background) on the part subset [14] of the Labeled Faces in the Wild (LFW) dataset [13]. We use the network structure in Fig. 2 in both sets of experiments, with the only difference being that we apply a zero-mean transform to patch channels prior to encoding in the BSDS experiments. This choice was simply made to increase dictionary efficiency in the case of contour detection, where absolute color is likely less important. For experiments on the LFW dataset, we directly encode raw patches.

6.1   Contour Detection

Figure 4 shows contour detection results on example images from the test set of the 500 image version [8] of the BSDS [12]. Figure 5 shows the precision-recall curve for our contour detector as benchmarked against human-drawn ground-truth. Performance is comparable to the heavily-engineered state-of-the-art global Pb (gPb) detector [8].

Note that both gPb and SCG [15] apply a spectral clustering procedure on top of their detector output in order to generate a cleaner globally consistent result. In both cases, this extra step provides a performance boost. Table 1 displays a more nuanced comparison of our contour detection performance with that of SCG before globalization. Our detector performs comparably to (local) SCG. We expect that inclusion of a sophisticated spectral integration step [25] will further boost our contour detection performance, but leave the proof to future work.

It is also worth emphasizing that our system is the only method in Table 1 that relies on neither hand-crafted filters (global Pb, SCG) nor hand-crafted features (global Pb, Structured Edges). Our system is learned entirely from data and even relies on a *generatively trained* representation as a critical component.

Additional analysis of our results yields the interesting observation that the second layer of our multipath network appears crucial to texture understanding. Figure 6 shows a comparison of contour detection results when our system is restricted to use only layer 1 versus results when the system uses the sparse representation from both layers 1 and 2. Inclusion of the second layer (deep sparse coding) essentially allows the classification stage to learn an off switch for texture edges.

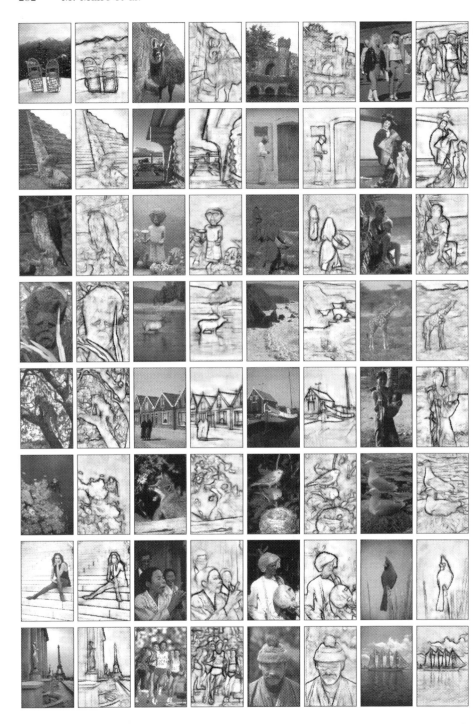

Fig. 4. Contour detection results on BSDS500. We show images and corresponding contours produced via reconstructive sparse code transfer. Contours are displayed prior to applying non-maximal suppression and thinning for benchmarking purposes.

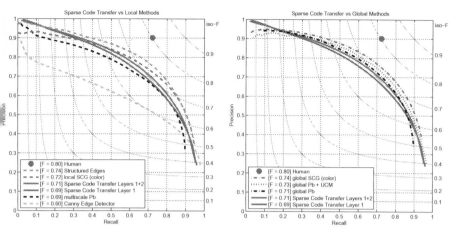

Fig. 5. Contour detection performance on BSDS500. Our contour detector (solid red curve) achieves a maximum F-measure ($\frac{2 \cdot Precision \cdot Recall}{Precision + Recall}$) of 0.71, similar to other leading approaches. Table 1 elaborates with more performance metrics. *Left:* We show full precision-recall curves for algorithms that, like ours, predict boundary strength directly from local image patches. Of these algorithms, sparse code transfer is the only one free of reliance on hand-designed features or filters. Note that addition of the second layer improves our system's performance, as seen in the jump from the blue to red curve. *Right:* Post-processing steps that perform global reasoning on top of locally detected contours can further boost performance. Application of spectral clustering to multiscale Pb and local SCG yields superior results shown as global Pb and global SCG, respectively. Further transforming global Pb via an Ultrametric Contour Map (UCM) [26] yields an additional boost. Without any such post-processing, our local detector offers performance equivalent to that of global Pb.

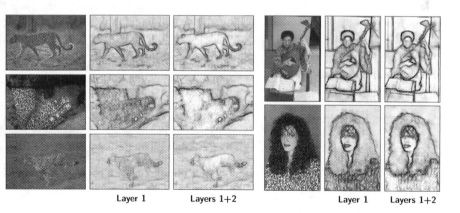

| Layer 1 | Layers 1+2 | Layer 1 | Layers 1+2 |

Fig. 6. Texture understanding and network depth. From left to right, we display an image, the contours detected using only the sparse representation from the layer 1 dictionaries in Fig. 2, and the contours detected using the representation from both layers 1 and 2. Inclusion of the second layer is crucial to enabling the system to suppress undesirable fine-scale texture edges.

Table 1. Contour benchmarks on BSDS500. Performance of our sparse code transfer technique is competitive with the current best performing contour detection systems [8,15,16]. Shown are the detector F-measures when choosing an optimal threshold for the entire dataset (ODS) or per image (OIS), as well as the average precision (AP). The upper block of the table reports scores prior to application of spectral globalization, while the lower block reports improved results of some systems afterwards. Note that our system is the only approach in which both the feature representation and classifier are entirely learned.

	Performance Metric			Hand-Designed		Spectral
	ODS F	OIS F	AP	Features?	Filters?	Globalization?
Human	0.80	0.80	–	–	–	–
Structured Edges [16]	**0.74**	**0.76**	**0.78**	yes	no	no
local SCG (color) [15]	0.72	0.74	0.75	no	yes	no
Sparse Code Transfer Layers 1+2	0.71	0.72	0.74	**no**	**no**	no
Sparse Code Transfer Layer 1	0.69	0.71	0.72	**no**	**no**	no
local SCG (gray) [15]	0.69	0.71	0.71	no	yes	no
multiscale Pb [8]	0.69	0.71	0.68	yes	yes	no
Canny Edge Detector [27]	0.60	0.63	0.58	yes	yes	no
global SCG (color) [15]	**0.74**	**0.76**	0.77	yes	yes	yes
global Pb + UCM [8]	0.73	**0.76**	0.73	yes	yes	yes + UCM
global Pb [8]	0.71	0.74	0.65	yes	yes	yes

6.2 Semantic Labeling of Faces

Figure 7 shows example results for semantic segmentation of skin, hair, and background classes on the LFW parts dataset using reconstructive sparse code transfer. All results are for our two-layer multipath network. As the default split of the LFW parts dataset allowed images of the same individual to appear in both training and test sets, we randomly re-split the dataset with the constraint that images of a particular individual were either all in the training set or all in the test set, with no overlap. All examples in Fig. 7 are from our test set after this more stringent split.

Note that while faces are centered in the LFW part dataset images, we directly apply our algorithm and make no attempt to take advantage of this additional information. Hence, for several examples in Fig. 7 our learned skin and hair detectors fire on both primary and secondary subjects appearing in the photograph.

7   Conclusion

We demonstrate that sparse coding, combined with a reconstructive transfer learning framework, produces results competitive with the state-of-the-art for contour detection. Varying the target of the transfer learning stage allows one to port a common sparse representation to multiple end tasks. We highlight

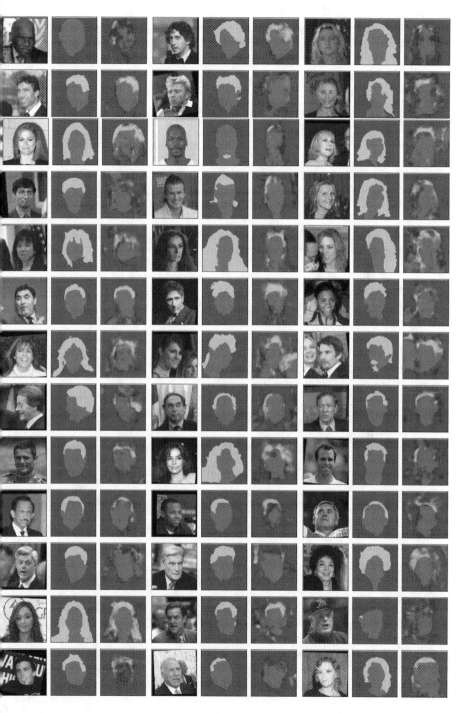

Fig. 7. Part labeling results on LFW. *Left:* Image. *Middle:* Ground-truth. Semantic classes are skin (green), hair (red), and background (blue). *Right:* Semantic labeling predicted via reconstructive sparse code transfer (Color figure online).

semantic labeling of faces as an additional example. Our approach is entirely data-driven and relies on no hand-crafted features. Sparse representations similar to the one we consider also arise naturally in the context of deep networks for image recognition. We conjecture that multipath sparse networks [6] can produce shared representations useful for many vision tasks and view this as a promising direction for future research.

Acknowledgments. ARO/JPL-NASA Stennis NAS7.03001 supported Michael Maire's work.

References

1. Le, Q.V., Ranzato, M., Monga, R., Devin, M., Chen, K., Corrado, G.S., Dean, J., Ng, A.Y.: Building high-level features using large scale unsupervised learning. In: ICML (2012)
2. LeCun, Y., Kavukcuoglu, K., Farabet, C.: Convolutional networks and applications in vision. In: ISCAS (2010)
3. Krizhevsky, A., Sutskever, I., Hinton, G.E.: ImageNet classification with deep convolutional neural networks. In: NIPS (2012)
4. Zeiler, M.D., Taylor, G.W., Fergus, R.: Adaptive deconvolutional networks for mid and high level feature learning. In: ICCV (2011)
5. Yu, K., Lin, Y., Lafferty, J.: Learning image representations from the pixel level via hierarchical sparse coding. In: CVPR (2011)
6. Bo, L., Ren, X., Fox, D.: Multipath sparse coding using hierarchical matching pursuit. In: CVPR (2013)
7. Zeiler, M.D., Fergus, R.: Visualizing and understanding convolutional networks. In: Fleet, D., Pajdla, T., Schiele, B., Tuytelaars, T. (eds.) ECCV 2014, Part I. LNCS, vol. 8689, pp. 818–833. Springer, Heidelberg (2014)
8. Arbeláez, P., Maire, M., Fowlkes, C., Malik, J.: Contour detection and hierarchical image segmentation. PAMI **33**(5), 898–916 (2011)
9. Elad, M., Aharon, M.: Image denoising via sparse and redundant representations over learned dictionaries. IEEE Trans. Image Process. **15**(12), 3736–3745 (2006)
10. Pati, Y.C., Rezaiifar, R., Krishnaprasad, P.S.: Orthogonal matching pursuit: recursive function approximation with applications to wavelet decomposition. In: Asilomar Conference on Signals, Systems and Computers (1993)
11. Rubinstein, R., Zibulevsky, M., Elad, M.: Efficient implementation of the K-SVD algorithm using batch orthogonal matching pursuit (2008)
12. Martin, D., Fowlkes, C., Tal, D., Malik, J.: A database of human segmented natural images and its application to evaluating segmentation algorithms and measuring ecological statistics. In: ICCV (2001)
13. Huang, G.B., Ramesh, M., Berg, T., Learned-Miller, E.: Labeled faces in the wild: a database for studying face recognition in unconstrained environments (2007)
14. Kae, A., Sohn, K., Lee, H., Learned-Miller, E.: Augmenting CRFs with Boltzmann machine shape priors for image labeling. In: CVPR (2013)
15. Ren, X., Bo, L.: Discriminatively trained sparse code gradients for contour detection. In: NIPS (2012)
16. Dollár, P., Zitnick, C.L.: Structured forests for fast edge detection. In: ICCV (2013)

17. Martin, D., Fowlkes, C., Malik, J.: Learning to detect natural image boundaries using local brightness, color and texture cues. PAMI **26**(5), 530–54 (2004)
18. Shi, J., Malik, J.: Normalized cuts and image segmentation. PAMI **22**(8), 888–905 (2000)
19. Malik, J., Belongie, S., Leung, T., Shi, J.: Contour and texture analysis for image segmentation. IJCV **43**(1), 7–27 (2001)
20. Ren, X., Fowlkes, C.C., Malik, J.: Figure/ground assignment in natural images. In: Leonardis, A., Bischof, H., Pinz, A. (eds.) ECCV 2006. LNCS, vol. 3952, pp. 614–627. Springer, Heidelberg (2006)
21. Lim, J., Zitnick, C.L., Dollár, P.: Sketch tokens: a learned mid-level representation for contour and object detection. In: CVPR (2013)
22. Mairal, J., Leordeanu, M., Bach, F., Hebert, M., Ponce, J.: Discriminative sparse image models for class-specific edge detection and image interpretation. In: Forsyth, D., Torr, P., Zisserman, A. (eds.) ECCV 2008, Part III. LNCS, vol. 5304, pp. 43–56. Springer, Heidelberg (2008)
23. Yang, J., Wang, Z., Lin, Z., Shu, X., Huang, T.: Bilevel sparse coding for coupled feature spaces. In: CVPR (2012)
24. Aharon, M., Elad, M., Bruckstein, A.: K-SVD: an algorithm for designing overcomplete dictionaries for sparse representation. IEEE Trans. Signal Process. **54**(11), 4311–4322 (2006)
25. Maire, M., Yu, S.X., Perona, P.: Progressive multigrid eigensolvers for multiscale spectral segmentation. In: ICCV (2013)
26. Arbeláez, P.: Boundary extraction in natural images using ultrametric contour maps. In: POCV (2006)
27. Canny, J.: A computational approach to edge detection. PAMI **8**(6), 679–698 (1986)

A Message Passing Algorithm for MRF Inference with Unknown Graphs and Its Applications

Zhenhua Wang[1,2], Zhiyi Zhang[2]([✉]), and Nan Geng[2]

[1] School of Computer Science, The University of Adelaide, Adelaide, Australia
[2] College of Information Engineering, Northwest A&F University,
Yangling District, China
zhhsun@outlook.com, {zhangzhiyi,nangeng}@nwsuaf.edu.cn

Abstract. Recent research shows that estimating labels and graph structures simultaneously in Markov random Fields can be achieved via solving LP problems. The scalability is a bottleneck that prevents applying such technique to larger problems such as image segmentation and object detection. Here we present a fast message passing algorithm based on the mixed-integer bilinear programming formulation of the original problem. We apply our algorithm to both synthetic data and real-world applications. It compares favourably with previous methods.

1 Introduction

Many computer vision applications involve predicting structured labels like sequence and trees. A potential function is typically defined to measure the consistency between structured label candidates and observations, and maximising the potential function over the labelling space discloses the structured label estimation. An example is the semantic image segmentation (pixel labelling) task which requires assigning each pixel or superpixel a label representing the corresponding object category. Labels of all pixels form a sequence. A typical potential function for this task is a sum of all unary potentials and pairwise potential potentials, where each unary term measures the consistency between the pixel label and the photometric information of the pixel, and each pairwise term evaluates the consistency between the labels of neighbouring pixels [1].

Markov random fields (MRFs) provide a compact representation of the dependency among structured variables. Each random variable is typically represented by a node in the MRF graph, and the dependency between a pair of variables is encoded by an edge in the graph. A vacancy of edge between two nodes indicates that the associated variables are independent conditioned on observing the statuses of all rest variables. In this sense, the graph structure of MRF is essential in modelling the structured prediction problems. Despite maximising the potential function is NP-hard in general, approximations can be found efficiently by carrying out message passing [2] on MRF graphs.

To determine the structure of MRF graphs, one usually chooses to optimise the information gain [3]. Alternatively, rules based on heuristics or domain

© Springer International Publishing Switzerland 2015
D. Cremers et al. (Eds.): ACCV 2014, Part IV, LNCS 9006, pp. 288–302, 2015.
DOI: 10.1007/978-3-319-16817-3_19

knowledge can be used. For example, in image segmentation, one usually uses grid graphs with edges reflecting pixel adjacency; in human activity recognition with multiple persons, one can use tree structured graphs that span shortest Euclidean distances across all people. However, determining graphs heuristically or based on domain knowledge is not principle and is prone to input variance. First of all, if we create graphs by defining rules derived from domain knowledge, the rules are always too problem-oriented to be generally applicable. Second, unwanted edges can be easily introduced by using heuristics. For example, in human activity recognition, graphs generated according to the near-far relationship between people can be undesirable because two persons might be interacting even when they are far away from each other (passing basketball for instance). Due to these reasons, digging adaptive graphs directly from inputs is interesting.

Inferring graphs and labels directly and simultaneously from data has shown to be favourable comparing with using fixed hand-engineered graphs in human action recognition [4,5]. However, the related inference problem is highly challenging. Lan et al. [4] propose an approach to the problem which alternates between finding the best label for a fixed graph using loopy belief propagation, and finding the best graph for a fixed set of labels via solving a LP. A rounding scheme is used to decode the structures from LP solutions. Recently, Wang et al. [5] showed that the problem of finding labels and graphs jointly can be formulated as a bilinear programming (BLP) problem, which they then relaxed to a LP problem. A branch and bound (B&B) method was then developed to improve the quality of the solution using the LP as bounds, which essentially involves solving a number of LPs. Unfortunately, this B&B method is extremely time-consuming even for small graphs, meaning that an early-stop is usually used which results in a sub-optimal solution. To enable inferring graphs and labels simultaneously on large-scale problems, we propose a message passing-style algorithm in this paper. We formulate the inference as a *mixed integer bilinear programming problem* [6]. Then we derive the *partial-dual* (the term is probably first used in [7]) of the mixed integer bilinear programming problem. To solve the dual problem, we fix a majority of variables in the partial-dual and the reduced problem can be solved *analytically*. This approach can be viewed as a message passing process which extends Globerson's MPLP algorithm [8] to MRF inference with unknown graphs. We apply our algorithm to both synthetic data and real computer vision tasks including semantic image segmentation and human action recognition. Our algorithm is competitive with the state-of-the-art on accuracy while is much faster.

The rest of the paper is organised as follows. In Sect. 2 we show our formulation of the inference problem. Next in Sect. 3 we describe our message passing algorithm. Then we compare our algorithm with other methods on synthetic data in Sect. 4. Finally in Sect. 5 we show the applications of our algorithm on semantic image segmentation and human activity recognition.

2   Mixed Integer Bilinear Programming Formulation

Let $\mathcal{V} = \{1, 2, \ldots, n\}$ be the node set; $\mathcal{E} = \{(i,j)|i,j \in \mathcal{V}, i < j\}$ be the set containing all possible edges; $y_i \in \mathcal{Y}$ denote the discrete random variable corresponding to node i; and $\mathbf{y} = [y_i]_{i \in \{1,2,\ldots,n\}}$ be a collective representation of all random variables. Introducing binary variables $z_{ij} \in \{0,1\}, \forall (i,j) \in \mathcal{E}$ to represent if an edge (i,j) exist ($z_{ij} = 1$) or not ($z_{ij} = 0$), and letting $\mathbf{z} = [z_{ij}]_{i,j \in \mathcal{V}, i<j}$ be a collective representation of all z_{ij} variables formed by collecting all z_{ij} variables in the order of enumerating all possible i and j indices in turn. Following [5], inferring graphs and labels simultaneously can be formulated as the following:

$$\max_{\mathbf{y},\mathbf{z}} \sum_{i \in \mathcal{V}} \theta_i(y_i) + \sum_{(i,j) \in \mathcal{E}} \theta_{ij}(y_i, y_j) z_{ij},$$

$$\text{s.t.} \sum_{(i,j) \in \mathcal{E}} \mathbb{1}(i = k \text{ or } j = k) z_{ij} \leq h, \forall k \in \mathcal{V}. \tag{1}$$

Here $\theta_i(y_i), \theta_{ij}(y_i, y_j)$ denote unary and pairwise potentials respectively, $\mathbb{1}(\cdot)$ is an indicator function that gives 1 if the condition inside the brackets is true, and gives 0 otherwise. The constraints control the sparsity of the estimated graph by enforcing the maximum degree of the graph less than a constant h. When $\{z_{ij}\}_{(i,j) \in \mathcal{E}}$ is given, *i.e.* we known the graph structure, the above problem recovers the traditional MRF inference problem.

Formulation. Introducing binary variables $\mu_i(y_i) \in \{0,1\}$ $\forall i \in \mathcal{V}$, and binary variables $\mu_{ij}(y_i, y_j)$ $\forall (i,j) \in \mathcal{E}, y_i, y_j$. Let $\boldsymbol{\mu}_1 = [\mu_i(y_i)]_{i \in \mathcal{V}, y_i \in \mathcal{Y}}, \boldsymbol{\mu}_2 = [\mu_{ij}(y_i, y_j)]_{i<j, y_i, y_j \in \mathcal{Y}}$ be the collective representations of all $\mu_i(y_i), \mu_{ij}(y_i, y_j)$ variables respectively by collecting all $\mu_i(y_i)$ and $\mu_{ij}(y_i, y_j)$ variables in the order of enumerating all possible $i, j \in \mathcal{V}, y_i, y_j \in \mathcal{Y}$ in turn. Problem (1) can be equivalently written as

$$\max_{\boldsymbol{\mu}_1, \boldsymbol{\mu}_2, \mathbf{z}} \sum_{i \in \mathcal{V}} \sum_{y_i} \mu_i(y_i) \theta_i(y_i) + \sum_{(i,j) \in \mathcal{E}} \sum_{y_i, y_j} \mu_{ij}(y_i, y_j) \theta_{ij}(y_i, y_j) z_{ij}$$

$$\text{s.t.} \sum_{y_i} \mu_i(y_i) = 1 \ \forall i \in \mathcal{V},$$

$$\sum_{y_i, y_j} \mu_{ij}(y_i, y_j) = 1 \ \forall (i,j) \in \mathcal{E},$$

$$\sum_{y_i} \mu_{ij}(y_i, y_j) = \mu_j(y_j) \ \forall (i,j) \in \mathcal{E}, y_j,$$

$$\sum_{y_j} \mu_{ij}(y_i, y_j) = \mu_i(y_i) \ \forall (i,j) \in \mathcal{E}, y_i,$$

$$\sum_{(i,j) \in \mathcal{E}} \mathbb{1}(i = k \text{ or } j = k) z_{ij} \leq h, \forall k \in \mathcal{V}, \tag{2}$$

which can be relaxed into a mixed integer bilinear programming problem:

$$\max_{\boldsymbol{\mu}_1, \boldsymbol{\mu}_2, \mathbf{z}} \sum_{i \in \mathcal{V}} \sum_{y_i} \mu_i(y_i) \theta_i(y_i) + \sum_{(i,j) \in \mathcal{E}} \sum_{y_i, y_j} \mu_{ij}(y_i, y_j) \theta_{ij}(y_i, y_j) z_{ij}$$

$$\text{s.t.} \ (\boldsymbol{\mu}_1, \boldsymbol{\mu}_2, \mathbf{z}) \in \mathcal{M}, \tag{3}$$

where $\mathcal{M}$ is a space defined as

$$
\mathcal{M} = \left\{ \boldsymbol{\mu}, \mathbf{z} \left| \begin{array}{l} \sum_{y_i} \mu_i(y_i) = 1, \forall i \in \mathcal{V}, \\ \sum_{y_i, y_j} \mu_{ij}(y_i, y_j) = 1, \forall (i,j) \in \mathcal{E}, \\ \sum_{y_i} \mu_{ij}(y_i, y_j) = \mu_j(y_j), \forall (i,j) \in \mathcal{E}, y_j, \\ \sum_{y_j} \mu_{ij}(y_i, y_j) = \mu_i(y_i), \forall (i,j) \in \mathcal{E}, y_i, \\ \sum_{(i,j) \in \mathcal{E}} \mathbb{1}(i = k \text{ or } j = k) z_{ij} \le h, \forall k \in \mathcal{V}, \\ \mu_i(y_i) \in [0,1], \forall i \in \mathcal{V}, y_i, \\ \mu_{ij}(y_i, y_j) \in [0,1], \forall (i,j) \in \mathcal{E}, y_i, y_j, \\ z_{ij} \in \{0,1\}, \forall (i,j) \in \mathcal{E}. \end{array} \right. \right\} \tag{4}
$$

Note our mixed integer bilinear formulation is exactly the same as the bilinear relaxation in [5] except that $z_{ij} \in \{0,1\}$ in our problem as compared with $z_{ij} \in [0,1]$ in the bilinear formulation in [5]. As a result, our relaxation (3) is tighter than the bilinear relaxation. As we will see later, the formulation leads to not only very fast algorithm scales to large inference problem, but also the closed-form solution for updating beliefs.

3   The Message Passing Algorithm

Message passing, also known as belief propagation is a strategy to perform inference on probabilistic graphical models, e.g. MRFs. The success of message passing algorithms lies in splitting the original inference problem into small sub-problems according to the structure of the problem (known as factorisation), where each sub-problem can be efficiently solved via propagating messages among nodes.

Compared with traditional message passing algorithms performed on MRF graphs with known structures, our message passing algorithm has two differences. Firstly, it does not require knowing the graph structure of MRF. Instead, the algorithm automatically estimates the graph structure and labelling simultaneously in a unique framework. Secondly, we derive a partial-dual of the original inference problem and perform the messaging passing in the partial-dual space. In comparison with existing algorithms for MRF inference with unknown graphs, our algorithm is significantly faster because it iteratively solves the sub-problems of the partial-dual problem which have analytical solutions.

3.1   The Partial-Dual Problem

It turns out that the following problem is equivalent to the problem (3):

$$
\max_{\mathbf{z}} \; \min_{\boldsymbol{\beta}} \; \sum_{i \in \mathcal{V}} \max_{y_i} \sum_{j \in \mathcal{V} \setminus \{i\}} \max_{y_j} \beta_{ji}(y_j, y_i) + \theta_i(y_i)
$$

$$
\text{s.t.} \; \sum_{(i,j) \in \mathcal{E}} \mathbb{1}(i = k \text{ or } j = k) z_{ij} \le h, \forall k \in \mathcal{V},
$$

$$
z_{ij} \in \{0,1\} \; \forall (i,j) \in \mathcal{E},
$$

$$
\beta_{ij}(y_i, y_j) + \beta_{ji}(y_j, y_i) = \theta_{ij}(y_i, y_j) z_{ij} \; \forall (i,j) \in \mathcal{E}, y_i, y_j. \tag{5}
$$

Remember $\mathbf{z}$ are the primal variables that represent the graph structure. Here $\boldsymbol{\beta} = [\beta_{ij}(y_i, y_j)]_{i \neq j, y_i, y_j}$ are the dual variables. Despite the existence of the primal variables $\mathbf{z}$, for a fixed $\mathbf{z}$ this problem is called the partial-dual problem of (3) because it is actually a Lagrangian dual of the primal problem (3) when $\mathbf{z}$ are known.

The derivation is briefed as follows. First we fix all structure variables $\mathbf{z}$ and the problem (3) becomes a linear programming problem of $\boldsymbol{\mu}$, for which we next derive a Lagrangian dual using the technique presented by Globerson *et al.* in [8]. Then we remove redundant constraints and variables, leaving only the dual variables $\boldsymbol{\beta}$. At last $\mathbf{z}$ are reset as free variables and we get (5). In comparison with the primal version (3), the dual problem contains far fewer constraints. However, solving such a problem is still difficult. We next present our message passing algorithm that solves (5) approximately but efficiently.

3.2   The Algorithm

In order to solve (5), we adopt an iterative strategy. Concisely, during each iteration we fix all the primal and dual variables in (5) except for the variables related to one selected edge. The reduced problem is solved analytically. This process is repeated until a max-number of iterations is reached.

Problem reduction. Let $\mathcal{E}^*$ denote the current edge estimation, and let $\mathbf{z}^*$ denote the corresponding solution of structure variables. During each iteration a node pair (i, j) is selected. By fixing all variables unchanged except for variables related to (i, j), *i.e.* z_{ij}, $\beta_{ij}(y_i, y_j)$ and $\beta_{ji}(y_j, y_i)$ $\forall y_i, y_j$, the problem (5) becomes

$$\max_{z_{ij} \in \{0,1\}} \quad \min_{\boldsymbol{\beta}_{ij}, \boldsymbol{\beta}_{ji}} \quad q(\boldsymbol{\beta}_{ij}, \boldsymbol{\beta}_{ji})$$

$$\text{s.t.} \ \beta_{ij}(y_i, y_j) + \beta_{ji}(y_j, y_i) = \theta_{ij}(y_i, y_j) z_{ij} \ \forall y_i, y_j,$$

$$\sum_{(r,s) \in \mathcal{E}^*} \mathbb{1}(r = k \text{ or } s = k) z_{rs}^* - z_{ij}^* + z_{ij} \leq h \ \forall k \in \{i, j\},$$

$$\beta_{ij}(y_i, y_j), \beta_{ji}(y_j, y_i) \in [0, 1] \ \forall y_i, y_j. \tag{6}$$

Here $\boldsymbol{\beta}_{ij} = [\beta_{ij}(y_i, y_j)]_{\forall y_i, y_j}, \boldsymbol{\beta}_{ji} = [\beta_{ji}(y_j, y_i)]_{\forall y_j, y_i}$, and the objective function

$$q(\boldsymbol{\beta}_{ij}, \boldsymbol{\beta}_{ji}) = \max_{y_i}[\lambda_i^{-j}(y_i) + \max_{y_j} \beta_{ji}(y_j, y_i) + \theta_i(y_i)] +$$

$$\max_{y_j}[\lambda_j^{-i}(y_j) + \max_{y_i} \beta_{ij}(y_i, y_j) + \theta_j(y_j)], \tag{7}$$

where λ_i^{-j}, λ_j^{-i} are compact representations of the following:

$$\lambda_i^{-j}(y_i) = \sum_{k \in \mathcal{V} \setminus \{i,j\}} z_{ki}^* \max_{y_k} \beta_{ki}(y_k, y_i), \tag{8}$$

$$\lambda_j^{-i}(y_j) = \sum_{k \in \mathcal{V} \setminus \{i,j\}} z_{kj}^* \max_{y_k} \beta_{kj}(y_k, y_j). \tag{9}$$

As in [8], we define

$$\lambda_{ki}(y_i) = \max_{y_k} \beta_{ki}(y_k, y_i) \tag{10}$$

as the message passing from node k to node i. According to (8) and (9), $\lambda_i^{-j}(y_i)$ is an accumulation of messages passing from all neighbouring nodes (except for j) to i when it takes the label y_i, and $\lambda_j^{-i}(y_j)$ is an accumulation of messages passing from all neighbouring nodes (except for i) to j when it takes the label y_j. As we will see later, these messages carry essential information needed for updating the current solutions.

Update via message passing. Because z_{ij} is a binary variable, we choose to exhaustively search over $z_{ij} \in \{0, 1\}$. We have the following proposition:

Proposition 1. *For any particular* z_{ij}, *the problem* (6) *actually has analytical solutions: minimising* $q(\boldsymbol{\beta}_{ij}, \boldsymbol{\beta}_{ji})$ *yields the following results*

$$\beta_{ij}(y_i, y_j) = \tfrac{1}{2}[\lambda_i^{-j}(y_i) + \theta_{ij}(y_i, y_j)z_{ij} + \theta_i(y_i) - \lambda_j^{-i}(y_j) - \theta_j(y_j)], \quad (11)$$

$$\beta_{ji}(y_j, y_i) = \tfrac{1}{2}[\lambda_j^{-i}(y_j) + \theta_{ij}(y_i, y_j)z_{ij} + \theta_j(y_j) - \lambda_i^{-j}(y_i) - \theta_i(y_i)]. \quad (12)$$

Proof. Let $\hat{z}_{ij}$ denote a fixed value of z_{ij}. According to Eq. (7), the following inequality holds:

$$q(\boldsymbol{\beta}_{ij}, \boldsymbol{\beta}_{ji}) \geq \max_{y_i, y_j}\{\lambda_i^{-j}(y_i) + \lambda_j^{-i}(y_j) + \beta_{ji}(y_j, y_i) + \beta_{ij}(y_i, y_j) + \theta_i(y_i) + \theta_j(y_j)\} =$$

$$\underbrace{\max_{y_i, y_j}\{\lambda_i^{-j}(y_i) + \lambda_j^{-i}(y_j) + \theta_{ij}(y_i, y_j)\hat{z}_{ij} + \theta_i(y_i) + \theta_j(y_j)\}}_{LB}. \quad (13)$$

Hence LB is a lower bound of $q(\boldsymbol{\beta}_{ij}, \boldsymbol{\beta}_{ji})$. Plug the $\boldsymbol{\beta}_{ij}, \boldsymbol{\beta}_{ji}$ given (11) and (12) into Eq. (7), we have:

$$q(\boldsymbol{\beta}_{ij}, \boldsymbol{\beta}_{ji}) = \max_{y_i, y_j}[\lambda_i^{-j}(y_i) + \frac{1}{2}\max_{y_j}(\lambda_j^{-i}(y_j) + \theta_{ij}(y_i, y_j)\hat{z}_{ij} + \theta_j(y_j) - \lambda_i^{-j}(y_i) -$$

$$\theta_i(y_i)) + \theta_i(y_i)] + \max_{y_i, y_j}[\lambda_j^{-i}(y_j) + \frac{1}{2}\max_{y_i}(\lambda_i^{-j}(y_i) + \theta_{ij}(y_i, y_j)\hat{z}_{ij} +$$

$$\theta_i(y_i) - \lambda_j^{-i}(y_j) - \theta_j(y_j)) + \theta_j(y_j)]. \quad (14)$$

$$\implies q(\boldsymbol{\beta}_{ij}, \boldsymbol{\beta}_{ji}) =$$

$$\max_{y_i, y_j}[\lambda_i^{-j}(y_i) + \frac{1}{2}(\lambda_j^{-i}(y_j) + \theta_{ij}(y_i, y_j)\hat{z}_{ij} + \theta_j(y_j) - \lambda_i^{-j}(y_i) - \theta_i(y_i)) + \theta_i(y_i)] +$$

$$\max_{y_i, y_j}[\lambda_j^{-i}(y_j) + \frac{1}{2}(\lambda_i^{-j}(y_i) + \theta_{ij}(y_i, y_j)\hat{z}_{ij} + \theta_i(y_i) - \lambda_j^{-i}(y_j) - \theta_j(y_j)) + \theta_j(y_j)]. \quad (15)$$

$$\implies q(\boldsymbol{\beta}_{ij}, \boldsymbol{\beta}_{ji}) = \max_{y_i, y_j}\{\lambda_i^{-j}(y_i) + \lambda_j^{-i}(y_j) + \theta_{ij}(y_i, y_j)\hat{z}_{ij} + \theta_i(y_i) + \theta_j(y_j)\}, \quad (16)$$

which means that LB can be reached with $\boldsymbol{\beta}_{ij}, \boldsymbol{\beta}_{ji}$ given by (11) and (12). Since we are minimising the objective in (6) over $\boldsymbol{\beta}_{ij}, \boldsymbol{\beta}_{ji}$, the proof is complete.

$\square$

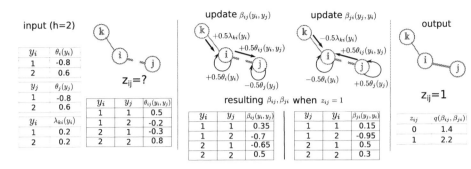

Fig. 1. Updating z_{ij} via message passing for a toy example with three nodes $\{i,j,k\}$. Here $h = 2$. The required information includes potentials $\theta_i(y_i), \theta_j(y_j), \theta_{ij}(y_i, y_j) \forall y_i, y_j$, and the messages propagated from all other nodes to i, j, i.e. $\lambda_{ki}(y_i) \forall y_i$. The middle diagram visualise the computation of $\beta_{ij}(y_i, y_j)$ and $\beta_{ji}(y_j, y_i)$. Arrows denote message or potential flows when $z_{ij} = 1$. The function values of $q(\beta_{ij}, \beta_{ji})$ are given by the table at the bottom of the right diagram. The value of z_{ij} is the one in $\{0,1\}$ that gives larger $q(\beta_{ij}, \beta_{ji})$ and does not violate any sparsity constraints in (1).

Note when $z_{ij} = 0$, setting $\beta_{ij}(y_i, y_j) = 0$, $\beta_{ji}(y_j, y_i) = 0$ also solves the optimisation problem (6). In such case, we just use this trivial solution due to two reasons. First, the computation of (11) and (12) can be avoided. Second, this trivial solution gives zeros messages between (i, j), which is coherent with the fact that there is no edge between node i and node j.

Let $\{\beta_{ij}^0, \beta_{ji}^0\}$, $\{\beta_{ij}^1, \beta_{ji}^1\}$ denote the solution of (6) when z_{ij} equals 0 and 1 respectively. To get the final solution, we need to know the optimal value of z_{ij}. Since we are maximising over z_{ij}, the optimal z_{ij} is 1 if two conditions are met: (1) $q(\beta_{ij}^0, \beta_{ji}^0) < q(\beta_{ij}^1, \beta_{ji}^1)$; (2) all sparsity constraints in (6) are not violated when setting $z_{ij} = 1$. Otherwise we let $z_{ij} = 0$. Updating z_{ij} via this method is illustrated in Fig. 1. If the optimal value of z_{ij} is 1, we compute $\beta_{ij}(y_i, y_j), \beta_{ji}(y_j, y_i)$ according to (12); otherwise we set $\beta_{ij}(y_i, y_j), \beta_{ji}(y_j, y_i)$ to 0. Then we can update messages $\lambda_{ij}(y_j)$ and $\lambda_{ji}(y_i)$ according to (10). Note in practice, it is not necessary to store β values explicitly as all information we need for further computation is included in messages. During each iteration, we randomly select an edge (i, j) and solve the associated problem (6) exactly. Then we evaluate the objective in (1) using the current solution as inputs. If the current solution improves this objective, it is kept otherwise we discard it and consider the next (i, j). As shown in Fig. 1, computing z_{ij} and $\{\beta_{ij}, \beta_{ji}\}$ can be viewed as a process of passing messages to nodes i and j from other nodes. Hence we call this algorithm partial-dual based message passing (PDMP). More details about our algorithm can be found in Algorithm 1. Note the decoding, *i.e.* determining the labelling **y** is achieved via maximising the so-called node beliefs over the labelling space of each node.

Currently the PDMP algorithm supports pairwise potentials only. However, with a modification of the sparsity constraints (*e.g.* restricting the total number

---

Algorithm 1. PDMP Algorithm.

Require: potentials θ, h, max iteration number $tmax$.
Output: estimated $\mathbf{y}^*$ and $\mathbf{z}^*$.
1: **Initialise:** $\lambda_{ij}(y_j) \leftarrow 0$, $\lambda_{ji}(y_i) \leftarrow 0$, $z_{ij} \leftarrow 0$, $t \leftarrow 0$, $o_t \leftarrow -\infty$.
2: **while** $t < tmax$ **do**
3:     **for** each $(i,j) \in \mathcal{E}$ (pick (i,j) randomly without repetition) **do**
4:         compute $\beta^1_{ij}(y_i, y_j)$, $\beta^1_{ji}(y_j, y_i)$ via (12).
5:         $\beta^0_{ij}(y_i, y_j) \leftarrow 0$, $\beta^0_{ji}(y_j, y_i) \leftarrow 0$, $z_{ij} \leftarrow 1$.
6:         **if** $q(\beta^0_{ij}, \beta^0_{ji}) < q(\beta^1_{ij}, \beta^1_{ji})$ and $\mathbf{z}$ is feasible **then**
7:             $\beta_{ij}(y_i, y_j) \leftarrow \beta^1_{ij}(y_i, y_j)$, $\beta_{ji}(y_j, y_i) \leftarrow \beta^1_{ji}(y_j, y_i)$.
8:         **else**
9:             $\beta_{ij}(y_i, y_j) \leftarrow \beta^0_{ij}(y_i, y_j)$, $\beta_{ji}(y_j, y_i) \leftarrow \beta^0_{ji}(y_j, y_i)$, $z_{ij} \leftarrow 0$.
10:        **end if**
11:        update messages $\lambda_{ij}(y_j)$, $\lambda_{ji}(y_i)$ via (10).
12:    **end for**
13:    compute node beliefs: $b_i(y_i) \leftarrow \sum_{k \in \mathcal{V} \setminus \{i\}} z_{ki} \lambda_{ki}(y_i) + \theta_i(y_i)$.
14:    decode: $\mathbf{y} \leftarrow [y_i]$ with $y_i \leftarrow \max_{y_i} b_i(y_i)$.
15:    $o_{t+1} \leftarrow \sum_{i \in \mathcal{V}} \theta_i(y_i) + \sum_{(i,j) \in \mathcal{E}} \theta_{ij}(y_i, y_j) z_{ij}$.
16:    **if** $o_t < o_{t+1}$ **then**
17:        $\mathbf{y}^* \leftarrow \mathbf{y}$, $\mathbf{z}^* = [z_{uv}] \; \forall (u,v) \in \mathcal{E}$.
18:    **end if**
19:    $t \leftarrow t + 1$.
20: **end while**
21: return $\mathbf{z}^*$ and $\mathbf{y}^*$.

---

of super-edges), a similar message passing algorithm for graphs with arbitrary cliques can be obtained.

4   Running Time Comparison

We compare the running time of our PDMP algorithm against the following methods:

- Lan the method proposed in [4] which alternatingly implement two steps: (1) fix graph structure and solve a MRF inference problem (with known graph); (2) fix labels and solve a LP problem. See [4] for more details.
- LP solves a linear programming relaxation [5] of the inference problem (2). The LP problems are solved using the Mosek toolbox [9].
- LP+B&B the branch and bound method proposed in [5]. The bounds are computed via solving the LP relaxation.

We generate synthetic data using a method similar to [10]. The node potentials are uniformly sampled from $\mathcal{U}(-1, 1)$, while the edge potentials are created as a product of a coupling strength and a distance $\mathrm{dis}(y_i, y_j)$ between labels y_i, y_j. The coupling strength is sampled from $\mathcal{U}(-1, 1)$. Four types of distance functions are used including linear: $\mathrm{dis}(y_i, y_j) = |y_i - y_j|$, quadratic: $\mathrm{dis}(y_i, y_j) = (y_i - y_j)^2$,

Table 1. Comparison of running time (by seconds) on synthetic data generated by using different distance functions. For each distance function the best is highlighted.

	Ising	Linear	Quadratic	Potts
LP	17	12	11	11
Lan [4]	2	1	1	1
LP+B&B [5]	570	402	403	403
PDMP (ours)	**0.01**	**0.007**	**0.007**	**0.007**

Ising: $\text{dis}(y_i, y_j) = y_i y_j$, Potts: $\text{dis}(y_i, y_j) = \mathbb{1}(y_i = y_j)$. We compare the average running time of solving twenty different synthetic examples with the number of nodes fixed to be 30. We let the sparsity parameter $h = 2$. The results are shown in Table 1. Clearly our PDMP algorithm is the fastest, while the LP+B&B is the slowest.

5   Applications

We apply the proposed method to semantic image segmentation and human activity recognition. To our knowledge, this is the first work that estimates labels and graph structures simultaneously in semantic image segmentation.

5.1   Semantic Image Segmentation

Given an over-segmented image, the task here is to assign each super-pixel in the over-segmentation a label to express its object category.

Table 2. Methods for image segmentation. The column G gives the approach used to create graph structures, and the column *inference* lists the methods used to solve the inference problem. Here BP means belief propagation, *Adj* stands for *Adjacent*. Note the first two methods can also use the $-\log$ potential functions used by Lan and PDMP. However, the performance is not as good as using the exp potentials.

	$\phi_2(y_i, y_j)$	$\phi_3(y_i, y_j)$	G	inference
CRF–Adj	$\exp(-\|c_i - c_j\|_2)$ if $y_i = y_j$, $1 - \exp(-\|c_i - c_j\|_2)$ if $y_i \neq y_j$	$\exp(-\|q_i - q_j\|_2)$ if $y_i = y_j$, $1 - \exp(-\|q_i - q_j\|_2)$ if $y_i \neq y_j$	Adj	BP
CRF–MST	same as CRF–Adj	same as CRF–Adj	2D MST	BP
Lan	$-\log(\|c_i - c_j\|_2)$ if $y_i = y_j$, 0 if $y_i \neq y_j$	$-\log(\|q_i - q_j\|_2)$ if $y_i = y_j$, 0 if $y_i \neq y_j$	Lan [4]	Lan [4]
PDMP	same as Lan	same as Lan	PDMP	PDMP

A number of datasets are publicly available. In this paper we use the KITTI dataset [11]. The original dataset contains both 2D images (1240×380) and 3D laser data taken by a vehicle in different urban scenes. Since 2D information is more general in practice, we discard 3D information in our experiments.

There are 70 labelled images made by [12] as groundtruth. The original labelling contains 10 classes: road, building, vehicle, people, pavement, vegetation, sky, signal, post/pole and fence. As in [13], the 10 classes are mapped to five more general classes that are: ground (road and pavement), building, vegetation, and objects (vehicle, people, signal, pole and fence). Following [12,13], the labelled images are divided into two parts containing 45 and 25 images respectively. The first part is used for training while the second part is used for testing.

A MRF based image segmentation strategy is adopted here. Each image $\mathbf{x}$ is over-segmented into small regions (super-pixels) at first using SLIC toolbox [14]. The super-pixels and their relations are represented by a graph $G = (\mathcal{V}, \mathcal{E})$ with the edge set $\mathcal{E}$ *unknown*. Each node $i \in \mathcal{V}$ in the MRF graph denotes a label y_i of the related super-pixel i. Each edge $(i, j) \in \mathcal{E}$ in the MRF graph encodes the dependency between the associated labels y_i, y_j. Let $\phi_1(y_i), \phi_2(y_i, y_j), \phi_3(y_i, y_j)$ denote the node feature, the edge feature in relevant to colour, and the edge feature in relevant to super-pixel location respectively. The potential function (parameterised by $\mathbf{w} = [w_1, w_2, w_3]$) is

$$F(\mathbf{x}, \mathbf{w}; \mathbf{y}, G) = \sum_{i \in \mathcal{V}} w_1 \phi_1(y_i) + \sum_{(i,j) \in \mathcal{E}} w_2 \phi_2(y_i, y_j) + w_3 \phi_3(y_i, y_j). \quad (17)$$

Maximising F over $\mathbf{y}$ and G uncovers the label estimation of all super-pixels. We test four methods: (1) CRF–Adjacency (Adj); (2) CRF–Minimum spanning tree (MST); (3) Lan; (4) PDMP. These methods are summarised by Table 2.

Features. To compute the node feature ϕ_1, we use the method employed in [13]: for each super-pixel, image features are extracted; then a classifier is trained on the extracted features; with the trained classifier, a score vector is computed for each super-pixel with each score representing the confidence of labelling the super-pixel by a particular label candidate. Let $\mathbf{c}_i$, $\mathbf{q}_i$ denote the LAB colour, the 2D position of the super-pixel i respectively. The definitions of ϕ_2 and ϕ_3 for different methods are given in Table 2. For Lan and PDMP methods, in order to estimate graph structures, the $-\log$ distance is used rather than Potts. This distance allows to filter highly impossible edges out, *e.g.* the ones with super-pixels far away from each other and distinct in colour. Though $-\log$ feature can be used by other methods, the results are worse than using the exp potentials.

Graph construction. CRF-MST and CRF-Adj use pre-constructed graphs. CRF-MST uses MST computed based on weights that equal the sum of two values: (1) ℓ_2 norm of the difference between the 2D locations of two super-pixels; (2) ℓ_2 norm of the difference between the LAB colour vectors of two super-pixels. CRF-Adj uses graphs consistent with super-pixel adjacency–if two super-pixels are adjacent, their nodes are connected by an edge. For the other two methods, the graphs are estimated together with labels using different inference methods.

Inference. Since the first two methods use fixed graphs, *i.e.* G is known, belief propagation (BP) can be used to estimate labels. For the last two methods, it is easy to formulate (17) into (1). Hence graphs and labels can be estimated

Table 3. Segmentation accuracy and time (by seconds) on KITTI dataset. For each column the best is highlighted. Column *overall* reports the overall segmentation accuracy, and column *mean* shows the accuracy as an average of accuracies of different classes. Among the methods that estimate graphs and labels simultaneously, our PDMP method is much faster than Lan.

	Ground	Objects	Building	Vegetation	Sky	Overall	Mean	Time
CRF–Adj	96.3 %	63.9 %	**87.7 %**	90.5 %	91.3 %	84.4 %	85.9 %	0.516
CRF–MST	96.3 %	67.8 %	84.6 %	**96.5 %**	97.7 %	86.2 %	88.6 %	**0.023**
Lan [4]	**97.9 %**	71.3 %	83.7 %	87.6 %	97.4 %	85.1 %	87.6 %	7.323
PDMP (ours)	97.6 %	**73.1 %**	87.3 %	95.1 %	**98.3 %**	**88.3 %**	**90.3 %**	3.357

simultaneously using Lan and PDMP approaches respectively. Note using LP or LP+B&B to do inference in this experiment are computationally prohibitive.

Regarding to the model parameter $\mathbf{w}$, the first two approaches use the maximum pseudo likelihood (MPL) method [15] to learn $\mathbf{w}$, while Lan and PDMP use empirically selected $\mathbf{w} = [1, 0.1, 0.2]$. The quantitative results are shown in Table 3. Overall our PDMP method performs much better than all rest methods on accuracy, and is much faster than Lan which estimates graphs as well. Notably, the methods using fixed MRF graphs are much faster than Lan and PDMP since their inference problem is much easier than the problem (1). Visualisation of some segmentation results by different methods is provided in Fig. 2. It can be seen that the estimated graphs (e) are more coherent with the layout of objects than tree-structured graphs (c) and adjacency graphs (b). A closer look at the figure suggests that our PDMP algorithm finds less undesirable edges than Lan, *e.g.* the connection between the vegetation and the white box in the right-most column.

5.2   Human Activity Recognition

We now consider the task of recognising human group activities. For clarity, the term *activity* is used to describe the behaviour of a group of people, while the term *action* refers to the behaviour of an individual. Let $\mathcal{A}$ denote the activity set. Given an image and n body detections, let $\mathbf{x}_0$ denote the descriptor for the whole image, $\mathbf{x}_1, \mathbf{x}_2, \ldots, \mathbf{x}_n$ denote descriptors for each of n persons, $\mathbf{y} = [y_1, y_2, \ldots, y_n]$ ($y_i \in \mathcal{A}$) represent the corresponding action variables, and $a \in \mathcal{A}$ represent the activity variable for the image. Let $G = (\mathcal{V}, \mathcal{E})$ denote a graph spanning all action variables. The potential function $f_{\mathbf{w}}(\mathbf{x}; a, \mathbf{y}, G)$ (proposed in [4]) is given by

$$f_{\mathbf{w}}(\mathbf{x}; a, \mathbf{y}, G) = \mathbf{w}_0^\top \boldsymbol{\phi}_0(\mathbf{x}_0, a) + \sum_i (\mathbf{w}_1^\top \boldsymbol{\phi}_1(\mathbf{x}_i, y_i) + \mathbf{w}_2^\top \boldsymbol{\phi}_2(a, y_i)) +$$
$$\sum_{(j,k) \in \mathcal{E}} \mathbf{w}_3^\top \boldsymbol{\phi}_3(\mathbf{x}_j, \mathbf{x}_k, y_j, y_k, a). \tag{18}$$

Here $\boldsymbol{\phi}_0, \boldsymbol{\phi}_1, \boldsymbol{\phi}_2, \boldsymbol{\phi}_3$ are image-activity feature, image-action feature, action-activity feature and action-action feature defined in [4][1], $\mathbf{w}_0, \mathbf{w}_1, \mathbf{w}_2, \mathbf{w}_3$ are

---

[1] To compute these features, we need low-level image descriptors. All evaluating methods using the potential function (18) use the same descriptors extracted by us.

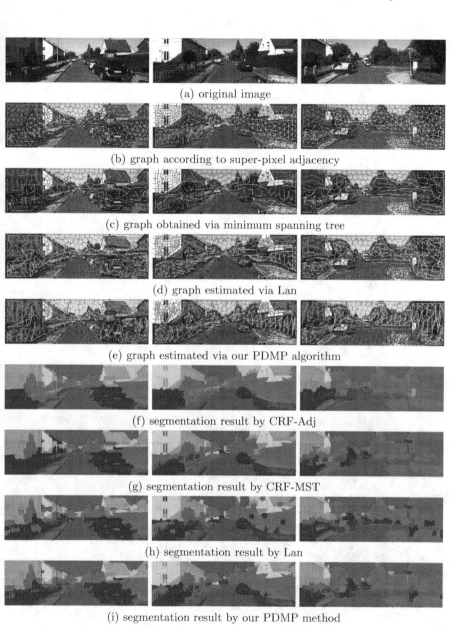

(a) original image

(b) graph according to super-pixel adjacency

(c) graph obtained via minimum spanning tree

(d) graph estimated via Lan

(e) graph estimated via our PDMP algorithm

(f) segmentation result by CRF-Adj

(g) segmentation result by CRF-MST

(h) segmentation result by Lan

(i) segmentation result by our PDMP method

Fig. 2. Visualisation of estimated graphs ((b)–(e)) and labels ((f)–(i)) in the image segmentation task. Note a red edge indicates that the label predictions for the associated nodes are different, while edges in other colours indicate identical label predictions (one colour corresponds to one class). Colour code for segmentation results: ▓ *ground*, ▓ *building*, ▓ *vegetation*, ▓ *objects*, ▓ *sky*. Our PDMP results are the best in general (Color figure online).

Table 4. Results on CAD dataset by different methods. Here *time* means the average running time by seconds. For each column the best is hilighted.

	Cross	Wait	Queue	Walk	Talk	Overall	Mean	Time
MCSVM	44.1%	47.2%	94.6%	64.9%	94.0%	68.9%	69.0%	**0.001**
SSVM	45.0%	47.2%	95.3%	**65.2%**	96.1%	71.6%	69.8%	0.002
Lan [4]	55.9%	59.7%	94.6%	62.2%	**99.5%**	75.6%	74.4%	0.062
LP [5]	**60.7%**	60.4%	93.6%	47.3%	**99.5%**	75.0%	72.3%	0.044
LP+B&B [5]	55.9%	**61.8%**	**95.7%**	55.4%	**99.5%**	75.4%	73.7%	0.425
PDMP (ours)	59.3%	59.7%	94.6%	60.8%	**99.5%**	**76.2%**	**74.8%**	0.002

model parameters to be learned during training via latent structured SVM (structured SVM is not applicable since the training problem is non-convex), see [4] for details.

To find the best a, we need to maximise (18) over $a, G, \mathbf{y}$. One can formulate this problem into a form (1) (*c.f.* [4]), which can be solved using our PDMP algorithm or the inference methods described at the beginning of Sect. 4.

Two additional methods are employed as baselines. The first one is the multi-class SVM (MCSVM): we train a multi-class SVM classifier with linear kernel using HoG descriptor extracted from the minimum bounding box area of all human body detections. The second one is structured SVM (SSVM), for which

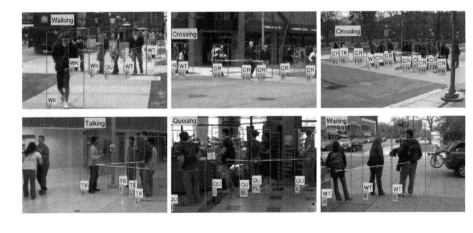

Fig. 3. Visualisation of prediction results on the CAD dataset by PDMP. Activity and action predictions are shown as the texts in cyan and yellow boxes respectively. The human body pose is shown in green boxes. The estimated graph structures are visualised by cyan lines. Abbreviations: cross–CR, walk–WK, wait–WT, Queue–QU, talk–TK, front–F, left–L, right–R, back–B, front-left–FL, front-right–FR, back-left–BL (Color figure online).

we train a structured SVM [16] to discriminate activities. The potential function used for this method is a special case of (18) by fixing G as MST computed based on 2D distance between body detections. To related inference problem is solved via BP.

We show the results in Table 4. Our PDMP method outperforms all other methods. Please notice using fixed graphs (SSVM) performs much worse than estimating graphs from data (Lan, LP, LP+B&B, PDMP), which verifies the importance of inferring MRF graphs. Comparing with Lan, LP and LP+B&B, our PDMP method performs better because (1) PDMP solves (3) which is tighter than the relaxations used by its competitors; (2) during each iteration PDMP solves a sub-problem of the partial-dual problem (5) exactly. Visualisation of a few recognition results by the PDMP approach is given in Fig. 3.

6   Conclusion

We proposed an algorithm to solve MRF inference with unknown graphs. The algorithm is based on the mixed integer bilinear programming formulation, from which we derived its partial-dual and approximately solved the partial dual via message passing. The algorithm scales good to large inference problems without sacrificing performance. We compared our method with existing methods on both synthetic data and real problems. Improvements have been made using our inference technique.

Acknowledgement. We thank Qinfeng Shi for his suggestion on the exposition of this paper. We thank Cesar Dario Cadena Lerma for his help on using the KITTI dataset. This work was supported by a grant from the National High Technology Research and Development Program of China (863 Program) (No. 2013AA10230402), and a grant from the Fundamental Research Funds of Northwest A&F University (No. QN2013056).

References

1. Shotton, J., Winn, J., Rother, C., Criminisi, A.: Textonboost for image understanding: Multi-class object recognition and segmentation by jointly modeling texture, layout, and context. IJCV **81**, 2–23 (2009)
2. Pearl, J.: Reverend bayes on inference engines: A distributed hierarchical approach. In: AAAI, pp. 133–136 (1982)
3. Nowozin, S., Rother, C., Bagon, S., Sharp, T., Yao, B., Kohli, P.: Decision tree fields. In: ICCV (2011)
4. Lan, T., Wang, Y., Mori, G.: Beyond actions: Discriminative models for contextual group activities. In: NIPS (2010)
5. Wang, Z., Shi, Q., Shen, C., van den Hengel, A.: Bilinear programming for human activity recognition with unknown mrf graphs. In: CVPR (2013)
6. Adams, W.P., Sherali, H.D.: Mixed-integer bilinear programming problems. Math. Program. **59**, 279–305 (1993)
7. Hiroshi, K.: Bilinear Programming: Part I. An Algorithm for Solving Bilinear Programs. Technical Report No. 71-9, Operations Research House, Stanford University (1971)

8. Globerson, A., Jaakkola, T.: Fixing max-product: Convergent message passing algorithms for map lp-relaxations. In: NIPS (2007)
9. Andersen, E., Andersen, K.: Mosek (version 7). Academic version (2013). www.mosek.com
10. Ravikumar, P., Lafferty, J.: Quadratic programming relaxations for metric labeling and markov random field map estimation. In: ICML (2006)
11. Geiger, A., Lenz, P., Urtasun, R.: Are we ready for autonomous driving? The kitti vision benchmark suite. In: CVPR, pp. 3354–3361 (2012)
12. Sengupta, S., Greveson, E., Shahrokni, A., Torr, P.H.: Urban 3d semantic modelling using stereo vision. In: International Conference on Robotics and Automation, pp. 580–585 (2013)
13. Cadena, C., Košecká, J.: Semantic segmentation with heterogeneous sensor coverages. In: International Conference on Robotics and Automation (2014)
14. Vedaldi, A., Fulkerson, B.: VLFeat: An open and portable library of computer vision algorithms (2008). http://www.vlfeat.org/
15. Koller, D., Friedman, N.: Probabilistic Graphical Models: Principles and Techniques. MIT Press, Cambridge (2009)
16. Tsochantaridis, I., Joachims, T., Hofmann, T., Altun, Y.: Large margin methods for structured and interdependent output variables. JMLR **6**, 1453–1484 (2006)

Face and Gestue, Tracking

Joint Estimation of Pose and Face Landmark

Donghoon Lee[✉], Junyoung Chung, and Chang D. Yoo

Department of Electrical Engineering, KAIST, Daejeon, Korea
iamdh@kaist.ac.kr

Abstract. This paper proposes a parallel joint boosting method that simultaneously estimates poses and face landmarks. The proposed method iteratively updates the poses and face landmarks through a cascade of parallel random ferns in a forward stage-wise manner. At each stage, the pose and face landmark estimates are updated: pose probabilities are updated based on previous face landmark estimates and face landmark estimates are updated based on previous pose probabilities. Both poses and face landmarks are simultaneously estimated through sharing parallel random ferns for the pose and face landmark estimations. This paper also proposes a triangular-indexed feature that references a pixel as a linear weighted sum of three chosen landmarks. This provides robustness against variations in scale, transition, and rotation. Compared with previous boosting methods, the proposed method reduces the face landmark error by 7.1 % and 12.3 % in the LFW and MultiPIE datasets, respectively, while it also achieves pose estimation accuracies of 78.6 % and 94.0 % in these datasets.

1 Introduction

Computer vision applications such as face recognition [3,28,29], facial expression recognition [8], age estimation [16,17], and gaze estimation [24] are garnering significant attention, and achieving high performance in these applications remains difficult with variations in poses, expressions, and occlusions. In order to obtain more robustness, localizing the fiducial face landmark points is considered to be a key pre-processing step in many applications [3,24,28,29]. However, accurate face landmark estimation itself is a difficult problem. Among the obstacles to obtaining accurate face landmarks, pose variations that involve 3D non-rigid deformation when projecting a 3D face on a 2D space is particularly difficult to manage, but it must be overcome for accurate estimation [9].

Most previous face landmark estimation methods do not use the pose information and, when they do, the pose is estimated prior to the face landmark estimation [9], which is referred to as the two-step method in this paper. The intuition behind the two-step method is that the face landmark depends on the pose, and a more precise location for the face landmark can be obtained using a pose-conditional landmark estimator. We observed that the face landmark information could also improve the accuracy of the pose estimate. In order to utilize this, the poses and face landmarks should be estimated simultaneously.

© Springer International Publishing Switzerland 2015
D. Cremers et al. (Eds.): ACCV 2014, Part IV, LNCS 9006, pp. 305–319, 2015.
DOI: 10.1007/978-3-319-16817-3_20

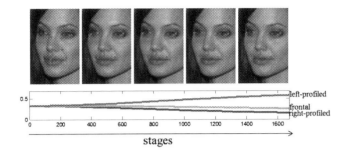

Fig. 1. Application results of parallel joint boosting to face landmarks and pose estimations in different stages. The pose probabilities and face landmark estimates are gradually updated with increases in the number of stages.

In this paper, a parallel joint boosting method to simultaneously estimate the pose and face landmarks is proposed. The proposed method has been motivated by gradient boosting [14] and LogitBoost [15], which have been used to estimate face landmarks [4] and poses, respectively. The proposed method combines gradient boosting and LogitBoost through a single weak regressor and then iteratively updates both estimates in a forward stage-wise manner as illustrated in Fig. 1. In each stage, the face landmark estimates are updated based on the pose probability that is estimated in the previous stage, while the pose probabilities are updated based on the face landmarks obtained in the previous stage. Each stage consists of a number of weak regressors, and each weak regressor that assumes a particular pose is learned.

The remainder of this paper is organized as follows. Section 2 reviews selected related work, and the details of the proposed method are described in Sect. 3. The experimental and comparative results are reported in Sects. 4 and 5, respectively. The conclusions are presented in Sect. 6.

2   Related Work

Previous methods have attempted to manage large pose variations using appearance-based models [5,7,20,21], morphable-model [2,3], and template matching [25,30] using parametric shape constraints. Although various strategies and improvements have been proposed over the past few decades, these methods have poor generalizability against unseen samples and suffer from slow training speeds. An alternative approach uses a part-based model [1,23,32] that considers the landmark estimation problem as a part detection problem.

Regression based methods [4,6,27] have been actively proposed where shape constraints are achieved in non-parametric manners, and they have exhibited promising results for both of accuracy and computation time.

Cao *et al.* [4] proposed a cascade regression method that uses random ferns as weak learners. The foundation of their method is representing the regressed shape as a linear combination of all training shapes. It was demonstrated that the aggregation of random ferns results in a robust estimator with real-time operation.

Dantone *et al.* proposed a pose-inspired method with conditional random forests, where each conditional random forest is an expert regressor of each pose [9]. Their algorithm works in two-steps: estimate the head pose using regression forest and estimate the landmarks conditional to the head pose using conditional regression forests. The limitation of the two-step approach is that misclassification in poses cannot be managed well.

However, we found that poses and face landmarks should be estimated iteratively because they affect each other's improvement in accuracy. Furthermore, sharing parallel random ferns enables simultaneous estimation of poses and face landmarks in one structure.

3   Joint Estimation of Poses and Face Landmarks

This section provides a brief overview of two boosting methods: gradient boosting for face landmark estimation and LogitBoost for pose estimation. The proposed method for joint estimation of poses and face landmarks is also described.

3.1   Boosting Methods

Gradient Boosting. Gradient boosting provides a foundation for a number of face landmark estimation methods [4,11]. Gradient boosting formulates the face landmark estimation problem as an additive cascade regression as follows:

$$\mathbf{s}^t = \mathbf{s}^{t-1} + r^t(\mathbf{I}; \alpha^t), \tag{1}$$

where $\mathbf{s}^t$ is the face landmark estimate at the t-th stage, $\mathbf{I}$ is an input image, and $r^t(\cdot; \cdot)$ is a weak regressor at the t-th stage parameterized by α^t. The final estimate at stage T is given by $\mathbf{s}^T = \mathbf{s}^0 + \sum_{t=1}^{T} r^t(\mathbf{I}; \alpha^t)$.

Given training samples, $\{\hat{\mathbf{s}}_i, \mathbf{I}_i\}_{i=1}^{N}$, and the regressor parameters, $\{\alpha^t\}_{t=1}^{T}$, are learned through minimizing the empirical loss, $\Psi(\cdot, \cdot)$, in a greedy forward stage-wise manner, as follows:

$$\alpha^t = \operatorname*{argmin}_{\alpha^t} \frac{1}{N} \sum_{i=1}^{N} \Psi(\hat{\mathbf{s}}_i, \mathbf{s}_i^t), \tag{2}$$

$$= \operatorname*{argmin}_{\alpha^t} \frac{1}{N} \sum_{i=1}^{N} \Psi(\hat{\mathbf{s}}_i, \mathbf{s}_i^{t-1} + r^t(\mathbf{I}_i; \alpha^t)). \tag{3}$$

A reasonable choice of loss function, $\Psi(\cdot, \cdot)$, for the face landmark estimation is:

$$\Psi(\hat{\mathbf{s}}, \mathbf{s}) = ||\hat{\mathbf{s}} - \mathbf{s}||, \tag{4}$$

which is typically considered to be a performance measure.

In this paper, a random fern with L split functions, $\{f_l\}_{l=1}^L$, is considered to be a weak regressor, and it partitions the feature space into 2^L disjoint bins, $\{\mathbf{R}_b\}_{b=1}^{2^L}$. Equation 3 is reduced to:

$$\delta\bar{\mathbf{s}}_b = \underset{\delta\bar{\mathbf{s}}_b}{\mathrm{argmin}} \frac{1}{N} \sum_{i=1}^N ||\delta\mathbf{s}_i - r^t(\mathbf{I}_i; f_l, \delta\bar{\mathbf{s}}_b)||, \tag{5}$$

$$= \frac{1}{1 + \beta / \sum_{i=1}^N \mathbf{1}_{R_b}(f(\mathbf{I}_i))} \frac{\sum_{i=1}^N \delta\mathbf{s}_i \mathbf{1}_{R_b}(f(\mathbf{I}_i))}{\sum_{i=1}^N \mathbf{1}_{R_b}(f(\mathbf{I}_i))}. \tag{6}$$

Here, $\alpha = \{\{f_l\}_{l=1}^L, \{\delta\bar{\mathbf{s}}_b\}_{b=1}^{2^L}\}$ and $\{\delta\bar{\mathbf{s}}_b\}_{b=1}^{2^L}$ are bin outputs, $\mathbf{1}_R(\cdot)$ is a binary indicator function, $\delta\mathbf{s} = ||\hat{\mathbf{s}} - \mathbf{s}||$, and β is a shrinkage parameter.

LogitBoost. LogitBoost [15] is a statistical boosting method for classification and has been used for pose estimations [31]. Given J number of pose classes, LogitBoost considers the following relationships between the pose probability, π_j, and the logistic function, H_j, as follows:

$$\pi_j = \frac{e^{H_j}}{\sum_{i=1}^J e^{H_i}}, \tag{7}$$

$$H_j = \log \pi_j - \frac{1}{J} \sum_{i=1}^J \log \pi_i. \tag{8}$$

Here, H_j has a cascade regression form similar to gradient boosting, which is given below:

$$H_j^t = H_j^{t-1} + h_j^t(\mathbf{I}; \beta^t), \tag{9}$$

which gives $H_j^T = H_j^0 + \sum_{t=1}^T h^t(\mathbf{I}; \beta^t)$ at the T-th stage. At each stage, LogitBoost fits an individual weak regressor, h_j^t, for each pose using the weighted least-squares of $z_j = \frac{y_j - \pi_j}{w_j}$ to feature with the weights $w_j = \pi_j(1 - \pi_j)$. Here, y_j is a binary indicator that indicates the j-th pose.

The random fern is usually used as a weak regressor, and the solution to the weighted least-squares regression problem using the random fern is given as follows:

$$\delta\bar{h}_{b,j} = \alpha \frac{\sum_{i=1}^N w_{i,j} z_{i,j} \mathbf{1}_{R_b}(f(\mathbf{I}_i))}{\sum_{i=1}^N w_{i,j} \mathbf{1}_{R_b}(f(\mathbf{I}_i))}. \tag{10}$$

Here, $\{\delta\bar{h}_{b,j}\}_{b,j=1}^{2^L, J}$ are bin outputs and α is a shrinkage parameter. The shrinkage process based on β is omitted (refer to Eq. 6)

For more details about LogitBoost, we suggest that readers refer to [15].

Algorithm 1. Joint boosting evaluation

1: **Input:** Image $\mathbf{I}$, weak regressors $\{f^t, \delta \bar{\mathbf{s}}^t, \delta \bar{\mathbf{h}}^t\}_{t=1}^T$
2: Initialize $\mathbf{s}^0$, H_j^0
3: **for** $t = 1$ to T **do**
4:      $b \leftarrow f^t(\mathbf{I})$ ▷ *Compute bin index*
5:      $\mathbf{s}^t \leftarrow \mathbf{s}^{t-1} + \delta \bar{\mathbf{s}}_b^t$
6:      $H_j^t \leftarrow H_j^{t-1} + \delta \bar{h}_{b,j}^t$ for $\forall j$
7: **end for**
8: $\pi_j^T \leftarrow \dfrac{e^{H_j^T}}{\sum_{j=1}^J e^{H_j^T}}$, for $\forall j$
9: **Output:** Face landmark estimates $\mathbf{s}^T$, pose probability π_j^T

3.2   Parallel Joint Boosting

Assuming that poses and face landmarks are closely coupled, we conjecture that the following procedures should be considered in order to improve both estimates: (1) estimation of face landmarks should use the pose information and (2) estimations of the poses should use face landmark information. Procedures (1) and (2) should be conducted in an iterative manner, such that both estimates are updated at each iteration. The proposed method includes both procedures. The details of the proposed method are described in the following.

Joint Boosting. In the joint boosting method, gradient boosting and LogitBoost are combined through a single set of random ferns. When one set of random ferns to implement the gradient boosting and a separate set of random ferns to implement LogitBoost share a common split function, then the gradient boosting and LogitBoost can be combined using a single set of random ferns. Gradient boosting and LogitBoost, which are based on random ferns, have been proposed in the past for face landmark estimations [4] and pose estimations [31], respectively. However, neither has been used simultaneously or jointly.

Algorithm 1 describes an evaluation procedure using the joint boosting. The random fern of the joint boosting is parameterized by $\{f^t, \delta \bar{\mathbf{s}}^t, \delta \bar{h}^t\}_{t=1}^T$, which are the split functions, gradient boosting bin outputs, and LogitBoost bin outputs, respectively. Gradient boosting for face landmark estimations and LogitBoost for pose estimations share a common split function, f, and distinguish themselves through separate bin outputs. Consequently, the poses and face landmarks can be simultaneously estimated through carefully selecting the split function. Note that the bin outputs, $\delta \bar{\mathbf{s}}$ and $\delta \bar{h}$, can be obtained using Eqs. 6 and 10, respectively.

We adopted landmark-indexed features[1] [4,13] and simple decision stumps in order to design the split functions. Landmark-indexed features have been successfully applied to both pose [13] and landmark [4] estimations. At each stage,

---

[1] Landmark-indexed features are also known as shape-indexed features [4] and pose-indexed features [13]. We use the term landmark-indexed feature for consistency in this paper.

Algorithm 2. Parallel joint boosting evaluation: soft

1: **Input:** Image $\mathbf{I}$, weak regressors $\{f^{t|k}, \delta\bar{\mathbf{s}}^{t|k}, \delta\bar{\mathbf{h}}^{t|k}\}_{t,k=1}^{T,J}$
2: Initialize $\mathbf{s}^0$, H_j^0
3: **for** $t = 1$ to T **do**
4:     **for** $k = 1$ to J **do**
5:         $b \leftarrow f^{t|k}(\mathbf{I})$ ▷ *Compute bin index*
6:         $\delta\mathbf{s}^{t|k} \leftarrow \delta\bar{\mathbf{s}}_b^{t|k}$
7:         $H_k^{t|k} \leftarrow H_k^{t-1} + \delta\bar{h}_{b,j}^{t|k}$, for $\forall j$
8:         $\pi_j^{t|k} \leftarrow \dfrac{e^{H_j^{t|k}}}{\sum_{j=1}^J e^{H_j^{t|k}}}$, for $\forall j$
9:     **end for**
10:     $\mathbf{s}^t \leftarrow \mathbf{s}^{t-1} + \sum_{k=1}^J \pi_k^{t-1} \delta\mathbf{s}^{t|k}$
11:     $\pi_j^t \leftarrow \sum_{k=1}^J \pi_k^{t-1} \pi_j^{t|k}$, for $\forall j$
12:     $H_j^t \leftarrow \log \pi_j^t - \frac{1}{J} \sum_{j=1}^J \log \pi_j^t$, for $\forall j$
13: **end for**
14: $\pi_j^T \leftarrow \dfrac{e^{H_j^T}}{\sum_{j=1}^J e^{H_j^T}}$, for $\forall j$
15: **Output:** Face landmark estimates $\mathbf{s}^T$, pose probability π_j^T

---

the landmark-indexed features are extracted based on previous face landmark estimates, and previous face landmark estimates are used for the pose estimations. The details of the landmark-indexed features that we used are described in Sect. 3.3.

Parallel Expansion. The intuition behind the parallel joint boosting is to use the pose probabilities in the previous stage to improve the accuracies of the face landmark estimates. In the parallel joint boosting, each stage consists of J number of parallel random ferns, and each random fern assumes a particular pose and is pose-conditionally learned.

We model face landmarks, $\mathbf{s}$, as a mixture of J pose-conditional landmarks, $\{s^{|k}\}_{k=1}^J$, with the pose-probability weights, π^k, as follows:

$$\mathbf{s} = \sum_{k=1}^J \pi^k \mathbf{s}^{|k}. \tag{11}$$

The parallel joint boosting consists of $T \times J$ weak regressors with the parameters, $\{f^{t|k}, \delta\bar{s}^{t|k}, \delta\bar{h}^{t|k}\}_{t,k=1}^{T,J}$, and are formulated based on the mixture model.

The overall procedure of the parallel joint boosting is described in Algorithm 2, and the details of each stage of the parallel joint boosting are described here.

1. The face landmark estimates, $\mathbf{s}^t$, are updated based on the previous face landmark estimates, $\mathbf{s}^{t-1}$, J number of pose-conditional face landmark updates, $\delta\bar{s}^{t|k}$, and corresponding pose probabilities, π_k^{t-1}, in the previous stage using the equation: $\mathbf{s}^t = \mathbf{s}^{t-1} + \sum_{k=1}^J \pi_k^{t-1} \delta\bar{s}^{t|k}$.

Algorithm 3. Parallel joint boosting evaluation: hard

1: **Input:** Image $\mathbf{I}$, weak regressors $\{f^{t|k}, \delta\bar{\mathbf{s}}^{t|k}, \delta\bar{\mathbf{h}}^{t|k}\}_{t,k=1}^{T,J}$
2: Initialize $\mathbf{s}^0$, H_j^0
3: **for** $t = 1$ to T **do**
4:     $k \leftarrow \operatorname{argmax}_k \pi_k^{t-1}$
5:     $b \leftarrow f^{t|k}(\mathbf{I})$ ▷ *Compute bin index*
6:     $\mathbf{s}^t \leftarrow \mathbf{s}^{t-1} + \pi_k^{t-1}\delta\bar{\mathbf{s}}_b^{t|k}$
7:     $H_j^t \leftarrow H_j^{t-1} + \delta\bar{h}_{b,j}^{t|k}$, for $\forall j$
8: **end for**
9: $\pi_j^T \leftarrow \dfrac{e^{H_j^T}}{\sum_{j=1}^J e^{H_j^T}}$, for $\forall j$
10: **Output:** Face landmark estimates $\mathbf{s}^T$, pose probability π_j^T

---

2. The pose probabilities are simultaneously updated using the equation: $\pi_j^t = \sum_{k=1}^J \pi_k^{t-1}\pi_j^{t|k}$. Here, $\pi_j^{t|k}$ is obtained using the relationship between the pose probability and logistic function, $H_j^{t|k}$, given in Eq. 7. $H_j^{t|k}$ can be computed using the equation, $H_j^{t|k} = H_j^{t-1} + \delta\bar{h}_{b,j}^{t|k}$.

This method is called the "soft" decision method, and it is distinguished from the "hard" decision method as follows.

The hard decision method is described in Algorithm 3. The computation cost in the evaluation procedure of the soft decision method lineally increases with J. The hard decision method updates the posse and face landmarks in a greedy manner, while the soft decision method processes all random ferns even when the associated probability is close to zero. Through choosing the most probable pose and corresponding pose-conditional random fern at every stage, the computational cost in the evaluation procedure is irrelevant to J.

The bin outputs for the face landmark estimations of the pose-conditional weak regressor can be obtained through solving the minimization problem weighted by the pose-probability estimates that were obtained in the previous stage, π_j^{t-1}, and these are reduced to:

$$\delta\bar{\mathbf{s}}_b^{t|k} = \frac{\sum_{i=1}^N \pi_k^{t-1}\delta\mathbf{s}_i^t \mathbf{1}_{R_b^{t|k}}\left(f^{t|k}(\mathbf{I}_i)\right)}{\sum_{i=1}^N \pi_k^{t-1}\mathbf{1}_{R_b^{t|k}}\left(f^{t|k}(\mathbf{I}_i)\right)}. \tag{12}$$

Here, the shrinkage process based on β is omitted (refer to Eq. 6).

The bin outputs for the pose estimations can be obtained through applying Eq. 10 to all parallel ferns.

$$\delta\bar{h}_j^{t|k} = \alpha\frac{\sum_{i=1}^N \pi_k^{t-1}w_{i,j}z_{i,j}\mathbf{1}_{R_b}\left(f^{t|k}(\mathbf{I}_i)\right)}{\sum_{i=1}^N \pi_k^{t-1}w_{i,j}\mathbf{1}_{R_b}\left(f^{t|k}(\mathbf{I}_i)\right)}. \tag{13}$$

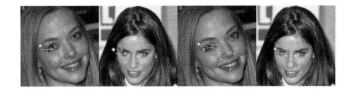

Fig. 2. Triangular-indexed features reference a point with a linear combination of randomly generated weight vectors that are constrained to $\sum_i w_i = 1$. Any point in the face region can be represented invariant to shape deformation and scaling.

3.3 Triangular-Indexed Features

Regression-based methods typically require a high number of iterations for accurate landmark estimations; thus, for real-time operations, the update should be based on features that require low computational costs, such as the pixel intensity difference between two points as used in [11,22]. In order to gain geometric invariance, local coordinates are used to index a pixel point through determining its local coordinates references from the closest landmark [4]. This feature is invariant to scale variations face transitions, and its efficacy has been proven through achieving state-of-the-art performance in real-time operations [4]. However, this feature is limited by the large pose variations in yaw and roll axes that deform the pixel: single reference landmarks cannot counter pixel displacements due to large pose variations. This feature requires regular similarity transformations to the mean shape in the regression, which can hinder real-time operations. In order to overcome this problem, Cao *et al.* [4] used a two-step framework to obtain features that are robust to large pose variations.

In the proposed triangular-indexed feature, the pixel point is indexed as a linear weighted sum of three landmarks what form a triangular mesh on the face. The linear weighted sum of the arbitrarily chosen landmarks can represent almost every point in the face and it is invariant to large pose estimations. The triangular-indexed features do not require similarity transformations; hence, its computation is cheap. Triangular mesh templates can be generated through selecting three landmarks manually or randomly offline that will used throughout the iteration. Then, a weight vector, $\mathbf{w} \in \mathbb{R}^3$, is randomly sampled in the following manner: sample $w_1 \sim U(0,1)$ where $U(0,1)$ is the uniform distribution; and sample $w_2 \sim U(0,1)$ and $w_3 \sim U(0,1)$ such that $E[w_2] = E[w_3] = 0$; and then, normalize the weights to make the sum to 1. This procedure can be interpreted as randomly selecting a pixel point nearby landmark $\mathbf{l}_1$ in order to bind the location inside the face region and to index the coordinates to three landmarks including $\mathbf{l}_2$ and $\mathbf{l}_3$ to gain geometric invariance. Figure 2 depicts a triangular-indexed feature compared with [4] shown in the images on the left. Finally, a pixel point, $\mathbf{p} \in \mathbb{R}^2$, is generated through estimating $\mathbf{p} = \sum_i w_i \mathbf{l}_i$. In contrast to [4], we considered the pose probabilities, $\pi|_{j=1}^J$, as weights and computed the weighted correlation with δs. The computational complexity was reduced from $O(P^2)$ to $O(P)$ through adopting the fast correlation computation introduced in [4].

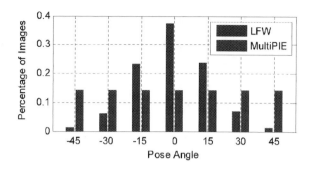

Fig. 3. Distributions of the poses in the LFW and MultiPIE. LFW consists of mostly frontal images, while MultiPIE consists of images in various poses.

4 Experiments

The objectives of our experiments were two-fold: to compare the proposed method with the state-of-the-art methods and to demonstrate the efficacy of the joint estimation of poses and face landmarks. We conducted experiments on two benchmark datasets: Labeled Faces in the Wild (LFW) [19] and MultiPIE [18]. Our experiments focused on the evaluation of face landmark estimations because our key interest is in face landmark estimations.

4.1 Datasets

LFW. LFW contains 13,233 face images of 5,749 people and is remarkably challenging due to its constraint of the images of LFW being detected using the Viola-Jones face detector [26]. There were no pose annotations for the original LFW; therefore, we used the POSIT method [10] to obtain the approximate pose annotations, and they were quantized into three poses: left-profile, frontal, and right-profile.

MultiPIE. MultiPIE contains approximately 750,000 face images of 337 people with varying viewpoints, illumination conditions, and facial expressions. We considered 250 people collected from Session 1 with varying poses from $-45°$ to $45°$ with $15°$ intervals, under 19 illumination conditions and two facial expressions.

4.2 Implementation Details

The benchmark methods [9,27] often use the Viola Jones face detector to locate the face position. However, the detection often fails on profiled faces in Multi-PIE. Therefore, we simulated the output of the face detector through randomly providing a bounding box that overlaps a minimum of 80 % of the ground truth.

Because the code used in [4] was not distributed to publicly, we developed and implemented it ourselves. The parameters of our implementation were set

Table 1. Average error for landmark estimation on LFW.

Method	Error	Method	Error
Dantone [9]	0.0696	Cao-Ti	0.0563
Human [9]	0.0597	Soft-Li	0.0584
Ever. [12]	0.0963	Soft-Ti	**0.0552**
Yang [27]	0.0645	Hard-Li	0.0589
Cao-Li [4]	0.0594	Hard-Ti	**0.0552**

to be the same as [4], except the number of initial shapes for training data augmentation. We used 5 and 2 instead of 20 for the LFW and MultiPIE datasets, respectively, in order to adjust the number of training samples. In more detail, we set the number of stages to $T = 10$ and $K = 500$, the number of features to $P = 400$, the depth of the random fern to $F = 5$, and the shrinkage parameter to $\beta = 1000$.

In order to implement the parallel joint boosting, we adopted the two-stage cascade method proposed in [4], and we set the parameters to be the same as [4]. For the soft decision method, K was adaptively chosen as 166 and 71 for the LFW and MultiPIE, respectively, in order to to adjust the number of processed weak regressors in the evaluation. α was set to 0.005, and we manually designed 40 and 20 templates for the triangular-indexed features for LFW and MultiPIE, respectively.

5   Results

For the face landmark estimations, we measured the estimation errors as a fraction of inter-ocular distance, which is the distance between the ground truth and estimation normalized using the inter-ocular distance. For the pose estimations, the classification accuracies were reported. We performed five-fold cross validations, and we report the mean accuracy in both datasets.

5.1   Comparison Using LFW

We compared the proposed methods with the following methods: Dantone *et al.* [9], human manual annotation [9], Everingham *et al.* [12], Yang and Patras [27], and Cao *et al.* [4]. Furthermore, we employed the results reported in [9]. For [27], we used the results of Fig. 5 in [27], and [4] was implemented ourselves.

In order to evaluate the impact of the decision methods (soft or hard) and the triangular-indexed feature, we conducted experiments on all possible combinations: Cao-Li [4], Cao-Ti, Soft-Li, Soft-Ti, Hard-Li, and Hard-Ti. Here, Li and Ti indicate the landmark-indexed feature and triangular-indexed feature, respectively.

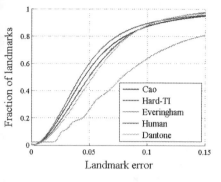

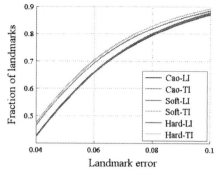

Fig. 4. Comparison between the benchmark methods and the proposed methods for the LFW.

Fig. 5. Comparison with Cao *et al.* [4] and the proposed methods for the LFW.

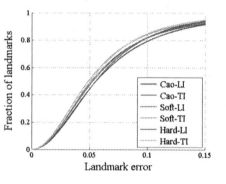

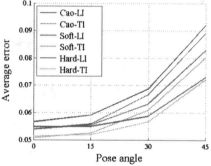

Fig. 6. Comparison with Cao *et al.* [4] and the proposed methods for the MultiPIE.

Fig. 7. Average error for the pose estimations ($0°$, $15°$, $30°$, and $45°$) for the MultiPIE.

Table 1 and Fig. 4 present the comparisons between the state-of-the-art methods and proposed methods. The proposed methods achieved remarkable performances and reduced the average error from the best current method [4] by 7 % with 78.6 % pose estimation accuracy. Surprisingly, both [4] and the proposed method outperformed the performance of human manual annotation performance.

Table 1 and Fig. 5 illustrate the detailed comparisons with Cao *et al.* [4] and the proposed methods. The parallel joint boosting method was insignificant on the LFW. This resulted from the LFW consisting of nearly frontal images as illustrated in Fig. 3. The triangular-indexed feature consistently improved the performance compared with the landmark-indexed feature [4].

Table 2. Errors for each face landmark point and the average errors estimated on MultiPIE.

Landmarks	Cao-Li [4]	Cao-Ti	Soft-Li	Soft-Ti	Hard-Li	Hard-Ti
Eyes	0.0547	0.0593	**0.0515**	0.0546	0.0526	0.0540
Nose	0.0859	0.0760	0.0794	0.0710	0.0787	**0.0703**
Mouth	0.0702	0.0647	0.0660	0.0605	0.0654	**0.0594**
Chin	0.0953	0.0922	0.0902	0.0880	0.0905	**0.0855**
Average	0.0715	0.0682	0.0671	**0.0638**	0.0670	**0.0627**

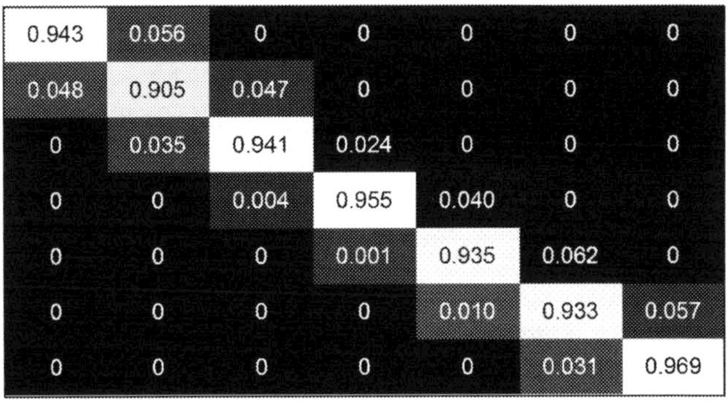

Fig. 8. The confusion matrix of the pose estimations for MultiPIE using Hard-Ti (values ≤0.001 have been omitted).

5.2   Comparison Using MultiPIE

The primary objective of the experiments using MultiPIE was to verify the effectiveness of the joint estimation of the poses and face landmarks. We compared the landmark estimation results of the previous gradient boosting method from [4] and the proposed method.

The face landmark estimation results for MultiPIE are illustrated in Fig. 6. The proposed hard and soft decision methods clearly outperformed Cao et al. [4] for both using the landmark-indexed features and the triangular-indexed features. Table 2 presents the errors for each face landmark point and the average error. The Hard-Ti method achieved the best performance for the nose, mouth, and chin, and it also achieved the minimum average error. The Hard-Ti method reduced the average error by 12.3 % compared with Cao-Li. When the feature was fixed to a landmark-indexed feature, the soft and hard decision methods reduced the average error by 6.2 % and 6.3 %, respectively. Using the triangular-indexed features for the Cao, Soft, and Hard methods reduced the average error by 4.6 %, 4.9 %, and 6.4 %, respectively. The most difficult point to estimate was the chin (0.0855 was the best result).

Figure 7 presents the average error for various poses. The Hard-Li and Hard-Ti methods exhibited more smooth curves compared with the Cao-Li and Cao-Ti

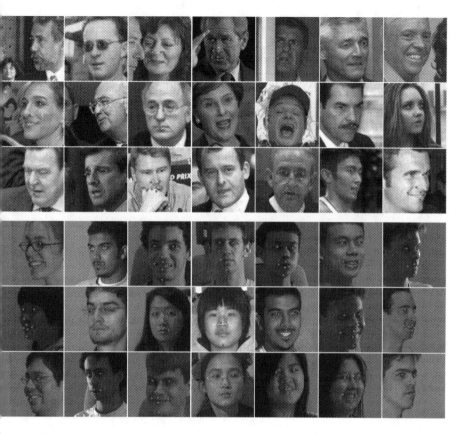

Fig. 9. Qualitative results for the LFW (top three rows) and MultiPIE (bottom three rows) datasets.

methods, which could be interpreted as the hard decision method being more robust to pose variations.

The confusion matrix of the pose estimations for the Hard-Ti method is depicted in Fig. 8. The average accuracy recorded was 94.6 %. Although we did not compare this performance with the other pose estimation methods because our primary focus was on face landmark estimations, the proposed method achieved reliable accuracy (Figs. 8 and 9).

6   Conclusion

We proposed a parallel boosted regression method for simultaneous estimation of poses and face landmarks. The proposed method enables the estimation of both poses and face landmarks simultaneously, and the method improved both estimations based on pose-conditional random ferns and triangular-indexed features. Experiments using the LFW database demonstrated that the proposed method achieves high performance in face landmark estimation, even better than the performance of human manual annotations. The results from the MultiPIE database demonstrated that the proposed model improves the performance of face landmark estimations in large pose variations and sufficiently supports our intuitive idea. The pose estimation results have also demonstrated reliable accuracy.

Acknowledgement. This work was supported by ICT R&D program of MSIP/IITP [14-824-09-014, Basic Software Research in Human-level Lifelong Maching Learning (Machine Learning Center)].

References

1. Belhumeur, P., Jacobs, D., Kriegman, D., Kumar, N.: Localizing parts of faces using a consensus of exemplars. In: CVPR (2011)
2. Blanz, V., Vetter, T.: A morphable model for the synthesis of 3d faces. In: Proceedings of the 26th Annual Conference on Computer Graphics and Interactive Techniques, pp. 187–194. ACM (1999)
3. Blanz, V., Vetter, T.: Face recognition based on fitting a 3d morphable model. TPAMI **25**, 1063–1074 (2003)
4. Cao, X., Wei, Y., Wen, F., Sun, J.: Face alignment by explicit shape regression. IJCV **107**, 177–190 (2014)
5. Cootes, T.F., Edwards, G.J., Taylor, C.J.: Active appearance models. TPAMI **23**, 681–685 (2001)
6. Cootes, T.F., Ionita, M.C., Lindner, C., Sauer, P.: Robust and accurate shape model fitting using random forest regression voting. In: Fitzgibbon, A., Lazebnik, S., Perona, P., Sato, Y., Schmid, C. (eds.) ECCV 2012, Part VII. LNCS, vol. 7578, pp. 278–291. Springer, Heidelberg (2012)
7. Cootes, T.F., Taylor, C.J., Cooper, D.H., Graham, J.: Active shape models-their training and application. Comput. Vis. Image Underst. **61**, 38–59 (1995)
8. Chew, S.W., Lucey, S., Lucey, P., Sridharan, S., Conn, J.F.: Improved facial expression recognition via uni-hyperplane classification. In: CVPR (2012)
9. Dantone, M., Gall, J., Fanelli, G., Van Gool, L.: Real-time facial feature detection using conditional regression forests. In: CVPR (2012)
10. Dementhon, D.F., Davis, L.S.: Model-based object pose in 25 lines of code. IJCV **15**, 123–141 (1995)
11. Dollár, P., Welinder, P., Perona, P.: Cascaded pose regression. In: CVPR (2010)
12. Everingham, M., Sivic, J., Zisserman, A.: Hello! my name is... buffy-automatic naming of characters in tv video. In: BMVC (2006)
13. Fleuret, F., Geman, D.: Stationary features and cat detection. J. Mach. Learn. Res. **9**, 1437 (2008)
14. Friedman, J.: Greedy function approximation: a gradient boosting machine. Ann. Stat. **29**, 1189–1232 (2001)
15. Friedman, J., Hastie, T., Tibshirani, R.: Additive logistic regression: a statistical view of boosting (with discussion and a rejoinder by the authors). Ann. Stat. **28**, 337–407 (2000)
16. Geng, X., Smith-Miles, K., Zhou, Z.H.: Facial age estimation by learning from label distributions. In: AAAI (2010)

17. Geng, X., Zhou, Z.H., Zhang, Y., Li, G., Dai, H.: Learning from facial aging patterns for automatic age estimation. In: Proceedings of the 14th Annual ACM International Conference on Multimedia, pp. 307–316. ACM (2006)
18. Gross, R., Matthews, I., Cohn, J., Kanade, T., Baker, S.: Multi-pie. Image Vis. Comput. **28**, 807–813 (2010)
19. Huang, G., Mattar, M., Berg, T., Learned-Miller, E., et al.: Labeled faces in the wild: a database forstudying face recognition in unconstrained environments. In: ECCV Workshop (2008)
20. Matthews, I., Baker, S.: Active appearance models revisited. IJCV **60**, 135–164 (2004)
21. Milborrow, S., Nicolls, F.: Locating facial features with an extended active shape model. In: Forsyth, D., Torr, P., Zisserman, A. (eds.) ECCV 2008, Part IV. LNCS, vol. 5305, pp. 504–513. Springer, Heidelberg (2008)
22. Ozuysal, M., Calonder, M., Lepetit, V., Fua, P.: Fast keypoint recognition using random ferns. TPAMI **32**, 448–461 (2010)
23. Smith, B.M., Zhang, L., Brandt, J., Lin, Z., Yang, J.: Exemplar-based face parsing. In: CVPR (2013)
24. Sugano, Y., Matsushita, Y., Sato, Y., Koike, H.: An incremental learning method for unconstrained gaze estimation. In: Forsyth, D., Torr, P., Zisserman, A. (eds.) ECCV 2008, Part III. LNCS, vol. 5304, pp. 656–667. Springer, Heidelberg (2008)
25. Tzimiropoulos, G., Zafeiriou, S., Pantic, M.: Robust and efficient parametric face alignment. In: ICCV (2011)
26. Viola, P., Jones, M.J.: Robust real-time face detection. IJCV **57**, 137–154 (2004)
27. Yang, H., Patras, I.: Sieving regression forest votes for facial feature detection in the wild. In: ICCV (2013)
28. Yi, D., Lei, Z., Li, S.Z.: Towards pose robust face recognition. In: CVPR (2013)
29. Yin, Q., Tang, X., Sun, J.: An associate-predict model for face recognition. In: CVPR (2011)
30. Yuille, A.L., Hallinan, P.W., Cohen, D.S.: Feature extraction from faces using deformable templates. IJCV **8**, 99–111 (1992)
31. Zhang, J., Zhou, S.K., McMillan, L., Comaniciu, D.: Joint real-time object detection and pose estimation using probabilistic boosting network. In: CVPR (2007)
32. Zhu, X., Ramanan, D.: Face detection, pose estimation, and landmark localization in the wild. In: CVPR, pp. 2879–2886. IEEE (2012)

Probabilistic Subpixel Temporal Registration for Facial Expression Analysis

Evangelos Sariyanidi$^{(\boxtimes)}$, Hatice Gunes, and Andrea Cavallaro

Centre for Intelligent Sensing, Queen Mary University of London, London, UK
{e.sariyanidi,h.gunes,a.cavallaro}@qmul.ac.uk

Abstract. Face images in a video sequence should be registered accurately before any analysis, otherwise registration errors may be interpreted as facial activity. Subpixel accuracy is crucial for the analysis of subtle actions. In this paper we present PSTR (Probabilistic Subpixel Temporal Registration), a framework that achieves high registration accuracy. Inspired by the human vision system, we develop a motion representation that measures registration errors among subsequent frames, a probabilistic model that learns the registration errors from the proposed motion representation, and an iterative registration scheme that identifies registration failures thus making PSTR aware of its errors. We evaluate PSTR's temporal registration accuracy on facial action and expression datasets, and demonstrate its ability to generalise to naturalistic data even when trained with controlled data.

1 Introduction

The automatic recognition of facial actions, activity and expressions is a fundamental building block for intelligent and assistive technologies for various domains including healthcare (*e.g.* pain analysis), driving (*e.g.* drowsiness detection), lip reading, animation (*e.g.* facial action synthesis) and social robotics [1,2]. Inaccurate temporal registration of face images is detrimental to facial action and expression analysis as local intensity and texture variations introduced by registration errors can be interpreted as facial activity [3]. Even small errors of 0.5 pixels can cause a larger variation than the one caused by facial actions (see Fig. 1a, and b). Registration errors have an adverse effect on other components of the systems that analyse facial activity in various contexts such as AU detection [4] and basic emotion recognition ([5] vs. [6]).

Facial expression recognisers [3,5,7–11] rely on *spatial* registration techniques, which ignore the consistency among subsequent video frames as they register each frame independently. The common approach is to register faces based on a set of facial landmarks. However, state-of-the-art landmark detectors cannot achieve

Electronic supplementary material The online version of this chapter (doi:10. 1007/978-3-319-16817-3_21) contains supplementary material, which is available to authorized users. Videos can also be accessed at http://www.springerimages.com/videos/978-3-319-16816-6.

D. Cremers et al. (Eds.): ACCV 2014, Part IV, LNCS 9006, pp. 320–335, 2015.
DOI: 10.1007/978-3-319-16817-3_21

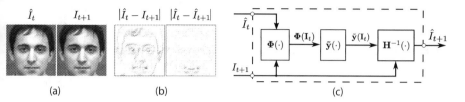

(a)   (b)   (c)

Fig. 1. (a) Two consecutive unregistered images $(\hat{I}_t, I_{t+1})$ with registration error $t_x = t_y = 0.5$ pixels. (b) Difference between the images of the pair in (a) before $(|\hat{I}_t, I_{t+1}|)$ and after $(|\hat{I}_t, \hat{I}_{t+1}|)$ registration. (c) Illustration of how the proposed framework registers two consecutive frames.

subpixel accuracy [12,13] and therefore subsequent frames cannot be registered with respect to each other. One deviation from the literature is the work of Jiang *et al.* [14], which crops the first frame based on landmarks and registers subsequent frames to the first frame using Robust FFT [15]. Although Robust FFT can maintain high registration accuracy, particularly for large registration errors, it does not achieve the desired subpixel accuracy.

We aim at providing accurate registration for spatio-temporal facial expression analysis. In particular, we consider registration via *homographic* transformation for suppressing the registration errors that occur due to rigid head or body movements, or the errors induced when cropping a face after face detection. We attribute local non-rigid registration errors to facial actions, and therefore leave these errors intact in order to enable their analysis in subsequent system layers (*e.g.* facial representation and classification). Specifically, we are interested in Euclidean registration as more general homographic transformations such as projective or affine transformation, do not necessarily preserve the shape of the face and can introduce distortions that alter the facial display.

In this paper we propose a Probabilistic Subpixel Temporal Registration (PSTR) framework that achieves high registration accuracy for Euclidean face registration. Influenced by the studies on motion perception [16], we propose a *motion representation* to implicitly encode the registration errors in a sequence. We then develop a *supervised probabilistic model* that takes the motion representation and estimates the registration errors in a sequence using the information encoded in the representation. We finally develop an *iterative registration framework* that has the supervised probabilistic model in its core. This framework formulates registration as an optimisation problem, and relies on the probabilistic nature of the supervised model to achieve convergence and terminate the optimisation. The framework benefits further from the probabilistic nature of the model and identifies its own errors.

The contribution of this work is three-fold: the development of (i) a motion representation that is robust to illumination variations (Sect. 3), (ii) a probabilistic model that learns the relationships between the features of motion representation and the corresponding registration errors (Sect. 4), and (iii) a registration error estimator which enables PSTR to detect its own errors (Sect. 5).

2   Formulation

Let $\mathbf{S} = (I_1, I_2, \ldots, I_T)$ be a video sequence where $T \in \mathbb{N}^+$ and $I_1, I_2, \ldots, I_T$ are the consecutive frames. Our goal is to obtain a registered sequence $\hat{\mathbf{S}} = (\hat{I}_1, \hat{I}_2, \ldots, \hat{I}_T)$, *i.e.* a sequence where any two images $\hat{I}_i, \hat{I}_j$ are registered with respect to each other. To achieve this, we aim to perform pairwise registration among all consecutive image pairs in $\mathbf{S}$ starting from the first pair. We consider the first image I_1 as the reference image, denote it with $\hat{I}_1$ and register I_2 to $\hat{I}_1$. In general, $\mathbf{I}_t$ denotes a pair of images consisting of a reference (registered) image and an unregistered image as $\mathbf{I}_t = (\hat{I}_t, I_{t+1})$. The registration is performed for all pairs $\mathbf{I}_t$ for $t = 1, \ldots, T - 1$.

The registration of a pair $\mathbf{I}_t$ is illustrated in Fig. 1c. Firstly, the motion representation $\mathbf{\Phi}(\cdot)$ is extracted from the images in $\mathbf{I}_t$. Then, the features $\mathbf{\Phi}(\mathbf{I}_t)$ are fed into the registration error estimator $\tilde{\mathbf{y}}(\cdot)$. Finally, the estimated errors $\tilde{\mathbf{y}}(\mathbf{I}_t)$ and the unregistered image I_{t+1} are passed to a homographic back-transformation $\mathbf{H}^{-1}(\cdot)$, which outputs the registered image $\hat{I}_{t+1}$.

3   Motion Representation

Our work is influenced by the biology literature that studies motion perception [16,17], that is, the ability of inferring the speed and direction of objects in a dynamic scene. The main idea is to consider the registration errors among subsequent frames as a source of *motion*, and to discover this motion using motion perception models. Many motion perception models are developed by analysing the motion of a moving line [16,17]. Adelson and Bergen [16] showed that convolution with an appropriately designed spatio-temporal Gabor filter pair can be used to discover the speed and orientation of a moving line.

We first discuss how a Gabor filter pair can be used to identify the speed and orientation of a moving pattern. We then describe how to extract Gabor features that are robust to illumination variations. We finally develop a *motion representation* that extracts features using multiple Gabor filter pairs.

3.1   Gabor Motion Energy

Let us denote a $2D$ moving line with $f_l(x, y, t)$:

$$f_l(x, y, t) = c\delta \left(x \cos \theta_l - y \sin \theta_l - t v_l \right), \tag{1}$$

where θ_l defines the spatial orientation of f_l as well as the direction of motion; v_l defines the speed and c controls the luminance value of the line.

A $3D$ Gabor filter can be represented as in [18] (see the reference for a detailed discussion on parameters):

$$g_\phi(x, y, t) = \frac{\gamma}{2\pi\sqrt{2\pi}\sigma^2\tau} e^{\left(-\frac{\bar{x}^2 + \gamma\bar{y}^2}{2\sigma^2} - \frac{(t - \mu_t)^2}{2\tau^2} \right)} \cos\left(\frac{2\pi}{\lambda}(\bar{x} + v_g t + \phi) \right) \tag{2}$$

where $\bar{x} = x\cos(\theta_g) + y\sin(\theta_g)$ and $\bar{y} = -x\sin(\theta_g) + y\cos(\theta_g)$. The parameters θ_g and v_g define the orientation and speed of motion that the filter is tuned for. The parameter ϕ is the phase offset of the filter. It can be set to $\phi = 0$ to obtain an even-phased (cosine) filter g^e and $\phi = \frac{\pi}{2}$ to obtain an odd-phased (sine) filter g^o — the two filters together form a quadrature pair (g^e, g^o).

The convolution $f_l * g_\phi$ provides useful information towards understanding the motion of the line [16]. This can be illustrated for the $2D$ line f_l as follows. When a vertical bar $(\theta_l \approx \pi/2)$ moves with a speed $v_l = v_g > 0$, the convolution response gets maximal for $\theta_g = \theta_l$ and strictly smaller as $\theta_g \to -\pi/2$. The response is almost flat when $\theta_g = -\theta_l$. This behaviour is useful as it provides information about the speed and orientation of the motion, and can discriminate between forward and backward motion, *i.e.* it is selective in terms of direction as it yields no output for motion in opposite direction.

Although the convolution $f_l * g_\phi$ helps identifying the speed and orientation of the line, it also poses some difficulties [16]. Firstly, the convolution $f_l * g_\phi$ yields an oscillating output due to the trigonometric $\cos(\cdot)$ function, therefore it is hard to derive a meaningful conclusion by looking at a particular part of the response. Secondly, the convolution output is sensitive to luminance polarity, *i.e.* the response would change if we would invert the luminance of the bar [16]. To deal with these shortcomings, Adelson and Bergen [16] suggested to use *motion energy*, which is defined as:

$$E_{f,v_g,\theta_g}(x,y,t) = (f * g^e)^2 + (f * g^o)^2. \tag{3}$$

Instead of oscillating, the energy $E_f = E_{f,v_g,\theta_g}$ generates a uniform peak at the points where the line sits at any given time t. Furthermore, E_f is insensitive to luminance polarity, *i.e.* the response is not affected if we were to invert the luminance of the line with the background [16].

3.2 Pooling

The $3D$ convolution involved in the computation of E_f can yield a high dimensional output. This dimensionality must be reduced to improve computational performance and avoid the curse of dimensionality [19]. To this end, we perform pooling, which proved to be a biologically plausible [20–22] and computationally efficient [23] approach. We use two types of pooling, namely mean and maximum (max) pooling, denoted respectively with $\phi_f^\mu = \phi^\mu(\mathbf{E}_f)$ and $\phi_f^\cap = \phi^\cap(\mathbf{E}_f)$, where $\mathbf{E}_f$ is the volume of energy obtained by computing E_f for all $(x, y, t) \in \Omega$ where $\Omega = X \times Y \times T$ is the domain of the sequence f. We add another statistical descriptor, the standard deviation $\phi_f^\sigma = \phi^\sigma(\mathbf{E}_f)$. The three features can be computed as follows:

$$\phi_f^\mu = \frac{1}{|\Omega|}\int_\Omega E_f(\mathbf{x})d\mathbf{x}, \quad \phi_f^\cap = \max_{\mathbf{x}\in\Omega} E_f(\mathbf{x}), \quad \phi_f^\sigma = \sqrt{var(\mathbf{E}_f)} \tag{4}$$

where $|\Omega|$ denotes the volume of Ω and $\mathbf{x} = (x, y, t)$ is a point in space-time.

3.3   Contrast Normalisation

The energy E_f is sensitive to the average intensity value of f as Gabor filters are not zero mean [24]. Therefore, a contrast normalisation is essential for increasing the generalisation ability of the Gabor features.

Let $\mathbf{I} = \mathbf{I}(\mathbf{x}) = \mathbf{I}(x, y, t)$ be a sequence of a moving pattern. Consider two sequences $\mathbf{I}_i(\mathbf{x}), \mathbf{I}_j(\mathbf{x})$ which contain the same moving pattern as in $\mathbf{I}(\mathbf{x})$ but differ from $\mathbf{I}(\mathbf{x})$ with a linear illumination variation such as $\mathbf{I}_i(\mathbf{x}) = (\alpha_i t + \beta_i)\mathbf{I}(\mathbf{x})$, and $\mathbf{I}_j(\mathbf{x}) = (\alpha_j t + \beta_j)\mathbf{I}(\mathbf{x})$. Ideally, we would desire the features extracted for both patterns to be identical, $i.e.$ $\phi(\mathbf{I}_i) = \phi(\mathbf{I}_j)$. To map the features of $\phi(\mathbf{I}_i)$ and $\phi(\mathbf{I}_j)$ close together, we perform normalisation. On the one hand, if normalisation is performed on individual images ($e.g.$ z-normalisation, contrast-stretching, histogram equalisation) apparent motion along the sequence can be generated. On the other hand, a normalisation performed on the entire sequence may not necessarily map the features $\phi(\mathbf{I}_i)$ and $\phi(\mathbf{I}_j)$ close to one another. To overcome such problems, we define a new energy function, the *normalised energy* $\tilde{E}$. Normalisation is achieved by dividing each frame in an input sequence with a coefficient that is proportional to the illumination coefficient in the frame.

Let $I_i^{t_k}$ be an image from the sequence $\mathbf{I}_i$ at any fixed time t_k. We use the image $I_i^{t_k}$ to synthesise a static sequence $\mathbf{I}_i^{t_k}$ of length $(t_f - t_0)$ by repeating the same image throughout the time interval, $i.e.$ $\mathbf{I}_i^{t_k}(\mathbf{x}) \equiv \mathbf{I}_i(x, y, t_k) = (\alpha_i t_k + \beta_i)\mathbf{I}(x, y, t_k) = (\alpha_i t_k + \beta_i)\mathbf{I}^{t_k}(\mathbf{x})$. We can compute the energy of $\mathbf{I}_i^{t_k}$ as follows:

$$E_{\mathbf{I}_i^{t_k}}(\mathbf{x}) = \left[\int (\alpha_i t_k + \beta_i)\mathbf{I}^{t_k}(\mathbf{x} - \mathbf{u})g^e(\mathbf{u})d\mathbf{u}\right]^2 + \left[\int (\alpha_i t_k + \beta_i)\mathbf{I}^{t_k}(\mathbf{x} - \mathbf{u})g^o(\mathbf{u})d\mathbf{u}\right]^2$$

$$= (\alpha_i t_k + \beta_i)^2 \left\{\left[\int \mathbf{I}^{t_k}(\mathbf{x} - \mathbf{u})g^e(\mathbf{u})d\mathbf{u}\right]^2 + \left[\int \mathbf{I}^{t_k}(\mathbf{x} - \mathbf{u})g^o(\mathbf{u})d\mathbf{u}\right]^2\right\}$$

$$= (\alpha_i t_k + \beta_i)^2 E_{\mathbf{I}^{t_k}}(\mathbf{x}) \tag{5}$$

where $\mathbf{u} = \begin{bmatrix} u & v & w \end{bmatrix}$ is the convolution variable. Since for fixed t_k the term $\alpha_i t_k + \beta_i$ is constant, a feature $\phi_{\mathbf{I}_i^{t_k}}$ for $\phi \in \{\phi^\cap, \phi^\mu, \phi^\sigma\}$ can be computed through (4) as:

$$\phi_{\mathbf{I}_i^{t_k}} = \phi(\mathbf{E}_{\mathbf{I}_i^{t_k}}) = (\alpha_i t_k + \beta_i)^2 \phi(\mathbf{E}_{\mathbf{I}^{t_k}}) = (\alpha_i t_k + \beta_i)^2 \phi_{\mathbf{I}^{t_k}}. \tag{6}$$

Note that (6) includes $(\alpha_i t_k + \beta_i)$, which will cancel out the illumination term in the input sequence. Let us define the normalised energy $\tilde{E}$ for $\mathbf{I}_i$ as:

$$\tilde{E}_{\mathbf{I}_i}(\mathbf{x}) = \left[\frac{\mathbf{I}_i}{(\phi_{\mathbf{I}_i^t})^{\frac{1}{2}}} * g^e\right]^2 + \left[\frac{\mathbf{I}_i}{(\phi_{\mathbf{I}_i^t})^{\frac{1}{2}}} * g^o\right]^2$$

$$= \left[\int \frac{(\alpha_i w + \beta_i)\mathbf{I}(\mathbf{u})}{(\alpha_i w + \beta_i)(\phi_{\mathbf{I}^w})^{\frac{1}{2}}}g^e(\mathbf{x} - \mathbf{u})d\mathbf{u}\right]^2 + \left[\int \frac{(\alpha_i w + \beta_i)\mathbf{I}(\mathbf{u})}{(\alpha_i w + \beta_i)(\phi_{\mathbf{I}^w})^{\frac{1}{2}}}g^o(\mathbf{x} - \mathbf{u})d\mathbf{u}\right]^2$$

$$= \left[\int \frac{\mathbf{I}(\mathbf{u})}{(\phi_{\mathbf{I}^w})^{\frac{1}{2}}}g^e(\mathbf{x} - \mathbf{u})d\mathbf{u}\right]^2 + \left[\int \frac{\mathbf{I}(\mathbf{u})}{(\phi_{\mathbf{I}^w})^{\frac{1}{2}}}g^o(\mathbf{x} - \mathbf{u})d\mathbf{u}\right]^2. \tag{7}$$

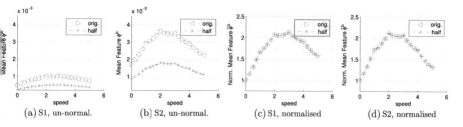

(a) S1, un-normal.　　(b) S2, un-normal.　　(c) S1, normalised　　(d) S2, normalised

Fig. 2. The un-normalised (ϕ^{μ}) and normalised ($\tilde{\phi}^{\mu}$) mean features extracted from moving face sequences of two subjects (S1, S2) for varying speeds.

The illumination coefficients are cancelled out by dividing each frame I_i^t in $\mathbf{I}_i$ with the feature of the synthesised sequence $\mathbf{I}_i^t$, *i.e.* $\phi_{\mathbf{I}_i^t}$. Based on the normalised energy, we define the normalised features $\tilde{\phi}^{\mu}, \tilde{\phi}^{\cap}, \tilde{\phi}^{\sigma}$ as:

$$\tilde{\phi}_f^{\mu} = \phi^{\mu}(\tilde{\mathbf{E}}_f), \quad \tilde{\phi}_f^{\cap} = \phi^{\cap}(\tilde{\mathbf{E}}_f), \quad \tilde{\phi}_f^{\sigma} = \phi^{\sigma}(\tilde{\mathbf{E}}_f) \tag{8}$$

where $\tilde{\mathbf{E}}_f$ is the normalised energy volume $\tilde{E}$ computed for a $\Omega = X \times Y \times T$.

A prominent illumination issue is gray-scale shift (*e.g.* due to imaging conditions or skin color differences), *i.e.* $\alpha_i = 0, \beta_i \neq 0$. The effect of normalisation against gray-scale shift is shown in Fig. 2. Moving sequences of various speeds are synthesised from the faces of two subjects (S1, S2). Each plot displays the variation of features with respect to the motion speed. The features of each sequence are computed for two cases: (1) original intensities (orig.) and (2) intensities multiplied with 0.5 (half). The un-normalised features $\phi(\cdot)$ are affected by both gray-scale variation (Fig. 2a and b) and inter-personal variation (Fig. 2a vs. b), whereas normalised features $\tilde{\phi}(\cdot)$ not only suppress gray scale shift completely (Fig. 2a and b), but also map the features of different subjects closer (Fig. 2c vs. d).

3.4 Motion in Various Speeds and Orientations

Although $E_{v,\theta}$ (or $\tilde{E}_{v,\theta}$) identifies the motion that it is tuned for, it cannot directly identify various speeds and orientations. For this reason, we construct a Gabor filter bank with filter pairs tuned to various speeds and orientations: $\mathbf{G} = \{(g_{v_i,\theta_j}^e, g_{v_i,\theta_j}^o) : v_i \in \{v_1, \ldots, v_{K_v}\}, \theta_j \in \{\theta_1, \ldots, \theta_{K_\theta}\}\}$.

The feature vector for a pair of consecutive images $\mathbf{I}$ is computed as follows. Firstly, $\tilde{\mathbf{E}}_{v_i,\theta_j}$ is computed for each pair g_{v_i,θ_j} in $\mathbf{G}$. Secondly, each $\tilde{\mathbf{E}}_{v_i,\theta_j}$ is partitioned into spatio-temporal slices $\tilde{\mathbf{E}}_{v_i,\theta_j}^{m,n}$. Next, the normalised feature of each slice $\tilde{\phi} = \phi(\tilde{\mathbf{E}}_{v_i,\theta_j}^{m,n})$ is computed for a single $\phi \in \{\phi^{\mu}, \phi^{\cap}, \phi^{\sigma}\}$ (*i.e.* a motion representations consists of only one feature type). Finally, the feature vector is obtained by concatenating all features $\tilde{\phi}$ computed for positive integers i, j, m, n such that $i \leq K_v, j \leq K_\theta, m \leq M, n \leq N$.

In the following sections, we will denote each feature with $\phi_k = \phi(\tilde{\mathbf{E}}_{v_i,\theta_j}^{m,n})$ and the final feature vector with $\mathbf{\Phi}(\mathbf{I}) = \begin{bmatrix} \phi_1 \ldots \phi_k \ldots \phi_K \end{bmatrix}$ where K is the size of the feature vector and k the feature index that can be computed as $k = (m-1)M + (n-1)N + (i-1)K_v + (j-1)K_\theta + 1$.

4   Estimating Registration Errors

To model the relations between the features $\Phi(\cdot)$ and corresponding registration errors, we use a *discrete* probabilistic model. A continuous model would require an assumption over the distribution of the features (*e.g.* Poisson, Gaussian), whereas the discrete model is trained straight from data without any assumption. Also, the proposed model can be trained in a single iteration and does not require the optimisation of parameters that would risk overfitting to a dataset.

4.1   Labeling

Since the probabilistic model we use is discrete, we define our labels to be also discrete. The misalignment between the images of a pair $\mathbf{y}(\mathbf{I})$ is defined as $\mathbf{y}(\mathbf{I}) = (\delta t_x, \delta t_y, \delta s, \delta \theta)$ where $\delta t_x, \delta t_y, \delta s$ and $\delta \theta$ are respectively the horizontal translation, vertical translation, scaling and rotation difference between the images of $\mathbf{I}$. We define $\Delta t_x, \Delta t_y, \Delta s$ and $\Delta \theta$, the sets that represent the range of each variation as $\Delta t_x = \{\delta t_x^-, \delta t_x^- + dt_x, \ldots, \delta t_x^+\}$, $\Delta t_y = \{\delta t_y^-, \delta t_y^- + dt_y, \ldots, \delta t_y^+\}$, $\Delta s = \{\delta s^-, \delta s^- + ds, \ldots, \delta s^+\}$ and $\Delta \theta = \{\delta \theta^-, \delta \theta^- + d\theta, \ldots, \delta \theta^+\}$. The first (*e.g.* δt_x^-) and last elements (*e.g.* δt_x^+) in each set represent the minimum and maximum value for each variation, and the increment values dt_x, dt_y, ds and $d\theta$ the difference between successive labels (*i.e.* the resolution of our labels). The set of all registration errors that our framework will deal with is referred to as the *label space* $\mathcal{L}$ and is defined as $\mathcal{L} = \Delta t_x \times \Delta t_y \times \Delta s \times \Delta \theta$.

Since we use a supervised model, we need training samples (pairs $\mathbf{I}^j$) and labels (registration errors $\mathbf{y}^j = \mathbf{y}(\mathbf{I}_j)$). Let $\mathcal{X}$ be a set containing N samples $\mathcal{X} = \{\mathbf{I}^1, \ldots, \mathbf{I}^N\}$, Φ be the set of features $\Phi = \{\mathbf{\Phi}^1, \ldots, \mathbf{\Phi}^N\}$ where $\mathbf{\Phi}^j = \mathbf{\Phi}(\mathbf{I}^j)$ and $\mathcal{Y}$ the set that contains the labels $\mathcal{Y} = \{\mathbf{y}^1, \ldots, \mathbf{y}^N\}$ where $\mathbf{y}^j \in \mathcal{L}$. A practical issue that needs to be addressed is how the samples $\mathbf{I}^j$ and their labels $\mathbf{y}^j$ will be obtained. Suppose that we have face sequences where we know that the subject does not display any head or body motion. Then, if we define a fixed face rectangle and crop the entire sequence based on this rectangle, the cropped sequence will contain only facial activity and no registration errors. To obtain one training sample $\mathbf{I}^j$, we firstly pick any two consecutive frames from the cropped sequence. Next, we apply a random Euclidean transformation to both frames. The label $\mathbf{y}^j$ can be easily computed from the random transformation. By picking frames that are temporally farther (rather than consecutive pairs), we can obtain pairs that involve larger facial activity and train a system that is more robust to large facial activity. Thus, using a number of face sequences, we can automatically synthesize as many training samples as we need.

4.2   Modeling

To model the relationships between the features extracted from the pairs $\mathbf{\Phi}^j$ and the corresponding registration errors $\mathbf{y}^j$, we define two discrete random variables $\mathbf{X}$ (for $\mathbf{\Phi}^j$) and $\mathbf{Y}$ (for $\mathbf{y}^j$).

Since $\mathbf{X}$ is discrete, we need to discretise the continuous feature vectors $\mathbf{\Phi}^j$. To this end we perform uniform quantisation over all features $\phi_k^j \in \mathbf{\Phi}^j$. We divide he space $[0, 1]$ into k bins and map each ϕ_k^j to an integer q such as $q = 1, 2, \ldots, Q$. 3efore this mapping, we normalise ϕ_k^j to map onto $[0, 1]$. The normalisation is)ased on the training dataset, specifically to the maximum and minimum values)f each feature k. Let $\min(\phi_k)$ and $\max(\phi_k)$ be defined as $\min(\phi_k) = \min\{\phi_k^p \in \mathbf{\Phi}^p : \mathbf{\Phi}^p \in \Phi\}$ and $\max(\phi_k) = \max\{\phi_k^p \in \mathbf{\Phi}^p : \mathbf{\Phi}^p \in \Phi\}$. We denote the bin index)f each feature ϕ_k^j with q_k^j and compute it as follows:

$$q_k^j = \arg_q \min \left\{ \left| \frac{\phi_k^j - \min(\phi_k)}{\max(\phi_k) - \min(\phi_k)} - \left(\frac{3q}{2} - 1 \right) \right| : q = 1, \ldots, Q \right\}, \quad (9)$$

vhere $\frac{3q}{2} - 1$ is the center of the bin with index q and $|\cdot|$ is the L_1 metric. We hall denote the quantised vector of all the features in $\mathbf{\Phi}^j$ with $\mathbf{q}^j = \mathbf{q}(\mathbf{I}^j) = q_1^j, q_2^j, \ldots, q_K^j)$, and the set that contains the quantised vectors extracted from all of the training samples in $\mathcal{X}$ with $\mathcal{Q} = \{\mathbf{q}^1, \ldots, \mathbf{q}^N\}$.

The random variable $\mathbf{X} = (X_1, \ldots, X_K)$ takes on values $\mathbf{q} = (q_1, \ldots, q_K)$ and $\mathbf{Y}$ takes on values $\mathbf{y} \in \mathcal{L}$. The registration errors and the Gabor features of image)airs are modelled jointly by computing the joint distribution $\mathbf{P}(\mathbf{X} = \mathbf{q}, \mathbf{Y} = \mathbf{y})$. 'or computational simplicity, we rely on the naive Bayes assumption and com-)ute the joint distribution as follows:

$$\mathbf{P}(\mathbf{X} = \mathbf{q}, \mathbf{Y} = \mathbf{y}) = \mathbf{P}(X_1 = q_1, \ldots, X_K = q_K \mid \mathbf{Y} = \mathbf{y})\mathbf{P}(\mathbf{Y} = \mathbf{y})$$
$$\approx \mathbf{P}(\mathbf{Y} = \mathbf{y}) \prod_{i=1}^{K} \mathbf{P}(X_k = q_k \mid \mathbf{Y} = \mathbf{y}). \quad (10)$$

To compute this distribution, we must compute the individual likelihood func-ions $\mathbf{P}(\mathbf{Y} = \mathbf{y} \mid X_k = q_k)$ for each $\mathbf{y} \in \mathcal{L}$. To this end, we adopt the frequency nterpretation of probability and learn each likelihood function from the train-ng samples. Let $\mathcal{U}$ and $\mathcal{V}$ be two sets defined respectively as $\mathcal{U} = \{q_k^j, \mathbf{y}^j : \mathbf{y} = $ $_j \wedge q_k = q_k^j, \mathbf{y}^j \in \mathcal{Y}, q_k^j \in \mathbf{q}^j \in \mathcal{Q}\}$ and $\mathcal{V} = \{\mathbf{y}^j : \mathbf{y} = \mathbf{y}^j, \mathbf{y}^j \in \mathcal{Y}\}$. The ikelihood can be computed as:

$$\mathbf{P}(X_k = q_k \mid \mathbf{Y} = \mathbf{y}) = \frac{|\mathcal{U}|}{|\mathcal{V}|}, \quad (11)$$

vhere $|\cdot|$ is the cardinality of the set. We assume the priors to be uniform $\mathbf{P}(\mathbf{Y} = \mathbf{y}) = 1/|\{\mathcal{L}\}|$ for each $\mathbf{y} \in \mathcal{L}$.

4.3   Estimation

)nce we learn the model $\mathbf{P}(\mathbf{X}, \mathbf{Y})$, the task of estimating the misalignment in a ;iven image pair $\mathbf{I}$ is fairly straightforward. We rely on Bayesian inference and ind the label $\mathbf{y} \in \mathcal{L}$ that maximises the posterior probability:

$$\mathbf{P}(\mathbf{Y} = \mathbf{y} \mid \mathbf{X} = \mathbf{q}) = \frac{\mathbf{P}(\mathbf{Y} = \mathbf{y})\mathbf{P}(\mathbf{X} = \mathbf{q} \mid \mathbf{Y} = \mathbf{y})}{\sum\limits_{\mathbf{y}_l \in \mathcal{L}} \mathbf{P}(\mathbf{Y} = \mathbf{y}_l)\mathbf{P}(\mathbf{X} = \mathbf{q} \mid \mathbf{Y} = \mathbf{y}_l)}. \quad (12)$$

The posterior probability is computed for all $\mathbf{y} \in \mathcal{L}$, and the registration error)etween the images of a pair $\mathbf{I}$ is finally estimated by selecting the label $\mathbf{y} \in \mathcal{L}$ hat maximises the above posterior probability as follows:

$$\tilde{\mathbf{y}}(\mathbf{I}) = \arg_{\mathbf{y} \in \mathcal{L}} \max \mathbf{P}(\mathbf{Y} = \mathbf{y} \mid \mathbf{X} = \mathbf{q}(\mathbf{I})). \quad (13)$$

Algorithm 1. Estimating registration errors between two images

---

Input Unregistered pair $\mathbf{I} = (\hat{I}, I')$
Output Registration error estimation $\tilde{\mathbf{y}}^*$

1: $\tilde{\mathbf{y}}_1 \leftarrow \tilde{\mathbf{y}}(\mathbf{I}); \ \tilde{\mathbf{y}}^* \leftarrow \tilde{\mathbf{y}}_1; \ \tilde{I}_1 \leftarrow \mathbf{H}^{-1}(\tilde{\mathbf{y}}^*)I'$ ▷ Estimate, Update
2: **for** $i \leftarrow 1, T$ **do**
3:     **if** $\tilde{\mathbf{y}}_i = \underline{0}$ **then**
4:         **return** $\tilde{\mathbf{y}}^*$ ▷ Converged
5:     **end if**
6:     $\tilde{\mathbf{y}}_{i+1} \leftarrow \tilde{\mathbf{y}}((\hat{I}, \tilde{I}_i)) \oplus \tilde{\mathbf{y}}^*; \ \tilde{\mathbf{y}}^* \leftarrow \tilde{\mathbf{y}}_{i+1}; \ \tilde{I}_{i+1} \leftarrow \mathbf{H}^{-1}(\tilde{\mathbf{y}}_{i+1})I'$ ▷ Estimate, Update
7: **end for**
8: $i^* \leftarrow \arg_{i \in \{1,\dots,T\}} \max \mathbf{P}_{\underline{0}}((I, \tilde{I}_i))$
9: **return** $\tilde{\mathbf{y}}_{i^*}$ ▷ Best iteration

---

5   Registration

Ideally, a single estimation $\tilde{\mathbf{y}}(\cdot)$ of the model $\mathbf{P}(\cdot)$ would be sufficient for registering two images. However, in practice $\tilde{\mathbf{y}}(\cdot)$ may not approximate the actual errors $\mathbf{y}(\cdot)$ with high accuracy in a single estimation, especially for large registration errors. Therefore, we deal with this as an optimisation problem where the output is estimation of the registration error denoted with $\tilde{\mathbf{y}}^*$. Once we compute $\tilde{\mathbf{y}}^*$, we obtain the registered image $\hat{I}'$ through $\hat{I}' = \mathbf{H}^{-1}(\tilde{\mathbf{y}}^*)I'$ where $\mathbf{H}^{-1}$ is a Euclidean back-transformation. To compute $\tilde{\mathbf{y}}^*$, we perform estimation and back-transformation iteratively.

The overall procedure for registering a pair of images is summarised in Algorithm 1 — the $\oplus$ operator is defined for $\mathbf{y}_1, \mathbf{y}_2$ as $\mathbf{y}_1 \oplus \mathbf{y}_2 = (\delta_{x1} + \delta_{x2}, \delta_{y1} + \delta_{y2}, \delta_{s1}\delta_{s2}, \delta_{\theta1} + \delta_{\theta2})$. The optimisation terminates either by converging within the allowed number of iterations, or by reaching the maximum number of iterations and returning the error that is the 'closest' to convergence according to the *convergence probability* $\mathbf{P}_{\underline{0}}(\mathbf{I}) = \mathbf{P}(\mathbf{Y} = \underline{0} \mid \mathbf{X} = \mathbf{q}(\mathbf{I}))$. As was illustrated in Fig. 1c, the registration of the entire sequence is performed by registering the pairs $\mathbf{I}_t$ consecutively for all $t = 1, \dots, T - 1$.

5.1   Coarse-to-Fine Estimation

To achieve high accuracy, we keep the resolution of our label space $\mathcal{L}$ high by selecting small $dt_x, dt_y, ds, d\theta$ values. However, this increases the size of the space $|\mathcal{L}|$. Therefore, we adopt a coarse-to-fine approach that allows us to simultaneously achieve high registration accuracy and keep the label space dimensionality low. We train multiple models $\mathbf{P}^i(\cdot)$ with label spaces $\mathcal{L}_i$, *i.e.* $i = 1, \dots, K_{\mathcal{L}}$. The spaces are defined from coarse to fine — $\mathcal{L}_1$ is the coarsest and $\mathcal{L}_2, \mathcal{L}_3, \dots$ are increasingly finer spaces. We cascade the models $\mathbf{P}(\cdot)^i$ and apply Algorithm 1 to each model $\mathbf{P}(\cdot)^i$ sequentially. We obtain the final estimation by accumulating the error estimations of all models $\mathbf{P}(\cdot)^i$.

5.2   Identifying Failure

The convergence probability $\mathbf{P_0(I)}$ provides the confidence needed to verify whether the two images in $\mathbf{I}$ are registered correctly. To complete the verification, we compare $\mathbf{P_0(I)}$ with a threshold probability P_θ.

Consider that we have *positive* and *negative* sample pairs — a positive sample is a pair of two correctly registered images and a negative sample is a pair of two unregistered images. The task is to find a threshold probability P_θ that will enable separation with a high true positive rate and a low false positive rate. To this end, we compute the convergence probability $\mathbf{P_0}(\cdot)$ for all positive and negative samples.

We then compute a ROC curve by setting the threshold P_θ to various values by incrementing it with a small step size. We set the final threshold P_θ to a value that yields a false positive rate as low as 0.5 %. Then the registration of an image pair is verified if $\mathbf{P_0(I)} > P_\theta$ or otherwise it is assumed that the images of $\mathbf{I}$ are not registered correctly.

6   Experiments

6.1   Setup and Evaluation Measures

We evaluate PSTR for pair and sequence registration. We test the performance of each feature type in $\{\tilde{\phi}^\mu, \tilde{\phi}^\cap, \tilde{\phi}^\sigma\}$ for parameters $N, M = 2, 3$ (Sect. 3.4). The Gabor filter bank $\mathbf{G}$ is obtained with filters of 8 orientations and 5 speeds such that $v_i \in \{1, 2, \ldots, 5\}, \theta_j \in \{0°, 45°, \ldots, 360°\}$. All images are resized to 200×200. The bin number for quantisation Q (Sect. 4.2) is set to 8 after experimenting with the values $4, 6, 8, \ldots, 20$ and not observing performance gain for more than 8 bins. As shown in Table 1, we train four probabilistic models for different label spaces $\mathcal{L}_i$ (see Sect. 5). To show that we can increase accuracy through finer labels, we report two results: one obtained by excluding $\mathcal{L}_4$ (*i.e.* selecting $\mathcal{L}_3$ as the finest label space) and one by including $\mathcal{L}_4$.

For *pair registration*, we measure performance using the mean absolute error (MAE) ε^p computed separately for translation ($\varepsilon^p_{t_x}, \varepsilon^p_{t_y}$ in pixels), scaling (ε^p_s as a percentage %) and rotation (ε^p_θ in degrees) as follows. Let $\mathbf{I}_i$ be one of the pairs, *i.e.* $i = 1, \ldots, N_p$, and $\bar{\delta}^i_{t_x}$ be the horizontal translation error for i^{th} pair.

Table 1. Parameters that describe the label spaces $\mathcal{L}_1, \mathcal{L}_2, \mathcal{L}_3$ and $\mathcal{L}_4$.

	$\delta t_x^{-\dagger}$	$\delta t_x^{+\dagger}$	$\delta t_y^{-\dagger}$	$\delta t_y^{+\dagger}$	δs^{-*}	δs^{+*}	$\delta\theta^{-\ddagger}$	$\delta\theta^{+\ddagger}$	$dt_x^\dagger$	$dt_y^\dagger$	ds^*	$d\theta^\ddagger$
$\mathcal{L}_1$	-12	12	-12	12	0.85	1.15	-15	15	3	3	0.03	3
$\mathcal{L}_2$	-4	4	-4	4	0.94	1.06	-3	3	1	1	0.01	1
$\mathcal{L}_3$	-1.5	1.5	-1.5	1.5	0.99	1.01	-1	1	0.5	0.5	0.002	0.2
$\mathcal{L}_4$	-0.5	0.5	-0.5	0.5	0.998	1.002	-0.2	0.2	0.125	0.125	0.001	0.1

†Pixels, *percentage ratio, ‡degrees.

The MAE $\varepsilon_{t_x}^p$ is computed as $\varepsilon_{t_x}^p = \sum_i^{N_p} \bar{\delta}_{t_x}^i / N_p$. The MAEs $\varepsilon_{t_y}^p, \varepsilon_s^p$ and ε_θ^p are computed similarly. We additionally compare PSTR with (Robust) FFT [15] as it is a state-of-the-art registration technique already used for facial expression recognition [14]. PSTR cannot be compared with the registration methods of most facial action analysis systems as they crop faces across an ad-hoc rectangle defined through a number of fiducial points [7]. Similarly to Robust FFT [15], we compare PSTR with RANSAC registration using SURF [25] and MSER [26].

For *sequence registration*, we measure the average MAE over sequences (ε^s) separately for translation ($\varepsilon_{t_x}^s$, $\varepsilon_{t_y}^s$) scaling (ε_s^s) and rotation (ε_θ^s) computed as follows. Let $\mathbf{S}_i$ denote one of the N_s sequences where the length of each sequence is equivalently T. Let $\bar{\delta}_{t_x}^{i,j}$ denote the horizontal translation error of jth pair in i^{th} sequence. The average MAE for horizontal translation $\varepsilon_{t_x}^s$ is computed as $\varepsilon_{t_x}^s = \sum_i^{N_s} (\sum_j^{T-1} \bar{\delta}_{t_x}^i / (T-1)) / N_s$. The MAEs $\varepsilon_{t_y}^s, \varepsilon_s^s$ and ε_θ^s are computed similarly.

We use standard datasets for evaluation, namely the CK+, PIE [27] and SEMAINE [28] datasets. The training *for all* the experiments is performed on CK+ dataset. In the CK+ and PIE datasets there exist sequences with almost no head pose variation and body movement. We select 129 such sequences from CK+ dataset, and we use 112 of them for training and the remaining 17 for testing. The 112 training sequences include 1814 consecutive pairs, which are randomly transformed to synthesise as many pairs as needed (as described in Sect. 4.1). The 17 testing sequences include 244 consecutive pairs of images — random homographic transformations are applied to them to obtain the unregistered pairs and sequences.

To evaluate both the robustness against illumination variation and the usefulness of the failure identification ability of PSTR, we perform experiments on the PIE dataset, which contains rapid illumination variations. We demonstrate performance on 200 pairs obtained from 10 sequences of 10 subjects.

We also test PSTR for naturalistic expressions on the SEMAINE dataset. However, since naturalistic expressions include head/body motion, we are not able to obtain a ground truth for this dataset and therefore provide only qualitative results through a video (Sect. 6.4).

6.2 Pair Registration

The translation output of FFT is an integer with 1 pixel resolution. To evaluate subpixel registration performance, we perform registration with FFT at double the image size (400 × 400) and reduce the estimated translation to half, *i.e.* increase the translation resolution of the FFT method to 0.5 pixels. The translation resolution of PSTR is also limited at 0.5 pixels for $\mathcal{L}_3$ (Table 1).

Table 2 shows the pair registration errors of PSTR and the FFT method. PSTR outperforms FFT as well as RANSAC-based registration with SURF or MSER features. The mean (ϕ^μ) and standard deviation features (ϕ^σ) perform slightly better than max ($\phi^\cap$). Increasing the number of pooling regions N does not provide a major performance improvement for ϕ^μ and $\phi^\cap$, and therefore N

Table 2. Pair (left of double lines) and sequence (right of double lines) registration performance on CK+ dataset.

ϕ	N	$\varepsilon^p_{t_x}$ †		$\varepsilon^p_{t_y}$ †		ε^p_s *		ε^p_θ ‡		$\varepsilon^s_{t_x}$ †		$\varepsilon^s_{t_y}$ †		ε^s_s *		ε^s_θ ‡	
		$\mathcal{L}_{1\text{-}3}$	$\mathcal{L}_{1\text{-}4}$	$\mathcal{L}_{1\text{-}3}$	$\mathcal{L}_{1\text{-}4}$	$\mathcal{L}_{1\text{-}3}$	$\mathcal{L}_{1\text{-}4}$	$\mathcal{L}_{1\text{-}3}$	$\mathcal{L}_{1\text{-}4}$	$\mathcal{L}_{1\text{-}3}$	$\mathcal{L}_{1\text{-}4}$	$\mathcal{L}_{1\text{-}3}$	$\mathcal{L}_{1\text{-}4}$	$\mathcal{L}_{1\text{-}3}$	$\mathcal{L}_{1\text{-}4}$	$\mathcal{L}_{1\text{-}3}$	$\mathcal{L}_{1\text{-}4}$
ϕ^μ	2	.07	.08	.07	.08	.08	.05	.07	.03	.31	.23	.38	.26	.28	.19	.18	.06
$\phi^\cap$	2	.11	.08	.15	.09	.11	.06	.16	.03	.34	.23	.46	.26	.31	.18	.24	.08
ϕ^σ	2	.05	.08	.06	.07	.08	.05	.06	.02	.34	.23	.43	.24	.23	.18	.18	.06
ϕ^μ	3	.07	.06	.08	.07	.07	.04	.06	.02	.50	.60	.56	.79	.28	.78	.24	.25
$\phi^\cap$	3	.07	.06	.06	.07	.07	.04	.05	.02	.65	.53	.81	.60	.64	.40	.34	.27
ϕ^σ	3	.05	.06	.06	.07	.06	.04	.06	.02	.55	.54	.59	.56	.36	.41	.22	.28
FFT	–	.18		.26		.57		.17		–		–		–		–	
SURF	–	.24		.29		.10		.05		–		–		–		–	
MSER	–	.38		.37		.17		.09		–		–		–		–	

can be set to 2 to keep the dimensionality low. Note that we are able to reduce errors, particularly for scaling and rotation, by including the model trained with the finest label space $\mathcal{L}_4$. The average computation time for PSTR is approximately 5 seconds (on a conventional desktop computer with Intel^{TM}i5 processor), which is larger compared to Robust FFT, RANSAC-SURF and RANSAC-MSER methods whose average computation time is respectively 0.25, 0.33 and 0.46 seconds. The bottleneck for PSTR is convolution with $3D$ Gabor filters. The speed of PSTR can be increased if the Gabor representation can be replaced with a motion representation that is computationally more efficient.

In Fig. 3a, b we show examples from the SEMAINE dataset. Fig. 3a shows the difference between the images of a pair with mouth expression obtained after applying the mean errors of PSTR (for $\phi = \phi^\sigma$ and $N = 3$) and FFT to the second image in each pair (Fig. 3a). While the differences provided by FFT hardly help identifying the location of the expression, PSTR clearly shows where the expression occurs. Identifying the *absence* of facial activity is as important as detecting facial activity. We applied a similar test but for a pair with no facial activity (Fig. 3b). The differences provided by FFT generate spurious activity.

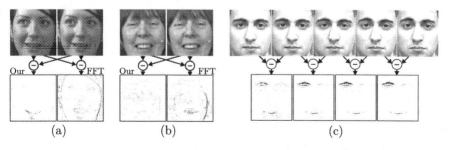

(a)   (b)   (c)

Fig. 3. (a) Difference between pair of images with a subtle mouth expression, after registering the images with PSTR and FFT; (b) Difference between images without expression; (c) Difference of each pair in a sequence after registration.

Table 3. Pair registration performance with illumination variation (PIE dataset).

Method	$\varepsilon_{t_x}^{p\,\dagger}$	$\varepsilon_{t_y}^{p\,\dagger}$	ε_s^{p*}	$\varepsilon_\theta^{p\ddagger}$	# Eliminated Pairs
PSTR	0.13	0.11	0.07	0.05	11 (automatically)
FFT	0.29	0.25	0.55	0.16	10 (manually)
SURF	0.75	0.80	0.52	0.29	44 (manually)
MSER	1.78	2.55	1.43	0.95	73 (manually)

Instead, the difference image of PSTR shows no signs of facial activity except from minor artifacts introduced by interpolation.

6.3   Identifying Failure

In the PIE dataset, the transition from 16th to 17th frame in all sequences involves a very sudden illumination variation, and causes PSTR, FFT and RANSAC-based methods to fail. PSTR identifies failures automatically.

Table 3 provides the MAE performance on the PIE dataset — the PSTR results are obtained with the parameters $\phi = \phi^\sigma, N = 2$ and label spaces $\mathcal{L}_{1-4}$. The typical symptom of failure in PIE experiments is large estimation error, in which case the mean error MAE gets very high even when only a single failure occurs. We therefore compute the MAE only over the pairs where registration did not fail. For our method, failure is identified using the threshold probability P_θ as described in Sect. 5.2 — the threshold is computed as $P_\theta = e^{-34}$ using samples synthesised from the CK+ dataset. For FFT and RANSAC, we manually eliminated the pairs with a translation error larger than 5 pixels. The rightmost column in Table 3 lists the number of pairs eliminated when computing the results.

Table 3 suggests that PSTR and FFT are robust against illumination variations as the performance of both methods on the PIE dataset is similar to their performance on CK+ dataset. The number of pairs where failure is expected (pairs obtained from the 16th and 17th frame) is 10. RANSAC-based methods failed in more than 10 pairs, whereas FFT failed only on the 10 pairs. PSTR also failed on these 10 pairs and identified these failures successfully. PSTR produced only 1 false negative by eliminating a correctly registered pair.

6.4   Sequence Registration

Sequence registration performance on CK+ dataset is given in Table 2 (right). Similarly to pair registration, we give two values at each cell — one obtained by including $\mathcal{L}_4$ and one by excluding $\mathcal{L}_4$. Expectedly, errors are slightly higher than in pair registration. The ground truth is common for all images in a sequence $\mathbf{S}_i$ (essentially all frames are mapped to the first frame), and since facial expressions display larger variation in a sequence than in a pair, errors are more likely to occur. Also, the exactness of ground truth cannot be guaranteed. Although we selected sequences with almost no head/body motion and limited sequence length to $T = 7$, minor motions might have been displayed by the subjects.

In Fig. 3c we show an example of a registered sequence from the CK+ dataset. The images on top are obtained after registration, and the ones on bottom are obtained by taking the difference between consecutive image pairs. The sequence contained a slowly evolving mouth expression and (right) eyebrow movement. The resulting difference images clearly illustrate the usefulness of PSTR — no matter how slowly the expression evolves, the difference images capture face actions and *only* face actions.

We provide a demo video that depicts the sequences after registration — the video is available as supplementary material and also on an online channel[1]. Although we perform training only with the controlled CK+ dataset, PSTR is able to perform accurate registration for naturalistic expressions with head/body and background motion (SEMAINE dataset) as well as sequences with rapid illumination variations (PIE dataset).

7 Conclusions

We presented a probabilistic framework for temporal face registration (PSTR) that achieves subpixel registration accuracy. The framework is based on a *motion representation* that measures registration errors between subsequent frames, a supervised *probabilistic model* that learns the registration errors from the proposed representation, and an iterative *registration error estimator*. We demonstrated on three publicly available datasets that the proposed framework not only achieves high registration accuracy but can also generalise to naturalistic data even when trained only with controlled data. Although as a proof of concept we evaluated the framework on facial action and expression data, the proposed method can be used for multiple application domains which require facial activity analysis. The source code of PSTR is available to the research community via http://cis.eecs.qmul.ac.uk/software.html.

Acknowledgement. The work of E. Sariyanidi and H. Gunes is partially supported by the EPSRC MAPTRAITS Project (Grant Ref: EP/K017500/1).

References

1. Vinciarelli, A., Pantic, M., Bourlard, H.: Social signal processing: survey of an emerging domain. Image Vis. Comput. **27**, 1743–1759 (2009)
2. Gunes, H., Schuller, B.: Categorical and dimensional affect analysis in continuous input: current trends and future directions. Image Vis. Comput. **31**, 120–136 (2013)
3. Valstar, M., Schuller, B., Smith, K., Eyben, F., Jiang, B., Bilakhia, S., Schnieder, S., Cowie, R., Pantic, M.: AVEC 2013 - the continuous audio/visual emotion and depression recognition challenge. In: Proceedings ACM International Workshop on Audio/Visual Emotion Challenge, pp. 3–10 (2013)

---

[1] The demo video is available on http://www.youtube.com/user/AffectQMUL.

4. Almaev, T., Valstar, M.: Local Gabor binary patterns from three orthogonal planes for automatic facial expression recognition. In: Proceedings International Conference on Affective Computing and Intelligent Interaction, pp. 356–361 (2013)
5. Zhao, G., Pietikäinen, M.: Boosted multi-resolution spatiotemporal descriptors for facial expression recognition. Pattern Recogn. Lett. **30**, 1117–1127 (2009)
6. Zhao, G., Pietikainen, M.: Dynamic texture recognition using local binary patterns with an application to facial expressions. IEEE Trans. Pattern Anal. Mach. Intell. **29**, 915–928 (2007)
7. Zeng, Z., Pantic, M., Roisman, G.I., Huang, T.S.: A survey of affect recognition methods: audio, visual, and spontaneous expressions. IEEE Trans. Pattern Anal. Mach. Intell. **31**, 39–58 (2009)
8. Jiang, B., Valstar, M., Martinez, B., Pantic, M.: Dynamic appearance descriptor approach to facial actions temporal modelling. IEEE Trans. Syst. Man Cybern. Part B **44**, 161–174 (2014)
9. Huang, X., Zhao, G., Zheng, W., Pietikäinen, M.: Towards a dynamic expression recognition system under facial occlusion. Pattern Recogn. Lett. **33**, 2181–2191 (2012)
10. Valstar, M.F., Pantic, M.: Combined support vector machines and hidden markov models for modeling facial action temporal dynamics. In: Lew, M., Sebe, N., Huang, T.S., Bakker, E.M. (eds.) HCI 2007. LNCS, vol. 4796, pp. 118–127. Springer, Heidelberg (2007)
11. Valstar, M., Jiang, B., Mehu, M., Pantic, M., Scherer, K.: The first facial expression recognition and analysis challenge. In: Proceedings IEEE International Conference Automatic Face Gesture Recognition, pp. 921–926 (2011)
12. Çeliktutan, O., Ulukaya, S., Sankur, B.: A comparative study of face landmarking techniques. EURASIP J. Image Video Process. **2013**, 13 (2013)
13. Zhu, X., Ramanan, D.: Face detection, pose estimation, and landmark localization in the wild. In: Proceedings IEEE Conference on Computer Vision and Pattern Recognition, pp. 2879–2886 (2012)
14. Jiang, B., Valstar, M., Pantic, M.: Action unit detection using sparse appearance descriptors in space-time video volumes. In: Proceedings IEEE International Conference on Automatic Face and Gesture Recognition, pp. 314–321 (2011)
15. Tzimiropoulos, G., Argyriou, V., Zafeiriou, S., Stathaki, T.: Robust FFT-based scale-invariant image registration with image gradients. IEEE Trans. Pattern Anal. Mach. Intell. **32**, 1899–1906 (2010)
16. Adelson, E.H., Bergen, J.R.: Spatio-temporal energy models for the perception of motion. J. Opt. Soc. Am. **2**, 284–299 (1985)
17. Kolers, P.A.: Aspects of Motion Perception. Pergamon Press, Oxford (1972)
18. Petkov, N., Subramanian, E.: Motion detection, noise reduction, texture suppression, and contour enhancement by spatiotemporal Gabor filters with surround inhibition. Biol. Cybern. **97**, 423–439 (2007)
19. Bellman, R.: Dynamic Programming. Princeton University Press, Princeton (1957)
20. Amano, K., Edwards, M., Badcock, D.R., Nishida, S.: Adaptive pooling of visual motion signals by the human visual system revealed with a novel multi-element stimulus. J. Vis. **9**, 1–25 (2009)
21. Pinto, N., Cox, D.D., DiCarlo, J.J.: Why is real-world visual object recognition hard? PLoS Comput. Biol. **4**, e27 (2008)
22. Webb, B.S., Ledgeway, T., Rocchi, F.: Neural computations governing spatiotemporal pooling of visual motion signals in humans. J. Neurosci. **31**, 4917–4925 (2011)

23. Boureau, Y.L., Ponce, J., LeCun, Y.: A theoretical analysis of feature pooling in visual recognition. In: International Conference on Machine Learning, pp. 111–118 (2010)
24. Fischer, S., Šroubek, F., Perrinet, L., Redondo, R., Cristóbal, G.: Self-invertible 2d log-Gabor wavelets. Int. J. Comput. Vis. **75**, 231–246 (2007)
25. Bay, H., Tuytelaars, T., Van Gool, L.: SURF: Speeded up robust features. In: Leonardis, A., Bischof, H., Pinz, A. (eds.) Computer Vision - ECCV 2006. LNCS, vol. 3951, pp. 404–417. Springer, Heidelberg (2006)
26. Matas, J., Chum, O., Urban, M., Pajdla, T.: Robust wide-baseline stereo from maximally stable extremal regions. Image Vis. Comput. **22**, 761–767 (2004)
27. Sim, T., Baker, S., Bsat, M.: The CMU pose, illumination, and expression database. IEEE Trans. Pattern Analysis and Machine Intelligence **25**, 1615–1618 (2003)
28. McKeown, G., Valstar, M., Cowie, R., Pantic, M., Schroder, M.: The SEMAINE database: annotated multimodal records of emotionally colored conversations between a person and a limited agent. IEEE Trans. Affect. Comput. **3**, 5–17 (2012)

Depth Recovery with Face Priors

Chongyu Chen[1,2], Hai Xuan Pham[3],
Vladimir Pavlovic[3], Jianfei Cai[4(✉)], and Guangming Shi[1]

[1] School of Electronic Engineering, Xidian University, Xi'an, China
[2] Institute for Media Innovation,
Nanyang Technological University, Singapore, Singapore
[3] Department of Computer Science, Rutgers University, New Brunswick, USA
[4] School of Computer Engineering,
Nanyang Technological University, Singapore, Singapore
asjfcai@ntu.edu.sg

Abstract. Existing depth recovery methods for commodity RGB-D sensors primarily rely on low-level information for repairing the measured depth estimates. However, as the distance of the scene from the camera increases, the recovered depth estimates become increasingly unreliable. The human face is often a primary subject in the captured RGB-D data in applications such as the video conference. In this paper we propose to incorporate face priors extracted from a general sparse 3D face model into the depth recovery process. In particular, we propose a joint optimization framework that consists of two main steps: deforming the face model for better alignment and applying face priors for improved depth recovery. The two main steps are iteratively and alternatively operated so as to help each other. Evaluations on benchmark datasets demonstrate that the proposed method with face priors significantly outperforms the baseline method that does not use face priors, with up to 15.1 % improvement in depth recovery quality and up to 22.3 % in registration accuracy.

1 Introduction

Commodity RGB-D sensors such as Microsoft Kinect [1] have received significant attention in the recent years due to their low cost and the ability to capture synchronized color images and depth maps in real time. They have been successfully used in many applications such as game or 3D teleconferencing [2–4]. However, the depth measurements provided by commodity RGB-D sensors are far from perfect and often contain severe artifacts such as noise and holes. In order to combat these artifacts, several methods [5–10] have been proposed to recover the depth from commodity RGB-D sensors. The common idea of these methods is to make use of spatial consistency in the depth map, temporal consistency or the guidance from the aligned color image.

 RGB-D sensors are often used in human-related applications such as teleconference, where the human face is the common focus of attention. Modeling the human face is also central to other application such as face detection, face recognition, and face tracking [11,12]. Accurate face reconstruction critically

© Springer International Publishing Switzerland 2015
D. Cremers et al. (Eds.): ACCV 2014, Part IV, LNCS 9006, pp. 336–351, 2015.
DOI: 10.1007/978-3-319-16817-3_22

depends on the quality of the measured depth and texture data. In the case of face modeling, the space of 3D face shapes is highly restrictive and can serve as an important guidance to improve the depth reconstruction. To the best of our knowledge, we are not aware of any existing work that utilizes face priors (or in general high-level semantic prior) in the depth recovery process. Incorporating a face prior can play significant role for depth recovery, especially at large camera-object distance. This is because the depth quality rapidly deteriorates as the face-camera distance increases, which makes the depth-based face reconstruction challenging. Using face priors could therefore extend the domain of the depth-based face reconstruction and analysis beyond the current limited camera ranges.

In this work, we propose to incorporate a general sparse 3D face model for depth recovery. However, it is non-trivial to derive effective face prior information for depth recovery from the sparse 3D model. Several important challenges arise in this context. On one hand, the 3D model needs to be deformed to align it with the input RGB-D data. Nevertheless, accurate alignment is hard to achieve due to the heterogeneous, quantized noise in the input data. On the other hand, if the alignment is not accurate, the extracted face priors might provide wrong guidance to the depth recovery. In addition, the 3D model is often sparse to support tractable computation, while the depth recovery requires a dense guidance. To address all these issues, we propose a joint optimization framework to iteratively and alternatively refine the depth and the face alignment that will, while reinforcing each other, lead to improved depth recovery and model registration. Extensive results show that our method with face priors clearly outperforms the baseline method that does not utilize face priors.

The rest of this paper is organized as follows. Section 2 presents the existing works related to the proposed method, including the depth recovery framework and the 3D face model used in this paper. Section 3 describes the technical details of the proposed method. Finally, Sect. 4 shows the experimental results and Sect. 5 concludes this paper.

2   Background

In this section we present a baseline model for depth recovery based on a global energy minimization framework and also discuss a sparse 3D deformable shape prior model. These models form the basis of our joint sparse prior-guided depth recovery framework, which will be discussed in Sect. 3.

2.1   Depth Recovery Framework

For depth recovery, several global approaches based on convex optimizations [7,9] have been proposed in recent years, which achieve improved recovery accuracy compared to the local approaches based on filtering techniques [5,13–15]. In this paper, we use a simplified version of the depth recovery framework proposed by Chen et al. [9] as the baseline method due to its general form and practical effectiveness.

In [9], depth recovery is formulated as an energy minimization problem. Given a color image I and its corresponding (noisy) depth map Z, the depth map is recovered by solving

$$\min_{U} \lambda E_d(U, Z) + E_r(U), \tag{1}$$

where U is the recovered depth map, λ is the trade-off parameter, E_d is the data term, and E_r is the regularization term. Both E_d and E_r are quadratic functions. In particular, the data term is defined as

$$E_d(U, Z) = \frac{1}{2} \sum_{i \in \Omega_d} \omega_i \left(U(i) - Z(i)\right)^2, \tag{2}$$

and the regularization term is defined as

$$E_r(U) = \frac{1}{2} \sum_{i \in \Omega_s} \sum_{j \in \Omega_i} \alpha_{ij} (U(i) - U(j))^2, \tag{3}$$

where i stands for pixel index (e.g., $i = (i_x, i_y)$), Ω_d is the set of pixels with valid depth measurements, Ω_s is the set of pixels with sufficient surroundings, and Ω_i is the set of neighboring pixels of pixel i. To be consistent with the empirical accuracy model of Kinect depth measurements [16], the distance-dependent weight ω_i is defined as

$$\omega_i = \begin{cases} \left(\frac{Z_{\max} - Z(i)}{Z_{\max} - Z_{\min}}\right)^2 & Z(i) \in [Z_{\min}, Z_{\max}], \\ 0, & \text{otherwise} \end{cases} \tag{4}$$

where $Z_{\min} = 500$ mm and $Z_{\max} = 5000$ mm are the minimum and maximum reliable working distances for Kinect [1]. The weight α_{ij} is designed according to the color and depth similarities between pixel i and pixel j (please refer to [9] for details).

The effectiveness of this framework stems, in part, from the convexity of Eq. (1), implied by the specific forms of Eqs. (2) and (3). This additive energy formulation also makes it possible to include additional terms dependent on the prior 3D shape prior.

2.2   Face Shape Model and Its Deformation

Statistical models such as Active Shape Models (ASMs) [17] and Active Appearance Models (AAMs) [18,19] have become a common and effective approach to face modeling for the purpose of face pose, shape or deformation estimation and tracking. These methods were originally designed to work with monocular color image input, and there have been efforts to incorporate the depth data into these techniques, such as the work in [20] where the authors utilized the depth frame as an additional texture to the traditional color texture in their ASM framework. In [21], the author extend the AAM framework by fitting the 3D shape to the point cloud using the Iterative Closest Point (ICP) procedure separately after each AAM optimization iteration. The biggest disadvantage of these methods is the fact that their performance depends heavily on the data which they learn the statistical models from.

Another approach for face modeling is to use 3D deformable models as in [22–27]. In these works, the 3D face model is controlled by a set of static shape deformation units (SUs) and action deformation units (AUs). SUs represent the face biometry of an individual, whereas facial expressions are modeled by action units, which are person-independent.

One such model is Candide-3, a generic wireframe model (WFM) developed by J. Ahlberg [28]. The Candide-3 WFM is a sparse model, consisting of 113 vertices and 184 triangles constructed from these vertices that define its surface, as shown in Fig. 2(a). Every vertex $p(k) \in \Re^3$, $k \in \Omega_p$ (e.g., $\Omega_p = \{1, \ldots, 113\}$), of the 3D shape model is formed according to a low-dimensional subspace model:

$$p(k) = p_0(k) + S(k)\sigma + A(k)\alpha, \tag{5}$$

where $p_0(k)$ are the base coordinates of the vertex (corresponding to a reference neutral expression face), $S \in Re^{3 \times K_S}$ and $A \in Re^{3 \times K_A}$ are, respectively, the shape and action deformation bases (matrices) associated with the vertex. $\sigma \in \Re^{K_S}$ is the vector of shape deformation parameters and $\alpha \in \Re^{K_A}$ is the vector for action deformation parameters. For the Candide-3 model, $K_S = 14$ and $K_A = 7$. In this work, without loss of generality, we are only interested in the static shape deformation under the neutral face expression ($\alpha = 0$). Thus, the general transformation of a vertex given global rigid rotation R and translation t is defined as:

$$p(k) = R(p_0(k) + S(k)\sigma) + t. \tag{6}$$

The geometry of the model is therefore determined by the base (average) shape p_0, the models of deformation S, and is parameterized by the (rigid and non-rigid) deformation vector $u = [\theta_x, \theta_y, \theta_z, t_x, t_y, t_z, \sigma^T]^T$, where θ_x, θ_y, θ_z are three rotation angles of R, t_x, t_y, t_z are three translation values corresponding to three axes x, y and z. In the rest of this work, for brevity, we will use notation P to denote all vertices $p(k)$ in a shape $P = \{p(k), k \in \Omega_p\}$ and will often write $P = P(u) = R(P_0 + S\sigma) + t$ to indicate the full deformed 3D shape according to the model in (6).

A number of other 3D deformable face modeling approaches have refined this model, e.g., blendshape-based models using an interactive (bilinear) SU/AU composition [12]. Nevertheless, Candide-3 model has the benefit of being sparse and simple, yet general enough, thus lowering the computational burden while still being able to serve as a shape *prior* in the depth recovery process. For instance, a similar model was used in Pham et al. [29] who introduced an on-line tracking framework based on Candide-3, which operates on RGB-D streams. Their tracker performs acceptably even on low quality input, for examples when the point cloud is sparse, the texture and/or point cloud is noisy. We therefore restrict our attention to this spare family of 3D face shape models for our problem at hand.

In this work we extend the framework of [29] to include depth refinement in the initialization pipeline, thus improve the overall performance of both depth recovery and shape model fitting to a static neutral pose of test subject.

3   Proposed Method

Given a color image I and its corresponding (aligned) noisy depth map Z as input, our goal is to obtain a good depth map of the face region using the face priors derived from the general 3D deformable model. The pipeline of the proposed method is shown in Fig. 1. The first two components in Fig. 1 are pre-processing steps to roughly clean up the depth data and roughly align the general face model to the input point cloud. The last two components in Fig. 1 are the core of our proposed framework. For component of the guided depth recovery, we fix the face prior and use it to update the depth, while for the last component, we fix the depth and update the face prior. The last two components alternatively and iteratively operate until convergence.

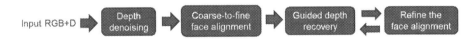

Fig. 1. The pipeline of the proposed method.

3.1   Energy Model for Depth Recovery with Face Priors

To incorporate the face shape prior into the depth recovery process, we propose to recover the depth map U by solving the following optimization problem:

$$\min_{U,u} E_r(U) + \lambda_d E_d(U) + \lambda_f E_f(U, u), \qquad (7)$$

where u represents the parameters of the face model defined in Sect. 2.2, E_r and E_d are the regularization term and the data term as shown in Eq. (1), E_f is the term designed for the face prior (to be defined below), and λ_d and λ_f are the trade-off parameters.

The definition of E_d follows that of [9], defined in Eq. (2). For E_r defined in Eq. (3), we use the weights α_{ij}:

$$\alpha_{ij} = \frac{\beta_{ij}}{\sum_{j \in \Omega_i} \beta_{ij}}, \qquad (8)$$

with

$$-\log \beta_{ij} \propto \frac{\|i - j\|^2}{2l_s^2} + \frac{\|I(i) - I(j)\|^2}{2l_I^2} + \frac{(Z(i) - Z(j))^2}{2l_z^2}, \qquad (9)$$

which are essentially the weights used in joint trilateral filtering [15], with l_s, l_I, and l_z the lengthscale constants.

We define the novel face prior E_f term as

$$E_f(U, u) = \sum_{i \in \Omega_f} \eta_i \left(U(i) - T_f(P(u), i) \right)^2, \tag{10}$$

where Ω_f is the set of pixels with the face prior, and T_f is a function that transforms the sparse face model P defined through a latent deformation u to a dense depth map compatible with U. This term is critical to the recovery process and we will describe it in detail in the next section.

3.2   Shape Prior for Depth Recovery

Considering that the guidance from the sparse vertices of the Candide model may be too weak to serve as the prior for the full (dense) depth map U, we need to generate a dense synthetic depth map Y from the aligned face prior $P(u)$ using an interpolation process. It is possible to define different interpolation functions according to desired dense surface properties. In computer graphics, such models may use non-uniform rational basis spline (NURBS) to guarantee surface smoothness. Here, for the purpose of a shape prior we choose a simple piece-wise linear interpolation. This process is denoted as

$$Y = \mathrm{lerp}(P(u)). \tag{11}$$

Figure 2 shows an example of the generated dense depth map from the sparse shape P.

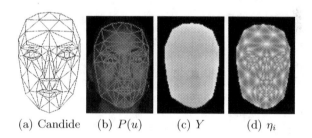

(a) Candide   (b) $P(u)$ (c) Y (d) η_i

Fig. 2. The synthetic depth map Y and its weights $\eta_i (i \in \Omega_f)$. (a) The base shape of Candide-3 Wireframe Model. (b) The 3D wireframe model $P(u)$ drawn upon the texture frame. (c) The synthetic depth map Y generated from the 3D wireframe model. (d) The weights distribution associated with the synthetic dense depth map, where brighter means a larger weight.

To mitigate the effects of the piece-wise flat dense patches due to the linear interpolation, we introduce a weighting scheme defined through weights η_i in (10). In particular, for each pixel $Y(i)$, we use a normalized weight that is adaptive to the pixel's distances from the neighboring vertices of the sparse shape P. Let (a_i, b_i, c_i) be the barycentric coordinates of pixel i inside a triangle defined by its three neighboring vertices of P. Then, its weight is computed as

$$\eta_i = \sqrt{a_i^2 + b_i^2 + c_i^2}, \ i \in \Omega_f. \tag{12}$$

This suggests that the pixels corresponding to model vertices have the highest weight of 1 while the weights decline towards the center of each triangular patch. An illustration of the weights is given in Fig. 2(c), where bright pixels represent large weights.

3.3 Energy Optimization

From the definitions of the energy functions in Eq. (7), it can be seen that the overall optimization of U remains a convex task, for a given fixed prior P. However, the optimization of the face model parameter set u might not be convex since it involves rigid and non-rigid deformation. Therefore, to tackle the global optimization task which includes both the depth U and the deformation u recovery, we resort to a standard recursive alternate optimization process. In other words, we will first optimize u while keeping U fixed, and then optimize U for the fixed deformation u.

Specifically, we divide problem (7) into three well studied subproblems: depth recovery, rigid registration, and non-rigid deformation. The subproblem of depth recovery is solved with fixed u,

$$\hat{U} = \arg\min_{U} E_r(U) + \lambda_d E_d(U) + \lambda_f E_f(U). \tag{13}$$

With U now fixed, the rigid registration between the shape prior P and the point cloud U is solved by an ICP approach, while the non-rigid deformation of the face model is found by solving

$$\hat{\sigma} = \arg\min_{\sigma} E_f(\sigma), \tag{14}$$

where σ represents the shape unit (SU) parameters of Candide model.

We here assume that the solution to (14) is only related to the sparse face vertices P and is therefore independent of the interpolation process or the pixel-wise weights. Therefore, the optimal σ can be obtained by solving

$$\hat{\sigma} = \arg\min_{\sigma} \sum_{k \in \Omega_p} \left(R(p_0(k) + S(k)\sigma) + t - V(k) \right)^2, \tag{15}$$

where V represents the points in the input point cloud that correspond to the model vertices. The correspondences are found by a point-to-point ICP. The overall optimization procedure for solving (7) is summarized in Algorithm 1.

Algorithm 1. The proposed solving procedures

Input: Color image I and its corresponding depth map Z of the user's face, the trade-off factors λ_d and λ_f, and the stopping thresholds ϵ_1 and ϵ_2.

Output: The refined depth map U and the model parameters u which consists of rotation angles θ, translation vector t, and SU parameters σ.

Preparation:

Estimate the initial model parameters θ_0, t_0, and σ_0 from I and Z;

Compute the weights ω_i and η_i for each pixel i;

$u_0 \leftarrow [\theta_0, t_0, \sigma_0^T]^T$, $\sigma_1 \leftarrow \mathbf{0}$, $U_0 \leftarrow Z$, $U_1 \leftarrow \mathbf{0}$, $n \leftarrow 1$;

while $not\ (\|\sigma_n - \sigma_{n-1}\|_2^2 \le \epsilon_1\ and\ \|U_n - U_{n-1}\|_2^2 \le \epsilon_2)$ **do**

$\quad U_n = \arg\min_U E_r(U) + \lambda_d E_d(U) + \lambda_f E_f(U, u_{n-1})$;

$\quad$ Construct a point cloud from U_n;

$\quad$ Solve ICP for θ_n (i.e. R_n), t_n and the correspondences V;

$\quad \sigma_n = \arg\min_\sigma \|R_n(P_0 + S\sigma) + t_n - V\|^2$;

$\quad u_n \leftarrow [\theta_n, t_n, \sigma_n^T]^T$;

$\quad n \leftarrow n + 1$;

end

3.4   Implementation

The proposed guided depth recovery assumes starting with a roughly aligned face model. To get this rough registration, several pre-processing steps are added before solving the optimization problem (7), as shown in Fig. 1. For depth denoising, we use the baseline method [9] to reduce the noise of the input depth map.

The preparation step shown in Algorithm 1 is a coarse-to-fine procedure. In the coarse alignment, we use a classical face detector [30] to detect the face and an ASM alignment algorithm [31] to extract 2D landmark points. After we convert these 2D landmark points to 3D points according to the pre-processed depth map, the SVD-based registration method [32] is used to roughly align the Candide-3 model to the RGB-D data. An example of such coarse alignment is shown in Fig. 3(a). Then, in the refining alignment, the small set of correspondences from the coarse alignment is used as regularization to the standard point-to-plane ICP optimization [33]. In particular, we solve

$$\min_{R,t} \sum_{i \in \Omega_p} \left((Rp_0(i) + t - d(i))^T n(i) \right)^2 + w_a \sum_{j=1}^{6} \|Rp_0(j) + t - d(j)\|^2 \quad (16)$$

to update rotation R and translation t, where $d(i)$ is the correspondence from the data point cloud for vertex $p(i)$ and $n(i)$ is the normal vector at $d(i)$. The first term in (16) is the point-to-plane distance function of all vertices of the 3D shape; minimizing this energy function has the effect of sliding the wireframe model over the surface of the data point cloud. The second term in (16) is the point-to-point distance function of six anchor point pairs as in [29] with weight w_a, where the six anchor points are the six eye and mouth corner vertices of the Candide model, and $d(j)$ are kept fixed as the six correspondences of eye and mouth corners used in the previous SVD-based registration step. Minimizing the second term helps prevent the shape model from moving away too much. At the end, some heuristics on search for the corresponding nose and chin tips are performed to estimate initial values of shape deformation parameters σ_0 before entering the main optimization loop. Figure 3 gives an intuitive illustration for this coarse-to-fine alignment.

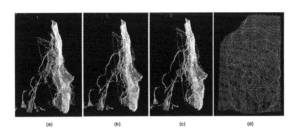

Fig. 3. The coarse-to-fine face alignment. (a) The alignment after SVD-based pose estimation. (b) The alignment refined by the point-to-plane ICP with regularization. (c) and (d) The alignment after estimating initial shape deformation parameters.

4   Experiments

In this section, we conduct experiments to evaluate the performance of the proposed method. We first use the BU4D Facial Expression Database [34] for quantitative evaluation. Considering that Kinect is the most popular commodity RGB-D sensor, we add some Kinect-like artifacts according to [16] to the depth maps generated from the BU4D database. By using synthetic data, we are able to obtain the ground truth for quantitative evaluation. We also show qualitative results on a real-world data captured by Kinect sensor[1].

4.1   Generating Data Sets for Quantitative Evaluations

According to [16], distance-dependent noise and quantization error are the two main characteristics of the data captured by Kinect. We simulate these two artifacts in our experiments. In particular, the distance-dependent noise is computed by

$$Z'(i) = Z_0(i) + n(i), \tag{17}$$

where i stands for pixel index, Z_0 is the depth map generated from the face model, $n(i)$ is a random sample of a Gaussian distribution $N(0, cZ_0^2(i))$, and $c = 1.43 \times 10^{-5}$ is Kinect-oriented constant [16]. The quantization artifact is simulated by quantizing the noisy depth map using quantization steps computed from the camera parameters of Kinect. An example of adding Kinect-like artifacts is shown in Fig. 4.

---

[1] More results can be found at http://www.ntu.edu.sg/home/asjfcai/.

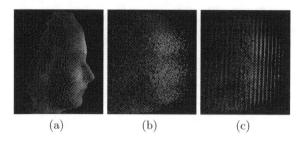

(a)   (b)   (c)

Fig. 4. An example of adding Kinect-like artifacts. (a) The noise-free depth map. (b) The depth map with distance-dependent noise. (c) The depth map with both noise and quantization error.

4.2   Quantitative Evaluations

To show the effectiveness of our idea of utilizing the prior face information, we compare the proposed method with the baseline method [9]. For a fair comparison, the parameters l_s, l_I, l_z, and λ_d are set according to [9] for both the proposed and the baseline methods. For the proposed method, we empirically set $\epsilon_1 = 0.5$ and $\epsilon_2 = 3$. It should be noted that the proposed method is not sensitive to these parameters because its performance will be similar when the parameters change within a reasonable range. Considering that the reliability of the input depth map decreases as the distance increases, we use a relatively small value for λ_f at close distances, and a relative large value at far distances. According to our experience, $[0.1, 0.5]$ is a reasonable range of λ_f for the distance between 1.2 m and 2.0 m.

BU4D database contains more than 600 3D face expression sequences. For the evaluation of depth recovery, we re-render them as RGB-D data sets and only use the frame of neutral expression because the action units are not considered in our depth reconstruction task. Each depth map is rendered at four different camera distances: 1.2 m, 1.5 m, 1.75 m, and 2.0 m. There are 220 sets of RGB-D data with a neutral expression as the 1st frame, which are used in our experiments.

Figure 5 shows the mean absolute error (MAE) of the recovered depth map for each data set. Since we focus on face fidelity, the MAE is computed only using the depth values inside the face region. It can be seen that, in most cases, the proposed method achieves higher recovery accuracy compared to the baseline method, which suggests that the face prior is helping the depth recovery. Figure 6 gives a representative comparison between the baseline and the proposed methods. In Fig. 6(a) and (b), we color the differences between the recovered depth maps and the ground truth, where dark blue represents small difference and other colors represent large differences. It is shown that the baseline method cannot well handle the case of rich texture. Some large errors around the eyes' region are good examples for this case. In contrast, the face priors used in the proposed method can reduce such artifact and thus leads to higher recovery quality. In Fig. 6(c), we use the light blue color to represent the region where the proposed method achieves higher recovery quality, and yellow color to represent

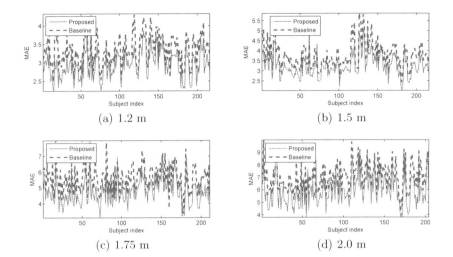

(a) 1.2 m

(b) 1.5 m

(c) 1.75 m

(d) 2.0 m

Fig. 5. The depth MAE results on data sets rendered at different camera distances, (a) 1.2 m, (b) 1.5 m, (c) 1.75 m, and (d) 2.0 m.

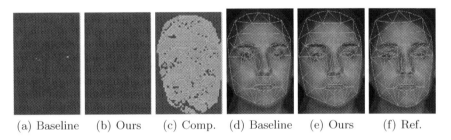

(a) Baseline   (b) Ours   (c) Comp.   (d) Baseline   (e) Ours   (f) Ref.

Fig. 6. Representative results of depth recovery and face registration. (a) The difference map for the result of the baseline method, where dark blue represents small errors and light blue represents large errors. (b) The difference map for the result of the proposed method. (c) The comparison between the baseline and the proposed methods. The light blue color indicates the region where the proposed method achieves lower recovery error and the yellow color indicates the region where the baseline method is better. (d) The registration result of fitting the model to the depth map recovered by the baseline method. (e) The registration result of the proposed method. (f) The registration result of fitting the model to the noise-free depth map, which is used as the reference.

the region where the baseline method is better. The case shown in Fig. 6(c) is representative for most data sets. Therefore, the proposed method generally achieves higher recovery quality compared to the baseline method.

Besides the recovery error, we also evaluate the registration accuracy. To get the reference registration and shapes, we fit the 3D face model to noise-free data. The face model is also fitted to the depth maps obtained by different methods. We then compare the fitting result with the reference registration. A visual comparison between the registration results is shown in Fig. 6(d)–(f). Figure 7 gives

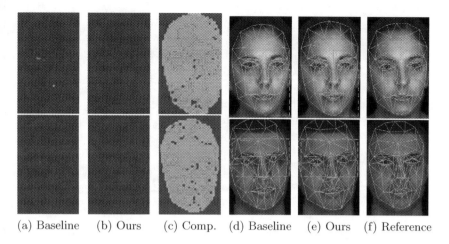

(a) Baseline   (b) Ours   (c) Comp.   (d) Baseline   (e) Ours   (f) Reference

Fig. 7. Representative results of depth recovery and face registration on the datasets rendered at 1.75 m. For the depth recovery results, the baseline method produces some severe recovery error around the eyes and the nose, while the proposed method can effectively reduce the noise in these regions. For the face registration results, the proposed method produces a better fitting around the face boundary compared to the baseline method.

more visual comparisons. We can see that the proposed method produces a more accurate face registration compared to the baseline method, especially in the eyes' region and around the face boundary.

Table 1. Quantitative evaluations of the proposed method using 4 metrics. The results obtain by the baseline and the proposed methods are separated by "/". The improvement of the proposed method over the baseline method is shown in percentages.

Dataset	Mean depth MAE	2D translation error	2D landmark error	3D shape error
1.20 m	3.33/2.97 (10.8 %)	0.75/0.59 (21.3 %)	1.17/1.02 (12.8 %)	2.24/1.87 (16.5 %)
1.50 m	3.76/3.29 (12.5 %)	0.52/0.44 (15.4 %)	0.99/0.85 (14.1 %)	2.30/1.93 (16.1 %)
1.75 m	5.58/4.79 (14.2 %)	0.54/0.44 (18.5 %)	1.07/0.89 (16.8 %)	2.60/2.02 (22.3 %)
2.00 m	7.04/5.98 (15.1 %)	0.57/0.46 (19.3 %)	1.09/0.93 (14.7 %)	3.03/2.46 (18.8 %)

Quantitative evaluations of the depth quality and registration accuracy are shown in Table 1. Besides the mean MAE for the recovery error, three metrics are used to compute the registration error. The 2D translation error is the 2D Euclid distance between the center of the fitted face model and the center of the reference model in the image plane. After aligning two 2D face models by aligning their centers, we compute the mean distance between the 2D landmarks of the fitted model and that of the reference model and denote it as 2D landmark error.

The 3D shape error is computed by scaling the difference between 3D models, i.e., $err_{3D} = \|P_{\text{fit}} - P_{\text{ref}}\|/N_M$, where P_{fit} is the model that fits to the recovered depth map and P_{ref} is the reference model that fits to the noise-free depth map. It can be seen that the proposed method achieves an improvement of recovery accuracy up to 15.1 %, and the improvement of recovery accuracy exhibits a generally increasing trend with the distance. This is because the quality of the input depth map keeps decreasing with the increase of the distance and the baseline method only uses the input depth map as the data term. The improvement of the proposed method in registration accuracy is also significant, up to 22.3 %. It indicates that a better recovered depth map is helpful for the face alignment.

4.3 Experiments on Real Data

For the experiments on real data, we use Kinect to capture several RGB-D frames of a mannequin and a male subject at distances ranging from 1.0 m to 2.0 m. The results of the proposed and the baseline methods are then visually compared because we do not have the true face geometry.

Figure 8 shows the registration (red wireframe) and depth recovery (white cloud) results of the mannequin at distances 1.50 m and 1.68 m. Figure 9 shows some similar results for the male subject. It is shown that the proposed method clearly outperforms the baseline method. The depth maps in these tests were

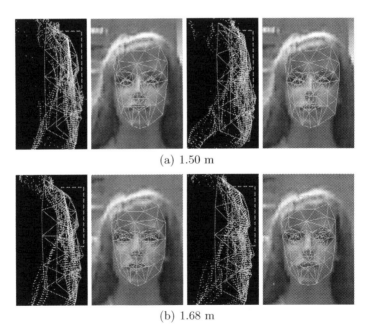

(a) 1.50 m

(b) 1.68 m

Fig. 8. The results on real Kinect data of a mannequin, which are shown in both 2D and 3D. In each figure, the result of the baseline method is on the left-hand side, while the result of the proposed method is on the right-hand side.

captured at a relatively large distance from the sensor and, as a consequence, using the baseline alone is insufficient to reconstruct the depth maps properly. Specifically, the depth maps recovered by the baseline method are flat on the upper half of the face in Fig. 8, mainly at the forehead and noseline areas. On the other hand, the proposed method guided by the face prior is able to reconstruct more reasonable depth maps in those areas, which, e.g., follows the natural shape of a forehead. This also affects the final registration quality, although to a somewhat lesser extent than in the BU4D synthetic data. We attribute this to the discrepancy between the depth noise model used in BU4D experiments and that in the real data, as well as the additional noise in the color/texture channels.

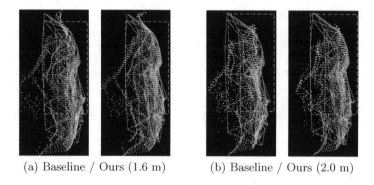

(a) Baseline / Ours (1.6 m)   (b) Baseline / Ours (2.0 m)

Fig. 9. The results on real Kinect data of a male subject.

5   Conclusion

The major contributions of this paper are twofold. First, we introduce the idea of using face priors in depth recovery, which has not been studied in literature before. Second, we formulate the problem as a joint optimization and develop an effective solution for it. Experimental results on a benchmark dataset show that, despite the coarse and sparse face prior model, properly taking into account the face priors brings in up to 15.1 % of improvement in depth quality, which can be essential for applications such as 3D telepresence and teleconference. It can be expected that more accurate face priors will bring in more improvements. Moreover, the proposed method also leads to better registration accuracy, up to 22.3 % of improvement, suggesting that the proposed method can also help other RGB-D face analysis tasks such as face tracking.

Acknowledgement. This research, which is carried out at BeingThere Centre, is mainly supported by the Singapore National Research Foundation under its International Research Centre @ Singapore Funding Initiative and administered by the IDM Programme Office. This research is also partially supported by the 111 Project (No. B07048), China.

References

1. Mutto, C., Zanuttigh, P., Cortelazzo, G.: Microsoft Kinect^{TM} range camera. In: Mutto, C., Zanuttigh, P., Cortelazzo, G. (eds.) Time-of-Flight Cameras and Microsoft Kinect^{TM}. SpringerBriefs in Electrical and Computer Engineering, pp. 33–47. Springer, Boston (2012)
2. Maimone, A., Fuchs, H.: Encumbrance-free telepresence system with real-time 3D capture and display using commodity depth cameras. In: International Symposium Mixed Augmented Reality (ISMAR), pp. 137–146. IEEE, Basel, Switzerland (2011)
3. Kuster, C., Popa, T., Zach, C., Gotsman, C., Gross, M.: Freecam: a hybrid camera system for interactive free-viewpoint video. In: Proceedings of the Vision, Modeling, and Vision (VMV), Berlin, Germany, pp. 17–24 (2011)
4. Zhang, C., Cai, Q., Chou, P., Zhang, Z., Martin-Brualla, R.: Viewport: a distributed, immersive teleconferencing system with infrared dot pattern. IEEE Multimedia 20, 17–27 (2013)
5. Min, D., Lu, J., Do, M.: Depth video enhancement based on weighted mode filtering. IEEE Trans. Image Process. 21, 1176–1190 (2012)
6. Richardt, C., Stoll, C., Dodgson, N.A., Seidel, H.P., Theobalt, C.: Coherent spatiotemporal filtering, upsampling and rendering of RGBZ videos. Comp. Graph. Forum 31, 247–256 (2012)
7. Yang, J., Ye, X., Li, K., Hou, C.: Depth recovery using an adaptive color-guided auto-regressive model. In: Fitzgibbon, A., Lazebnik, S., Perona, P., Sato, Y., Schmid, C. (eds.) ECCV 2012, Part V. LNCS, vol. 7576, pp. 158–171. Springer, Heidelberg (2012)
8. Zhao, M., Tan, F., Fu, C.W., Tang, C.K., Cai, J., Cham, T.J.: High-quality Kinect depth filtering for real-time 3D telepresence. In: IEEE International Conference on Multimedia and Expo (ICME), pp. 1–6 (2013)
9. Chen, C., Cai, J., Zheng, J., Cham, T.J., Shi, G.: A color-guided, region-adaptive and depth-selective unified framework for Kinect depth recovery. In: International Workshop Multimedia Signal Processing (MMSP), pp. 8–12. IEEE, Pula, Italy (2013)
10. Qi, F., Han, J., Wang, P., Shi, G., Li, F.: Structure guided fusion for depth map inpainting. Pattern Recogn. Lett. 34, 70–76 (2013)
11. Li, H., Yu, J., Ye, Y., Bregler, C.: Realtime facial animation with on-the-fly correctives. ACM Trans. Graph. 32, 42:1–42:10 (2013)
12. Cao, C., Weng, Y., Zhou, S., Tong, Y., Zhou, K.: FaceWarehouse: a 3D facial expression database for visual computing. IEEE Trans. Vis. Comput. Graph. 20, 413–425 (2014)
13. Tomasi, C., Manduchi, R.: Bilateral filtering for gray and color images. In: International Conference on Computer Vision (ICCV), pp. 839–846. IEEE, Bombay, India (1998)
14. Petschnigg, G., Szeliski, R., Agrawala, M., Cohen, M., Hoppe, H., Toyama, K.: Digital photography with flash and no-flash image pairs. ACM Trans. Graph. 23, 664–672 (2004)
15. Lai, P., Tian, D., Lopez, P.: Depth map processing with iterative joint multilateral filtering. In: Picture Coding Symposium (PCS), pp. 9–12. IEEE, Nagoya, Japan (2010)
16. Khoshelham, K., Elberink, S.O.: Accuracy and resolution of Kinect depth data for indoor mapping applications. Sensors 12, 1437–1454 (2012)

17. Cootes, T., Taylor, C., Cooper, D., Graham, J.: Active shape models - their training and applications. Comput. Vis. Image Underst. **61**, 39–59 (1995)
18. Cootes, T., Edwards, G., Taylor, C.: Active appearance models. IEEE Trans. Pattern Anal. Mach. Intell. **23**, 681–684 (2001)
19. Matthews, I., Baker, S.: Active appearance models revisited. Int. J. Comput. Vis. **60**, 135–164 (2004)
20. Baltruaitis, T., Robinson, P., Matthews, I., Morency, L.P.: 3D constrained local model for rigid and non-rigid facial tracking. In: CVPR, pp. 2610–2617 (2012)
21. Wang, H., Dopfer, A., Wang, C.: 3D AAM based face alignment under wide angular variations using 2D and 3D data. In: ICRA (2012)
22. Cai, Q., Gallup, D., Zhang, C., Zhang, Z.: 3D deformable face tracking with a commodity depth camera. In: Daniilidis, K., Maragos, P., Paragios, N. (eds.) ECCV 2010, Part III. LNCS, vol. 6313, pp. 229–242. Springer, Heidelberg (2010)
23. Ahlberg, J.: Face and facial feature tracking using the active appearance algorithm. In: 2nd European Workshop on Advanced Video-Based Surveillance Systems (AVBS), London, UK, pp. 89–93 (2001)
24. DeCarlo, D., Metaxas, D.: Optical flow constraints on deformable models with applications to face tracking. Int. J. Comput. Vis. **38**, 99–127 (2000)
25. Dornaika, F., Ahlberg, J.: Fast and reliable active appearance model search for 3D face tracking. IEEE Trans. Syst. Man Cybern. **34**, 1838–1853 (2004)
26. Dornaika, F., Orozco, J.: Real-time 3D face and facial feature tracking. J. Real-time Image Proc. **2**, 35–44 (2007)
27. Orozco, J., Rudovic, O., Gonzàlez, J., Pantic, M.: Hierarchical on-line appearance-based tracking for 3D head pose, eyebrows, lips, eyelids and irises. Image Vis. Comput. **31**, 322–340 (2013)
28. Ahlberg, J.: An updated parameterized face. Technical report, Image Coding Group. Department of Electrical Engineering, Linkoping University (2001)
29. Pham, H.X., Pavlovic, V.: Hybrid on-line 3D face and facial actions tracking in RGBD video sequences. In: Proceedings of the International Conference on Pattern Recognition (ICPR) (2014)
30. Viola, P., Jones, M.: Rapid object detection using a boosted cascade of simple features. In: CVPR, pp. I-511–I-518 (2001)
31. Saragih, J.M., Lucey, S., Cohn, J.F.: Deformable model fitting by regularized landmark mean-shift. Int. J. Comput. Vis. **91**, 200–215 (2011)
32. Arun, K.S., Huang, T.S., Blostein, S.D.: Least-squares fitting of two 3D point sets. IEEE Trans. Pattern Anal. Mach. Intell. **9**, 698–700 (1987)
33. Low, K.: Linear least-squares optimization for point-to-plane ICP surface registration. Technical report TR04-004, Department of Computer Science, University of North Carolina at Chapel Hill (2004)
34. Yin, L., Chen, X., Sun, Y., Worm, T., Reale, M.: A high-resolution 3D dynamic facial expression database. In: 8th IEEE International Conference on Automatic Face Gesture Recognition, pp. 1–6. IEEE (2008)

Inlier Estimation for Moving Camera Motion Segmentation

Xuefeng Liang$^{(\boxtimes)}$, Cuicui Zhang, and Takashi Matsuyama

IST, Graduate School of Informatics, Kyoto University, Kyoto, Japan
{xliang,tm}@i.kyoto-u.ac.jp, zhang@vision.kuee.kyoto-u.ac.jp

Abstract. In moving camera videos, motion segmentation is often performed on the optical flow. However, there exist two challenges: (1) Camera motions lead to three primary flows in optical flow: translation, rotation, and radial flow. They are not all solved in existing frameworks under Cartesian coordinate system; (2) A moving camera introduces 3D motion, the depth discontinuities cause the motion discontinuities that severely confuse the motion segmentation. Meanwhile, the mixture of the camera motion and moving objects' motions make indistinctness between foreground and background. In this work, our solution is to find a low order polynomial to model the background flow field due to its coherence. To this end, we first amend the Helmholts-Hodge Decomposition by adding coherence constraints, which can handle translation, rotation, and radial flow fields under a unified framework. Secondly, we introduce an Incoherence Map and a progressive Quad-Tree partition to reject moving objects and motion discontinuities. Finally, the low order polynomial is achieved from the rest flow samples on two potentials in HHD. We present results on more than twenty videos from four benchmarks. Extensive experiments demonstrate a better performance in dealing with challenging scenes with complex backgrounds. Our method improves the segmentation accuracy of state-of-the-art by 10% ∼ 30%.

1 Introduction

With rapid increase of mobile cameras (handhold camera, wearable camera, etc), video analysis faces more challenges. One of them is that appearance motions are no longer simple in such scenes where multiple objects could move independently, in addition to the camera motion. It is named 3D motion. A common scheme in 3D motion segmentation is to use optical flow or trajectories as a cue. As optical flow can be directly used for clustering or to compensate for the camera motion, the pixelwise model are often used for segmentation [1–4].

However, here are two major drawbacks of using optical flow. (1) Camera motions in 3D scene cause three primary motion flows in optical flow: translation,

---

Electronic supplementary material The online version of this chapter (doi:10. 1007/978-3-319-16817-3_23) contains supplementary material, which is available to authorized users. Videos can also be accessed at http://www.springerimages.com/videos/978-3-319-16816-6.

© Springer International Publishing Switzerland 2015
D. Cremers et al. (Eds.): ACCV 2014, Part IV, LNCS 9006, pp. 352–367, 2015.
DOI: 10.1007/978-3-319-16817-3_23

rotation, and radial flow. The well accepted interpretation of the flow vector is based on Cartesian coordinate system with two bases x, y. Then, a motion vector in 2D is denoted by u, v. For translation, it can be interpreted as an invariant u/v that depends on depth and camera motion only. But for rotation and radial flow, the u/v changes with x, y changing on image plan too. Then, there is no invariant to interpret them under the Cartesian coordinate system. For example, Fig.1.(b) and Fig.4.(b) involve the radial flow and rotation, respectively. The direction and magnitude of flow vectors are changing w.r.t the change of x, y. To our best knowledge, no scheme could well handle all these three flows based on dense flow field. (2) Optical flow depends on the object's distance from the camera. A varied depth causes a different magnitude of the flow. This may make a clustering algorithm to label backgrounds at different depths as separate objects although they are static in the real world. In Fig.1.(b), there is a significant motion discontinuity between the stopped car and the far away background. To handle motion discontinuities, other works need auxiliary information (e.g. color, edge energy) to merge small segments into one as a post-processing.

As the flow filed of the static background (inlier) in optical flow is caused by the camera motion, it should be globally coherent. But, existing optical flow algorithms give much error at the depth discontinuity, and make those flows incoherent with the camera motion. For a moving object in 3D scene, its flow field (outlier), however, is caused by not only its own motion but also the camera motion. So, an outlier consists of both incoherent and coherent flows w.r.t. the camera motion. Thus, the coherence in optical flow can be a cue for 3D motion segmentation. In this work, our object is to find an appropriate polynomial for inlier modeling according to its coherence, which requires no prior knowledge and post-processing. To this end, the first challenge is how to put three primary motion flows into one scheme. Helmholtz-Hodge decomposition (HHD) was initially developed to characterize the rotation and radial flow by curl-divergence regularization. HHD can decompose an arbitrary motion field into *curl-free* and *divergence-free* components through finding their unique corresponding scalar and vector potentials no matter the motion is coherent or not. To ensure the coherence, we amend conventional HHD by adding two constraints: piece-wise smoothness, and global minimization. Nevertheless, the obtained two potentials consist of the major coherent inlier and a little coherent outliers. To better estimate inlier, we introduce an Incoherence Map (IM) by subtracting the projection of two potentials from optical flow. It intuitively depicts the outliers and motion discontinuities. Moreover, a progressive Quad-Tree partition is proposed for precisely labeling outliers and motion discontinuities on IM, and rejecting them from two potentials. Therefore, outliers is completely excluded in inlier estimation. The motion discontinuities are also excluded, but do not affect the coherent flows at the fields with different depths. Afterwards, our object can be achieved by approximating the low order polynomials using rest samples on two potentials.

Other approaches for 3D motion segmentation can be categorized as (1) using optical flow, and (2) trajectories clustering. Chen and Bajic [1] proposed an outlier rejection filter that explicitly filters motion vectors by checking their similarity in a pre-defined window. Chen and Bajic [2], and Qian and Bajic [3] proposed a joint

354   X. Liang et al.

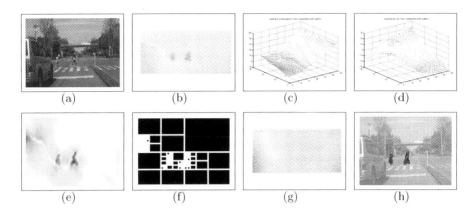

(a)   (b)   (c)   (d)

(e)   (f)   (g)   (h)

Fig. 1. (a) A traffic scene where two kids are running from left to right. A car stops at the left side. The camera is moving towards the stop line. (b) The original optical flow. Besides two outliers, here exists a significant flow discontinuity between the left side car and far away background. (c) The potential of divergence-free component. (d) The potential of curl-free component. (e) Incoherence Map *IM*. (f) Progressive Quad-Tree Partition on IM to reject the outliers, motion discontinuities, and noise. (g) The estimated inlier. It has been rather coherent. (h) Result of 3D motion segmentation. It detects outliers only.

global motion estimation, which iteratively update the inlier model by segmenting outliers out. Although these methods have achieved great progress in dealing with independent motions, they are very likely to over-segment objects due to the motion bias introduced by camera motion [2]. Narayana et al. [4] proposed a method using the direction of motion flow only. It works well for 2D translation, but has difficulty with rotation and radial flow. Brox and Malik [5] segment trajectories by computing the pairwise distances between all trajectories and finding a low-dimensional embedding using spectral clustering. Later, Ochs and Brox [6] improved the spectral clustering by using higher order interactions that consider triplets of trajectories. Elqursh and Elgammal [7] proposed an online extension of spectral clustering by considering trajectories from multiple frames. But, they require a post-processing for merging. Kwak et al. [8] use a Bayesian filtering framework that combines block-based color appearance models with separate motion models for segmentation. However, they require a special initialization procedure in the first frame.

In contrast, our method is a frame-to-frame scheme, requires neither trajectories from multiple frames nor special initialization and post-processing. In additional, it handles all three primary flows in one scheme, and works on a rather wide bank of videos.

2   Modeling Inlier of Optical Flow

2.1   Models of Optical Flow and 3D Motion Segmentation

Let X, Y, Z denote the horizontal, vertical and depth axes in Cartesian coordinate of a real world, and let x, y denote the corresponding coordinates in the image plane. The image plane is located at the focal length: $Z' = f$. In 3D scene, the camera motion has two components: a translation $T = (T_X, T_Y, T_Z)$ and a rotation $R = (R_X, R_Y, R_Z)$. They are always coherent (continues and smooth in both direction and magnitude) in a short time interval $\triangle t$. Then, the resulting 2D optical flow u and v in the x and y image axes are [9]

$$
\begin{bmatrix} u \\ v \end{bmatrix} = \begin{bmatrix} -f(\dfrac{T_X}{Z} + R_Y) + x\dfrac{T_Z}{Z} + yR_Z - x^2\dfrac{R_Y}{f} + xy\dfrac{R_X}{f} \\ -f(\dfrac{T_Y}{Z} - R_X) + y\dfrac{T_Z}{Z} - xR_Z + y^2\dfrac{R_X}{f} - xy\dfrac{R_Y}{f} \end{bmatrix}.
\tag{1}
$$

Beside constant f, camera motion T and R, and image coordinates x and y, it is noted from Eq.(1) that u and v are functions with depth Z too. Thus, an ideal optical flow field $(\mathcal{OF})$ in 3D scene is a collection of 2D $\mathcal{OF}$s of n static planar surfaces in background (named *inlier*, $\mathcal{F}_{in}$) and $\mathcal{OF}$s of m foreground moving objects (named *outlier*, $\mathcal{F}_{out}$). We can formulate them as

$$
\mathcal{OF} = \mathcal{F}_{in} + \mathcal{F}_{out},
\tag{2}
$$

where $\mathcal{F}_{in} = [\mathcal{F}_{in}(B_1)\, \mathcal{F}_{in}(B_2)\ldots\mathcal{F}_{in}(B_n)]$, $\mathcal{F}_{out} = [\mathcal{F}_{out}(O_1)\, \mathcal{F}_{out}(O_2)\ldots\mathcal{F}_{out}(O_m)]$, B_i denotes a static planar surface and O_j denotes a moving object. Please note that $\mathcal{F}_{out}(O_j)$ is incoherent with $\mathcal{F}_{in}$ because its own motion does not match the camera motion.

Theoretically speaking, each $\mathcal{F}_{in}(B_i)$ or $\mathcal{F}_{out}(O_j)$ could be approximated by a polynomial. Thus, entire $\mathcal{OF}$ could be also approximated by a high order polynomial $\mathcal{P}$.

$$
\mathcal{OF} = [\mathcal{F}_{in}(B_1)\ldots\mathcal{F}_{in}(B_n)\, \mathcal{F}_{out}(O_1)\ldots\mathcal{F}_{out}(O_m)] \approx \mathcal{P},
\tag{3}
$$

where high order is required due to the outliers, motion discontinuities caused by depth discontinuities, and noise.

To segment 3D motion, many studies tried to model outliers directly. Moving objects, however, can be either rigid or non-rigid, outlier modeling is a nontrivial task. Instead of complex modeling and auxiliary constrains, we model inlier by a general approach in this work other than modeling outliers. As the inlier is caused by camera motion, each $\mathcal{F}_{in}(B_i)$ must be coherent, and can be modeled by a simple polynomial $\mathcal{P}_i$. But Eq.(1) shows $\mathcal{F}_{in}(B_i)$ is a function with Z in translation and radial flow fields. Modeling $\mathcal{F}_{in}$ is still difficult.

Most optical flow algorithms share a common assumption of local motion smoothness, and apply an optimization to minimize the global error. The difference among them only focuses on implementations of the optimization. This strategy is ideally designed for the motion of one planar surface. But, it is also applied on the object's boundaries, where depths vary, because algorithms do not know where the depth discontinuities are. For inlier $\mathcal{F}_{in}$, at the place where depth variation is not significant, optical flow algorithms give rather smooth flow field and connect motion fields of two adjacent planar surfaces. By the same token, algorithms often give much errors at the place having significant depth discontinuity. These incorrect flows are incoherent with camera motion, but are minority in $\mathcal{F}_{in}$. Then, $\mathcal{F}_{in}$ can be reformulated as

$$\mathcal{F}_{in} = a_1 \mathcal{F}_{in}^{coherent} + b_1 \mathcal{F}_{in}^{incoherent}, \qquad a_1 >> b_1, \qquad (4)$$

where a and b are quantity coefficients.

The primary reason of the moving objects standing out in a moving camera video is that their motions are incoherent with camera motion and result in significant variances on optical flow field $\mathcal{OF}$. Besides, $\mathcal{F}_{out}$ is partially caused by camera motion as well, which is coherent with $\mathcal{F}_{in}$, but is minority. Now, $\mathcal{F}_{out}$ can be reformulated as

$$\mathcal{F}_{out} = a_2 \mathcal{F}_{out}^{coherent} + b_2 \mathcal{F}_{out}^{incoherent}, \qquad b_2 >> a_2. \qquad (5)$$

One major difficulty in 3D motion segmentation is induced by the mixed flow field of camera motion and moving objects' motions. These dependent motions lead to indistinctness of the difference between inlier $\mathcal{F}_{in}$ and outliers $\mathcal{F}_{out}$. To segment outliers from inlier, our object, therefore, becomes finding an appropriate polynomial

$$\mathcal{P}' \approx a_1 \mathcal{F}_{in}^{coherent} + a_2 \mathcal{F}_{out}^{coherent}, \qquad (6)$$

which rejects incoherence $(b_1 \mathcal{F}_{in}^{incoherent} + b_2 \mathcal{F}_{out}^{incoherent})$ in inlier and outliers.

2.2   Three Primary Motion Flows and Their Potentials

Equation (1) shows motion vectors in $\mathcal{OF}$ caused by camera motion can be decomposed into two components: V_T and V_R representing camera translation and rotation, respectively.

$$V_T = \left[\frac{xT_Z - fT_X}{Z}, \frac{yT_Z - fT_Y}{Z} \right]^T, \; V_R = \begin{bmatrix} yR_Z - x^2\dfrac{R_Y}{f} + xy\dfrac{R_X}{f} - fR_Y \\ -xR_Z + y^2\dfrac{R_X}{f} - xy\dfrac{R_Y}{f} + fR_X \end{bmatrix}.$$

To simplify analysis, motion vectors caused by camera motion can be further decomposed into three primary components:

1. V_{T_X} caused by camera translation on image plan $\mathbb{X}(x, y)$:

$$V_{T_X} = \left[-\frac{fT_X}{Z}, -\frac{fT_Y}{Z} \right], \; \arctan(V_{T_X}) = \frac{T_X}{T_Y}, \; |V_{T_X}| = \frac{f}{Z}\sqrt{T_X^2 + T_Y^2}. \qquad (7)$$

It is noted that the direction of flow is independent on the depth Z, and the magnitude is inversely proportional to the depth Z. Eq.(7) indicates that if the depth variation is not significant in 3D scene (e.g. the static background is rather far from the camera), the coherence of both direction and magnitude is preserved. If background is pretty close to the camera, the depth discontinuity will lead to motion discontinuity that is incoherent with camera motion.

2. V_{T_Z} caused by camera translation along Z axis. It presents a radial flow field with the origin at the focus-of-expansion.

$$V_{T_Z} = \left[\frac{xT_Z}{Z}, \frac{yT_Z}{Z}\right], \quad \arctan(V_{T_Z}) = \frac{x}{y}, \quad |V_{T_Z}| = \frac{T_Z}{Z}\sqrt{x^2 + y^2}. \quad (8)$$

It is noted that the flow direction is dependent on neither the depth Z nor camera motion, but only determined by image plan coordinates x and y. The magnitude is also inversely proportional to the depth Z. Analogically, the coherent flow field is maintained at the place having less depth variation. But, the incoherence occurs at the place having significant depth discontinuity. Please see Fig.1.(b) as an example.

3. V_R caused by camera rotation along an axis parallel with the camera optical axis Z. Please note that camera rotation, which rotates along image axes x or y in a short time interval $\triangle t$, could be simulated as a translation. In this work, we consider camera rotation perpendicular to the image plan only.

$$V_R = [yR_Z, -xR_Z], \quad \arctan(V_R) = -\frac{y}{x}, \quad |V_R| = R_Z\sqrt{x^2 + y^2}. \quad (9)$$

It is noted that both direction and magnitude of V_R are independent on depth Z, but dependent on image plan coordinates x and y. This indicates that a 3D motion segmentation can reduce to a 2D motion segmentation while camera solely rotates perpendicular to the image plan. Obviously, the coherence of flow field is preserved.

Consequently, an arbitrary optical flow field $\mathcal{OF}$ can be represented by a combination of above three primary flows as:

$$\mathcal{OF} = \alpha V_{T_X} + \beta V_{T_Z} + \gamma V_R,$$

where α, β and γ are quantity coefficients.

Analogically, Prof. Helmholtz explained that the motion of a volume element in 3D space consists of: *1) expansion or contraction, 2) rotation, and 3) translation. The expansion/contraction (radial flow field) can be represented as the gradient of a scalar potential function because it is irrotational. The rotation can be represented as the curl of a vector potential function since it is incompressible. Translation, however, being neither compressible nor rotational can be represented as either the gradient of a scalar potential, or the curl of a vector potential* [10]. It is named by *Helmholtz-Hodge Decomposition* (HHD) [11]. According to HHD, any flow field in our work consists of two components:

1. **Curl-free component** representing divergence (radial flow) and translation because they are irrotational.

$$\theta = \nabla \cdot \mathcal{OF} = V_{T_Z} + V_{T_X}$$

2. **Divergence-free component** representing curl (rotation) and translation because they are incompressible.

$$\vec{\omega} = \nabla \times \mathcal{OF} = V_{T_R} + V_{T_X}$$

Go a step further, curl-free and divergence-free components can be expressed as the curl of a vector potential $\overrightarrow{W}$ and the gradient of a scalar potential E,

$$\mathcal{OF} = \nabla E + \nabla \times \overrightarrow{W}. \tag{10}$$

where $E(x) = -\frac{1}{4\pi}\int\frac{\theta(x')}{|x-x'|}dx'$, $\overrightarrow{W}(x) = -\frac{1}{4\pi}\int\frac{\overrightarrow{\omega}(x')}{|x-x'|}dx'$, and $x \in \mathbb{R}^3$. However, θ and $\overrightarrow{\omega}$ are what we expect. In reality, E and $\overrightarrow{W}$ are computed by energy minimization,

$$\min F(E) = \min \int (\mathcal{OF} - \nabla E)^2, \ \min G(\overrightarrow{W}) = \min \int (\mathcal{OF} - \nabla \times \overrightarrow{W})^2.$$

Theoretically speaking, HHD can decompose an arbitrary motion flow field into curl-free component ∇E and divergence-free component $\nabla \times \overrightarrow{W}$, no matter it is coherent or not. But, we expect coherent potentials for approximating the coherent flow field caused by camera motion, see Eq.(6). To ensure the coherence, our work amended the conventional HHD by adding the first constraint: 1) piece-wise smooth $\mathcal{S}$. Meanwhile, we make an assumption $\mathcal{F}_{in} > \mathcal{F}_{out}$, and add the second constraint: 2) global minimization at entire motion flow field Ω, which ensures the optimization to minimize the inlier, other than the outliers.

$$\begin{aligned} \arg\min_{\mathcal{S}} F(E) &= \arg\min_{\mathcal{S}} \int_{\Omega} (\mathcal{OF} - \nabla E)^2 d\Omega, \\ \arg\min_{\mathcal{S}} G(\overrightarrow{W}) &= \arg\min_{\mathcal{S}} \int_{\Omega} (\mathcal{OF} - \nabla \times \overrightarrow{W})^2 d\Omega. \end{aligned} \tag{11}$$

Please see Fig.1(c) and (d), they are the divergence-free and curl-free potentials respectively. Therefore, these two potential E and $\overrightarrow{W}$ could be our object: coherent surfaces which can be formulated by low order polynomial $\mathcal{P}'$.

2.3 Incoherence Map and Incoherence Labeling

Due to the global optimization and piece-wise smooth constraint, our amended implementation keeps most coherent flow (95% ∼ 99%) into two potentials, but definitely rejects incoherent flow $\mathcal{F}_{in}^{incoherent}$ and $\mathcal{F}_{out}^{incoherent}$. Then, the majority of outliers, motion discontinuities and noise, which are not decomposed into ∇E and $\nabla \times \overrightarrow{W}$, will rest in a remainder. Please note that two potentials still contain a small quantity of $\mathcal{OF}_{out}^{coherent}$. They cannot be directly used for the inlier estimation. Thus, we use this remainder to draw an *Incoherence Map* (IM) to label incoherent flows in $\mathcal{OF}$.

First, we estimate the coherent flow field presented in the curl-free and divergence-free components by a linear combination as:

$$\mathcal{V} = \alpha(\nabla E) + \beta(\nabla \times \overrightarrow{W}), \tag{12}$$

where $\mathcal{V} \subseteq \mathcal{OF}$, α and β are quantity coefficients that indicate how much ∇E and $\nabla \times \overrightarrow{W}$ are involved in $\mathcal{OF}$. We use a distance to determine α and β.

$$d_\theta = \int \frac{|\mathcal{OF} - \nabla E|}{|\mathcal{OF}|}, \qquad d_\omega = \int \frac{|\mathcal{OF} - \nabla \times \overrightarrow{W}|}{|\mathcal{OF}|}, \tag{13}$$

where d_θ represents the distance between the curl-free component and the optical flow field, and d_ω represents the distance between the divergence-free component and the optical flow field. Then, α and β are determined as following:

- While $d_\theta < 0.5$ and $d_\omega > 0.5$, it implies the optical flow looks more like a radial flow field (curl-free component).
- While $d_\theta > 0.5$ and $d_\omega < 0.5$, it implies the optical flow looks more like a rotation field (divergence-free component).
  Under above two cases,

$$\alpha = \frac{d_\theta}{d_\theta + d_\omega}, \qquad \beta = \frac{d_\omega}{d_\theta + d_\omega}.$$

- While $d_\theta < 0.5$ and $d_\omega < 0.5$, it means both components are similar to the optical flow, and implies a translation. Then,

$$\alpha = 0.5, \qquad \beta = 0.5.$$

Afterwards, we can draw Incoherence Map from remainder by

$$IM = \mathcal{OF} - \alpha(\nabla E) - \beta(\nabla \times \overrightarrow{W}). \tag{14}$$

Please see Fig.1.(e), it clearly reveals the outliers, depth discontinuities and computation error.

IM makes outliers and motion discontinuities labeling much easier. However, Eq.(12) and Eq.(14) show that IM consists of a small portion of inlier as well. To ensure the accurate labeling, we introduce a *Progressive Quad-Tree Partition* on IM. The basic idea is that it partition IM into quadrants recursively if a quadrant is not coherent. The partition is called by the following two conditions:

1. the variance of a sub-quadrant $var(\Omega_i)$ is greater than $t * var(\Omega)$;
2. the mean of a sub-quadrant $mean(\Omega_i)$ is greater than $mean(\Omega)$.

where var and $mean$ calculate the variance and mean of flow direction and magnitude, respectively. t is a threshold. Ω is the entire IM. The condition 1 is for detecting the motion discontinuities including the boundaries of outliers and noise, where the flow value changes violently. The condition 2 is for detecting outliers' body, where the outliers' flow differs from inlier's flow because inlier has been almost canceled by two potentials in IM. Partition performs until no region can be split further. The smallest regions represent outliers, motion discontinuities and noise. The rest larger regions represent the coherent inlier, and will be involved in inlier approximation in next section.

The threshold t determines how the Quad-Tree partitions IM. Since local deformations usually vary on different IMs, it is rather difficult to find the best partition using one threshold. We, therefore, define a set of thresholds in a descending order, and introduce a progressive Quad-Tree partition. The t is initially set to 1, and reduces with a step 0.05 for next partition. The procedure stops when the difference between the current Quad-Tree QT' and the previous one QT is less than a convergence value ε. The updated QT' is used for labeling incoherence in IM. The pseudo-code is

Data: IM
Result: Labeled incoherence
$t = 1$; $QT = 0$;
Split(Ω);
while $|QT' - QT| > \varepsilon$ **do**
    for *each quadrant* Ω_i **do**
        if $var(\Omega_i) > t * var(\Omega) \parallel mean(\Omega_i) > mean(\Omega)$ **then**
            Split(Ω_i);
            Go to for loop;
        end
    end
    Update QT' and QT;
    $t = t - 0.05$;
end
Mark all smallest blocks as incoherence;

Algorithm 1. Progressive Quad-Tree Partition

Figure 1.(f) shows the result of progressive Quad-Tree partition which effectively labels outliers and depth discontinuities on IM.

2.4 Inlier Estimation

Multi-parametric models had been conducted to recover the inlier [12]. They were designed for camera motions ranging from simple translation to complex perspective transformation. But, the limitation is that a prior knowledge of motion structure is required to select an appropriate model. Nevertheless, this prior knowledge is not always available in real data. By contrast, we employ a general solution, polynomial surface fitting, using d-order polynomial

$$\mathcal{P} = a_{d0}x^d + a_{0d}y^d + \cdots + a_{ij}x^iy^j + \cdots + a_{10}x + a_{01}y + a_{00}, \quad (15)$$

to estimate inlier $\mathcal{F}_{in}$ from two potentials E and $\overrightarrow{W}$. The advantage is that it requires no prior knowledge.

It is known that high order terms in Eq.(15) present the high frequency signals (incoherence: outliers, motion discontinuities and noise in this work). Thanks to IM and algorithm 1, the incoherence has been labeled and rejected in process afterwards. As explained in Eq.(6) and Eq.(11), our object is to find low order polynomial $\mathcal{P}'$ which expresses the coherent inlier. The inlier estimation, eventually, can be performed by sampling the rest flows on two potentials E and $\overrightarrow{W}$. Since outliers and noise are completely excluded, surface fitting utilizes nearby samples to approximate the inlier. Thus, the result is rather coherent with the camera motion. For motion discontinuities, surface fitting interpolates the samples at both sides of discontinuity to approximate the violent flow change. So, the result also presents the trend of rapid flow change. But the gradient of

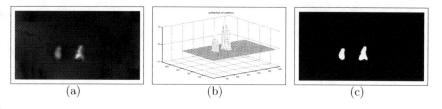

(a)   (b)   (c)

Fig. 2. (a) The outliers map from Eq.(17). The flow discontinuities have become very weak. (b) The potential of outliers. (c) The labeled outliers.

the change becomes less than the one on original $\mathcal{OF}$. In our work, a polynomial of $d = 5$ is employed to produce coherent and accurate potentials E' and $\overrightarrow{W}'$ using the samples after rejecting incoherence. The final inlier is estimated by a linear combination where α, β have been determined in section 2.3,

$$\mathcal{F}'_{in} = \alpha \nabla E' + \beta \nabla \times \overrightarrow{W}'. \tag{16}$$

Figure 1.(g) shows the estimated inlier. It demonstrates that our method approximates the inlier rather coherent, and the outliers have been excluded effectively.

3   Outliers Detection

With estimated inlier, outliers $\mathcal{F}_{out}$ can be detected directly by subtracting the $\mathcal{F}'_{in}$ from the original optical flow $\mathcal{OF}$,

$$\mathcal{F}_{out} \cong \mathcal{OF} - \mathcal{F}'_{in}. \tag{17}$$

Please see Fig.2.(a). However, low order polynomial surface fitting has a defect that it better fits the data with dense samples but goes wild at the edges of the original domain Ω due to lack of adequate samples. To reduce the error, the result is filtered by the mean-curvature of the original potential. The final segmentation is obtained subsequently by assigning binary labels on the true outliers. We will use the segmentation result to evaluate the performance of proposed method in experiments. Figure 2.(c) and (b) show the detected outliers and their potentials, respectively. Figure 1.(h) shows the 3D segmentation result.

4   Experiments

The performance of proposed method is evaluated on four benchmark datasets: Hopkins [13], Berkeley Motion Segmentation [5], Complex Background [4], and SegTrack [14]. The Hopkins dataset contains video sequences along with the features extracted and tracked in all the frames, which has three categories: checkerboard, car, and people sequences. Since checkerboard sequences do not correspond to natural scenes. We just use one sequence (1R2TCR) to show the effectiveness of our method in dealing with cameras rotation. The Berkeley dataset is derived from the Hopkins dataset, which consists of 26 moving camera videos: car, people, and Marple sequences. This dataset has full pixel-level annotations on multiple objects for a few frames sampled throughout the video. Since Marple sequences mainly contain static scenes or the objects are static, it is little challenging for our method. Thus, they are not involved in the experiments. Complex Background and SegTrack datasets contain extremely challenging scenes, where the background motion is much more complex than other datasets. They also provide full pixel-level annotations on multiple objects at each frame within each video. These two datasets are employed to highlight the advantage of our method.

We first illustrate the performance of the proposed method on three sequences that consist of camera translation, rotation and zoom in/out, respectively. Then we compare our method with state-of-the-art [4] on all four datasets. Optical flow is calculated using Brox's method [15] and optimized by [16].

4.1   Performance on Three Typical Sequences

We demonstrate the performance of our method on three typical sequences:*cars2*, *1R2TCR*, and *drive* that involve varied camera motions.

[1] **Cars2 Sequence:** This sequence is from the Berkeley dataset. Three cars are translating in the scene. The camera is translating too, please see Fig.3.

[2] **1R2TCR-Checkerboard Sequence:** This data is from the Hopkins dataset. The basket is rotating, and the box is translating from left to the right. The camera is rotating, please see Fig.4.

[3] **Drive sequence:** This sequence is from the Complex Background dataset. A car is turning to left at the corner. The camera is zooming in, please see Fig.5.

For more examples, please refer the supplemental material.

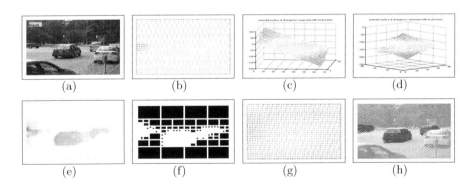

Fig. 3. (a) Cars2 sequence. (b) The original optical flow. Camera motion is translation. (c), (d) Two potentials of E and W. (e) IM. (f) Progressive Quad-Tree Partition on IM. (g) The estimated inlier. (h) Segmentation result.

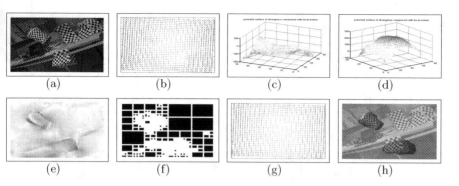

Fig. 4. 1R2TCR sequence. Please refer to Fig.3 for the description of subfigures.

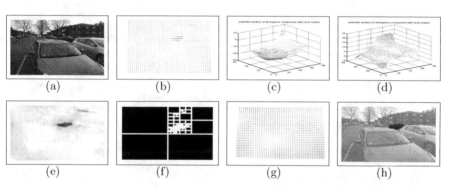

Fig. 5. Drive sequence. Please refer to Fig.3 for the description of subfigures.

4.2   Comparison with State-of-the-art

The proposed method is compared with the latest dense motion field based approach [4], which present two versions: (1) FOF, which uses optical flow information only, and (2) FOF+color+prior, which combines optical flow, color appearance and a prior model to improve the accuracy. We reported the F-measure of ours, FOF and FOF+color+prior presented in their paper in Table 1. F-measure is employed because it considers both the precision P_r and the recall R_c of the test to compute the score as [17]:

$$F = \frac{2 \times R_c \times P_r}{R_c + P_r}.$$

Table 1 shows that our method outperform FOF and FOF+color+prior on almost all videos: it raises the F-measure by 10 % – 30 % on *Cars* 2, 3, 4, 7, and *People* 1 sequence in the Berkely dataset; around 10 % on the *drive, parking*, and *store* sequences in the Complex Background dataset; and more than 20 % on the *parachutte* and *monkeydog* sequences in the SegTrack dataset. This result is quite appealing even on videos containing extremely challenging scenes, such as the

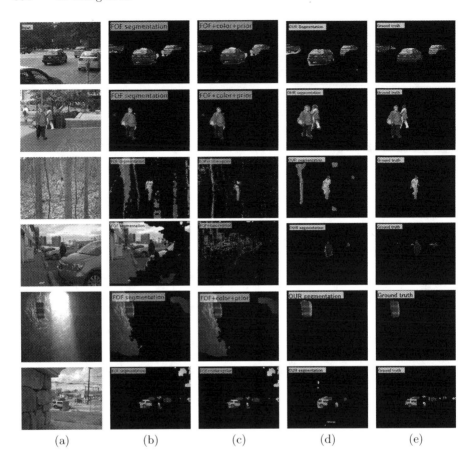

Fig. 6. Segmentation results of FOF, FOF-color and ours on challenging scenes: (a) input sequences, from top to bottom: cars2, people2, forest, store, parachute, traffic, (b) FOF, (c) FOF+color+prior, (d) our segmentation, (e) ground-truth segmentation.

ones with occlusions, complex backgrounds, and noises. A few other results are shown in Fig.6, where the last column is the ground truth. In most cases, our segmentation agrees with the ground truth more than existing methods.

Other relevant works are Ochs *et al.* [6], Elqursh and Elgammal [7] and Kwak *et al.* [8]. These methods analysis trajectories using multiple frames, and some also need special initialization at the first frame. Thus, they are not directly comparable to inlier and outliers accuracy measure. Both our method and FOF are based on optical flow, and a frame-to-frame method requiring neither initialization nor prior knowledge. Therefore, we only compare our method with FOF in this paper only.

Although, the proposed method achieves inspiring performance, extensive experiences shows it may fail in the following cases:

Table 1. F-measures of FOF method [4], and ours.

Sequences	FOF	FOF+color	Our	Sequences	FOF	FOF+color	Our
Cars1	47.81	50.84	**76.38**	drive	30.13	61.80	**83.03**
Cars2	46.37	56.60	**83.23**	forest	19.48	31.44	**35.81**
Cars3	67.18	73.57	**87.47**	parking	43.47	73.19	**83.57**
Cars4	38.51	47.96	**84.52**	store	28.46	70.74	**80.10**
Cars5	64.85	70.94	**84.92**	traffic	66.08	71.24	**71.77**
Cars6	78.09	84.34	**85.81**	—	—	—	—
Cars7	37.63	42.92	**86.10**	birdfall2	68.68	75.69	**76.23**
Cars8	87.13	87.61	**90.78**	girl	75.73	**81.95**	78.06
Cars9	68.99	66.38	**77.52**	parachute	51.49	54.36	**86.72**
Cars10	53.98	50.84	**54.93**	cheetah	12.68	22.31	**55.77**
People1	56.76	69.53	**80.14**	penguin	14.74	20.71	**21.71**
People2	85.35	88.40	**89.91**	monkeydog	10.79	18.62	**45.45**

- Motions of moving objects are very weak comparing with the camera motion. In this case, the outliers are more likely to be decomposed by HHD because they are pretty coherent with the inlier, and can not appear in IM. Such as the *cars* 1, 9 and 10 sequences and *forest* contain some objects' motions which are very small.
- A few isolated static objects stand alone in a texture-free background while camera is moving. In this case, our method may mistake these isolated static objects as moving objects.
- The outlier is greater than inlier. In this case, HHD fails to decompose the inlier because of the global minimization.

We have to point out that the accuracy of the optical flow affects the performance of our method as well. The *girl* sequence shows such an example. It captures a fast running girl in the sports yard. Some frames are blurred terribly, and have severe noisy optical flows. In this case, only optical flow is not sufficient. That's why FOF+color+prior utilizes additional information (color appearance) and prior models to improve the performance. In addition, both methods appear less accurate on the three sequences (*cheetah, penguin, monkeydog*) in the Seg-Track dataset. The reason is they have multiple moving objects, but the ground truth intended for tracking one primary object as the foreground, causing all methods appear less accurate.

5 Conclusions

We have presented a general framework for 3D motion segmentation on a wide bank of moving camera videos. This framework solved two problems: 1) the amended HHD can handle the coherent inlier of all three primary motion flows (translation, rotation, and radial flow), 2) the proposed Incoherence Map and progressive Quad-Tree precisely label the outliers, motion discontinuities and noise. The afterward inlier estimation is achieved by approximating low order polynomials using the rest samples on two potentials in HHD. This compensates the depth discontinuity in the 3D motion. We have evaluated our approach on four benchmark datasets. Extensive experiments showed a rather comparable performance than state-of-the-art. In the future work, more coherent information (e.g. colors, the direction only) might further help our method for segmentation.

Acknowledgement. This work is supported by: Japan Society for the Promotion of Science, Scientific Research KAKENHI for Grant-in-Aid for Young Scientists (ID:25730113).

References

1. Chen, Y.M., Bajic, I.V.: Motion vector outlier rejection cascade for global motion estimation. IEEE Signal Process. Lett. **17**, 197–200 (2010)
2. Chen, Y.M., Bajic, I.V.: A joint approach to global motion estimation and motion segmentation from a coarsely sampled motion vector field. IEEE Trans. Circ. Syst. Video Technol. **21**, 1316–1328 (2011)
3. Qian, C., Bajic, I.V.: Global motion estimation under translation-zoom ambiguity. In: Proceedings of IEEE PacRim, pp. 46–51 (2013)
4. Narayana, M., Hanson, A., Learned-Miller, E.: Coherent motion segmentation in moving camera videos using optical flow orientations. In: ICCV (2013)
5. Brox, T., Malik, J.: Object segmentation by long term analysis of point trajectories. In: Daniilidis, K., Maragos, P., Paragios, N. (eds.) ECCV 2010, Part V. LNCS, vol. 6315, pp. 282–295. Springer, Heidelberg (2010)
6. Ochs, P., Malik, J., Brox, T.: Segmentation of moving objects by long term video analysis. IEEE Trans. Pattern Anal. Mach. Intell. (TPAMI) **36**(6), 1187–1200 (2014)
7. Elqursh, A., Elgammal, A.: Online moving camera background subtraction. In: Fitzgibbon, A., Lazebnik, S., Perona, P., Sato, Y., Schmid, C. (eds.) ECCV 2012, Part VI. LNCS, vol. 7577, pp. 228–241. Springer, Heidelberg (2012)
8. Kwak, S., Lim, T., Nam, W., Han, B., Han, J.H.: Generalized background subtraction based on hybrid inference by belief propagation and bayesian filtering. In: ICCV, pp. 2174–2181 (2011)
9. Irani, M., Rousso, B., Peleg, S.: Recovery of ego-motion using image stabilization. In: CVPR (1994)
10. Helmholtz, H.: On integrals of the hydrodynamical equations, which express vortex-motion. Philos. Mag. J. Sci. **33**, 485–512 (1867)
11. Bhatia, H., Norgard, G., Pascucci, V., Bremer, P.T.: The helmholtz-hodge decomposition - a survey. IEEE Trans. Vis. Comput. Graph. (TVCG) **19**, 1386–1404 (2013)
12. Su, Y., Sun, M.T., Hsu, V.: Global motion estimation from coarsely sampled motion vector field and the applications. IEEE Trans. Circuits System and Video Technology **15**, 232–242 (2005)
13. Tron, R., Vidal, R.: A benchmark for the comparison of 3D motion segmentation algorithms. In: CVPR (2007)

14. Tsai, D., Flagg, M., Rehg, J.M.: Motion coherent tracking with multi-label mrf optimization. In: BMVC (2010)
15. Brox, T., Bruhn, A., Papenberg, N., Weickert, J.: High accuracy optical flow estimation based on a theory for warping. In: Pajdla, T., Matas, J.G. (eds.) ECCV 2004. LNCS, vol. 3024, pp. 25–36. Springer, Heidelberg (2004)
16. Liang, X., McOwan, P., Johnston, A.: A biologically inspired framework for spatial and spectral velocity estimations. J. Opt. Soc. Am. A **28**, 713–723 (2011)
17. Dembczynski, K., Jachnik, A., Kotlowski, W., Waegeman, W., Hullermeier, E.: Optimizing the F-measure in multi-label classication: Plug-in rule approach versus structured loss minimization. In: International Conference on Machine Learning (ICML), pp. 1130–1138 (2013)

Real-Time Tracking of Multiple Objects by Linear Motion and Repulsive Motion

Lejun Shen[1]([✉]), Zhisheng You[2], and Qing Liu[1]

[1] Chengdu Sport University, Chengdu, China
sljcool@sina.com
[2] Sichuan University, Chengdu, China

Abstract. Successful multi-object tracking requires consistently maintaining object identities and real-time performance. This task becomes more challenging when objects are indistinguishable from one another. This paper presents a Bayesian framework for maintaining the identities of multiple objects. Our semi-independent joint motion model (SIMM) solves the coalescence and identity switching problem in real time. This joint motion model is a non-parametric mixture model that simultaneously captures linear motion and repulsive motion. Linear motion is a constant velocity model, while repulsive motion is described by a repulsive potential in MRF. By maintaining multimodality from multiple motion models, we can infer the appropriate motion model using image evidence and consequently avoid many identity switching errors. Moreover, we develop a new sampling method that does not suffer from the curse of dimensionality because of the availability of high-quality samples. Experimental results show that our approach can track numerous objects in real time and maintain identities under difficult situations.

1 Introduction

Multi-object tracking is important for many applications, such as video surveillance, robotics, radar-based tracking of aircraft, and sports video analysis. It is a relatively easy task when objects are distinguished from one another. In practical tracking applications, however, some objects are indistinguishable, such as similar looking people in surveillance videos [29], players of the same team in broadcast sport videos [15], and unlabelled measurements in radar tracking [26]. This paper aims to maintain the identities of multiple indistinguishable objects in real time.

The ambiguity caused by indistinguishable objects is one of the main difficulties encountered in multi-object tracking [6]. When objects present nonlinear motion, tracking becomes even more difficult, involving two subproblems: the *coalescence problem* (trackers associate more than one trajectory with some objects while losing track of others) and the *identity switching problem* (two

Electronic supplementary material The online version of this chapter (doi:10. 1007/978-3-319-16817-3_24) contains supplementary material, which is available to authorized users.

© Springer International Publishing Switzerland 2015
D. Cremers et al. (Eds.): ACCV 2014, Part IV, LNCS 9006, pp. 368–383, 2015.
DOI: 10.1007/978-3-319-16817-3_24

intersecting trajectories exchange identities). The coalescence problem can be solved by exclusion constraints: (C1) detection response (measurement) should be assigned to at most one trajectory, or (C2) two objects cannot occupy the same space. Constraint (C1) is known as *data association* [16,17,27]. Constraint (C2) is known as *Markov random field (MRF) motion* [10,30] in image plane or physical exclusion [13] in 3D world space. Once the coalescence problem is resolved, the identity switching problem becomes crucial, as discussed in the following paragraphs.

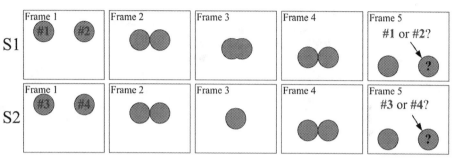

Fig. 1. We assign two identities to the two indistinguishable objects in frame 1. The correct identity of the object indicated by question mark depends on the motion model we *selected*, as shown in Fig. 2.

A linear motion model is commonly used in multi-object tracking, i.e., a constant velocity model or motion affinity using the assumption of linear motion. As shown in [6,20,29], however, the linear motion model is often plagued by nonlinear motion patterns in real scenes. This problem can be shown by a simple example: sequence S1 in Fig. 1, where two indistinguishable objects are marked ♯1 and ♯2 in frame 1. After frames 2, 3, and 4, what is the correct identity of the object indicated by the arrow in frame 5 ? Linear motion indicates that the identity is ♯1 (see H1 in Fig. 2), but the image evidence points to the identity as ♯2 because full occlusion does not occur in frame 3. The absence of full occlusion implies that no intersection happens, making the nonlinear motion model the preferred tool for disambiguating the object identities shown in S1.

The nonlinear motion model is also used in multi-object tracking. The MRF motion model is a typical representative and is often used to describe the repulsive force of objects (hereinafter called *repulsive motion*). It can better explain the directional changes in S1, but repulsive motion also presents the identity switching problem. Consider sequence S2 in Fig. 1. S2 also has 5 consecutive frames showing the continuous motions of two objects marked ♯3 and ♯4 in frame 1. After frames 2, 3, and 4, what is the correct identity of the object indicated by the arrow in frame 5? The repulsive motion model indicates that the correct identity is ♯4. The full occlusion in frame 3 may mean that intersection (H3 in Fig. 2) and departure (H4 in Fig. 2) are equally possible, but H3 can better explain the sequence in accordance with the inertia law of physics. Therefore, the linear motion model is the preferred tool for maintaining the identities of objects presented in S2.

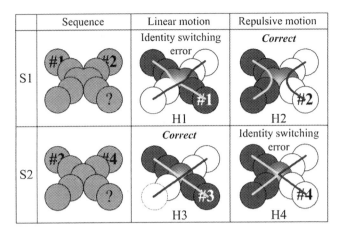

Fig. 2. Tracking results of linear motion and repulsive motion models. Our method can naturally evolve a correct motion model from multiple models (color figure online).

How to select the correct motion model (i.e. repulsive motion model in S1 and linear motion model in S2)? We use a Bayesian framework that adaptively selects an appropriate motion model. We generate multiple hypotheses according to multiple motion models, evaluate the likelihood of these hypotheses giving rise to observed data, maintain the multiple hypotheses, and infer the correct identity using the motion model that is consistently supported by the observed data.

The first contribution of this paper is a semi-independent joint motion model (Sect. 3.1). It is a non-parametric mixture model, which takes into account the repulsive force between objects, as well as their inertial force. This mixed motion model removes the ambiguity caused by indistinguishable objects. Moreover, it maintains multimodality (or multiple hypotheses), thereby evolving an correct motion model and avoiding identity switching errors (Sect. 3.2).

The second contribution of this paper is an efficient sampling method that does not suffer from the curse of dimensionality. The advantage of Monte Carlo simulation is that the accuracy of the Monte Carlo estimator does not depend on the dimensionality of a problem. High accuracy may be achieved with a relatively small number of high-quality samples. We design a tractable importance distribution to generate high-quality samples (Sect. 3.3). Therefore, our method scales well even under difficult situations (e.g. severe occlusion).

2   Related Works

Multi-object tracking methods can be divided into two categories. The first uses only current and past information to estimate the current state [3,4,10,12,17,19, 22,23,25,26,30]. It is well suited for real-time applications, but cannot recover from failure, because data association decisions are based only on past information. These decisions, once made, are fixed and may later be revealed as suboptimal. Maintaining multiple hypotheses can delay data association decision making until enough information has been obtained to derive the optimal solution. The capability of maintaining multiple distributions (p_L and p_R in this paper) is the key difference between our method and others. We use a non-parametric mixture model [25] to facilitating identity maintenance where the standard particle filter fails. Besides, we propose a novel importance distribution to avoid the curse of dimensionality.

The second category of multi-object tracking also uses future information to estimate the current state within a given time window [2,6,13,15,16,21,27–29]. It more effectively overcomes the ambiguities caused by long-time occlusions and false or missed detections. Initialization and termination are fully automatic [24]. The accuracy of object detectors, however, remains far from perfect. Detectors may generate unreliable detection responses if an object is fully or partially occluded by others. These detection errors propagate to the tracking (or data association) module and consequently cause identity switching error. For example, the comparison of S1 and S2 shows that the key difference is frame 3 (highlighted in red in Fig. 2). The missed or inaccurate detection response at frame 3 damages this key evidence and introduce identity ambiguity. Tracking-by-detection approaches suffers from this ambiguity. To avoid this problem, we use image patch, instead of detection response in the observation model, because image-patch based observation model capture the difference between S1 and S2.

The nonlinear motion model has been used in multi-object tracking applications, such as social behavior of people (path planning [20], moving groups [3], game context features [15]) and knowledge about scenes (motion patterns [29], entry/exit points [27]). By contrast, MRF motion model does not require the knowledge of scenes or targets. Khan et al. [10] modeled the interaction between objects by MRF motion model, and Yu et al. [30] proposed a set of collaborative trackers to solve the coalescence problem. Lanz [12] proposed a hybrid joint-separable filter, which is similar to our approach. Qu et al. [23] proposed a distributed architecture. Khan et al. demonstrated the failure mode of MRF motion when basic assumption (C2) is violated. High-order motion models can avoid this failure [23]. In Sect. 3.2, we discuss why (C2) causes failure and how to improve it using our SIMM approach.

Data association is naturally a discrete problem and trajectory estimation is a continuous problem [2]. The inference in discrete-continuous (hybrid) model is NP-hard [14]. The MRF motion model is described in a continuous state space and its repulsive potential is also a continuous function [10,30]. This continuous nature makes designing a tractable importance distribution possible. Our importance distribution Q^{simm} drastically reduces computational effort (Sect. 3.3).

Khan et al. [9] use multiple nearly independent trackers (a real-time version of [10]). Hess et al. [7] devised a pseudo-independent log-linear filter. They used previous states $\hat{x}_{t-1}$ of other objects to compute interaction features between objects. This simplification requires less computation but leads to identity switching error when severe occlusion presents because of the sample impoverishment. Our importance distribution Q^{simm} generate high-quality samples and consequently avoid sample impoverishment.

The mixture of multiple motion models is not a new idea. Isard et al. used a manual transition matrix in mixed-state CONDENSATION [8]. Yu et al. used a binary performance indicator to switch between motion models [31]. Oh et al. used a semi-Markov transition matrix learned from data [18]. Kwon et al. decomposed the motion of an object into two kinds of motions [11]. We do not manually set a transition matrix [8], nor empirically set a threshold of performance indicator [31], nor learn model parameters from data [6,7,15,18,20]. Our model parameters (m_0 and m_1) are fixed all the time. The particle sets can naturally evolve a correct motion model from multiple motion models according to image evidence.

3   Semi-Independent Multi-object Tracking

3.1   Problem Formulation

Multi-object tracking can be formalized as a sequential Bayesian estimation problem. We denote the state of the ith object at time t by $x_{i,t}$, the joint state by $X_t = \{x_{1,t}, x_{2,t}, ..., x_{M,t}\}$, the local observation of $x_{i,t}$ by $y_{i,t}$, and the joint observation by $Y_t = \{y_{1,t}, y_{2,t}, ..., y_{M,t}\}$, with M number of objects.

For computational efficiency, we assume that joint observation model $p(Y_t|X_t)$ can be factorized with respect to each individual object.

$$p(Y_t|X_t) = \prod_i p(y_{i,t}|x_{i,t}) \tag{1}$$

To maintain multiple distributions of multiple motion models, we formulate joint motion model $p(X_t|X_{t-1})$ as a mixture model, i.e.,

$$p(X_t|X_{t-1}) = \left(m_0 + m_1 c_G \prod_{j>i} \varphi(x_{i,t}, x_{j,t}) \right) \prod_i p(x_{i,t}|x_{i,t-1}) \tag{2}$$

where m_0 and m_1 are the mixture weights with $m_0 + m_1 = 1$. c_G is a normalization factor. $p(x_{i,t}|x_{i,t-1})$ is a constant velocity model. $\varphi(x_{i,t}, x_{j,t})$ denotes the repulsive potential that solves the coalescence problem. With the use of different parameter values, the motions of multiple objects may be completely independent ($m_0 = 1$, $m_1 = 0$), dependent ($m_0 = 0$, $m_1 = 1$) [10,30], or *semi-independent* ($m_0 = m_1 = 0.5$ in this paper). The intuition behind this model is that a target $x_{i,t}$ behaves in accordance not only with its own past state $x_{i,t-1}$ with weight m_0, but also with the behaviors of other targets $x_{j,t}$ with weight m_1.

This semi-independent joint motion model is the key novelty of this paper. The component ($m_0 + m_1 c_G \prod_{j>i} \varphi(x_{i,t}, x_{j,t})$) is designed to disambiguating object identities (Sect. 3.2). The component $\prod_i p(x_{i,t}|x_{i,t-1})$ outside the bracket is the key to real-time performance and scalability (Sect. 3.3). After using the assumption [12] that the joint distributions are approximated via the outer product of their marginal components $p(X_{t-1}|Y_{t-1}) = \prod_i p(x_{i,t-1}|Y_{t-1})$, Eqs. (1) and (2) lead to an multi-object tracking framework as follows.

Prediction:

$$p(x_{i,t}|Y_{t-1}) = \int p(x_{i,t}|x_{i,t-1})p(x_{i,t-1}|Y_{t-1})dx_{i,t-1} \qquad (3)$$

where $p(x_{i,t}|x_{i,t-1})$ is a constant velocity model.

Updating:

$$p_L(x_{i,t}|y_{i,t}) = c_i p(y_{i,t}|x_{i,t})p(x_{i,t}|Y_{t-1}) \qquad (4)$$

where c_i represents normalization factors and p_L denotes the posterior of linear motion.

Joint updating:

$$p_{MRF}(X_t|Y_t) = c_G \prod_{j>i} \varphi(x_{i,t}, x_{j,t}) \prod_i p_L(x_{i,t}|y_{i,t}) \qquad (5)$$

where p_{MRF} denotes the joint distribution of MRF.

Marginalization:

$$p_R(x_{i,t}|Y_t) = \int p_{MRF}(X_t|Y_t)dx_{\neg i,t} \qquad (6)$$

where $x_{\neg i,t}$ represents vector X_t with the ith component removed and p_R denotes the posterior of repulsive motion.

Mixture of distributions:

$$p(x_{i,t}|Y_t) = m_0 p_L(x_{i,t}|y_{i,t}) + m_1 p_R(x_{i,t}|Y_t) \qquad (7)$$

Please see our supplementary material (*.pdf) for complete mathematical derivations.

3.2   Mixture Model

We discuss how posterior distributions p_L and p_R collaboratively maintain object identities.

Likelihood ambiguity occurs if multiple interacting objects are identical in appearance (e.g., the tennis balls in Fig. 3). The observation model is useless in inferring the object identities. This ambiguity causes multiple modes in distribution $p_L(x_2)$ at t = 70 and consequently leads to the coalescence problem. By contrast, $p_R(x_2)$ has a single peak from t = 56 to t = 80 even when $p_L(x_2)$ has multiple modes. Therefore, *repulsive potential $\varphi(\cdot)$ eliminates the likelihood ambiguity that originates from the observation model.* As a result, x_2 maintains the correct identity throughout the interaction. Note that *no* complete occlusion occurs in S1 and the nearest distance between two true trajectories is 4 pixels (overlap ratio 74.8 %) at t = 67.

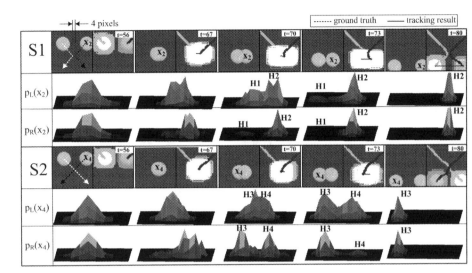

Fig. 3. The source image and tracking result of S1 are shown in the 1st row. The posterior of linear motion p_L and repulsive motion p_R are shown in the 2nd and 3rd row. Please see the text and our supplementary material for more details.

Identity ambiguity occurs if assumption (C2) is violated [10]. *Complete occlusion leads to the identity ambiguity* in S2, subsequently causing the multimodality of $p_R(x_4)$ at $t = 70$ (Fig. 3). In other words, two hypotheses exist: x_4 is associated with left-hand side peak H3 and right-hand side peak H4. This multimodality is maintained from $t = 67$ to $t = 78$ by mixture model (2). Finally, H3 is consistently supported by the observations in this time interval. Meanwhile, H4 is pruned away by $\varphi(\cdot)$. As a result, x_4 derives the correct identity at $t = 78$. By contrast, the traditional MRF motion model votes only H4, resulting in identity switching error. In this situation, *linear motion helps solve the identity ambiguity that stems from MRF motion.*

In summary, both linear motion and repulsive motion are indispensable to identity maintenance. Maintaining multimodality delays data association decision making until enough observations are collected.

3.3 Monte Carlo Implementation

We present a novel Monte Carlo implementation of the tracking framework in Sect. 3.1.

Curse of dimensionality. Computer vision systems are confronted with demands to track numerous objects in dense scenarios. In Eq. (5), the dimension of joint state X_t is high. Exploring a high-dimensional joint state space is generally computationally intensive. Fortunately, high-dimensional problems can be efficiently solved by Monte Carlo simulation if high-quality samples are available. The factorization property of Eq. (1) and the continuous nature of $\varphi(\cdot)$

enable the convenient use of importance sampling. In particle filter literature, the optimal importance distribution is $Q^{opt}(X_t|Y_t, X_{t-1})$. Transition prior (or joint proposal distribution in [10])

$$Q^{transition-prior} = \prod_i \int p(x_{i,t}|x_{i,t-1})p(x_{i,t-1}|Y_{t-1})dx_{i,t-1} \qquad (8)$$

is inefficient. We propose a novel importance distribution

$$Q^{simm} = \prod_i p_L = \prod_i p(y_{i,t}|x_{i,t}) \int p(x_{i,t}|x_{i,t-1})p(x_{i,t-1}|Y_{t-1})dx_{i,t-1} \qquad (9)$$

to approximate optimal importance distribution Q^{opt}. Q^{simm} provides us high-quality joint state samples because it incorporates current observations $y_{i,t}$.

Suppose that $p(x_{i,t-1}|Y_{t-1})$ at the previous time step is approximated by a set of N weighted particles:

$$p(x_{i,t-1}|Y_{t-1}) \approx \left\{ x_{i,t-1}^n, \pi_{i,t-1}^n \right\}_{n=1}^N \qquad (10)$$

where N is the number of particles, n is the index of samples, and $\pi_{i,t-1}^n$ is the weight of the nth particle.

Prediction. The prediction is generated by a proposal density that incorporates current detection responses D_t and transition prior $p(x_{i,t}|x_{i,t-1})$ [19].

$$q_i = (1 - \lambda)p(x_{i,t}|x_{i,t-1}) + \lambda g(x_{i,t}, D_t) \qquad (11)$$

where $p(x_{i,t}|x_{i,t-1})$ is a constant velocity model, $g(x_{i,t}, D_t) \sim N(x_{i,t} - D_t; \sigma^2)$ denotes the normal distribution evaluated for the distance between D_t and $x_{i,t}$. q_i improves tracker robustness and reduces model drift. A lower value of λ implies a suppression of false positive detection.

Updating. We derive the posterior of linear motion according to observation model $p(y_{i,t}|x_{i,t})$:

$$p_L(x_{i,t}|y_{i,t}) \approx \left\{ x_{i,t}^n, L_{i,t}^n = p(y_{i,t}|x_{i,t}^n) \right\}_{n=1}^N \qquad (12)$$

where $L_{i,t}^n$ is the linear motion weight of the nth particle.

Joint updating. We draw K un-weighted samples

$$p_L(x_{i,t}|y_{i,t}) \approx \left\{ x_{i,t}^{k*}, B_k(i) \right\}_{k=1}^K \qquad (13)$$

by resampling from Eq. (12) for $i = 1, ..., M$. $B_k(i)$ refers to the index of the particle in (12) at the kth sampling [22]. Storing the index of its parent is unnecessary in the standard particle filter, but it is useful in later procedures. We approximate Q^{simm} by combining M independent un-weighted samples to one joint state sample:

$$Q^{simm} \approx \left\{ X_t^{k*}, B_k \right\}_{k=1}^K \qquad (14)$$

where $X_t^{k*} = \left(x_{1,t}^{k*}, ..., x_{M,t}^{k*}\right)$, $B_k = (B_k(1), ..., B_k(M))$, and K is the number of joint state samples. Then, $p(X_t|Y_t)$ is approximated by

$$p_{MRF}(X_t|Y_t) \approx \left\{ X_t^{k*}, B_k, w_t^k = \prod_{j>i} \varphi(x_{i,t}^{k*}, x_{j,t}^{k*}) \right\}_{k=1}^{K} \tag{15}$$

where w_t^k is the weight of the kth joint state sample and the repulsive potential function is defined as

$$\varphi(x_i, x_j) = \exp\left(-\alpha \times \left(\frac{overlap(x_i, x_j)^2}{area(x_i)area(x_j)}\right)^2\right) \tag{16}$$

where $overlap(x_i, x_j)$ is the number of pixels that overlap between x_i and x_j , and $area(x_i)$ is the number of pixels of x_i. Note that (16) is currently implemented in the image-plane, but it can be easily used in 2D-ground-plane, 3D-world-space or pose-space after replacing (16) with a new function.

In visual tracking, the most computationally expensive operation is likelihood evaluation (12). The computational cost of resampling (13) is much lower than likelihood evaluation (12). For example, the computational time is 0.15 ms per sample in Eq. (12) and 0.004 ms per sample in Eq. (13). To generate 4000 joint state samples, traditional importance sampling needs 600 ms (=4000*0.15). Our joint updating needs only 46 ms (=200*0.15+4000*0.004) if K = 200. Moreover, the resampling preserves the support of distribution, and therefore avoids sample impoverishment.

Marginalization. An advantage of Monte Carlo simulation is that some computations are particularly easy. Marginalization is a good example. We can obtain marginal samples x^i by sampling (x^i, u^i) from augmented distribution $p(x, u)$, and disregard the u^i component [1]. In Eq. (6), $x_{\neg i,t}$ is an auxiliary variable. Given (15), $P_R(x_{i,t}|Y_t)$ can be easily obtained by ignoring $x_{\neg i,t}$

$$p_R(x_{i,t}|Y_t) \approx \left\{ x_{i,t}^{k*}, B_k(i), w_t^k \right\}_{k=1}^{K} \tag{17}$$

Mixture of distributions. The posterior of linear motion (12) and repulsive motion (17) cannot be directly mixed because N, the number of particles, is not equal to K, the number of joint state samples. We accumulate and normalize the weights according to $B_k(i)$:

$$p_R(x_{i,t}|Y_t) \approx \left\{ x_{i,t}^n, R_{i,t}^n = \sum_{B_k(i)=n} w_t^k \bigg/ \sum_{k=1}^{K} w_t^k \right\}_{n=1}^{N} \tag{18}$$

where $R_{i,t}^n$ is the repulsive motion weight of the nth particle.

Equation (18) is a normalized histogram representation of Eq. (17). Once histogram (18) has been computed, dataset (17) can be discarded, which can be advantageous if $K >> N$. Second, the transfer from Eqs. (17) to (18) does not change the expectation of Monte Carlo estimation. Third, computing mixture model (7) is easy.

$$p(x_{i,t}|Y_t) \approx \left\{ x_{i,t}^n, \pi_{i,t}^n = m_0 \times L_{i,t}^n + m_1 \times R_{i,t}^n \right\}_{n=1}^N \qquad (19)$$

Note that Eqs. (9), (14), (15), (18), (19) are new ideas of this paper. Normalization (c_i and c_G) is very important in our algorithm, which help us to improve the inference of data association decision-making. We explicitly implemented them (line 19 and 20 in Algorithm 1).

Algorithm 1. semi-independent joint motion model (SIMM) particle filter

---

1: Input: $\left\{ x_{i,t-1}^n, \pi_{i,t-1}^n \right\}_{n=1}^N$
2: **for** $i = 1$ to M **do**
3:    Resample $\{x_{i,t-1}^n\}_{n=1}^N$ from $\left\{ x_{i,t-1}^n, \pi_{i,t-1}^n \right\}_{n=1}^N$
4:    Sample $\{x_{i,t}^n\}_{n=1}^N$ from q_i, by Eq. (11)
5:    $L_{i,t}^n = p(y_{i,t}|x_{i,t}^n),\ for\ n = 1, ..., N$, by Eq. (12)
6:    $R_{i,t}^n = 0,\ for\ n = 1, ..., N$
7: **end for**
8: **for** $k = 1$ to K **do**
9:    $w = 1.0$
10:   Sample index $B(i)$ from the discrete distribution given by $\left\{ x_{i,t}^n, L_{i,t}^n \right\}_{n=1}^N,\ for\ i = 1, ..., M$, by Eq. (9) or (14)
11:   **for** $i = 1$ to M **do**
12:      **for** $j = i + 1$ to M **do**
13:         $w = w \times \varphi(x_{i,t}^{B(i)}, x_{j,t}^{B(j)})$, by Eq. (15)
14:      **end for**
15:   **end for**
16:   $R_{i,t}^{B(i)} = R_{i,t}^{B(i)} + w,\ for\ i = 1, ..., M$, by Eq. (18)
17: **end for**
18: **for** $i = 1$ to M **do**
19:   Normalize weights $L_{i,t}^n,\ for\ n = 1, ..., N$
20:   Normalize weights $R_{i,t}^n,\ for\ n = 1, ..., N$
21:   $\pi_{i,t}^n = m_0 \times L_{i,t}^n + m_1 \times R_{i,t}^n,\ for\ n = 1, ..., N$, by Eq. (19)
22: **end for**

---

4 Experiments

We evaluate our approach on six sequences: four synthetic video sequences (S1, S2, S3, and S4) and two public video sequences (PETS2009 S2L1 and UBC Hockey). We compare our method with one data association method (MC-JPDAF [26]) and four MRF motion methods: MCMC-based particle filter (MCMC) [10], Mean Field Monte Carlo (MFMC) [30], Distributed Multiple Object Tracking (DMOT) [23] and Psuedo-Independent Log-Linear Filters (PILLFs) [7]).

Experimental setup. We use 6000 particles, propagate 10 samples to the next time step, and discard 25 % to burn-in in MCMC; $N = 400$ and 5 iterations are run in MFMC; $N = 400$ and 6 iterations are run in DMOT. We use $K = 4000$, $N = 400$ and $\lambda = 0.05$ in our method.

The observation model of MC-JPDAF is the distance between the particle and the associated detection using Gaussian distribution. MCMC, MFMC, DMOT, and our method use the same observation model, where $p(y_{i,t}|x_{i,t})$ is the Bhattacharyya distance between HSV color histograms, and the same potential (16) with $\alpha = 16$.

In PILLFs, we use a constant velocity model and use two feature functions. The appearance feature f_1 is the Bhattacharyya distance between HSV color histograms and the interaction feature f_2 is (16). For fair comparisons, we do not use the error-driven discriminative training in [7]. Hence, the feature weights are fixed and equal $w_1 = w_2 = 0.5$.

In the PETS2009 dataset, we use a publicly available pedestrian detector [5]. In the UBC Hockey sequence, the detector is taken from [19]. In the synthetic sequences, the tracker is manually initialized in the first frame and an image background subtraction is used to detect BLOB-like objects.

4.1   Identity Switching Error

Identity switching is one of many important metrics in multi-object tracking [27]. This metric quantitatively evaluates the intrinsic ability of a tracking algorithm. It can be easily recognized if the "ID of target" does not equal the "ID of tracker" in Fig. 4.

Severe occlusion (S3). The most serious occlusion of 9 objects is that they merge into a single measurement (Fig. 4). This sequence challenges many existing methods, because 8 objects are fully occluded at t = 53. MC-JPDAF has no identity switching error bacause objects move with the linear motions. MCMC, MFMC, and DMOT fail because their basic assumption (C2) is violated. PILLFs fail because it uses previous states $\hat{x}_{t-1}$ to compute interaction features, not all the particles.

As shown in Table 1, MCMC, MFMC, DMOT and PILLFs all effectively work for S1, which fits their basic assumption (C2). MC-JPDAF effectively works for S2 and S3, which fit the linear motion assumption that underlies this algorithm. Table 1 shows that our tracking framework produces better results than Linear model (MC-JPDAF), MRF model (MFMC, MCMC, DMOT) and Log-Linear model (PILLFs), because our motion model (2) is less dependent on a single assumption than are the other models.

VAR1 is a variant of our method with $\lambda = 0.2$. The high value of λ makes it suffers from the unreliable detection responses. VAR2 is a variant of our method with $m_0 = 0$, which blocks the contribution of linear motion model and suffers from identity switching problem in S2.

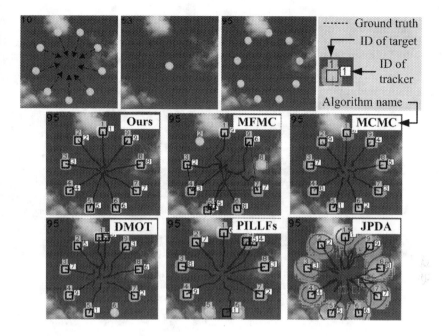

Fig. 4. Source images and tracking results for S3 (severe occlusion). Refer to text and supplementary material for more details.

Table 1. Counting of identity switching errors on 4 sequences.

Method	Sequences			
	S1	S2	S3	PETS2009 S2L1
MFMC [30]	0	1	>1	>1
MCMC [10]	0	1	>1	>1
MC-JPDAF [26]	1	0	0	>1
DMOT [23]	0	1	>1	>1
PILLFs [7]	0	1	>1	>1
Andriyenko et al. [2]	-	-	-	10
Yang et al. [29]	-	-	-	0
Segal et al. [24]	-	-	-	4
VAR1 ($\lambda = 0.2$)	1	0	>1	0
VAR2 ($m_0 = 0$)	0	1	>1	>1
Ours ($\lambda = 0.05$, $m_0 = 0.5$)	0	0	0	0

S2L2 sequence from PETS2009. It has 795 frames with a resolution of 768×576 and contains various occlusions, such as a long-time partial occlusion (t = 36 to 368, ID = 4,5), abrupt changes in direction (or repulsive motion) (e.g., t = 21 to 44, ID = 3), linear motion (e.g., t = 77 to 134, ID = 3), full occlusion

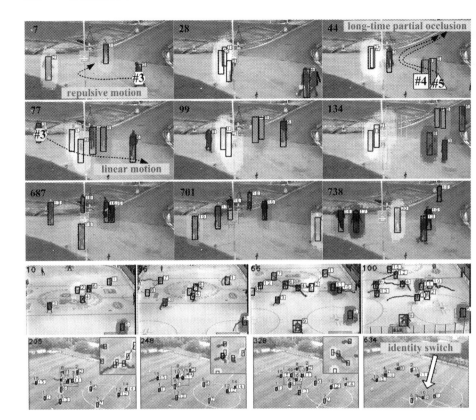

Fig. 5. Tracking results for PETS2009 S2L1 (1st, 2nd and 3rd rows), hockey [19] (4th row), and soccer game (5th row) sequences. Identity switching error is indicated by arrows. Refer to text and supplementary material for more details.

between objects, and occlusion with a road sign. We use $\lambda = 0.05$ to avoid model drift. The higher λ (VAR1) works well because objects are distinguishable.

In the soccer game sequence (Fig. 5), severe occlusion presents from t = 233 to 300 between two identical players. Our method has identity switching errors, which will be discussed in the Sect. 5.

4.2   Computation Speed

All the experiments are implemented in C++ and run on an Intel Core2 Duo 1.66 GHz PC.

Severe occlusion (S3). In Table 2, R is the quotient of Max. divided by Min. The large value of R indicates poor scalability. The minimal computation time of MC-JPDAF occurs at frame 10 with 512 data association hypotheses. The maximal computation time occurs at frame 54 with 17,572,114 hypotheses, because the gating procedure is disabled. Thus, MC-JPDAF suffers from the curse of

Table 2. Minimal, maximal, and average computation time (millisecond per frame) in S3 with R = Max./Min.

Method	Min.	Max.	Avg.	R
MFMC [30]	5.6	7910.5	2506.7	1412.5
MCMC [10]	49.5	62.8	53.1	1.2
MC-JPDAF [26]	1.7	2878.6	168.8	1693.3
DMOT [23]	5.6	25.3	9.5	4.5
PILLFs [7]	6.8	15.2	7.8	2.2
Ours	7.0	22.1	10.5	3.2

dimensionality. Moreover, the computational time of MFMC is high, because MFMC uses message passing and the MRF is a fully connected graph at frame 53 in S3. DMOT and FILLPs scales well.

Long-time random sequence (S4). A total of $M = 36$ objects (20×20 pixels) randomly walk in this video. It is a challenge because the dimension of the joint state is very high. Many complex interactions occur, including nonlinear motion before/within/after occlusion, and long-time occlusion. Our method ($N = 300$, $K = 4000$) can track 36 objects at 8.6 fps.

In our method, K is an empirically small constant and fixed all the time. Thus, our method scales well as the state space dimension M increases. Given the detector output, the speed of our method is 12 fps for PETS2009 S2L1 and 18.2 fps for UBC Hockey. Our executable program can be found in the supplementary material.

5 Conclusion

We have described and demonstrated a scalable real-time tracking framework for maintaining the identities of multiple indistinguishable objects. The motion model that is consistently supported by the observed data facilitates the inference of the correct object identities. Repulsive motion eliminates the ambiguity from observation models, but exhibits identity switching problems when complete occlusion occurs. Linear motion helps solve this problem. We use a mixture model to simultaneously capture these two motions and maintain multimodality. The proposed joint motion model is less dependent on a single assumption than are the other methods. Moreover, the factorization property and continuous nature of MRF motion enables the design of a tractable importance distribution, which generates high-quality samples and ensures the scalability of the algorithm.

The limitation of our method is that the identity ambiguity, caused by both complete and long-term occlusion between indistinguishable objects, cannot be reliably resolved because neither the observation model nor the motion model can provide sufficient evidence for inferring identities (Fig. 5).

Acknowledgments. This work was supported by National Natural Science Foundation of China (61001195) and Technology Research and Development Program of Sichuan Province of China (2010JY0078). We would like to thank anonymous reviewers of this paper for helpful comments.

References

1. Andrieu, C., De Freitas, N., Doucet, A., Jordan, M.: An introduction to MCMC for machine learning. Mach. Learn. **50**, 5–43 (2003)
2. Andriyenko, A., Schindler, K., Roth, S.: The Discrete-continuous optimization for multi-target tracking. In: Computer Vision and Pattern Recognition (2012)
3. Bazzani, L., Cristani, M., Murino, V.: Decentralized particle filter for joint individual-group tracking. In: Computer Vision and Pattern Recognition (2012)
4. Breitenstein, M.D., Reichlin, F., Leibe, B., Koller-Meier, E., Van Gool, L.: Online multiperson tracking-by-detection from a single, uncalibrated camera. IEEE Trans. Pattern Anal. Mach. Intell. **33**, 1820–1833 (2011)
5. Dalal, N., Triggs, B.: Histograms of oriented gradients for human detection. In: Computer Vision and Pattern Recognition (2005)
6. Dicle, C., Camps, O.I., Sznaier, M.: The way they move: tracking multiple targets with similar appearance. In: International Conference on Computer Vision (2013)
7. Hess, R., Fern, A.: Discriminatively trained particle filters for complex multi-object tracking. In: Computer Vision and Pattern Recognition (2009)
8. Isard, M., Blake, A.: A mixed-state condensation tracker with automatic model-switching. In: International Conference on Computer Vision (1998)
9. Khan, Z., Balch, T., Dellaert, F.: Efficient particle filter-based tracking of multiple interacting targets using an MRF-based motion model. In: International Conference on Intelligent Robots and Systems (2003)
10. Khan, Z., Balch, T., Dellaert, F.: MCMC-based particle filtering for tracking a variable number of interacting targets. IEEE Trans. Pattern Anal. Mach. Intell. **27**, 1805–1819 (2005)
11. Kwon, J., Lee, K.M.: Visual tracking decomposition. In: Computer Vision and Pattern Recognition (2010)
12. Lanz, O.: Approximate bayesian multibody tracking. IEEE Trans. Pattern Anal. Mach. Intell. **28**, 1436–1449 (2006)
13. Leibe, B., Schindler, K., Cornelis, N., Van Gool, L.: Coupled object detection and tracking from static cameras and moving vehicles. IEEE Trans. Pattern Anal. Mach. Intell. **30**, 1683–1698 (2008)
14. Lerner, U., Parr, R.: Inference in hybrid networks: Theoretical limits and practical algorithms. In: Proceedings of the Seventeenth Conference on Uncertainty in Artificial Intelligence (2001)
15. Liu, J., Carr, P., Collins, R.T., Liu, Y.: Tracking sports players with context-conditioned motion models. In: Computer Vision and Pattern Recognition (2013)
16. Milan, A., Schindler, K., Roth, S.: Detection-and trajectory-level exclusion in multiple object tracking. In: Computer Vision and Pattern Recognition (2013)
17. MacCormick, J., Blake, A.: A probabilistic exclusion principle for tracking multiple objects. Int. J. Comput. Vision **39**, 57–71 (2000)
18. Oh, S., Rehg, J., Balch, T., Dellaert, F.: Learning and inferring motion patterns using parametric segmental switching linear dynamic systems. Int. J. Comput. Vis. **77**, 103–124 (2008)

19. Okuma, K., Taleghani, A., de Freitas, N., Little, J.J., Lowe, D.G.: A boosted particle filter: multitarget detection and tracking. In: Pajdla, T., Matas, J.G. (eds.) ECCV 2004. LNCS, vol. 3021, pp. 28–39. Springer, Heidelberg (2004)
20. Pellegrini, S., Ess, A., Schindler, K., Van Gool, L.: You'll never walk alone: Modeling social behavior for multi-target tracking. In: International Conference on Computer Vision (2009)
21. Perera, A., Srinivas, C., Hoogs, A., Brooksby, G., Hu, W.: Multi-object tracking through simultaneous long occlusions and split-merge conditions. In: Computer Vision and Pattern Recognition (2006)
22. Pitt, M., Shephard, N.: Filtering via simulation: auxiliary particle filters. Int. j. comput. vis. **94**, 590–599 (1999)
23. Qu, W., Schonfeld, D., Mohamed, M.: Real-time distributed multi-object tracking using multiple interactive trackers and a magnetic-inertia potential model. IEEE Trans. Multimedia **9**, 511–519 (2007)
24. Segal, A.V., Reid, I.: Latent data association: bayesian model selection for multitarget tracking. In: International Conference on Computer Vision (2013)
25. Vermaak, J., Doucet, A., Prez, P.: Maintaining multimodality through mixture tracking. In: International Conference on Computer Vision (2003)
26. Vermaak, J., Godsill, S., Perez, P.: Monte carlo filtering for multi target tracking and data association. IEEE Trans. Aerosp. Electron. Syst. **41**, 309–332 (2005)
27. Wu, B., Nevatia, R.: Detection and tracking of multiple, partially occluded humans by bayesian combination of edgelet based part detectors. Int. J. Comput. Vision **75**, 247–266 (2007)
28. Xing, J., Ai, H., Lao, S.: Multi-object tracking through occlusions by local tracklets filtering and global tracklets association with detection responses. In: Computer Vision and Pattern Recognition (2009)
29. Yang, B., Nevatia, R.: Multi-target tracking by online learning of non-linear motion patterns and robust appearance models. In: Computer Vision and Pattern Recognition (2012)
30. Yu, T., Wu, Y.: Collaborative tracking of multiple targets. In: Computer Vision and Pattern Recognition (2004)
31. Yu, T., Wu, Y.: Decentralized multiple target tracking using netted collaborative autonomous trackers. In: Computer Vision and Pattern Recognition (2005)

6-DOF Model Based Tracking via Object Coordinate Regression

Alexander Krull$^{(\boxtimes)}$, Frank Michel, Eric Brachmann, Stefan Gumhold,
Stephan Ihrke, and Carsten Rother

TU Dresden, Dresden, Germany
alexander.krull@tu-dresden.de

Abstract. This work investigates the problem of 6-Degrees-Of-Freedom (6-DOF) object tracking from RGB-D images, where the object is rigid and a 3D model of the object is known. As in many previous works, we utilize a Particle Filter (PF) framework. In order to have a fast tracker, the key aspect is to design a clever proposal distribution which works reliably even with a small number of particles. To achieve this we build on a recently developed state-of-the-art system for single image 6D pose estimation of known 3D objects, using the concept of so-called 3D object coordinates. The idea is to train a random forest that regresses the 3D object coordinates from the RGB-D image. Our key technical contribution is a two-way procedure to integrate the random forest predictions in the proposal distribution generation. This has many practical advantages, in particular better generalization ability with respect to occlusions, changes in lighting and fast-moving objects. We demonstrate experimentally that we exceed state-of-the-art on a given, public dataset. To raise the bar in terms of fast-moving objects and object occlusions, we also create a new dataset, which will be made publicly available.

1 Introduction

In this paper we address the problem of tracking the pose of a previously known rigid object from a RGB-D video stream in real-time. The object pose is typically expressed relative to the camera and has 6-DOF, three for orientation and three for position. A solution to this problem has great impact in many application fields, ranging from augmented reality, human-computer interaction, to robotics. However, given constraints on high precision, real-time, as well as robustness to real world situations, such as occlusions and changes in lighting conditions, this is still an open problem.

Building on the results of multiple decades of research on object tracking, very recently several researchers have re-investigated pose estimation [4,14,21] and tracking approaches [8,16,18] in order to exploit new RGB-D sensor technology and to ensure real-time support through GPU based implementations. For the

---

Electronic supplementary material The online version of this chapter (doi:10. 1007/978-3-319-16817-3_25) contains supplementary material, which is available to authorized users.

© Springer International Publishing Switzerland 2015
D. Cremers et al. (Eds.): ACCV 2014, Part IV, LNCS 9006, pp. 384–399, 2015.
DOI: 10.1007/978-3-319-16817-3_25

tracking problem the PF framework [12] has become a preferred choice as it can model multi-modal probability densities that are essential for successful tracking of objects with occlusions.

As described in more detail in Sect. 3.2 the PF framework incrementally traces the posterior probability density of the 6D pose through a set of samples from the 6D Euclidean Group SE(3)[1]. Key ingredients to the PF are a model for the relative motion of the object over time, as well as an observation model for the image formation process. In single image pose estimation approaches, like [4], solely the observation model is used. An important difficulty in the application of the PF framework to 6D pose tracking is the high dimensionality of the state space, as each particle represents a 6D pose estimate. This either demands for a huge number of particles prohibiting real-time systems or for an importance sampling approach (compare [10]) based on a proposal distribution that effectively approximates the posterior probability distribution. Any pose estimation approach can be used to implement a proposal distribution as shown by Stückler et al. in [24], where a multi-resolution surfel representation of the tracked object was utilized.

In this work we demonstrate the combination of the PF framework with the recently developed concept of object coordinate regression which has achieved state of the art results for one shot estimation of camera pose [22] or object pose [4]. The object coordinate regression framework is detailed in Sect. 3.1. It exploits random forests to automatically learn optimal features from RGB-D training images. Brachmann et al. [4] have shown that such learning based approaches can efficiently deal with changes in illumination and with partial occlusions. Given this distinction between a training and test phase, our system works as follows. Given a potentially large selection of 3D objects, here 4, and 20 in [4], as well as example images of background, we first train a random forest. At test time, we know which object we want to track and use the output of the forest only for this particular object. Note, a straightforward extension, not evaluated in this work, is to jointly do multiple object detection and tracking. In this work, we carefully extend the work [4] to the 6D pose tracking problem. Our main contributions are:

- A new model-based 6D pose tracking framework, based on the concept of predicting 3D object coordinates, which helps to generalize better to real-world settings of fast-moving objects, occlusions and changes in lighting.
- The technically new aspect is a two-way procedure for optimally using the output of the object coordinate regression framework to determine the proposal distribution of the tracker.
- A new, challenging 6D pose tracking data set that will be publicly available.
- A system that exceeds state of the art results on 6D model-based tracking.

2   Related Work

Almost two decades ago the PF has been introduced for 2D visual tracking by Isard and Blake [15]. Based on a statistical observation model and a motion

---

[1] The group of rigid body transformations.

model the PF approximates the posterior distribution of the object's position in a non parametric form, using a set of samples. Ten years later Pupilli et al. [20] adapted the framework to 6-DOF camera tracking using edge features. Shortly later Klein et al. [16] presented an implementation that utilized the GPU for the evaluation of its observation model, which usually is the bottleneck in PF applications. The GPU implementation enabled them to deal with hidden edges while allowing a speedup [16].

The number of necessary particles and therefore the runtime can be reduced by guiding particle sampling with a proposal distribution. Ideally the proposal distribution is very close to the posterior distribution. Furthermore, it needs to exploit both the observation model and the motion model in order to improve over the standard PF as well as over one shot pose estimation. Bray et al. [5] improved hand pose tracking with a proposal distribution, which was defined as the mixture of two distributions both represented as a particle ensemble. The first particle ensemble is constructed in the default manner by applying the motion model to the sampled posterior distribution of the previous frame. The second ensemble is constructed by moving the resulting particles further to local optima and using them as centers of a mixture of normal distributions. Teuliere et al. [26] used a similar approach to edge-based tracking of simple objects from luminance images. Corresponding approaches for 3D pose tracking from RGB-D videos can be found in [7,9,18].

A PF that has to operate on the 6D Euclidean group SE(3) brings some theoretical challenges. The definition of probability distributions and calculation of average rotations is not straight forward. A theoretical analysis of these issues can be found in [6] and [17]. While earlier methods relied on simple random walk motion models, Choi et al. [9] used autoregressive models that assume a more or less constant pose velocity and were thus able to deal with faster motion.

With the availability of RGB-D sensors, the question of the best image features for the observation model has sparked recent research. Stückler et al. [24] use RGB-D images to learn 3D surfel maps of objects and use them in a PF operating on RGB-D. Choi et al. [8] present in their recent work a highly optimized GPU implementation that uses a traditional mesh representation. Their observation model is based on comparing rendered images and observations using color as well as depth features. Learning of the best features in a random forest has been successfully applied to pose estimation of articulated objects [25], camera pose [22] and object poses [4]. In these approaches a random forest is trained to predict part or object probabilities and in the latter two approaches also coordinates in a reference coordinate system of the background scene or the learned objects. During detection the output of this discriminative model is used as input to an optimization procedure for the 3D-pose with respect to an observation model. Brachmann et al. [4] improve over this basic concept by beneficially incorporating the predicted object probabilities and coordinates into the observation model, which is formulated in form of an energy.

In this work we build a PF tracking framework with the energy based observation model of [4] and carefully design a proposal distribution that intelligently exploits the input RGB-D image as well as the output of the trained discriminative model. In this way we combine the robustness of the discriminative model with respect to changes in illumination and the robustness of the PF framework with respect to occlusions. Furthermore, we use a two-way PF that builds on similar ideas as annealed PF approaches as previously proposed in [16] and [2]. The random forest approach is in spirit similar to boosting based approaches that have been examined in the area of tracking in the works [1,13,19,27]. Finally, our approach also uses GPU rendering features to efficiently evaluate the observation model.

3 Method

Given a stream of RGB-D images of a moving object our goal is to estimate in each frame t the object pose H_t. We assume that a 3D model of the corresponding object is available. We define the pose H_t as the transformation that maps a point from the local coordinate system of the object to the coordinate system of the camera. We cast pose estimation as a tracking problem and solve it with a PF framework. In Sect. 3.1 we introduce a regression forest, that predicts object probabilities and local object coordinates. This output is used in several steps of our approach. Then, we briefly reiterate the basic PF framework (Sect. 3.2). We follow with a description of our motion model (Sect. 3.3) and our definition of particle likelihood (Sect. 3.4). Finally, in Sect. 3.5 we describe how we adapt sampling of particles according to a proposal distribution which concentrates on image areas where high particle likelihood is expected. This is the main component to facilitate efficient and robust pose tracking.

3.1 Discriminative Prediction of Object Probabilities and Object Coordinates from a Single RGB-D Image

In order to assess the likelihood of particles (Sect. 3.4), and to concentrate hypotheses sampling on promising image areas (Sect. 3.5) we utilize a discriminative function. This function takes local image patches as input and estimates the following two outputs for the center pixel of each patch: the probability $p(c)$ of the pixel belonging to object c, and its coordinate $\mathbf{y}_c$ in the object coordinate system. We follow exactly the setup of [4] to achieve this mapping densely for each pixel of the current frame t using decision forests.

Note that we train the forest jointly for multiple objects although, in this work, we consider tracking one pre-specified object c only. During test time, discriminative predictions are only calculated for object c. Other objects, which the forest might know, are not considered. However, the same forest can provide predictions for different objects, so that training has to be done only once. In the following we give a short summary on training and prediction.

Training. We train an ensemble $\mathcal{T}$ of decision trees T^j. Each tree is trained separately using a set of object images as well as neutral background images. Object images are segmented and show object c in different poses. Each pixel within a segmentation mask is furthermore annotated with its object coordinate $\mathbf{y}_c$. Trees operate on simple scale-invariant depth and RGB difference features [22].

During training we select for each node one feature out of a randomly generated pool that maximizes the standard information gain defined on a discrete set of labels. These labels are obtained by separating object c into n_{cell} cells with a 3D grid resulting in n_{cell} discrete labels per object. One additional label is assigned to the background class.

We do not restrict tree depth but stop growing when less than a minimum number of pixels arrive at a node. At each leaf l^j we approximate the object probability $p(c|l^j)$ by the fraction of pixels at that leaf that belong to object c. The estimate of the object coordinate $\mathbf{y}_{c,l^j}$ is found by running mean-shift on all pixels of object c in leaf l^j and taking the largest mode.

Prediction. Each pixel of an input image is run through each tree in $\mathcal{T}$ and arrives at leafs $(l^1, \ldots, l^{|\mathcal{T}|})$. This results in a list of object probabilities $(p(c|l^1), \ldots, p(c|l^{|\mathcal{T}|}))$ and object coordinates $(\mathbf{y}_{c,l^1}, \ldots, \mathbf{y}_{c,l^{|\mathcal{T}|}})$ for each object c. The object probabilities of all trees are combined with Bayes rule over all known objects and the background class to obtain the final $p(c)$ for each pixel [4].

3.2 PF for 3D Pose Tracking

A PF approximates the current posterior distribution $p(H_t|Z_{1:t})$ of the pose H_t at time t given all previous observations $Z_{1:t}$. In each time step t the posterior distribution is represented by a set of samples $S_t = \{H_t^1, \ldots, H_t^N\}$, which are referred to as particles. Each particle has two velocity vectors $\mathbf{v}_t$ and $\mathbf{e}_t$ attached. They correspond to the previous translational and rotational motion respectively.

The PF requires an observation model and a motion model. The former describing the likelihood $p(Z_{t+1}|H_{t+1})$ of an observation given a pose. The latter describing the probability $p(H_{t+1}|H_t, \mathbf{v}_t, \mathbf{e}_t)$ of a pose given the previous pose H_t as well as the last velocity vectors. With each new frame $t+1$ a new set of particles S_{t+1} is found in three steps:

1. **Sampling:** For each particle H_t^i an intermediate particle $\hat{H}_{t+1}^i$ is sampled according to the motion model $p(\hat{H}_{t+1}^i|H_t^i, \mathbf{v}_t^i, \mathbf{e}_t^i)$. New velocities $\mathbf{v}_{t+1}^i$ and $\mathbf{e}_{t+1}^i$ are calculated (see supplemental note for details) using H_t^i and $\hat{H}_{t+1}^i$.
2. **Weighting:** Each intermediate particle is assigned a weight π_{t+1}^i, which is proportional to the likelihood $p(Z_{t+1}|\hat{H}_{t+1}^i)$ of the observed data given the pose $\hat{H}_{t+1}$.
3. **Resampling:** Finally, the set $S_{t+1} = \{H_{t+1}^1, \ldots, H_{t+1}^N\}$ of unweighted particles (with their attached velocities), is randomly drawn from $\{\hat{H}_{t+1}^1, \ldots, \hat{H}_{t+1}^N\}$ using probabilities proportional to the weights π_{t+1}^i.

The number of particles required to approximate the 6D posterior distribution can be drastically reduced if the sampling is concentrated in areas where one expects the true pose of the object. This is done using a proposal distribution $q(H_{t+1}|H_t, \mathbf{v}_t, \mathbf{e}_t)$ in the sampling step instead of the original motion model. To compensate for the fact that we sample from a different distribution, the calculation of weights has to be adjusted according to Eq. (19) in [10]:

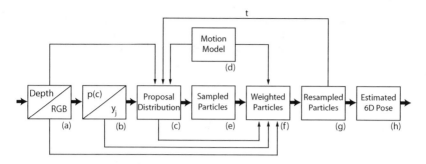

Fig. 1. Our tracking pipeline. For each frame t the RGB-D image(a) is processed by the forest to predict object probabilities and local object coordinates(b). We use the observed depth from the original image, the forest predictions and the particles from the last frame together with our motion model(d) to construct our proposal distribution(c). Particles are sampled(e) according to the proposal distribution, then weighted(f) and resampled(g). Our final pose estimate is calculated as mean of the resampled particles(h).

$$\pi_{t+1}^i \propto p(Z_{t+1}|\hat{H}_{t+1}^i) \frac{p(\hat{H}_{t+1}^i|H_t^i, \mathbf{v}_t^i, \mathbf{e}_t^i)}{q(\hat{H}_{t+1}^i|H_t^i, \mathbf{v}_t^i, \mathbf{e}_t^i)} \tag{1}$$

In the following we describe the specifics of our implementation of the PF framework: the motion model, the observation likelihood, and finally, our main contribution, the construction of our proposal distribution. An overview of our tracking pipeline can be found in Fig. 1.

3.3   Our Motion Model

The motion model describes which movements of the object are plausible between two frames. Generally speaking, we assume our object roughly continues its previous motion, and that an additional random normally distributed translation is applied to our pose together with a random rotation around the center of the object. More specifically we assume the rotation to be around a uniformly chosen random axis and the angle of the rotation to be normally distributed. We will introduce a continuous probability distribution on SE(3) representing such a random motion. It will be reused in the context of our proposal distribution as described in Sect. 3.5.

Let R_t and T_t be the homogeneous 4x4 matrix representations of the rotational and translational component of the pose $H_t = T_t R_t$. We model the change of the pose between two time steps t and $t + 1$ separately for both components: $H_{t+1} = T_{t+1}R_{t+1}$ with $T_{t+1} = \Delta_t^T T_t$, $R_{t+1} = \Delta_t^R R_t$ where Δ_t^T and Δ_t^R are 4x4 translation and rotation matrices, representing the change in the rotational and translational component respectively. Note that Δ_t^R contains the relative rotation around the object center and not the camera center. Translational change is defined as:

$$\Delta_t^T = T(\lambda_T \mathbf{v}_t + \boldsymbol{\omega}_T) \tag{2}$$

The vector $\boldsymbol{\omega}_T$ contains independent zero centered Gaussian noise with σ_T^2 variance. The symbol λ_T stands for a damping parameter. It determines how much the previous translation, described by the velocity vector $\mathbf{v}_t$ is continued. Finally, $T(\mathbf{v})$ shall be the translation matrix corresponding to the translation vector $\mathbf{v}$. The rotational change is defined as:

$$\Delta_t^R = R(\boldsymbol{\omega}_R \theta) R(\lambda_R \mathbf{e}_t) \tag{3}$$

The symbol $\boldsymbol{\omega}_R$ stands for a random unit vector that defines the rotation axis of the random movement. Here θ is a Gaussian distributed zero centered random variable determining the rotation angle[2]. Its variance is σ_R^2. The symbol λ_R stands for a damping parameter. It determines how much the previous rotation, described by the rotational velocity vector $\mathbf{e}_t$ is continued. Finally, $R(\mathbf{e})$ shall stand for the rotation matrix corresponding to the rotation vector[3] $\mathbf{e}$.

Based on the model described above we can calculate the probability density $p(H_{t+1}|H_t, \mathbf{v}_t, \mathbf{e}_t)$ for a transition to pose H_{t+1} given the previous pose H_t. We approximate our motion model using the following density function $f(H_{t+1}; H_t^{pred}, \Sigma^{mm}, \kappa^{mm})$, which is described at the end of this section:

$$p(H_{t+1}|H_t, \mathbf{v}_t, \mathbf{e}_t) \approx f(H_{t+1}; H_t^{pred}, \Sigma^{mm}, \kappa^{mm}) \tag{4}$$

This function describes the probability of an arbitrary pose H_{t+1} with respect to the predicted pose H_t^{pred}, which is found by extrapolating previous motion given by the velocity vectors $\mathbf{v}_t$ and $\mathbf{e}_t$. The probability distribution depends on the variance in the translational component through Σ^{mm} and the variance of the rotational component through κ^{mm}. The diagonal matrix $\Sigma^{mm} = I\sigma_T^2$, the term $\kappa^{mm} = 1/\sigma_R^2$ and

$$H_t^{pred} = T(\lambda_T \mathbf{v}_t) T_t R(\lambda_R \mathbf{e}_t) R_t \tag{5}$$

The density function $f(H; H', \Sigma, \kappa)$ corresponds to the random motion described in Eqs. (2) and (3):

$$f(H; H', \Sigma, \kappa) = f_n(\mathbf{v}^{diff}; \mathbf{0}, \Sigma) f_{vm}(\theta^{diff}; 0, \kappa)\phi(\theta^{diff}) \tag{6}$$

It consists of a zero centered multivariate normal distribution $f_n(\mathbf{v}^{diff}; \mathbf{0}, \Sigma)$ and a zero centered von Mises distribution $f_{vm}(\theta^{diff}; 0, \kappa)$. While the vector $\mathbf{v}^{diff}$ denotes the translational difference between H' and H, the symbol θ^{diff} stands for the angle of the difference rotation. The normal distribution models the translational noise $\boldsymbol{\omega}_T$ introduced in Eq. (2). The von Mises distribution in Eq. (6) is a close approximation for a wrapped normal distribution, it models the Gaussian rotational noise introduced by θ in Eq. 3. Note that the random rotation axis $\boldsymbol{\omega}_R$ of Eq. (3) has no influence on the density, since each rotation axis has equal probability. Also note that an additional factor $\phi(\theta^{diff})$ is necessary

---

[2] Please note, that because of its circular nature, applying rotations with the normally distributed angles θ will result in angles distributed in the interval between 0 and 2π according to a wrapped normal distribution. Such a distribution is difficult to handle and we will use a von Mises distribution as approximation.

[3] Direction and length of a rotation vector correspond to rotation axis and rotation angle, respectively.

to map the 1D density over angles onto the group of rotations SO(3). A more detailed discussion of $\phi(\theta^{diff})$ can be found in the supplemental note.

3.4 Our Observation Likelihood

We use a likelihood formulation based on the energy $E(H)$ from [4]:

$$p(Z_{t+1}|H) \propto \exp(-\alpha E(H)) \tag{7}$$

where α is a control parameter determining how harshly larger energy values should be punished. The energy term is a weighted sum of three components $E^{depth}(H)$, $E^{coord}(H)$ and $E^{obj}(H)$. Detailed equations can be found in [4]. The depth component $E^{depth}(H)$ punishes deviations between the observed and rendered depth images within the object mask. The other two components are concerned with the output of the forest. The coordinate component $E^{coord}(H)$ punishes deviations between each pixels true object coordinates for pose H and the object coordinates predicted by the forest. The object component $E^{obj}(H)$ punishes deviation between the ideal segmentation obtained by rendering and the soft segmentations predicted by the trees in form of $p(c|l^j)$.

In contrast to [4], we use a simple modification of the depth term, that copes better with occlusion. Depth values that lie in front of the object can be explained by occlusion. This is not the case for depth values that lie behind the object. Our modified depth term accounts for this by reducing the threshold of possible punishment for values in front of the object. A detailed description can be found in the supplemental note.

3.5 Our Proposal Distribution

Our proposal distribution allows our method to cope with unexpected motion and occlusion, while maintaining high accuracy. It allows us to approximate the posterior distribution $p(H_t|Z_{1:t})$ more accurately with a small number of particles. The construction of our proposal distribution is described in the following, and subsumed in Fig. 2.

A proposal distribution describes the sampling of a new particle $\hat{H}^i_{t+1}$ on the basis of an old particle H^i_t. We define the proposal distribution $q(H_{t+1}|H_t, \mathbf{v}_t, \mathbf{e}_t)$ for the particle H^i_t as a mixture of two parts (Fig. 2(o)):

$$q(H^i_{t+1}|H^i_t, \mathbf{v}^i_t, \mathbf{e}^i_t) = (1 - \alpha^{prop})f(H^i_{t+1}; H^{i,pred}_t, \Sigma^{prop}, \kappa^{prop})$$
$$+ \alpha^{prop}f(H^i_{t+1}; H^{est}_{t+1}, \Sigma^{prop}, \kappa^{prop}) \tag{8}$$

The mixture is governed by the weight α^{prop}. Both parts reuse the density function defined in Eq. (6) with variance parameters Σ^{prop} and κ^{prop}, which can be found in the supplemental note. The first part of Eq. (8) is centered on $H^{i,pred}_t$ which is the extrapolation of the current particle H^i_t according to our motion model as described in Eq. (5). Hence, $H^{i,pred}_t$ differs for each particle H^i_t. The second part of Eq. (8) is centered on a preliminary estimate H^{est}_{t+1} which is

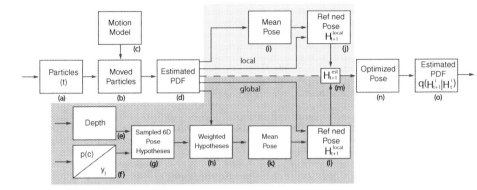

Fig. 2. To construct our proposal distribution we first calculate a continuous representation of the prior distribution for the pose at the current frame (a-d). Next we determine two pose estimates H_{t+1}^{local} (light gray) and H_{t+1}^{global} (dark gray). The local estimate is calculated based on a local search on propagated solutions via the motion model (i-j). The global estimate is based on the pose sampling scheme from [4] (e-l). We choose the particle with the lower energy and use it as starting point for a final optimization (n). Our final proposal distribution $q(H_{t+1}^i|H_t^i)$ for particle H_t^i is a mixture of two components (o): one centered on H_t^i and one on the newly found particle in (n). This figure represents component (c) of Fig. 1.

found based on the output of our discriminative function (Sect. 3.1). It does not depend on H_t^i, but is shared among all particles.

Regarding H_{t+1}^{est}, we will discuss two different ways to quickly obtain a good estimate: One way finds a local estimate H_{t+1}^{local}, the other way finds a global estimate H_{t+1}^{global}. While a proposal distribution based on a local estimate is sufficient in most cases, it may fail in situations with fast unexpected motion. The global estimate on the other hand depends on the quality of the discriminative prediction and may at times give noisy results. As a consequence, we apply a combination of the two approaches:

$$H_{t+1}^{est} = \mathrm{argmin}_{H \in \mathcal{H}} E'(H); \mathcal{H} = \{H^{local}, H^{global}\} \qquad (9)$$

Note, that this is our main technical contribution. Energy $E'(H)$ will be defined below. The preliminary estimate H_{t+1}^{est} is optimized (Fig. 2(n)) using a general purpose optimizer (details can be found in the supplemental note).

The remainder of this section is concerned with the calculation of H_{t+1}^{local} and H_{t+1}^{global}. First, however, we discuss how we represent prior knowledge used in both estimates.

Prior Knowledge. The proposal distribution should be an estimate of the posterior $p(H_{t+1}|Z_{1:t+1})$. Both of our estimates should thus include not only knowledge taken from the current observation i.e. the likelihood and results from the discriminative function, but also information from the previous particle set i.e. the prior. To include the prior we perform the following preparatory steps. We take the last set of particles $S_t = \{H_t^1, \ldots, H_t^N\}$ and move each particle according to the motion model (Fig. 2(a–c)). The result is an extrapolated set of particles

$\tilde{S}_{t+1} = \{\tilde{H}_{t+1}^1, \ldots, \tilde{H}_{t+1}^N\}$. In order to obtain a continuous representation we reuse the distribution $f(H; H^{center}, \Sigma, \kappa)$ (Eq. (6)). We fit $f(H; H^{center}, \Sigma, \kappa)$ to the set $\tilde{S}_{t+1}$ (Fig. 2(d)). The resulting parameters are $\tilde{H}^{center}, \tilde{\Sigma}, \tilde{\kappa}$. For details on the fitting procedure, please refer to the supplemental note. The distribution $f(H; \tilde{H}^{center}, \tilde{\Sigma}, \tilde{\kappa})$ is a representation of the knowledge we have about the pose at the current time $t + 1$ without considering the current observation Z_{t+1}. It is a representation of the prior.

Local Estimate. To find H_{t+1}^{local}, we use $\tilde{H}^{center}$ (Fig. 2(i)) as starting point for refinement as described in [4] (Fig. 2(j)). This refinement is done by repeatedly finding inlier pixels. Their predicted object coordinates together with the observed depth values enable a rough but quick optimization using Kabsch algorithm. In order to include prior knowledge in the refinement we change the objective function to:

$$E'(H) = \alpha E(H) - \ln f(H; \tilde{H}^{center}, \tilde{\Sigma}, \tilde{\kappa}) \qquad (10)$$

Because of this adjustment of the objective function the resulting H_{t+1}^{local} becomes a local maximum a posteriori (MAP) estimate.

Global Estimate. Calculation of the global estimate H_{t+1}^{global} is based on a sampling scheme similar to the one in [4]. We sample a set of m particles $\tilde{H}^i$ (Fig. 2(e–g)). Details can be found in the supplemental note. Then, the particles $\tilde{H}^i$ are weighted using the distribution $f(H; \tilde{H}^{center}, \tilde{\Sigma}, \tilde{\kappa})$ (Fig. 2(h)). Finally, their weighted mean is calculated (Fig. 2(k)) and used as initialization for the refinement (Fig. 2(l)), again using $E'(H)$ from Eq. (10) as objective function. This yields H_{t+1}^{global}.

4   Experiments

Some RGB-D object tracking datasets have been published in recent years. For example, Fanelli et al. [11] recorded a dataset to track human head poses using a Kinect camera. Song and Xiao [23] used a Kinect camera to record 100 RGB-D video sequences of arbitrary objects but do only provide 2D bounding boxes as ground truth. For our purpose, we found only one relevant dataset from Choi and Christensen [8]. It consists of 3D object models and synthetic test sequences.

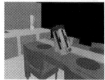
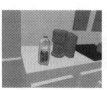
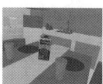
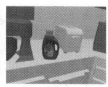

Kinect Box   Milk   Orange Juice   Tide

Fig. 3. Example images of the dataset provided by Choi and Christensen [8].

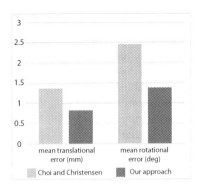

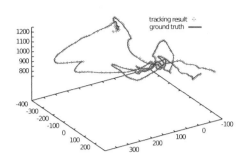

Fig. 4. Averaged translation and rotation RMSE on the dataset of [8].

Fig. 5. Reconstructed motion trajectory (green) for one sequence of our dataset (Cat, sequence 1). Ground truth is depicted blue for comparison (Color figure online).

For further evaluation, we recorded a new more challenging and realistic dataset on which we compared our approach. Additionally, we conduct experiments to demonstrate that our proposal distribution achieves superior results when unexpected object motion occurs.

Dataset of Choi and Christensen [8]. The dataset of Choi and Christensen [8] provides four textured 3D models and four synthetic test sequences (1000 RGB-D frames). To generate the test sequences, each of the four objects was placed in a static texture-less 3D scene and the camera was slowly moved around the object. The authors provide the ground truth camera trajectory which is error-free since it was generated through rendering. Figure 3 shows one image of each sequence.

To gather the training data for our random forest we rendered RGB-D images of each model. We sampled the full view sphere of the model regularly with fixed distance and including in-plane rotation. For the background set we used renderings from multiple 3D scenes from Google warehouse. We trained three decision trees with a maximum feature patch size of 20 pixel meter and $n_{cell} = 125$ discrete labels per object. We trained the trees for all 4 objects jointly. For each testing sequence the object to be tracked is assumed to be known, and predictions are only made for this object. Our PF uses 70 particles. The complete list of parameters is included in the supplemental note.

While testing we follow the evaluation protocol of Choi and Christensen [8] and compute the Root Mean Square Error (RMSE) of the translation parameters X,Y and Z and the rotation parameters Roll, Pitch and Yaw. We average the translational RMSE over three test runs, the coordinates (X,Y and Z), as well as over the four objects to obtain one translational error measure. We do the same for rotational RMSE. We compare to the numbers provided in [8] which also include results for the tracking implementation of the Point Cloud Library (PCL) [3]. We base our comparison on the results in [8] achieved with 12800 particles, for which the lowest error is reported.

Table 1. Comparison of the translation error (X,Y,Z), rotation error (Roll, Pitch, Yaw) and computation time on the synthetic dataset of Choi and Christensen [8] with results from our method, [8] and the PCL.

Objects	Tracker	RMSE						
		X (mm)	Y (mm)	Z (mm)	Roll (deg)	Pitch (deg)	Yaw (deg)	Time (ms)
Kinect box	PCL	43.99	42.51	55.89	7.62	1.87	8.31	4539
	Choi and Christensen	1.84	2.23	1.36	6.41	0.76	6.32	166
	Our	**0.83**	**1.67**	**0.79**	**1.11**	**0.55**	**1.04**	143
Milk	PCL	13.38	31.45	26.09	59.37	19.58	75.03	2205
	Choi and Christensen	0.93	1.94	1.09	3.83	**1.41**	3.26	**134**
	Our	**0.51**	**1.27**	**0.62**	**2.19**	1.44	**1.90**	135
Orange juice	PCL	2.53	2.20	1.91	85.81	42.12	46.37	1637
	Choi and Christensen	0.96	1.44	1.17	1.32	**0.75**	1.39	**117**
	Our	**0.52**	**0.74**	**0.63**	**1.28**	1.08	**1.20**	129
Tide	PCL	1.46	2.25	0.92	5.15	2.13	2.98	2762
	Choi and Christensen	0.83	1.37	1.20	**1.78**	**1.09**	**1.13**	**111**
	Our	**0.69**	**0.81**	**0.81**	2.10	1.38	1.27	116

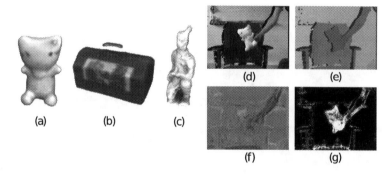

Fig. 6. (a)-(c) Our objects from left to right Cat, Toolbox, Samurai. (d) color frame and (e) depth frame recorded with the commercially available Kinect camera.(f) Probability map and (g) predicted 3D object coordinates from a single tree mapped to the RGB-cube for the object Cat.

Our method results in an average translational RMSE of 0.83 mm compared to 1.36 mm for [8], i.e. we achieve a 38 % lower translational error (PCL: 18.7 mm). For the average rotational RMSE we report 1.38 deg compared to 2.45 deg in [8], which is 43 % lower (PCL: 29.6 deg). We achieve these results while keeping the computation time on our system[4] comparable to the one reported in [8]. Figure 4 depicts the average RMSE over all objects. Detailed results including run-times can be found in Table 1.

Our dataset. The dataset which was provided by [8] is problematic for several reasons: testing sequences are generated synthetically without camera noise, and without occlusion. The objects are placed in a texture-less and static environment.

---

[4] Intel Core i7-3820 CPU @ 3.6GHz with a Nvidia GTX 550 TI GPU.

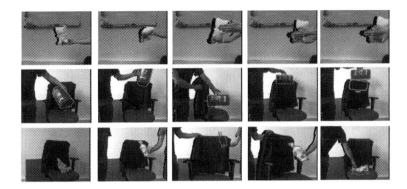

Fig. 7. Example images from our dataset. Blue object silhouettes depict ground truth and green silhouettes depict the estimated poses. The first four columns show correctly estimated poses and the last column missed poses (Color figure online).

In a static scene, a tracking method can in theory use the entire image to estimate the motion of the camera instead of estimating the motion of the object. Furthermore, the camera is moved around the object. The statistics of object motion when the camera is moved are very different from a situation where the camera is static and the object is moved. E.g., a complete vertical flip of the object is unlikely in the first scenario.

Table 2. Accuracy measured on our dataset. Comparison of our full proposal distribution to the local proposal distribution and to [4]. Evaluation is done based on all frames and on every third frame of the image sequences.

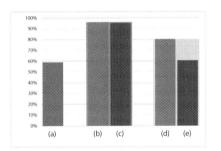

Fig. 8. Average accuracy over all sequences for (a) [4]. Our full proposal distribution using (b) all frames and (d) every third frame of the sequence. Our local proposal distribution using (c) all frames (e) every third frame of the sequence.

Objects	Sequence	Ratio of frames used	Method		Brachmann et al.
			Our Approach		
			full proposal distribution	local proposal distribution	
			Accuracy	Accuracy	Accuracy
Cat	1	100%	100%	89%	66.8%
		33%	91.5%	90.4%	
	2	100%	99.4%	100%	44.2%
		33%	94.9%	87.8%	
Samurai	1	100%	96.3%	96.7%	72%
		33%	68.6%	52.4%	
	2	100%	92.3%	98.1%	33.7%
		33%	55.4%	29.1%	
Toolbox	1	100%	88.8%	88.5%	54.7%
		33%	81.2%	68.2%	
	2	100%	100%	100%	59.4%
		33	89.9%	34.5%	

To address these issues we introduce our own dataset which consists of three objects. The objects were scanned in using Kinect, and six RGB-D testing sequences were recorded (350+ frames each). The objects are moved quickly in front of a static camera and are at times strongly occluded. Ground truth poses were manually labeled by hand annotation followed by ICP. In Fig. 7 five

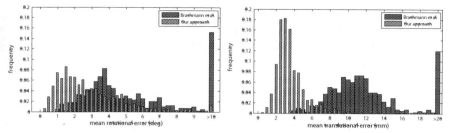

Fig. 9. Histogram of rotational and translational errors for our approach in comparison to [4], which is a single frame pose estimation framework.

images of each object are shown. For our dataset we trained decision trees as discussed in the previous section, but with renderings of our scanned-in objects, and a set of arbitrary RGB-D office images as background set. We keep all other training parameters as in the previously described experiment. We compare our approach to the one shot pose estimation from [4]. We exactly adhere to their training setup and parameters (3 trees, maximum patch size 20 pixel meter, 210 hypotheses per frame, Gaussian noise on training data). We measure accuracy as in [4] as the fraction of frames where the object pose was estimated correctly.

While our approach achieves 96.2 % accuracy on average over all sequences the approach of [4] only estimates 58.9 % of the poses correctly. Even though [4] is inherently robust to occlusion, the heavy occlusions in our dataset still cause it to fail. In contrast, our approach is able to estimate most poses correctly by using information from previous frames. The results are depicted in Fig. 8 (a) and (b). Additionally, we computed rotational and translational distances to the ground truth for both methods. The distribution of errors for one sequence is depicted in Fig. 9. The plots again show the large number of outlier estimations of [4] (rightmost bins). The plots also reveal that concerning correct poses, our approach leads to much more precise estimations.

To show that our full proposal distribution (Sect. 3.5) increases the robustness of our method we conducted the following experiment: We define a simplified variant of the proposal distribution, which is based only on H_{t+1}^{local} to which we also apply the final optimization. We term this variant *local proposal distribution*. We use it together with 120 particles since it needs less computation time. For this experiment, we artificially increase motion in our test sequences by using only every third frame. As before, we measure the number of correctly estimated poses. In this challenging setup the full proposal distribution achieves 80.3 % accuracy on average while the local proposal distribution achieves only 60.4 % accuracy. The results are depicted in Fig. 8 (b)–(e). Table 2 provides detailed information for the achieved accuracy on all sequences.

Figure 5 shows the estimated object motion path for one sequence with fast motion. The plot illustrates precision and robustness of our approach.

5   Conclusion

We have introduced a novel method applying the concept of 3D object coordinate regression to 6-DOF pose tracking. We utilize predicted object coordinates in a proposal distribution, making our method very robust with regard to fast movements in combination with occlusion. We have evaluated our method on the dataset by Coi and Christensen and demonstrated that it yields superior results. The method was additionally evaluated using a new dataset, specially designed for RGB-D 6-DOF pose tracking, which will be made available to the community.

Acknowledgement. This work has partially been supported by the European Social Fund and the Federal State of Saxony within project VICCI (#100098171).

We thank Daniel Schemala for development of the manual pose annotation tool, we used to generate ground truth data.

References

1. Avidan, S.: Ensemble tracking. IEEE Trans. PAMI **29**, 261–271 (2007)
2. Azad, P., Munch, D., Asfour, T., Dillmann, R.: 6-DoF model-based tracking of arbitrarily shaped 3D objects. In: IEEE ICRA, pp. 5204–5209 (2011)
3. Bersch, C., Pangercic, D., Osentoski, S., Hausman, K., Marton, Z.C., Ueda, R., Okada, K., Beetz, M.: Segmentation of textured and textureless objects through interactive perception. In: RSS Workshop on Robots in Clutter: Manipulation, Perception and Navigation in Human Environments (2012)
4. Brachmann, E., Krull, A., Michel, F., Gumhold, S., Shotton, J., Rother, C.: Learning 6D object pose estimation using 3D object coordinates. In: Fleet, D., Pajdla, T., Schiele, B., Tuytelaars, T. (eds.) ECCV 2014, Part II. LNCS, vol. 8690, pp. 536–551. Springer, Heidelberg (2014)
5. Bray, M., Koller-Meier, E., Van Gool, L.: Smart particle filtering for 3D hand tracking. In: IEEE International Conference on Automatic Face and Gesture Recognition, pp. 675–680 (2004)
6. Chiuso, A., Soatto, S.: Monte carlo filtering on lie groups. In: 39th IEEE Conference on Decision and Control, vol. 1, pp. 304–309 (2000)
7. Choi, C., Christensen, H.I.: 3D textureless object detection and tracking: an edge-based approach. In: IEEE/RSJ International Conference on IROS, pp. 3877–3884 (2012)
8. Choi, C., Christensen, H.I.: RGB-D object tracking: A particle filter approach on GPU. In: IEEE/RSJ International Conference on IROS, pp. 1084–1091 (2013)
9. Choi, C., Christensen, H.: Robust 3D visual tracking using particle filtering on the SE(3) group. In: 2011 IEEE ICRA, pp. 4384–4390 (2011)
10. Doucet, A., Godsill, S., Andrieu, C.: On sequential monte carlo sampling methods for bayesian filtering. Stat. Comput. **10**, 197–208 (2000)
11. Fanelli, G., Weise, T., Gall, J., Van Gool, L.: Real time head pose estimation from consumer depth cameras. In: Mester, R., Felsberg, M. (eds.) Pattern Recognition. LNCS, vol. 6835, pp. 101–110. Springer, Heidelberg (2011)
12. Gordon, N., Salmond, D., Smith, A.: Novel approach to nonlinear/non-gaussian bayesian state estimation. IEEE Radar Signal Process. **2**, 107–113 (1993)

13. Grabner, H., Bischof, H.: Online boosting and vision. IEEE CVPR **1**, 260–267 (2006)
14. Hinterstoisser, S., Lepetit, V., Ilic, S., Holzer, S., Bradski, G., Konolige, K., Navab, N.: Model based training, detection and pose estimation of texture-less 3D objects in heavily cluttered scenes. In: Lee, K.M., Matsushita, Y., Rehg, J.M., Hu, Z. (eds.) ACCV 2012, Part I. LNCS, vol. 7724, pp. 548–562. Springer, Heidelberg (2013)
15. Isard, M., Blake, A.: Contour tracking by stochastic propagation of conditional density. In: Buxton, B., Cipolla, R. (eds.) Computer Vision - ECCV 1996. LNCS, vol. 1064, pp. 343–356. Springer, Heidelberg (1996)
16. Klein, G., Murray, D.W.: Full-3D edge tracking with a particle filter. In: BMVC, pp. 1119–1128 (2006)
17. Kwon, J., Choi, M., Park, F.C., Chun, C.: Particle filtering on the euclidean group: framework and applications. Robotica **25**, 725–737 (2007)
18. McElhone, M., Stuckler, J., Behnke, S.: Joint detection and pose tracking of multi-resolution surfel models in RGB-D. In: IEEE ECMR, pp. 131–137 (2013)
19. Okuma, K., Taleghani, A., de Freitas, N., Little, J.J., Lowe, D.G.: A boosted particle filter: multitarget detection and tracking. In: Pajdla, T., Matas, J.G. (eds.) ECCV 2004. LNCS, vol. 3021, pp. 28–39. Springer, Heidelberg (2004)
20. Pupilli, M., Calway, A.: Real-time camera tracking using known 3d models and a particle filter. In: IEEE ICPR, vol. 1, pp. 199–203 (2006)
21. Rios-Cabrera, R., Tuytelaars, T.: Discriminatively trained templates for 3d object detection: a real time scalable approach. In: IEEE ICCV, pp. 2048–2055 (2013)
22. Shotton, J., Glocker, B., Zach, C., Izadi, S., Criminisi, A., Fitzgibbon, A.: Scene coordinate regression forests for camera relocalization in RGB-D images. In: IEEE CVPR, pp. 2930–2937 (2013)
23. Song, S., Xiao, J.: Tracking revisited using rgbd camera: unified benchmark and baselines. In: ICCV, pp. 233–240 (2013)
24. Stckler, J., Behnke, S.: Multi-resolution surfel maps for efficient dense 3D modeling and tracking. J. Vis. Commun. Image Represent. **25**, 137–147 (2014)
25. Taylor, J., Shotton, J., Sharp, T., Fitzgibbon, A.W.: The vitruvian manifold: Inferring dense correspondences for one-shot human pose estimation. In: IEEE CVPR, pp. 103–110 (2012)
26. Teuliere, C., Marchand, E., Eck, L.: Using multiple hypothesis in model-based tracking. In: IEEE ICRA, pp. 4559–4565 (2010)
27. Wu, B., Nevatia, R.: Detection and tracking of multiple, partially occluded humans by bayesian combination of edgelet based part detectors. Int. J. Comput. Vis. **75**, 247–266 (2007)

Poster Session 3

Probabilistic State Space Decomposition for Human Motion Capture

Prabhu Kaliamoorthi and Ramakrishna Kakarala[✉]

School of Computer Engineering, Nanyang Technological University,
Singapore, Singapore
prabhu.kaliamoorthi@gmail.com, ramakrishna@ntu.edu.sg

Abstract. Model-based approaches to tracking of articulated objects, such as a human, have a high computational overhead due to the high dimensionality of the state space. In this paper, we present an approach to human motion capture (HMC) that mitigates the problem by performing a probabilistic decomposition of the state space. We achieve this by defining a conditional likelihood for each limb in the articulated human model as opposed to an overall likelihood. The conditional likelihoods are fused by making certain conditional independence assumptions inherent in the human body. Furthermore, we extend the popular stochastic search methods for HMC to make use of the decomposition. We demonstrate with Human Eva I and II datasets that our approach is capable of tracking more accurately than the state-of-the-art systems using only a small fraction of the computational resources.

1 Introduction

Model-based methods for human motion capture (HMC) [1–6] rely on particle based systems that either perform global optimization within a restricted search volume or use a sequential Monte Carlo (SMC) style tracker. These are designed to be general optimization and tracking methods which are applied to HMC. However, articulated objects such as a human body, have a number of conditional independence properties. For example, one could assume that the head and the leg poses are conditionally independent given the pose of the torso. Existing particle based systems for HMC do not make use of these properties, i.e., they are incapable of extracting a good leg pose from a sample which has poor overall likelihood due to head pose. This is observed in Fig. 1a. Due to occlusion, these independence assumptions may not hold in a single view. However, most state of the art systems for HMC operate in a multi-view scenario, where these assumptions can be made to improve the tracking performance.

Partitioned sampling [7] is a technique that enables articulated object trackers to decompose the high dimensional state space. It has shown a 50 % reduction in the tracking overhead for an articulated hand [7] with fewer (4) degrees

Electronic supplementary material The online version of this chapter (doi:10.1007/978-3-319-16817-3_26) contains supplementary material, which is available to authorized users.

D. Cremers et al. (Eds.): ACCV 2014, Part IV, LNCS 9006, pp. 403–416, 2015.
DOI: 10.1007/978-3-319-16817-3_26

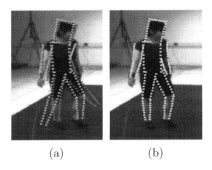

(a)   (b)

Fig. 1. Part (a) shows two poor overall poses which have a good fit for specific limbs, and (b) shows a new pose extracted from the two poor poses that has an overall good fit.

of freedom than a human (25–50). However, annealing based methods such as Annealed Particle Filter (APF [1]), Interacting Simulating Annealing (ISA [3]) have been claimed to perform better than partitioned sampling for high dimensional spaces such as those used in HMC. Though recent studies [4] indicate partitioned sampling to be a promising alternative for HMC, state of the art systems [3,4] do not make use of such a hierarchical decomposition, due to the lack of a systematic framework.

In this paper, we present a systematic approach to perform hierarchical decomposition. Though we apply our framework to HMC here, our method is a very general one, and it can be applied to other articulated objects such as a human hand or quadrupeds as well as other optimization problems that can be factorized. Our novel contributions are as follows. We describe a probabilistic framework to decompose the high dimensional state space of the HMC systems into subspaces of smaller dimension. The decomposition enables partitioned sampling type algorithms for HMC. We extend stochastic search methods (APF, ISA) to make use of the decomposition.

We validate the proposed method using the data from the Human Eva I and II datasets. Our results show that by decomposing the state space, we are able to capture complex human activity more accurately, using only a small fraction of the computational resources as the state-of-the-art systems [3,6,8].

2   Previous Work

There is a large body of research on HMC. Approaches such as [9,10] use local optimization for tracking. Despite showing promising results, local optimization based techniques are known to get stuck in incorrect hypotheses [8]. Hence these methods are expected to fail when the model is not exact, or if the image features are uncertain. Even if these assumptions do hold, these methods could still benefit from a decomposed search framework such as the one we propose here. Discriminative methods [11,12] that learn a mapping function between the image features and the human pose are known to require extensive training, and are expected to be sensitive to the appearance of the subject. Moreover, the generalization of these methods to novel poses not part of the training database is unclear.

More recently, HMC using pictorial structures [13] and belief propagation [14], which loosely assemble human parts to a plausible pose, have been proposed. However, these methods cannot ensure anatomically correct reconstruction of the human motion. Furthermore, they are confined to crude models of the subject and cannot be extended to more general surface meshes [2,3]. Our method enforces certain conditional independence assumptions similar to [14]. However, our approach is very different from [14] since we enforce hard rather than soft constraints between limbs, i.e., distances between connected limbs cannot change in our method. Furthermore, since the conditional independencies are induced by the kinematic model, our method has a different set of conditional independencies than model free methods such as [14].

Deutscher et al. [1] formulate HMC as a global optimization problem, and use randomized search algorithms that locate the global optimum in a restricted volume of the state space. Furthermore, they extend [1] their work using inspiration from genetic algorithms and perform crossover when generating new samples. Our method could be considered as an extension of this, where we perform crossover based on the fit of the individual parts. Gall et al. [3] describe a multi pass solution that perform a crude tracking with global optimization, which is later refined by a smoothing filter and local optimization. Sidenbladh et al. [15] describe a complete generative framework to model based HMC using the sequential Monte Carlo tracker. Our approach is compatible with these methods which are referred to as generative methods or analysis by synthesis framework in the literature. However, none of these methods have proposed a systematic framework to decompose the state space, which is the main focus of this paper.

In [6], authors describe a framework for the HMC of multiple subjects in parallel. This can be considered as a specific instance of our method where the likelihood for the two subjects are assumed to be independent. We show that by exploiting the conditional independence structure, the HMC of a single subject can be made more efficient. As a result, the general framework we present here can be used for the HMC of multiple subjects.

3   State Space Decomposition

3.1   Overview

Recent model-based methods for HMC [1–6], approach the problem as a dynamic maximum likelihood estimation of a high dimensional state space $\mathcal{X}$. In this paper, we make certain conditional independence assumptions about the likelihood, i.e., we assume the likelihood could be factorized into subspaces $\mathcal{X}_i, i \in \{1, \ldots, L\}$ of much smaller dimensions. The factorization is achieved by defining conditional likelihoods for each part rather than an overall likelihood as commonly done in model-based methods [3,4]. The conditional likelihoods are composed of a model to observation and an observation to model matching cost. However, since the conditional likelihoods are defined for each part, we

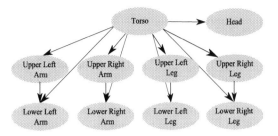

Fig. 2. The graphical model shows the conditional independence assumptions induced by the kinematic model.

decompose the observation probabilistically in order to define the conditional likelihoods. Using our conditional likelihoods, pose inference can be achieved using well known algorithms such as non-parametric belief propagation (NBP) [14]. However, this would result in a Bayesian particle based system that approximates the posterior with a set of samples. Since most Bayesian methods such as [7, 15] require a very high number of samples for HMC, we extend the stochastic search methods for inference instead of Bayesian techniques. In the rest of this section, we describe our method in detail.

3.2   Marginal Likelihood

We achieve decomposition by making a number of conditional independence assumptions. The assumptions are induced by the kinematic model used for tracking. Figure 2 shows a directed graphical model representing the conditional independence assumptions made. The decomposed subspaces $\mathcal{X}_i$ are simply the degrees of freedom (DOF) for the rigid objects represented by the nodes in Fig. 2. In order to illustrate model decomposition, let us consider the example of the lower left arm. After marginalizing the unrelated variables, the likelihood for the lower left arm and its parents is expressed as

$$P(lla, ula, tor) = P(lla|ula, tor)P(ula|tor)P(tor) \qquad (1)$$

where lla, ula and tor represent the pose parameters corresponding to the lower left arm, upper left arm, and the torso respectively. In order to obtain the likelihood of lla one can marginalize the above equation as below

$$P(lla = l) = \int P(lla = l, ula = u, tor = t)\, du\, dt \qquad (2)$$

The marginalization can be done numerically by a Monte Carlo approximation of the conditional likelihoods.

3.3   Conditional Likelihood

We use a variant of Oriented Chamfer Matching [16–18] in this work. However, the techniques that we discuss can be applied with other image features such as

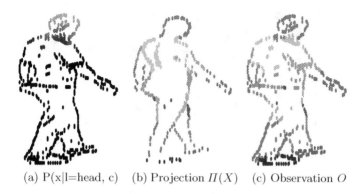

(a) P(x|l=head, c)   (b) Projection $\Pi(X)$ (c) Observation O

Fig. 3. The probability of the edge fragment given the part, $P(x|l,c)$, for head is shown in (a) (high probability in green and low probability in black). The edge fragments for the projection $\Pi(X)$ and the observation O, color coded according to the most probable label assignment $P(l|x,c)$ are shown in (b) and (c) respectively (Colour figure online).

those used in [3,4,6]. Let $\mathcal{P}$ be the space $\mathbb{R}^2 \times [0, \pi]$ representing oriented edge fragments. Let $O^c = \{o_i \in \mathcal{P}\}$ and $\Pi^c(X) = \{\pi_i \in \mathcal{P}\}$ represent the respective sets of observation and synthesized edge fragments for a specific camera c. The oriented chamfer distance between the two for the camera c is defined as

$$\psi^c(O^c, X) = \frac{1}{|O^c|} \sum_{o_i \in O^c} d(o_i, \Pi^c(X))$$

$$+ \frac{1}{|\Pi^c(X)|} \sum_{\pi_i \in \Pi^c(X)} d(\pi_i, O^c) \tag{3}$$

where $d : \mathcal{P} \times \mathcal{P}^N \to \mathbb{R}$, is a distance measure between an element in $\mathcal{P}$ and a set $\{\mathcal{P}\}$, $|O^c|$ and $|\Pi^c(X)|$ are the cardinalities of the sets O^c and $\Pi^c(X)$ respectively. It can be observed that ψ^c is composed of a model to observation and an observation to model matching term. The overall distance measure ψ is defined as the mean of the measure ψ^c from all cameras. The measure ψ provides a scalar cost that measures the overall match between the observation and the projection. In order to decompose it, we introduce a label l, which is distributed according to the L valued categorical distribution, formally, $l \sim Cat(L, p)$. The probability of the label indicates the degree of membership of an edge fragment to the individual rigid parts. Let us assume that the probability of the part given an edge fragment x in a camera c, $P(l|x,c)$, is known (described in Sect. 3.4). Assuming an uniform prior over the edge fragments given the camera, and using Bayes rule, one can obtain $P(x|l,c)$.

$$P(x|l,c) = \frac{P(l|x,c)}{\sum_x P(l|x,c)} \tag{4}$$

Since the possible values x can take is dependent upon c, here we assume the parameters for c and x are consistent, i.e., the probability $P(x,c)$ is non zero. Figure 3a shows the probability of the observed edge fragments for the head.

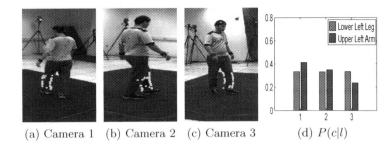

(a) Camera 1   (b) Camera 2   (c) Camera 3   (d) $P(c|l)$

Fig. 4. The probability of the camera given the part, $P(c|l)$, for the lower left leg and the upper left arm is shown. The edge fragments (in color) which are most likely to be from the upper left arm and the lower left leg are shown in green and cyan respectively.

In addition, assuming an uniform prior over the cameras and using Bayes rule, one can obtain the probability of the camera given the part as below

$$P(c|l) = \frac{\sum_x P(l|x,c)}{\sum_{x,c} P(l|x,c)} \tag{5}$$

$P(c|l)$ measures which camera is more likely to view a body part, and hence is more likely to help infer that part. Figure 4 shows $P(c|l)$ for the lower left leg and the upper left arm. It can be observed that for the lower left leg, which is equally visible in all three cameras, the measure $P(c|l)$ is equally distributed. Whereas, for the upper left arm which is nearly occluded in the third and second camera, the measure $P(c|l)$ is small for the third and second camera.

Using these probabilities the cost for a part l and camera c is expressed as

$$\phi_l^c(O^c, X) = E_{P(x=o_i|l,c)}[d(o_i, \Pi^c(X))] + E_{P(x=\pi_i|l,c)}[d(\pi_i, O^c)]] \tag{6}$$

where the first and the second term correspond to the observation to model and the model to observation matching cost respectively. Expressed differently, rather than summing the distance contribution from all the edge fragments as done in [16–18], we take a weighted sum with the weights estimated using Eq. 4. The total cost for the part l is expressed as the expectation of ϕ_l^c with respect to $P(c|l)$. Formally,

$$\phi_l(X) = E_{P(c|l)}[\phi_l^c(O^c, X)] \tag{7}$$

Modeling the likelihood to consider the visibility of the part is a novel aspect of our framework. Model-based methods in the current literature, take an average over all cameras to obtain the overall likelihood, which is equivalent to considering $P(c|l)$ to be uniform.

The conditional likelihood of a part given its parents is expressed as the cost for the respective part. Intuitively, treating the cost as conditional likelihood makes sense, since the cost for a part is conditioned on the value of the parameters for the parent links in the kinematic model. Formally,

$$- \log P(X_j|parents(X_j)) = \phi_l(X) + C \tag{8}$$

where X_j is a vector of parameters associated with the link j, $parents(X_j)$ is a vector of parameters for the ancestors of the link j (in the graphical model), and C is the normalization constant. For example, if j is considered to be the lla in Fig. 2, then the vector X_j would be the parameter for the 1D joint associated with the lla, and the vector $parents(X_j)$ would comprise of the parameters for the 9 DOF for the $torso$ (6) and the ula (3).

The formulation of the conditional likelihood in Eq. (8) is only an approximation due to occlusion. However, this is not a bad approximation since we take expectation over multiple cameras. Furthermore, since $P(c|l)$ is not uniform, the cost ϕ_l for the part l is more influenced by the view in which the part is not occluded.

3.4   Edge Fragment Prior

We estimate the prior probabilities for the observation edge fragments using the prior state estimate. A similar decomposition is performed in [6]. However, in our work the observation is a set of oriented edge fragments, whereas in [6] it is a silhouette. Let $\bar{X}$ be the prior estimate of the state. The edge fragments corresponding to the different parts can be separated by analyzing the part labels during the synthesis. Let $\Pi_l^c(\bar{X})$ represent a set of synthesized edge fragments corresponding to limb l and camera c. Let $\Pi^c(\bar{X})$ represent the complete set of synthesized edge fragments for camera c. The label probability for the observation edge fragment o_i is formally expressed as

$$
\log P(l|o_i, c) = C - \frac{1}{T} \begin{cases} \sum_{o \in O^c,\, p \in \Pi^c(\bar{X})} \frac{d_\mathcal{P}(o, p)}{|O^c||\Pi^c(\bar{X})|}, & \text{if } \Pi_l^c(\bar{X}) = \emptyset \\ d(o_i, \Pi_l^c(\bar{X})), & \text{otherwise} \end{cases} \tag{9}
$$

where T is a constant used to control the uncertainty and C is the normalization constant. The set $\Pi_l^c(\bar{X})$ is empty when the part l is occluded in the camera c. For such an occluded part, we define the probability to be a low nonzero value. Since setting a constant value can make it sensitive to the distance measure being used, we define it to be the mean distance between the set O^c and $\Pi^c(\bar{X})$. The function $d_\mathcal{P}$ is a distance metric between oriented edge fragments [16], which is typically a convex combination of the Euclidean metric and orientation distance.

The constant T has a significant impact on the edge prior. As T approaches ∞, the edge fragments become equally likely to be from any part and as T approaches 0, the edge fragments are assigned to a single part with high probability. In general, we observe that reducing T improves the search performance. This is expected since as T approaches 0, the edge prior is more informative. Therefore, the decomposed likelihood is influenced by both the model to observation and the observation to model matching cost. Whereas when T approaches ∞, as a result of a close to uniform edge prior, the observation to model matching cost in the decomposed likelihood is ineffective. However, when the observation is highly ambiguous, reducing T causes the tracker to get stuck in incorrect hypothesis. Hence T should be chosen as a trade-off between the two extremes.

The label probabilities for the projected model is defined as the Kronecker delta, since the part assignment is known with probability 1. Formally,

$$P(l = j | x = \pi_i, c) = \delta(\pi_i^l - j) \tag{10}$$

where π_i^l is the label corresponding to the projected model edge fragment π_i. The respective Fig. 3b and c show the most probable label assignment for the synthetic output and the observation for a specific camera.

3.5   Inference

We adapted the stochastic search procedures (APF [1], ISA [3]) to make use of the decomposed likelihoods. In this section, we describe the modifications we made. Stochastic search methods start with the predicted estimate of the state for the current frame (obtained using GP regression [3] or simple motion prediction strategies such as constant velocity or position [1]) and construct a sequence of layers. Each layer consists of a set of samples, each of which is a tuple consisting of the pose vector X^j and its respective normalized weight w^j. The index $j \in \{1, \ldots, N\}$, where N is the number of samples used in a layer. Sample weights w^j are obtained by evaluating the annealed likelihoods and normalizing as below

$$\log q^j = -\beta^l \, \psi(X^j), \quad w^j = \frac{q^j}{\sum_{k=1}^{N} q^k} \tag{11}$$

where β^l is the inverse annealing temperature for the layer chosen dynamically for each layer [1] or by a predetermined schedule [3]. In each layer, samples are selected according to their normalized weights. The selected samples are then perturbed by an adaptive diffusion kernel, and re-weighted to result in a normalized set of samples. At the end of the last layer, the expected state of the sample set is considered to be the estimate of the state.

The principal change we made to the procedure is in Eq. (11). The sample weights in the modified procedure are obtained by evaluating the annealed marginal likelihoods rather than the overall likelihood. Formally,

$$\log q_i^j = -\beta^l \, \psi_i(X_i^j), \quad w_i^j = \frac{q_i^j}{\sum_{k=1}^{N} q_i^k} \tag{12}$$

where the subscript i indicates that the sample weights are for the decomposed subspace and ψ_i is the corresponding negative log marginal likelihood obtained by numerical marginalization in Eq. (2). Using the decomposed weights, new samples are generated by re-sampling different X_i^js according to their respective w_i^js. They are finally combined to produce new samples X^j. This operation is similar to the crossover performed in [1], where the authors resample individual scalar values that makeup the state-space vector independently using the sample weights. However, we perform crossover based on the fit of the individual parts, i.e., cluster of scalar values (X_i^js) in the state space vector are resampled independently using different sample weights (w_i^j).

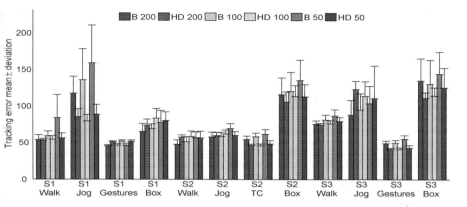

Fig. 5. Quantitative tracking results for Human Eva I dataset. It can be observed that our method (HD) performs competitively with 200 and 100 particles, and better than the baseline (B) with 50 particles.

4 Experiments and Results

In this section, we first validate the proposed method by comparing it to a baseline configuration using the Human Eva I dataset. Then, we compare the proposed method with the state of the art methods used in HMC [3,4,6,8] using the Human Eva II dataset. For Human Eva I, input from 3 RGB cameras and 2 grayscale cameras was used and for Human Eva II, input from all the 4 cameras was used for tracking. Similar to [4,8], we registered a set of markers provided by the ground truth for the first frame to the model, in order to measure tracking error. The marker location in subsequent frames were used to measure the error. For Human Eva II, the online evaluation system [4] was used to estimate the tracking error. We used the parameters described in [18] for the distance mesaure on oriented edge fragments.

We used a kinematic model made of 10 rigid links (L) and 25 DOF for Human Eva I. We used an extended kinematic model, with ankles, for Human Eva II resulting in 12 rigid links and 27 DOF. We used ISA configured with the parameters used in [3] as the baseline procedure for our experiments in the Human Eva I dataset. We used a likelihood based on OCM [16,17]. In our experiments, we found that for the torso, the cost ψ_{torso} is poorly constrained. Hence we added the cost corresponding to the parts directly connected to the torso such as the head, upper arms and the legs to ψ_{torso}, in order perform a stable inference. Figure 5 shows the time averaged mean error and deviation ($+1\sigma$) of 5 different runs for 12 different sequences in the Human Eva I dataset. In the figure, the baseline algorithm is referred to as **B** and the decomposed search is referred to as **HD**. The number of samples used per layer is displayed next to the name of the configuration for both the algorithms.

It can be noticed that the decomposition significantly improves the performance for sequences such as S1 Jog, S2 TC, S2 Box, S3 Gestures and S3 Box. However, for S3 Jog, it can be observed that it performs worse. Furthermore,

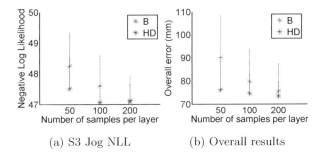

(a) S3 Jog NLL   (b) Overall results

Fig. 6. The negative log likelihood (NLL) for the S3 Jogging sequence and the overall tracking results of all the sequences for the six configurations are shown in sub-figures (a) and (b) respectively. Mean error is shown by the asterisk, mean error plus one standard deviation is shown by the bar.

it can be observed that tracking error is worse when higher number of samples are used for tracking. On analysis, we found that when using decomposed search the model got stuck in incorrect hypotheses. However, the incorrect hypothesis had a higher likelihood. This is observed in Fig. 6a, which shows the ensemble and time averaged negative log likelihood (NLL) for the S3 Jog sequence. It can be observed that the decomposed search still has a lower cost, i.e., it performs the task of search effectively. In general we observed that the decomposed search had a very wide effective search volume. Consequently, the decomposed tracker takes a different trajectory in comparison to the baseline version. We believe this results in marginally higher tracking error in sequences such as the S1 Gestures, S1 Box, and S2 Walk. However, these artifacts are caused by aspects such as poor model and observation, rather than the search procedure itself. This claim is further strengthened by the Human Eva II results that we present later which uses an accurate model and a relatively less noisy observation.

The overall mean error and deviation for all the 12 sequences is shown Fig. 6b. It can be noticed from the average performance, that both the mean error and the deviation are reduced in comparison to the baseline method. In addition, it can be noticed that the performance of the decomposed search is not significantly affected by the reduction in number of samples as opposed to the baseline method.

We compare our results with [3] for Human Eva II, since studies such as [6,8] use the implementation of [3]. Furthermore, the study in [4] uses an approximate model and hence it results in much higher tracking error than [3]. Rather than implementing the method in [3] ourselves, we compare our approach to the L1 results reported in [3], which is equivalent to our search procedure. We used the surface mesh provided with the Human Eva II dataset for tracking. Similar to [3], we reduced the mesh to have 4000 triangles to have an acceptable computational load.

A high speed approximate method using KD trees was used to synthesize oriented edge fragments from the surface mesh. Figure 3b shows the synthesized edge fragments, which can be observed to contain a few incorrect occluded

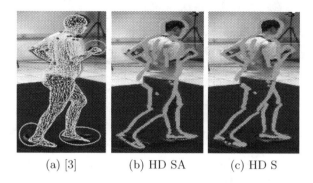

(a) [3]   (b) HD SA   (c) HD S

Fig. 7. Qualitative comparison of the tracked output for the subject S4, frame 580, camera 1. It can be observed that the leg pose estimated by our method is better than those reported in [3].

edge fragments. We obtained the probability in Eq. (10) from the skinning parameters [10] of the vertex. The distance $d_\mathcal{P}$ was robustified with the Geman-McClure function in order make the objective robust to outliers. Details of the

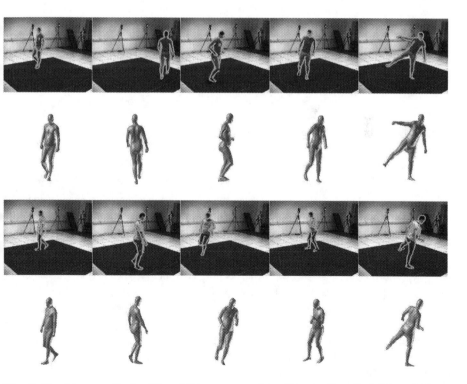

Fig. 8. Tracking results for S2 and S4 sequences from Human Eva II. Odd rows show the model output superimposed on the input from the camera, even rows show the 3d model.

Table 1. Our tracking results for the Human Eva II dataset are presented next to those reported in [3] for the subjects S2 and S4. The absolute and the relative error were obtained using the online evaluation system [4]. Best result in **bold**.

Frames		S2			S4		
		1-350	1-700	1-1202	2-350	2-700	2-1258
Absolute	[3]	41.5 ± 8.0	45.0 ± 12.9	43.8 ± 10.7	$34.6 \pm \mathbf{4.6}$	38.5 ± 6.9	38.1 ± 5.8
$\mu \pm \sigma$ (mm)	HD SA	$\mathbf{37.0 \pm 6.9}$	$\mathbf{41.7 \pm 9.1}$	42.4 ± 9.6	$\mathbf{31.2 \pm 5.4}$	$\mathbf{34.8 \pm 6.4}$	$\mathbf{36.3 \pm 5.7}$
	HD S	39.4 ± 7.6	44.6 ± 12.6	46.6 ± 12.9	31.6 ± 5.1	$35.3 \pm \mathbf{6.1}$	$37.1 \pm \mathbf{6.2}$
	B SA	$39.2 \pm \mathbf{6.8}$	44.7 ± 9.8	$44.2 \pm \mathbf{9.2}$	32.5 ± 5.9	36.7 ± 7.5	40.7 ± 9.9
Relative	[3]	$45.8 \pm \mathbf{9.0}$	48.4 ± 13.7	46.6 ± 11.4	43.9 ± 8.2	47.0 ± 10.6	45.3 ± 9.1
$\mu \pm \sigma$ (mm)	HD SA	$\mathbf{41.4 \pm 9.0}$	$\mathbf{43.4 \pm 8.9}$	$\mathbf{45.2 \pm 10.1}$	$\mathbf{32.0 \pm 5.9}$	$\mathbf{36.2 \pm 7.6}$	$\mathbf{38.2 \pm 7.4}$
	HD S	44.8 ± 10.3	47.9 ± 13.1	50.2 ± 14.3	$32.4 \pm \mathbf{5.7}$	$37.0 \pm \mathbf{7.3}$	39.0 ± 7.9
	B SA	45.0 ± 9.9	48.6 ± 10.7	48.4 ± 10.2	32.7 ± 6.5	38.3 ± 9	43.4 ± 13.5

Table 2. Number of samples used and the computation time on a standard PC. It can be observed that our method uses less than one-sixth of the number of samples used in [3].

Method	Samples	Computation time per frame
[3,6,8]	3750	76 s
ours	560	6 s

implementation such as the parameters used can be obtained from the source code supplied with the paper.

The decomposed search procedure was configured to use 8 layers and 70 samples per layer. The annealing schedule parameter α for the decomposed search was set to 0.2 and the adaptive diffusion parameter γ was set to 0.4 [3]. The parameter T described in Sect. 3.4 was set to 15. We used a constant position model [1] for prediction and a simple silhouette extraction method. The observation set O^c included oriented edge fragments from the silhouette and gray image in the foreground region. Table 1 summarizes the tracking results for the two sequences compared, where our method is referred to as **HD SA** (since it uses silhouette and appearance). It can be observed that our procedure performs better than [3] on most slots.

If the appearance of the subject is highly textured, the noise can be significantly higher than methods such as oriented chamfer matching can handle. In such a scenario the silhouette alone is the most reliable image feature. Hence we ran the above procedure with the observation set O^c containing oriented edge fragments from the silhouette alone. The results for this test are summarized in Table 1 as **HD S** (since it uses only silhouette). It can be observed that even without using appearance related features, our procedure results in comparable tracking performance as [3]. We provide the baseline results using ISA and OCM with the parameters used in [3], as **B SA** in the table. It can be observed that the proposed method **HD SA** is significantly better than the baseline.

Figure 7 shows the tracked result superimposed on the observation from the S4 sequence. It can be observed that the leg pose estimated by our method is slightly better than that in [3]. Figure 8 shows the tracked result for the S2 and S4 sequences from the Human Eva II dataset. Videos of the tracked and smoothed results, as well as the source code used to generate them, are available online [19].

The decomposition procedure we introduce in this paper marginally adds to the per sample overhead, but we found that this is insignificant in comparison to the rest of the processing. Since computational overhead to HMC is directly related to the number of samples used [4], it can be significantly reduced by using our method. The number of samples used for tracking and the computation time on a standard PC for the Human Eva II dataset is shown in Table 2. It can be observed from the table that the proposed method uses less than a sixth of the samples used in [3]. The computation time of our method is significantly lower both due to the decomposed search method which requires significantly lower number of samples and the OCM based likelihood, which can be realized at high speeds. Furthermore, the implementation in [3,6,8] uses a GPU based rendering. We did not use GPU acceleration in any form. We believe that by using a GPU based implementation of our method, HMC with the accuracy achieved in [3,6,8] would be possible at few frames per second.

5   Conclusion and Future Work

In this paper, we describe a probabilistic framework to decompose the high dimensional state space of the human motion capture system. We show that by defining conditional likelihood for each limb rather than an overall likelihood for the human model, a number of conditional independence assumptions can be made that enable the decomposition of the state space. We extend the state-of-the-art search method for HMC to make use of the decomposed subspaces. We demonstrate using the Human Eva I and II datasets that the decomposition framework significantly improves the tracking performance per sample, enabling the search technique to reach the tracking performance reported in the state of the art systems using only a fraction of the computational resources. In this work, we apply the decomposed search for the HMC of a single subject. In the future, we hope to apply our framework to multiple interacting subjects such as in [6], and for articulated hand tracking.

References

1. Deutscher, J., Reid, I.: Articulated body motion capture by stochastic search. IJCV **61**, 185–205 (2005)
2. Sigal, L., Balan, A.O., Black, M.J.: Combined discriminative and generative artic-ulated pose and non-rigid shape estimation, pp. 1337–1344. In: NIPS (2007)

3. Gall, J., Rosenhahn, B., Brox, T., Seidel, H.P.: Optimization and filtering for human motion capture. IJCV **87**, 75–92 (2010)
4. Sigal, L., Balan, A.O., Black, M.J.: HumanEva: Synchronized video and motion capture dataset and baseline algorithm for evaluation of articulated human motion. IJCV **87**, 4–27 (2010)
5. Pons-Moll, G., Baak, A., Gall, J., Leal-Taixé, L., Müller, M., Seidel, H.P., Rosenhahn, B.: Outdoor human motion capture using inverse kinematics and von Mises-Fisher sampling, pp. 1243–1250. In: ICCV (2011)
6. Liu, Y., Stoll, C., Gall, J., Seidel, H.P., Theobalt, C.: Markerless motion capture of interacting characters using multi-view image segmentation, pp. 1249–1256 . In: CVPR (2011)
7. MacCormick, J., Isard, M.: Partitioned sampling, articulated objects, and interface-quality hand tracking. In: Vernon, D. (ed.) ECCV 2000. LNCS, vol. 1843, pp. 3–19. Springer, Heidelberg (2000)
8. Gall, J., Stoll, C., de Aguiar, E., Theobalt, C., Rosenhahn, B., Seidel, H.P.: Motion capture using joint skeleton tracking and surface estimation, pp. 1746–1753. In: CVPR (2009)
9. Bregler, C., Malik, J.: Tracking people with twists and exponential maps, pp. 8–15. In: CVPR (1998)
10. Ballan, L., Cortelazzo, G.M.: Marker-less motion capture of skinned models in a four camera set-up using optical flow and silhouettes. In: 3DPVT (2008)
11. Agarwal, A., Triggs, B.: 3d human pose from silhouettes by relevance vector regression, pp. 882–888. In: CVPR (2004)
12. Bo, L., Sminchisescu, C.: Twin Gaussian processes for structured prediction. IJCV **87**, 28–52 (2010)
13. Andriluka, M., Roth, S., Schiele, B.: Monocular 3d pose estimation and tracking by detection, pp. 623–630. In: CVPR (2010)
14. Sigal, L., Isard, M., Haussecker, H.W., Black, M.J.: Loose-limbed people: estimating 3d human pose and motion using non-parametric belief propagation. IJCV **98**, 15–48 (2012)
15. Sidenbladh, H., Black, M.J., Fleet, D.J.: Stochastic tracking of 3D human figures using 2D image motion. In: Vernon, D. (ed.) ECCV 2000. LNCS, vol. 1843, pp. 702–718. Springer, Heidelberg (2000)
16. Liu, M.Y., Tuzel, O., Veeraraghavan, A., Chellappa, R.: Fast directional chamfer matching, pp. 1696–1703. In: CVPR (2010)
17. Shotton, J., Blake, A., Cipolla, R.: Multiscale categorical object recognition using contour fragments. TPAMI **30**, 1270–1281 (2008)
18. Kaliamoorthi, P., Kakarala, R.: Directional chamfer matching in 2.5 dimensions. IEEE Signal Process. Lett. **20**, 1151–1154 (2013)
19. https://sites.google.com/site/prabhukaliamoorthi/publications. Accessed 6 September (2014)

Spectral Graph Skeletons for 3D Action Recognition

Tommi Kerola, Nakamasa Inoue, and Koichi Shinoda$^{(\boxtimes)}$

Dept. of Computer Science, Tokyo Institute of Technology, Tokyo, Japan
{kerola,inoue}@ks.cs.titech.ac.jp, shinoda@cs.titech.ac.jp

Abstract. We present spectral graph skeletons (SGS), a novel graph-based method for action recognition from depth cameras. The contribution of this paper is to leverage a spectral graph wavelet transform (SGWT) for creating an overcomplete representation of an action signal lying on a 3D skeleton graph. The resulting SGS descriptor is efficiently computable in time linear in the action sequence length. We investigate the suitability of our method by experiments on three publicly available datasets, resulting in performance comparable to state-of-the-art action recognition approaches. Namely, our method achieves 91.4% accuracy on the challenging MSRAction3D dataset in the cross-subject setting. SGS also achieves 96.0 % and 98.8 % accuracy on the MSRActionPairs3D and UCF-Kinect datasets, respectively. While this study focuses on action recognition, the proposed framework can in general be applied to any time series of graphs.

1 Introduction

We live in a world where machines are able to either aid or completely replace humans in a large variety of tasks. Most such tasks are quite trivial and monotonic, but thanks to the advent of machine learning, we are at the verge of being able to demand satisfying performance even for more complex tasks. One such task is action recognition. If machines could robustly recognize and interpret human actions and gestures, the benefits would be vast for a number of areas, including games, health care and the security industry.

Classic approaches to action recognition based on simple color images face numerous difficulties due to intra-class variations of actions, background clutter and illumination variations. However, thanks to the emergence of cheap and affordable depth maps with devices such as the Microsoft Kinect, there has been a recent increase in research using 3D features [13]. Leveraging 3D cameras solves the problem of separating the action subject from the video background, and also eliminates irrelevant information such as illumination variance. Recently, due to the work of Shotton *et al.* [25], we have access to low-dimensional skeletons mapped to the human body. Out of the box, these skeletons are much more discriminative than the raw high-dimensional RGB-D data and allow the development of efficient methods for action recognition. However, while the 3D skeletons provide means of alleviating the action recognition task, they also

© Springer International Publishing Switzerland 2015
D. Cremers et al. (Eds.): ACCV 2014, Part IV, LNCS 9006, pp. 417–432, 2015.
DOI: 10.1007/978-3-319-16817-3_27

provide new challenges due to unstable joint positions resulting from tracking errors in the noisy depth maps.

A recurring question in machine learning is the one of how to best represent objects for handling the pattern learning task. Generally, the approaches to this problem can be divided into two: statistical and structural [2]. While statistical methods have received a great deal of attention in the past years, we ask ourselves if objects are not better represented by an explicit structure suitable to the task at hand. Considering that the human skeleton may be viewed as a graph in 3D space (see Fig. 2), is it feasible to believe that patterns such as actions may be well represented by a time series of such graphs? This question is our motivation for exploring the usage of graphs for action recognition.

In real life problems, graphs can be found everywhere. They occur in forms of *e.g.* social-and transportation networks, finite state machines, and also in domains such as brain fMRI and computer graphics [7]. Recent approaches for using graphs in machine learning include graph kernels [1,14,38], generalizations of signal processing frameworks to the graph domain [7,24], and also graph wavelets [5,6,12,20,22], such as the spectral graph wavelet transform [12]. While some difficulties and unsolved problems do remain, we believe that the future will hold even more promising new methods for the application of graphs in machine learning [2,7].

In this paper, we propose to use the spectral graph wavelet transform (SGWT) framework of Hammond *et al.* [12] for the depth map action recognition task. Our method encodes body joint positions from a skeleton tracker [25] and embeds these on a temporal skeleton graph in 3D space. Graph wavelets capture information about a signal at different scales, in four dimensions on the temporal skeleton graph; along both 3D joint positions and time. Further, spectral graph wavelets offer more flexibility than classical wavelets due to the freedom of graph design and selection of spectral kernels. To capture the sequential behavior of actions, we utilize a temporal pyramid pooling scheme [11,18,29] on the wavelet coefficients. This improves over approaches that consider only global information [17,34], since it allows us to capture differently segmented levels of temporal dependencies. Classification is finally performed using an off-the-shelf support vector machine (SVM). We name our action descriptor *spectral graph skeletons* (SGS), as it encodes the spectral content of a 3D skeleton sequence. Our proposed SGS descriptor has the following advantages:

– It is efficiently computable in $\mathcal{O}(T)$ time, where T is the number of frames in the action sequence. This makes it more computationally efficient than approaches that rely on solving heavy optimization problems [18,30].
– Its underlying spectral basis is mathematically well defined [12], enabling analysis about each part of the descriptor. On the contrary, methods such as sparse coding [18] produce bases that are not easily analyzable.

To the best of our knowledge, this is the first application of graph signal processing to the action recognition task in computer vision. While this paper focuses on recognition of actions, the framework can in general be applied to any time series of graphs.

The paper is organized as follows. Section 2 reviews related research in action recognition and graph signal processing. Section 3 provides a brief introduction to spectral graph wavelets. Our proposed method is then shown in Sect. 4, with related experiments in Sect. 5. Section 6 finally concludes the paper.

2 Related Work

2.1 3D Action Recognition

The advent of cheap 3D cameras such as the Kinect has enabled a great performance increase for action recognition tasks [17]. The availability of RGB-D data has considerably eased the task of segmenting an actor from its background; something that is normally quite challenging when using only RGB data. Related research in this field can be roughly divided into three categories: depth map-based, skeleton-based, and methods that utilize both.

Methods that make use of the raw depth map voxel data include Li *et al.* [17], who present a method where a bag of 3D points is sampled from 2D projections of salient depth map poses. Their results show that 3D action recognition clearly outperforms 2D approaches while additionally providing robustness against occlusions. Viera *et al.* [28] introduced space-time occupancy patterns (STOP), where the 3D points of the depth map are represented by a modified 4D histogram. Oreifej and Liu [21] learn a non-uniformly quantized 4D space, in which histograms of oriented 4D normals (HON4D) of the depth map are used for classification. Yang *et al.* [34] create DMM-HOG, which stacks orthogonally projected depth maps that are then applied to histograms of oriented gradients. Although depth map-based methods are able to capture information about shapes in great detail, they do however suffer from not knowing the correspondence between regions in the RGB-D data and the human body.

Other approaches rely only on the provided 3D skeletons. This includes DL-GSGC by Luo *et al.* [18], which uses sparse coding with constraints for group sparsity and feature geometry to increase the discriminative power. Together with max pooling and a temporal pyramid pooling scheme, their method also achieves an enhanced sequential representation structure. Zhao *et al.* [36] create SSS, which employs sparse coding and dictionary template learning to learn gestures based on distances between pairwise joints. Another method includes HOJ3D by Xia *et al.* [31], which applies linear discriminant analysis to create a time series of visual words (postures) that are then used as features in a hidden Markov model. Other methods use nearest-neighbor classifiers for classifying derivatives [35] (MP), or dimensionality-reduced relative measurements [33] (Eigenjoints) of 3D joint positions. Gowayyed *et al.* [11] create histograms of oriented displacements (HOD), where quantized angles of skeleton joints are applied to a temporal pyramid for handling temporal dependencies of actions. Ellis *et al.* [10] create a low latency scheme for classifying actions by finding canonical poses using multiple instance learning. While their method is efficiently computable, it is unsuitable for actions that have a strict temporal structure rather than a characteristic pose, such as the action *"drawing an x"*.

Finally, some works utilize both depth data and 3D skeletons simultaneously. Wang et al. [29] create an algorithm for selecting discriminative relative joint pairs that reduce ambiguity between action classes (AE). They also utilize a temporal pyramid, and classification is done using multiple kernel learning. Wang and Wu [30] develop MMTW for tackling temporal misalignment of actions by leveraging a discriminatively learned warping matrix for aligning action sequences before the classification step. Warping templates are learned one per class and classification is done using a latent structural SVM.

2.2   Signal Processing on Graphs

Recently, several techniques for generalizing classical signals processing (CSP) techniques to arbitrary graphs have been proposed [7]. Graph signal processing (GSP) provides graph analogs to classical Fourier transform tools, such as filtering, translation, convolution, etc.. CSP is restricted to signals in regular grids, but most natural signals do not follow this structure (e.g. sensor networks and anthropometric meshes). On the other hand, GSP allows processing signals on graphs that are directly adapted to the signal domain itself. By the increased freedom of graph design, we are able to extend CSP approaches to include additional information along e.g. extra added graph edges, ultimately increasing the descriptive power of the signal itself.

Several works have created wavelets on graphs using GSP [5,6,12,20,22]. One of the earliest works on graph wavelets include a method by Crovella and Kolaczyk [6] for analyzing computer traffic data on unweighted graphs. Hammond et al. [12] develop a spectral graph wavelet transform (SGWT), which allows analysis of localized signals on the graph Fourier spectrum of an undirected graph. We note that spectral graph wavelets can been seen related to sparse coding [27,32]. The spectral graph wavelets are however more efficiently computable, since they are based on a fixed mathematical structure (see Sect. 3).

In addition to these frameworks, applications of graph signal processing include edge-aware image processing [19], depth video coding [15], image compression [23], anomaly detection in wireless sensor networks [9], bridge structure health monitoring [3], brain functional connectivity analysis [16] and mobility pattern prediction [8]. To the best of our knowledge, GSP has not before been applied to action recognition; this paper presents the first such study.

3   Background of Spectral Graph Wavelets

We briefly review some theory of graph signal processing and spectral graph wavelets; see Shuman et al. [7] and Hammond et al. [12] for details. Let $\mathcal{G} = (\mathcal{V}, \mathcal{E})$ denote a graph with vertex set $\mathcal{V}$ and edge set $\mathcal{E}$ with $N = |\mathcal{V}|$ vertices. We let $\mathbf{W} \in \mathbb{R}^{N \times N}$ denote the weight matrix associated with $\mathcal{G}$, where $W(n, m) \in \mathbb{R}^+$ is the weight of the edge between vertices n and m, or 0 if there is no edge. Then $\mathbf{L} = \mathbf{D} - \mathbf{W}$ is the graph Laplacian matrix, where $\mathbf{D} = \text{diag}\{\mathbf{W1}\}$ is the diagonal degree matrix and $\mathbf{1}$ is the vector of all ones. We let $\{\lambda_\ell, \mathbf{u}_\ell\}_{\ell=0,\ldots,N-1}$ denote the eigenvalue and eigenvector pairs of $\mathbf{L}$. The spectrum of $\mathbf{L}$ carries a frequency interpretation [37], making it applicable for harmonic analysis on graphs. We will only consider undirected simple graphs, which makes all eigenvalues real and non-negative, since $\mathbf{L}$ is a real symmetric matrix [4].

A graph signal is a function $f : \mathcal{V} \to \mathbb{R}$ that assigns a value to each vertex. Such a signal can be represented as a vector $\mathbf{f} \in \mathbb{R}^N$ lying on a graph $\mathcal{G}$. By writing the eigendecomposition $\mathbf{L} = \mathbf{U\Lambda U}^T$, frequency analysis of $\mathbf{f}$ can be performed by taking the graph Fourier transform (GFT) $\widehat{f} = \mathbf{U}^T f$ [7]. Hammond et al. [12] define a spectral graph wavelet transform (SGWT) for graph signals on the eigenspectrum of $\mathbf{L}$.[1] Each spectral graph wavelet is realized by taking a kernel function $g : \mathbb{R}^+ \to \mathbb{R}^+$, scaling its domain by a scalar t, and finally localizing the result by convolving it with an impulse $\boldsymbol{\delta}_n \in \mathbb{R}^N$, which has value 1 at vertex n, and 0 everywhere else. A spectral graph wavelet $\boldsymbol{\psi}_{t,n} \in \mathbb{R}^N$ at scale t localized around vertex n can be written explicitly as

$$\psi_{t,n}(m) = \sum_{\ell=0}^{N-1} g(t\lambda_\ell)\mathrm{u}_\ell(n)\mathrm{u}_\ell(m), \; m = 1, \ldots, N \tag{1}$$

Given a graph signal $\mathbf{f}$, an SGWT coefficient is extracted by the inner product $\langle \boldsymbol{\psi}_{t,n}, \mathbf{f} \rangle$. The kernel g is chosen to act as the following band-pass filter [12]

$$g(x) = \begin{cases} x_1^{-\alpha}x^\alpha & \text{for } x < x_1 \\ s(x) & \text{for } x_1 \le x \le x_2 \\ x_2^\beta x^{-\beta} & \text{for } x > x_2 \end{cases} \tag{2}$$

where $\alpha = \beta = 2$, $x_1 = 1$, $x_2 = 2$ and $s(x)$ is a unique cubic spline that respects the curvature of g. Then, coefficients for smaller scales (small t) will localize high-frequency information around a vertex, while larger scales (large t) capture low-frequency information. The transform also includes a scaling kernel $h : \mathbb{R}^+ \to \mathbb{R}$, $h(x) = \gamma \exp(-(x/(0.6\epsilon))^4)$, for creating a scaling function $\boldsymbol{\phi}_n$ for stably representing low-frequency content in the graph [12]. Here, γ is set so that $h(0)$ equals the maximum value of g, and the design parameter $\epsilon = \lambda_{\max}/20$, where $\lambda_{\max}$ is an upper bound of the maximum eigenvalue of the graph Laplacian. The vector $\boldsymbol{\phi}_n$ is defined similarly to Eq. (1), with g replaced by h and setting $t = 1$.

Let M denote an integer such that the set of wavelet scales is $\{t_j\}_{j=1,\ldots,M}$. Then, the SGWT provides a transform with $M + 1$ scales; M wavelets and one scaling function. By gathering the wavelet and scaling function vectors in a transformation matrix $\mathbf{T} = [\boldsymbol{\psi}_{t_1,1}, \ldots, \boldsymbol{\psi}_{t_M,N}, \boldsymbol{\phi}_1, \ldots, \boldsymbol{\phi}_N]$, the transform coefficients can be expressed as a $(M + 1)N$-dimensional vector

$$\mathbf{c} = \mathbf{T}^T \mathbf{f} \tag{3}$$

We also note that the SGWT is an overcomplete transform, as it contains more wavelet coefficients than vertices in the graph. If a signal is representable

---

[1] Online source code available at http://wiki.epfl.ch/sgwt.

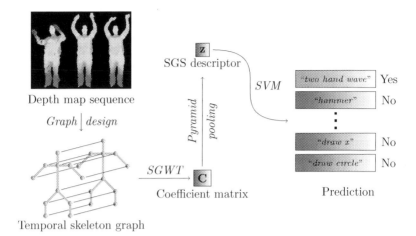

Fig. 1. Overview of the proposed action recognition system.

using only a few wavelet scales, then the SGWT can be viewed as quite similar to sparse coding [32], and each wavelet as an atom in a sparse dictionary [27]. However, since spectral graph wavelets are based on a fixed mathematical structure, they can be computed more efficiently, while sparse coding requires solving a heavy optimization problem [27]. It should be noted that while attempts to embed graph structure into the learned dictionary exists, this does not guarantee an efficient implementation [27]. Another advantage of spectral graph wavelets is that the explicit mathematical structure enables formal analysis of the effects of each wavelet basis.

In order to avoid explicit computation of the eigenspectrum of $\mathbf{L}$, which takes $\mathcal{O}(|\mathcal{V}|^3)$ time, the authors of the SGWT also introduce a method based on truncated Chebyshev polynomials for approximating the transform in $\mathcal{O}(|\mathcal{E}| + M|\mathcal{V}|)$ time [12]. Given a spectrum upper bound $\lambda_{\max}$, the approximation accesses $\mathbf{L}$ only through matrix-vector multiplications and is fast for sparse graphs. For the *normalized* graph Laplacian matrix $\mathcal{L} = \mathbf{D}^{-1/2}\mathbf{L}\mathbf{D}^{-1/2}$, there is a trivial upper bound $\lambda_{\max} = 2$ for the maximum eigenvalue, which is tight when the graph is bipartite [4]. We will use this approximation for all practical purposes in this paper. We further note that the approximation has been shown to be computable in a distributed manner [26].

4   Spectral Graph Skeletons

This section presents our method for 3D action recognition using the SGWT. A method overview can be seen in Fig. 1. We limit our study to the quite elementary graph gained from the tracked skeleton as described below. While it is plausible to believe that better performance might be achieved through combined usage of both depth maps and skeletons, we are in this study specifically interested in investigating the representative power of the skeleton as a graph.

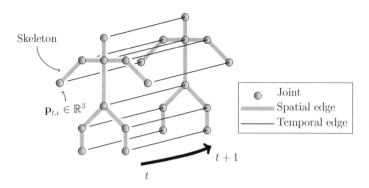

Fig. 2. Temporal skeleton graph, here shown partly by two temporally connected spatial skeleton graphs at frame t and $t+1$. Spatial edges between skeleton joints in the same frame and temporal edges between consequent frames in the action sequence are shown. Each joint i has a position $\mathbf{p}_{t,i} \in \mathbb{R}^3$. Note that the skeleton graph in this example is simplified for the purpose of illustration, and thus has fewer than the 20 joints given by Shotton *et al.* [25].

Joint Position Feature. For action recognition, we first acquire a sequence of T depth images from a depth camera, such as the Microsoft Kinect, with each pixel indicating the z-location of the corresponding area. Then, we obtain a tracked skeleton [25] with $J = 20$ joints of the human body for each frame of the depth image sequence, where the i-th joint at frame t has a 3D position $\boldsymbol{p}_{t,i} = [\mathrm{x}_i(t), \mathrm{y}_i(t), \mathrm{z}_i(t)]^T$ (see also Fig. 2). As body size differs between different human subjects, we use the limb normalization procedure of Zanfir *et al.* [35] for normalizing skeleton limb length, while still keeping limb angles and positions intact. As noted in previous research [18,29], the relative inter-joint positions give quite discriminative features. As the center hip joint of the tracked 3D skeleton is deemed quite stationary throughout actions, we create a relative position vector $\hat{\boldsymbol{p}}_{t,i} = \boldsymbol{p}_{t,i} - \boldsymbol{p}_{t,\text{center\_hip}}$ for describing the position of joint i.

Temporal Skeleton Graph. A tracked 3D skeleton at time t can be represented by a graph $\mathcal{G}_{\text{skel}}^{(t)} = (\mathcal{V}_{\text{skel}}^{(t)}, \mathcal{E}_{\text{skel}}^{(t)})$ with $|\mathcal{V}_{\text{skel}}^{(t)}| = J$ vertices. Consider the case where we have a sequence of T such skeleton graphs. The GFT on the graph Laplacian of a 1D ring graph produces an eigenbasis equal to the basis of the DFT on the real line [37]. Therefore, we link together each pair of consecutive skeleton graphs, and also the graph from the last frame together with the first frame in order to create a "ring" structure. Explicitly, we can write $\mathcal{E}_{\text{temporal}}^{(t)} = \{(v_{t,i}, v_{t',i}) : v_{t,i} \in \mathcal{V}_{\text{skel}}^{(t)}, v_{t',i} \in \mathcal{V}_{\text{skel}}^{(t')}\}$, $\mathcal{E}_{\text{spatial}}^{(t)} = \mathcal{E}_{\text{skel}}^{(t)}$, $\mathcal{E} = \bigcup_{t=1}^{T} \mathcal{E}_{\text{temporal}}^{(t)} \cup \mathcal{E}_{\text{spatial}}^{(t)}$, where $t' = (t \bmod T) + 1$. Then, using $\mathcal{E}$ and setting $\mathcal{V} = \bigcup_{t=1}^{T} \mathcal{V}_{\text{skel}}^{(t)}$, we can design a temporal skeleton graph $\mathcal{G} = (\mathcal{V}, \mathcal{E})$, $|\mathcal{V}| = TJ$, $|\mathcal{E}| = (|\mathcal{V}_{\text{skel}}| + |\mathcal{E}_{\text{skel}}|)T$, corresponding to the T frames long skeleton sequence, such that skeletons in consequent frames have their joints linked together by temporal edges. Spatial edges in $\mathcal{G}$ therefore correspond to directly connected physical limbs of the human body. See Fig. 2 for a visual explanation.

As graph signals are scalars by definition (see Sect. 3), we process each axis of the 3D space separately, defining a graph signal $\mathbf{f}_a$ on $\mathcal{G}$ so that $f_a(n) = \hat{p}_{t,i}(a)$ at vertex $n = J(t-1) + i$, where $a \in \{1, 2, 3\}$ is the coordinate axis of choice. Edge weights in the graph are set as follows. Since a signal along a temporal edge can be assumed to be strongly correlated between vertices, we set temporal edge weights to unity. Spatial edges, on the other hand, cannot be assumed to follow the same phenomenon. We instead assume that a signal along a spatial edge provides relevant information inversely proportional to the distance between a pair of joints. Spatial edge weights are therefore set by a radial basis function $\alpha \exp(-\|\hat{\mathbf{p}}_{t,i} - \hat{\mathbf{p}}_{t,j}\|_2^2/(2\sigma^2))$, $\forall(v_{t,i}, v_{t,j}) \in \mathcal{E}_{\text{skel}}^{(t)}$, which gives spatially closer joints a higher weight. Here, $\alpha = 1$ is a fusion factor for weights between the temporal and spatial domains. We believe this factor is formally necessary since we cannot assume that these spaces should use the same measure of distance. At this stage, we do not however have any theoretical means of determining α, so we set it to unity. Further, since we can assume that σ is not equal for all connected joint pairs in the skeleton, we define a pair-specific set $\Sigma_{\text{spatial}} = \{\frac{1}{3}\sum_a \sigma_{i,j,\text{spatial}}(a) : (v_i, v_j) \in \mathcal{E}_{\text{skel}}\}$, where $\boldsymbol{\sigma}_{i,j,\text{spatial}} \in \mathbb{R}^3$ is a vector describing the axis-wise standard deviation between joints i and j. The set Σ_{spatial} can easily be estimated from training data. Assuming normalized skeleton size, edge weights in $\mathcal{G}$ will thus become time invariant.

Using the SGWT with the normalized Laplacian matrix $\mathcal{L}$ for computational convenience, we extract wavelet coefficients from $\mathcal{G}$ at vertex n and scale t_j by calculating $\boldsymbol{\psi}_{t_j,n}^T \mathbf{F}$ as in Sect. 3, where $\mathbf{F} = [\mathbf{f}_1, \mathbf{f}_2, \mathbf{f}_3] \in \mathbb{R}^{N \times 3}$ is the matrix of concatenated axis-wise graph signals embedded on $\mathcal{G}$, and $\boldsymbol{\psi}_{t_j,n}$ is the spectral graph wavelet in Eq. (1). Consequently, each vertex will result in $M' = M + 1$ coefficients per axis, one for each wavelet scale (including the scaling kernel). The coefficients are represented by a coefficient matrix $\mathbf{C}$ similar to Eq. (3), but reshaped so that $\mathbf{C} \in \mathbb{R}^{T \times 3JM'}$. This will store the coefficients for each frame of the action sequence on each row.

Temporal Pyramid Pooling Scheme. In order to cope with varying action sequence length, we leverage a vector-valued pooling function $p : \mathbb{R}^{d \times 3JM'} \rightarrow \mathbb{R}^{3JM'}$ to create a feature vector $\mathbf{z} = p(\mathbf{C})$, where d is equal to the input matrix row count. The pooling function can for example be chosen as to do either absolute max or mean pooling along the temporal axis as

$$p_{\max}(\mathbf{C}) = \left[\max_t |C(t, i)|\right]_{i=1,\dots,3JM'} \tag{4}$$

$$p_{\text{mean}}(\mathbf{C}) = \left[\frac{1}{T}\sum_{t=1}^{T} |C(t, i)|\right]_{i=1,\dots,3JM'} \tag{5}$$

In the case of mean pooling, the resulting feature will encode the average acceleration for each axis and joint, windowed by SGWT kernels.

Similar to previous research [11, 18, 29], we create a temporal pyramid of coefficients for capturing the temporal order of actions. Let K denote the maximum

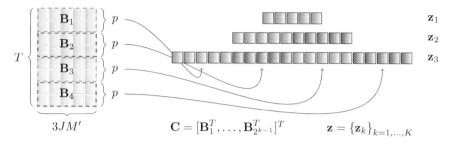

Fig. 3. Temporal pyramid pooling. Coefficient matrix $\mathbf{C}$ from a T frames long action sequence is pooled by a function $p : \mathbb{R}^{d \times 3JM'} \to \mathbb{R}^{3JM'}$ into $K = 3$ pyramid levels. The arrows illustrate the creation of the level 3 pyramid level vector $\mathbf{z}_3$. The final feature vector $\mathbf{z}$ is given by concatenation of the pyramid level vectors $\{\mathbf{z}_k\}_{k=1,...,K}$.

pyramid level. Then, the pooled feature vector at pyramid level $k \leq K$ is defined as $\mathbf{z}_k = [p(\mathbf{B}_1)^T, \ldots, p(\mathbf{B}_{2^{k-1}})^T]^T$, where $\{\mathbf{B}_i\}$ is a set of non-intersecting block matrices dividing $\mathbf{C}$ uniformly so that $\mathbf{C} = [\mathbf{B}_1^T, \ldots, \mathbf{B}_{2^{k-1}}^T]^T$. The final feature vector $\mathbf{z}$ is then a concatenation of the pyramid level vectors $\{\mathbf{z}_k\}_{k=1,...,K}$. A visual explanation of the temporal pyramid pooling scheme applied to $\mathbf{C}$ can be seen in Fig. 3.

If we assume that an action is most often performed using a limited part of the body (*e.g.* just the right hand), then most elements of $\mathbf{z}$ will become close to zero. We therefore reduce the $(2^K - 1)3JM'$-dimensional $\mathbf{z}$ using PCA. After applying PCA to $\mathbf{z}$, we ℓ^2-normalize and finally classify each action using a standard SVM. Our action descriptor encodes the spectral content of a sequence of skeletons. We thus name it *spectral graph skeletons* (SGS). As computing the SGWT approximation [12] in $\mathcal{O}(|\mathcal{E}| + M|\mathcal{V}|)$ time is the most costly part of the descriptor creation process, we have that for one action sequence, the descriptor is computable in $\mathcal{O}(T)$ time, treating parameters J, K, M constant.

Comparison with Previous Methods. While DMM-HOG [34] collapses the temporal variations into one axis, and thus suffers when temporal motion directionality is crucial, SGS is similar to STOP [28] and HON4D [21] in that we divide the space along the temporal axis. However, while STOP and HON4D only use the divided parts of the space separately, we combine them into a temporal pyramid like other works did [11,18,29] in order to capture both local and global information. MMTW [30] is able to find a non-uniform partition of the time axis that best captures discriminative parts of an action sequence, while our approach is more efficiently computable using only a uniformly partitioned temporal pyramid. Further, SGS is part of a group of methods that use relative joint positions [18,29,33,35,36]. While MP [35] and Eigenjoints [33] take relative velocity between joint pairs into account, SGS works well with just using the plain relative 3D positions. Since spectral graph wavelets can be seen related to sparse coding, as previously noted in Sect. 3, our approach is also similar to sparse coding methods [18,36], while being more efficiently computable.

Table 1. Recognition performance on the MSRAction3D dataset.

Method	Accuracy (%)
DL-GSGC [18]	96.7
MMTW [30]	92.7
MP [35]	91.7
SGS(p_{mean})	**91.4**
HOD [11]	90.2
HON4D [21]	88.9
AE [29]	88.2
SGS(p_{max})	**86.3**
SSS [36]	81.7
Canonical poses [10]	65.7
SGS (p_{mean}), no ring graph	87.6
SGS (p_{mean}), no SGWT	74.2

Table 2. Recognition performance on the MSRActionPairs3D dataset.

Method	Accuracy (%)
HON4D [21]	96.7
SGS(p_{mean})	**96.0**
SGS(p_{max})	**93.1**
AE [29]	82.2
DMM-HOG [34]	66.1

Table 3. Recognition performance on the UCF-Kinect dataset.

Method	Accuracy (%)
SGS(p_{mean})	**98.8**
SGS(p_{max})	**98.8**
MP [35]	98.5
Canonical poses [10]	95.9

5   Experiments

We test our proposed method on three publicly available datasets: MSRAction3D [17], MSRActionPairs3D [21] and UCF-Kinect [10]. The PCA dimension is set so that 98 % of the variance explained by the principal components is retained. For the SVM, we use a radial basis function (RBF) kernel. Both max (Eq. (4)) and mean (Eq. (5)) pooling are tried. Pyramid level K and the number of spectral graph wavelet scales M are decided by stratified cross-validation on the training set of each dataset.[2] We describe our results on the datasets that follow.

5.1   Datasets and Results

MSRAction3D. The MSRAction3D dataset [17] contains 10 subjects performing 20 different actions, of out which some are quite similar, such as "*draw x*" and "*draw circle*". Each subject performs each action up to three times; not necessarily in the same manner each time. Due to a large body of related research (see Sect. 2), this dataset has become quite a representative benchmark for 3D action recognition. Despite the availability of discriminative depth maps, this dataset remains quite challenging due to an abundance of visually similar actions as well as noisy joint positions. For fair comparison with previous research, we run

---

[2] In stratified cross-validation, the folds are selected so that the percentage of samples for each class in the dataset is preserved in each fold.

our experiments in the cross-subject setting, where samples from half of the subjects (*i.e.* subjects $1, 2, 3, 4, 5$) are used for training, and the rest for testing. This dataset contains some frames where the skeleton tracking fails, resulting in the joints to be erroneously located at the origin of the 3D coordinate system. We judge values to be missing only when the coordinates $(x, y, z) = (0, 0, 0)$, which Kinect outputs when the object is closer than 40 cm, or when no depth value could be found. For such missing values, the invalid joint positions are repaired using standard inter-frame linear interpolation.

The best parameters were $K = 4$ and $M = 50$ (decided by 5-fold cross-validation). PCA reduced the feature dimension from 45900 to 152. Results can be seen in Table 1. The confusion matrix is shown in Fig. 5. We see that mean pooling works better than max pooling, although both seem to be quite effective. Our SGS descriptor worked best with $K = 4$, but we note that even with $K = 1$ (no temporal pyramid), we got 83.5 % recognition accuracy. Note that $K > 4$ could not be tested due to insufficiently long sequences in the dataset. Our method is able to fully distinguish between visually similar actions such as "*draw x/circle*" (see Fig. 4) and achieves perfect accuracy for most actions. On the other hand, the method repeatedly mistakes the action "*hammer*" for "*draw x*". These two classes are both characterized by similar highly accelerating movements along all axes of the 3D space. While SGS is able to capture different ranges of acceleration, it has trouble capturing the small temporal order of how these accelerations occur, which is an important point of future work. Although our method gains comparable results to most previous researches, it is unable to achieve results comparable to the sparse coding approach DL-GSGC [18]. Note however that our method has the advantage of being computable in time linear in the sequence length, while DL-GSGC requires solving a computationally heavy optimization problem. Our method falls just short of MMTW [30], but it should be noted that while MMTW discriminatively learns a non-uniform warping of the time axis, our method works with a mere uniform division of the action sequence due to our temporal pyramid pooling scheme. Augmenting our temporal pyramid with non-uniform division is a probable point of future work.

To illustrate the significance of using the SGWT, Table 1 includes a result of using SGS without the SGWT, where temporal pyramid pooling is applied directly to the raw 3D coordinates. The table also shows that connecting the last skeleton with the first, creating a "ring graph" provides a slight improvement in performance.

Earlier work has also reported results on three separate action sets of MSRAction3D. The three action sets are defined to group visually similar action classes together [17], in order to test performance on small sets of similar actions. Our experiments follow this setup and results are shown in Table 4. Contrary to the previous experiment, max pooling is here seen slightly superior to mean pooling, indicating that the choice of max or mean pooling might depend on datasets. We can see that in this scenario with fewer action classes, our method achieves performance closer to DL-GSGC while being more efficiently computable.

MSRActionPairs3D [21]. This dataset was created to test performance for recognizing action pairs that are similar in motion, and differ in motion directionality

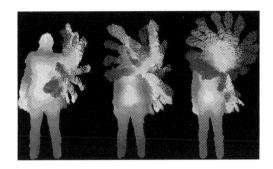

Fig. 4. Frontal view examples of the actions "*hammer*" (left), "*draw x*" (middle) and "*draw circle*" (right) in the MSRAction3D dataset.

Table 4. Recognition performance on the MSRAction3D dataset for the three different subject configurations on the three action sets as in Li *et al.* [17] Each cell shows accuracy (%). Test 1 uses the first 1/3 samples for training and the rest for testing. Test 2 uses the first 2/3 samples for training and the rest for testing. The cross-subject test follows the same setup as in Table 1.

Method	Test 1				Test 2				Cross-subject test			
	AS1	AS2	AS3	Avg	AS1	AS2	AS3	Avg	AS1	AS2	AS3	Avg
DL-GSGC [18]	100	98.7	100	99.6	100	98.7	100	99.6	97.2	95.5	99.1	97.3
SGS(p_{max})	**94.5**	**94.8**	**96.6**	**95.3**	**94.6**	**98.7**	**97.3**	**96.9**	**89.3**	**95.0**	**100**	**94.8**
SGS(p_{mean})	**96.6**	**90.8**	**98.0**	**95.1**	**98.6**	**96.0**	**98.6**	**97.7**	**88.4**	**91.6**	**100**	**93.3**
DMM-HOG [34]	97.3	92.2	98.0	95.8	98.7	94.7	98.7	97.4	96.2	84.1	94.6	91.6
STOP [28]	98.2	94.8	97.4	96.8	99.1	97.0	98.7	98.3	84.7	81.3	88.4	84.8
Eigenjoints [33]	94.7	95.4	97.3	95.8	97.3	98.7	97.3	97.8	74.5	76.1	96.4	82.3
HOJ3D [31]	98.5	96.6	93.5	96.2	98.6	97.9	94.9	97.2	88.0	85.5	63.5	79.0
Bag of 3D points [17]	89.5	89.0	96.3	91.6	93.4	92.9	96.3	94.2	72.9	71.9	79.2	74.7

only. An example of such an action pair is "*pick up box*" and "*put down box*". The dataset contains six action pairs performed by ten subjects, each subject performed each action three times. We run our experiments in the cross-subject setting, where the first five actors are used for training, and the rest for testing. The best parameters were $K = 5$ and $M = 1$ (decided by 5-fold cross-validation). PCA reduced the feature dimension from 3720 to 80. Results on MSRAction-Pairs3D can be seen in Table 2. Our method achieves comparable performance to HON4D [21], despite using only skeleton information. Additionally, HON4D discriminatively learns a non-uniform quantization of the 4D space, while our method works with only a simple uniform quantization along time using the temporal pyramid. We note that our method gets accuracy 56.6 % with $K = 1$ and 86.3 % with $K = 2$, confirming the importance of the temporal pyramid pooling scheme for recognizing motion directionality.

UCF-Kinect. The UCF-Kinect dataset [10] contains presegmented actions suitable for games, *e.g.* "*climb ladder*", "*leap*" and "*twist left*", with 1280 action

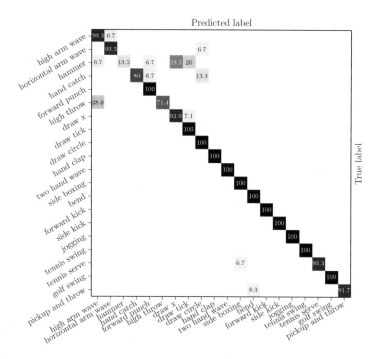

Fig. 5. Confusion matrix for using our method on the MSRAction3D dataset. Each cell shows classification accuracy (%) from white (0) to black (100) in the cross-subject setting. The average accuracy is 91.4 %.

sequences in total. 16 actions are performed by 16 subjects, with each subject performing each action five times each. Note that in this dataset the provided skeletons only have 15 joints. As the center hip joint is missing, we approximate it by the average of the left and right hip joint positions. We run our experiments in the same setting as Ellis *et al.* [10], reporting the average accuracy of 4-fold cross-validation. The best parameters were $K = 3$ and $M = 43$ (decided by 4-fold cross-validation). PCA reduced the feature dimension from 18480 to 127. Results on UCF-Kinect can be seen in Table 3. We can see that our method achieves superior performance compared to the original canonical pose approach [10], while performing slightly better than MP [35]. This shows that our proposed framework is suitable for recognition of game-related actions that make use of all tracked parts of the body.

5.2 Discussion

Since the graph Laplacian matrix $\mathcal{L}$ acts as a graph-analog to the classical Laplace operator [7], SGS is able to capture, per each joint and axis, the existence of ranges of acceleration. This range is determined by the SGWT kernel g. The window created by the SGWT kernel h in turn captures aggregated low-frequency information, such as the average position of the action in 3D space. We believe that SGS is able to distinguish between actions that can be characterized by different acceleration at each joint. On the other hand, this means that SGS potentially has trouble separating sets of actions that have the same such characteristics. This became evident in MSRAction3D, where "*hammer/draw x/draw tick*" exhibit a set of actions that when looked at along each axis, display similar ranges of acceleration around the same spatial location. In its basic form ($K = 1$), SGS is not able to capture the order in which ranges of accelerations occur, something which is important for actions bound by motion directionality, such as the ones in MSRActionPairs3D. While using the temporal pyramid ($K > 1$) effectively helps capturing such temporal order, we believe that a non-uniform partition of the time-axis might be required to fully capture action classes that exhibit a very locally dependent temporal order.

6   Conclusion

We have presented spectral graph skeletons (SGS), a novel graph-based method for action recognition from depth cameras. Our method leverages the SGWT framework [12] for creating an overcomplete representation of an action signal lying on a 3D skeleton graph. The graph wavelet coefficients are applied to a temporal pyramid pooling scheme, which creates a descriptor of an action sequence. For a T frames long action sequence, the SGS descriptor is efficiently computable in $\mathcal{O}(T)$ time. The power of our method was demonstrated by experiments on three publicly available datasets, resulting in performance comparable to state-of-the-art action recognition approaches.

While this early study of using graph wavelets for action recognition has shown some promising results, it is still in its infant stage. Several aspects of the method are subject to further exploration, such as investigating the possibility of constructing graphs directly on the raw depth data, using subgraphs instead of the whole skeleton, or the suitability of the descriptor for real-time recognition. We would like to emphasize that optimized selection of the wavelet kernel g in Sect. 3 could lead to increased performance and is therefore an important point of future work. One strategy could be to learn the kernel discriminatively from training data. The weight settings of temporal and spatial edges should also be looked at. Other frameworks for processing graph signals should also be explored, together with a more detailed analysis of the suitability of graph signals for action recognition. This paper has focused on action recognition, but the proposed framework is in general applicable to any time series of graphs.

Acknowledgement. The first author acknowledges the Japanese Government (Monbukagakusho:MEXT) scholarship support for carrying out this research.

References

1. Bunke, H., Riesen, K.: Recent advances in graph-based pattern recognition with applications in document analysis. Pattern Recogn. **44**, 1057–1067 (2011)

2. Bunke, H., Riesen, K.: Towards the unification of structural and statistical pattern recognition. Pattern Recogn. Lett. **33**, 811–825 (2012)
3. Chen, S., Cerda, F., Rizzo, P., Bielak, J., Garrett, J., Kovacevic, J.: Semi-supervised multiresolution classification using adaptive graph filtering with application to indirect bridge structural health monitoring. IEEE Trans. Signal Proc. **62**, 2879–2893 (2014)
4. Chung, F.R.: Spectral graph theory. CBMS Regional Conference Seriesin Mathematics, vol. 92, American Mathematical Society (1997)
5. Coifman, R.R., Maggioni, M.: Diffusion wavelets. Appl. Comput. Harmonic Anal. **21**, 53–94 (2006)
6. Crovella, M., Kolaczyk, E.: Graph wavelets for spatial traffic analysis. In: INFO-COM (2003)
7. Shuman, D.I., Narang, S.K., Frossard, P., Ortega, A., Vandergheynst, P.: The emerging field of signal processing on graphs: Extending high-dimensional data analysis to networks and other irregular domains. IEEE Signal Process. Mag. **30**, 83–98 (2013)
8. Dong, X., Ortega, A., Frossard, P., Vandergheynst, P.: Inference of mobility patterns via spectral graph wavelets. In: ICASSP (2013)
9. Egilmez, H.E., Ortega, A.: Spectral anomaly detection using graph-based filtering for wireless sensor networks. In: ICASSP (2014)
10. Ellis, C., Masood, S.Z., Tappen, M.F., Laviola Jr, J.J., Sukthankar, R.: Exploring the trade-off between accuracy and observational latency in action recognition. Int. J. Comput. Vis. **101**, 420–436 (2013)
11. Gowayyed, M.A., Torki, M., Hussein, M.E., El-Saban, M.: Histogram of oriented displacements (hod): describing trajectories of human joints for action recognition. In: IJCAI (2013)
12. Hammond, D.K., Vandergheynst, P., Gribonval, R.: Wavelets on graphs via spectral graph theory. Appl. Comput. Harmonic Anal. **30**, 129–150 (2011)
13. Han, J., Shao, L., Xu, D., Shotton, J.: Enhanced computer vision with Microsoft Kinect sensor: A review. IEEE Trans. Cybern. **43**, 1318–1334 (2013)
14. Hermansson, L., Kerola, T., Johansson, F., Jethava, V., Dubhashi, D.: Entity disambiguation in anonymized graphs using graph kernels. In: CIKM. ACM (2013)
15. Kim, W.S., Narang, S.K., Ortega, A.: Graph based transforms for depth video coding. In: ICASSP (2012)
16. Leonardi, N., Van De Ville, D.: Wavelet frames on graphs defined by fmri functional connectivity. In: ISBI (2011)
17. Li, W., Zhang, Z., Liu, Z.: Action recognition based on a bag of 3d points. In: CVPR Workshops (2010)
18. Luo, J., Wang, W., Qi, H.: Group sparsity and geometry constrained dictionary learning for action recognition from depth maps. In: ICCV (2013)
19. Narang, S.K., Chao, Y.H., Ortega, A.: Graph-wavelet filterbanks for edge-aware image processing. In: Statistical Signal Processing Workshop (SSP). IEEE (2012)
20. Narang, S.K., Ortega, A.: Perfect reconstruction two-channel wavelet filter banks for graph structured data. IEEE Trans. Signal Process. **60**, 2786–2799 (2012)
21. Oreifej, O., Liu, Z., Redmond, W.: Hon4d: Histogram of oriented 4d normals for activity recognition from depth sequences. In: CVPR (2013)
22. Ram, I., Elad, M., Cohen, I.: Generalized tree-based wavelet transform. IEEE Trans. Signal Process. **59**, 4199–4209 (2011)
23. Sandryhaila, A., Moura, J.M.F.: Nearest-neighbor image model. In: ICIP (2012)
24. Sandryhaila, A., Moura, J.M.F.: Discrete signal processing on graphs. IEEE Trans. Signal Process. **61**, 1644–1656 (2013)

25. Shotton, J., Sharp, T., Kipman, A., Fitzgibbon, A., Finocchio, M., Blake, A., Cook, M., Moore, R.: Real-time human pose recognition in parts from single depth images. Commun. ACM **56**, 116–124 (2013)
26. Shuman, D.I., Vandergheynst, P., Frossard, P.: Chebyshev polynomial approximation for distributed signal processing. In: DCOSS (2011)
27. Thanou, D., Shuman, D.I., Frossard, P.: Parametric dictionary learning for graph signals. In: IEEE GlobalSIP (2013)
28. Vieira, A.W., Nascimento, E.R., Oliveira, G.L., Liu, Z., Campos, M.F.M.: STOP: Space-Time Occupancy Patterns for 3D Action Recognition from Depth Map Sequences. In: Alvarez, L., Mejail, M., Gomez, L., Jacobo, J. (eds.) CIARP 2012. LNCS, vol. 7441, pp. 252–259. Springer, Heidelberg (2012)
29. Wang, J., Liu, Z., Wu, Y., Yuan, J.: Mining actionlet ensemble for action recognition with depth cameras. In: CVPR (2012)
30. Wang, J., Wu, Y.: Learning maximum margin temporal warping for action recognition. In: ICCV (2013)
31. Xia, L., Chen, C.C., Aggarwal, J.: View invariant human action recognition using histograms of 3d joints. In: CVPR Workshops (2012)
32. Yang, J., Yu, K., Gong, Y., Huang, T.: Linear spatial pyramid matching using sparse coding for image classification. In: CVPR (2009)
33. Yang, X., Tian, Y.: Eigenjoints-based action recognition using naive-bayes-nearest-neighbor. In: CVPR Workshops (2012)
34. Yang, X., Zhang, C., Tian, Y.: Recognizing actions using depth motion maps-based histograms of oriented gradients. In: ACM MM (2012)
35. Zanfir, M., Leordeanu, M., Sminchisescu, C.: The moving pose: An efficient 3d kinematics descriptor for low-latency action recognition and detection. In: ICCV (2013)
36. Zhao, X., Li, X., Pang, C., Zhu, X., Sheng, Q.Z.: Online human gesture recognition from motion data streams. In: ACM MM (2013)
37. Zhu, X., Rabbat, M.: Approximating signals supported on graphs. In: ICASSP (2012)
38. Zhu, X., Kandola, J., Lafferty, J., Ghahramani, Z.: Graph kernels by spectral transforms. In: Chapelle, O., Schoelkopf, B., Zien, A. (eds.) Semi-Supervised Learning, pp. 277–291. MIT Press (2006)

Robust Point Matching Using Mixture of Asymmetric Gaussians for Nonrigid Transformation

Gang Wang, Zhicheng Wang$^{(\boxtimes)}$, Weidong Zhao, and Qiangqiang Zhou

CAD Research Center, Tongji University,
Shanghai 201804, China
{gwang.cv,zqqcsu}@gmail.com
{zhichengwang,wd}@tongji.edu.cn

Abstract. In this paper, we present a novel robust method for point matching under noise, deformation, occlusion and outliers. We introduce a new probability model to represent point sets, namely asymmetric Gaussian (AG), which can capture spatially asymmetric distributions. Firstly, we use a mixture of AGs to represent the point set. Secondly, we use L_2-minimizing estimate (L_2E), a robust estimator to estimate densities between two point sets, to estimate the transformation function in reproducing kernel Hilbert space (RKHS) with regularization theory. Thirdly, we use low-rank kernel matrix approximation to reduce the computational complexity. Experimental results show that our method outperforms the comparative state-of-the-art methods on most scenarios, and it is quite robust to noise, deformation, occlusion and outliers.

1 Introduction

The point matching problem can be categorized into rigid and nonrigid matching depends on the transformation pattern. Generally, rigid transformation, containing translation, rotation and scaling, is relatively easy to estimate. By contrast, nonrigid transformation is hard to resolve since the transformation model is often unknown and difficult to model. Nonrigid transformation exists in numerous applications, including hand-written character recognition, facial-expression recognition and medical image registration.

However, there are many parameters in nonrigid transformation, causing several problems: (1) sensitive to noise, deformation, occlusion and outliers; (2) the trap of local minima; (3) high computational complexity. The nonrigid matching problem, in this sense, remains unsolved. Therefore, a point matching method should construct the complex transformation model with low computational complexity.

The Iterative Closest Point (ICP) algorithm [3] is one of the best known algorithms for point matching, because of its simplicity and low computational complexity. However, ICP requires a good initial position, *i.e.*, adequately close distance between the *Model* and the *Scene* point sets.

© Springer International Publishing Switzerland 2015
D. Cremers et al. (Eds.): ACCV 2014, Part IV, LNCS 9006, pp. 433–444, 2015.
DOI: 10.1007/978-3-319-16817-3_28

In order to address the limitations of ICP and improve the performance of matching, many interesting methods are proposed recently. Chui et al. [4] proposed a robust point matching algorithm named TPS-RPM. TPS-RPM is more robust than ICP to noise, deformation, occlusion and outliers.

Tsin et al. [20] proposed a correlation-based named kernel correlation (KC) point set registration method where the correlation of two kernel density estimates is used to formulate the cost function. Zheng et al. [21] proposed a robust point matching method for nonrigid shapes by preserving local neighborhood structures. Myronenko et al. [13,14] proposed another algorithm, namely the Coherence Point Drift (CPD), based on the motion coherence theory (MCT). CPD can get good results in a very short time when handling a large number of points.

Moreover, Jian et al. [7] proposed a robust point set registration approach using Gaussian mixture models (GMM), they leverage the closed-form expression for the L_2 distance between two Gaussian mixtures which represent the given point sets. Alternatively, Ma et al. [10] introduced L_2-minimizing estimate (L_2E) [17], a robust estimator in statistics, to the nonrigid transformation estimation problem. Then they proposed a robust point matching method named RPM-L_2E.

In this paper, we are present a novel robust point matching method. Briefly, the core of our method is using a mixture of asymmetric Gaussians (AG) to represent the density of the given point set. Then we use L_2E [17] to estimate the transformation parameters.

The rest of this paper organized as follows: A novel robust point matching method using mixture of asymmetric Gaussians and L_2-minimizing estimate for nonrigid transformation is presented in Sect. 2. Section 3 shows an optimal solution of our proposed method. The experiments and performance evaluation of our proposed method is shown in Sect. 4. In Sect. 5, we present a conclusion.

2   Method

2.1   Point Set Representation Using Mixture of Asymmetric Gaussians

We introduce a new probability model named Asymmetric Gaussian (AG) [8] which can capture spatially asymmetric distributions. AG is another form extending from Gaussian. It is shown that Gaussian has a symmetric distribution while AG has an asymmetric distribution by Fig. 1 where the density functions are plotted. Thus the distribution of AG is given by:

$$\mathscr{A}\left(x|\mu,\sigma^2,r\right) = \frac{1}{(2\pi\sigma^2)^{D/2}((r+1)/2)^D} \begin{cases} \exp\left(-\frac{|x-\mu|^2}{2\sigma^2}\right) & x \le \mu \\ \exp\left(-\frac{|x-\mu|^2}{2r^2\sigma^2}\right) & x > \mu \end{cases} \tag{1}$$

where D is the dimension of data, μ, σ^2 and r are parameters of AG where $r = 1$ means AG equaling to Gaussian.

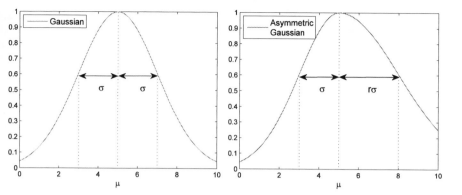

Fig. 1. Density functions of Gaussian and asymmetric Gaussian (AG).

Since the definition of the density model, it is easy to construct a mixture of AG which may be well approximate almost any density with a linear combination of local AGs. Then the overall density of the J-component mixture is given by:

$$p(x) = \sum_{j=1}^{J} w_j \mathscr{A}\left(x|\mu, \sigma^2, r\right) \tag{2}$$

where w_j is the weight of each component, and $\{w_j\}_{j=1}^{J}$ are mixing proportions satisfying $0 \leq w_j \leq 1$ and $\sum_{j=1}^{J} w_j = 1$.

Given two point sets: (1) the *Model* set $X_{M \times D} = (x_1, ..., x_M)^T$ which needs to be moved; (2) the *Scene* set $Y_{N \times D} = (y_1, ..., y_N)^T$ which is fixed. In this paper, we represent a discrete point set by a mixture of AGs where the number of AG components is equivalent to the number of points. Note that all AG components are weighted equally, and all point sets are normalized as distributions with zero mean and unit variance.

2.2 The Robust Point Matching Method

In this article, we select L_2E [17] to estimate the unknown parameters of the transformation between two AG mixtures. The estimation error of L_2E which maximizes the sum of the densities is less than the estimation error of maximum likelihood estimation (MLE) which maximizes the product of the densities. In nonrigid transformation, the transformation f can be solved by minimizing the following cost function:

$$F_{AG}\left(f, \sigma^2, r\right) = \frac{1}{(2\pi\sigma^2)^D ((r+1)/2)^{2D}} - \frac{2}{MN} \sum_{i=1}^{N} \sum_{j=1}^{M} \mathscr{A}\left(y_i - f(x_j)|0, \sigma^2 I, rI\right) \tag{3}$$

where f is the transformation model, $M \leq N$, and I is an identity matrix of size $D \times D$.

Following the idea of TPS-RPM [4], we use a slightly simpler form to estimate the transformation without considering outliers:

$$F_{AG}\left(f,\sigma^2,r\right) = \frac{1}{(2\pi\sigma^2)^D((r+1)/2)^{2D}} - \frac{2}{L}\sum_{l=1}^{L}\mathscr{A}\left(y_l - f\left(x_l\right)|0,\sigma^2 I, rI\right) \quad (4)$$

where L is the number of correspondences and $L \leq M$. y_l, which is recovered from Eq. 3 or other fitting models (e.g., Soft-assignment [4], Shape Context [2]), denotes the correspondence to x_l.

Here we introduce a special space, reproducing kernel Hilbert space (RKHS), and then finding the functional form of the transformation model f using calculus of variation. In RKHS, it is given the *Model* set $X \in \mathbb{R}^D$, the *Scene* set $Y \in \mathbb{R}^D$, and their correspondence set $S = \{(x_1, y_1), ..., (x_L, y_L)\}$. Then we define an RKHS $\mathscr{H}$ with a positive definite kernel function k. In this paper, we use the Gaussian kernel: $k\left(x_i, x_j\right) = \exp\left(-\beta\|x_i - x_j\|^2\right)$, where β is a constant. Thus we can define the kernel matrix K:

$$K = \begin{bmatrix} k\left(x_1, x_1\right) & \dots & k\left(x_1, x_L\right) \\ \vdots & \ddots & \vdots \\ k\left(x_L, x_1\right) & \cdots & k\left(x_L, x_L\right) \end{bmatrix} \quad (5)$$

The transformation function $f \in \mathscr{H}$ can be found by minimizing the following regularized least-squares [1,16]:

$$\varepsilon\left(f\right) = \min_{f \in H} F_{AG}\left(f, \sigma^2, r\right) + \frac{\lambda}{2}\|f\|_K^2 \quad (6)$$

where the first term is the empirical risk and the second term is the Tikhonov regularization [18], $\lambda > 0$ is a trade-off parameter, $\|\cdot\|_K$ denotes a norm in the RKHS. Tikhonov regularization form smoothly trades-off $\|f\|_K^2$ and the empirical risk and solves the ill-posed problem in point matching.

According to the representation theorem [12] and related study in [1,14], the solution of Eq. (6) to the Tikhonov regularization can be written in the following form:

$$f^*\left(\cdot\right) = \sum_{i=1}^{L} h_i K\left(x_i, \cdot\right) \quad (7)$$

for some $h_i \in \mathbb{R}^L$.

Substituting Eq. (7) into the cost function (4), we can therefore rewrite it with the Tikhonov regularization as

$$F_{AG}\left(H, \sigma^2, r\right) = \frac{2^D}{\left(\pi\sigma^2(r+1)^2\right)^D} - \frac{2^{(2+D)/2}}{L\left(\pi\sigma^2(r+1)^2\right)^{D/2}}\Gamma + \frac{\lambda}{2}tr\left(H^T K H\right) \quad (8)$$

where

$$\Gamma = \begin{cases} \exp\left(-\frac{\|Y - KH\|^2}{2\sigma^2}\right) & \text{if } y_i \leq (KH)_i \\ \exp\left(-\frac{\|Y - KH\|^2}{2r^2\sigma^2}\right) & \text{otherwise} \end{cases} \quad (9)$$

and $tr\,(\cdot)$ denotes the trace, $H = (h_1, ..., h_L)^T$ is an coefficient matrix of size $L \times D$.

2.3   Low-Rank Kernel Matrix Approximation

The matrix-valued kernel [12,19] plays an important role in the regularization theory, it provides an easy way to choose an RKHS. However, in this paper, the computational complexity of our method is $O(N^3)$, hopefully, low-rank kernel matrix approximation [11] can yield a large increase in speed with little loss in accuracy. Low-rank kernel matrix approximation $\widehat{K}$ is the closest τ-rank matrix approximation to K and satisfying L_2 and Frobenius norms.

Using eigenvalue decomposition of K, the approximation matrix can be rewritten as:

$$\widehat{K} = Q\Lambda Q^T \tag{10}$$

where Λ is a diagonal matrix of size $\tau \times \tau$ with τ largest eigenvalues and Q is an $L \times \tau$ matrix with the corresponding eigenvectors. The object function of our method therefore can be rewritten as:

$$F_{AG}\left(\widehat{H}, \sigma^2, r\right) = \frac{2^D}{\left(\pi\sigma^2(r+1)^2\right)^D} - \frac{2^{(2+D)/2}}{L\left(\pi\sigma^2(r+1)^2\right)^{D/2}}\widehat{\Gamma} + \frac{\lambda}{2}tr\left(\widehat{H}^T\widehat{K}\widehat{H}\right) \tag{11}$$

where

$$\widehat{\Gamma} = \begin{cases} \exp\left(-\frac{\|Y - U\widehat{H}\|^2}{2\sigma^2}\right) & \text{if } y_i \leq \left(U\widehat{H}\right)_i \\ \exp\left(-\frac{\|Y - U\widehat{H}\|^2}{2r^2\sigma^2}\right) & \text{otherwise} \end{cases} \tag{12}$$

and $U_{L \times \tau} = Q\Lambda$, parameter matrix $\widehat{H}$ of size $\tau \times D$ instead of the original matrix H.

3   Searching for an Optimal Solution

In this paper, the aforementioned cost function is convex in the neighborhood of the optimal position and, most importantly, always differentiable. Thus, the numerical optimization problem can be solved by employing some gradient-based optimization methods, such as quasi-Newton method [15]. The derivative of Eq. (11) with respect to the coefficient matrix $\widehat{H}$ is given by:

$$\frac{\partial F_{AG}}{\partial \widehat{H}} = \lambda U\widehat{H} + \frac{2\widehat{K}}{L\sigma^2(2\pi\sigma^2)^{D/2}((r+1)/2)^D} \begin{cases} V \circ (C \otimes 1) & \text{if } y_i \leq \left(U\widehat{H}\right)_i \\ \frac{1}{r^2}V \circ \left(\widehat{C} \otimes 1\right) & \text{otherwise} \end{cases} \tag{13}$$

where $V = U\widehat{H} - Y, C = \exp\left(diag\left(VV^T\right)/2\sigma^2\right), \widehat{C} = \exp\left(diag\left(VV^T\right)/2r^2\sigma^2\right)$ and 1 is an $1 \times D$ row vector of all ones. $\circ$ denotes the Hadamard product, $\otimes$ denotes the tensor product.

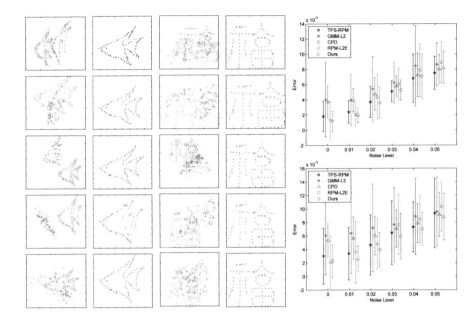

Fig. 2. Experiments on noise. The left figure of each group denotes initial point sets (the *Model* set: blue crosses, the *Scene* set: red circles), and the right figure denotes the registration result of our method. Note that increasing degrees of degradation from top to bottom. The rightmost figure (top: *fish*, bottom: *Chinese character*) is a performance comparison of our results (red circle) with the TPS-RPM (black pentagram), GMM-L_2 (green star), CPD (blue triangle) and RPM-L_2E (magenta square) methods. The error bars indicate the registration error means and standard deviations over 100 random trials (Color figure online).

Finally, we use deterministic annealing introduced by [4,7] which is a useful heuristic method to escape from the trap of local minima. The initialization value of σ^2, r and $\widehat{H}$ are 0.05, 9 and 0, respectively, and we set $\alpha = 0.95$, $\beta = 0.8$, $\lambda = 0.1$, and $\tau = 15$ for our method throughout this paper. Note that the termination condition of iteration is $\sigma^2 < 0.005$.

4   Experiments

In order to evaluate the performance of our method, we implemented it in Matlab and tested it on a laptop with Pentium CPU 2.4 GHz and 4 GB RAM. In this section, we first present the results of point sets qualitatively evaluate our method. Then we quantitatively evaluate our method via registration error which is the average Euclidean distance between the *Model* set and the *Scene* set, and compare our results with several comparative methods: TPS-RPM [4], GMM-L_2 [7], CPD [13,14] and RPM-L_2E [10], which are implemented using publicly available codes.

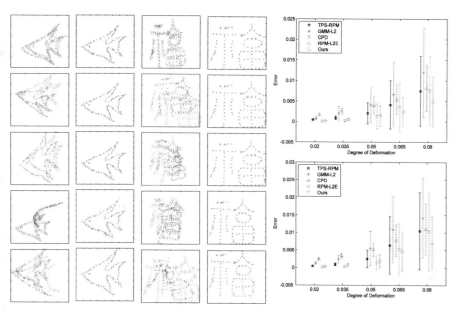

Fig. 3. Experiments on deformation. The left figure of each group denotes initial point sets (the *Model* set: blue crosses, the *Scene* set: red circles), and the right figure denotes the registration result of our method. Note that increasing degrees of degradation from top to bottom. The rightmost figure (top: *fish*, bottom: *Chinese character*) is a performance comparison of our results (red circle) with the TPS-RPM (black pentagram), GMM-L_2 (green star), CPD (blue triangle) and RPM-L_2E (magenta square) methods. The error bars indicate the registration error means and standard deviations over 100 random trials (Color figure online).

4.1 Synthetic Data

We have tested our method on the same data as in [4,10,21] named Chui-Rangarajan synthesized data sets. We chose four sets of the aforementioned data and designed them to evaluate the robustness of a method under 4 degradations: noise, deformation, occlusion and outliers. *Fish* and *Chinese character* shapes of data are used for point set registration, and there are 100 samples in each degradation level.

Noise. The noise, due to the processes of image acquisition and feature extraction are not accurate completely, arising from these processes and leading to the resulting feature points cannot be exactly matched [4]. The second and fourth columns of Fig. 2 show results of two shapes under the noise where its level from 0.01 to 0.05. Observing that when the noise level is large, two point sets are not aligned together perfectly. The rightmost column of Fig. 2 denotes the registration error of ours and the comparative methods on two shapes respectively. The registration results show that errors are becoming larger gradually as increasing

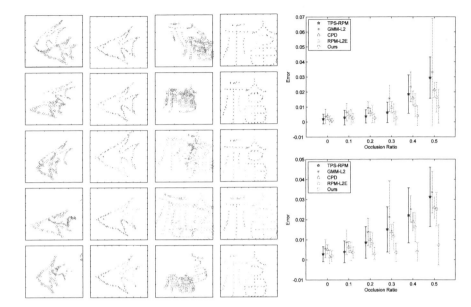

Fig. 4. Experiments on occlusion. The left figure of each group denotes initial point sets (the *Model* set: blue crosses, the *Scene* set: red circles), and the right figure denotes the registration result of our method. Note that increasing degrees of degradation from top to bottom. The rightmost figure (top: *fish*, bottom: *Chinese character*) is a performance comparison of our results (red circle) with the TPS-RPM (black pentagram), GMM-L_2 (green star), CPD (blue triangle) and RPM-L_2E (magenta square) methods. The error bars indicate the registration error means and standard deviations over 100 random trials (Color figure online).

the noise level. Our method and the other four methods have nearly means of registration errors, but our method is slightly more robust than the others by comparing their standard deviations.

Deformation. Nonrigid transformation is quite difficult than rigid. In our method, we use the Gaussian radial basis function (GRBF) to model the transformation. Observing that the registration results of our method are quite well, as shown in the top three rows of Fig. 3, but the fourth and fifth rows show some points drifted because of the large degree of deformation of the given *Model* set. Comparing our results with the other methods, as shown in the rightmost column of Fig. 3, means of errors of our method are less than TPS-RPM's, GMM-L_2's and CPD's clearly. When the degree of deformation is large, such as 0.065 and 0.08, our method outperforms RPM-L_2E.

Occlusion. Occlusion *a.k.a.*, missing points, some point features have no corresponding points in the other point set. In this paper, we follow the idea of TPS-RPM that the missing points are treated as outliers, where the outliers

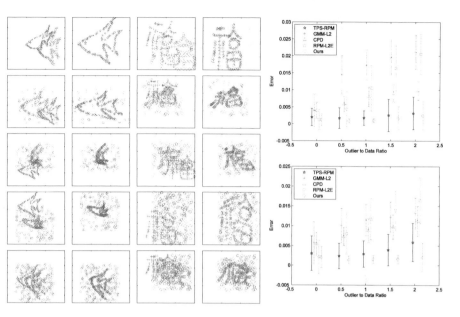

Fig. 5. Experiments on outliers. The left figure of each group denotes initial point sets (the *Model* set: blue crosses, the *Scene* set: red circles), and the right figure denotes the registration result of our method. Note that increasing degrees of degradation from top to bottom. The rightmost figure (top: *fish*, bottom: *Chinese character*) is a performance comparison of our results (red circle) with the TPS-RPM (black pentagram), GMM-L_2 (green star), CPD (blue triangle) and RPM-L_2E (magenta square) methods. The error bars indicate the registration error means and standard deviations over 100 random trials (Color figure online).

satisfy the normal distribution. Observing that input *Model* point set not only contains missing points, but also is deformed in several degrees, as shown in the first and third columns of Fig. 4. Results on the *fish* data, as shown in the second column of Fig. 4, show that almost extra points are aligned correctly. But on the *Chinese character* data, as shown in the fourth column of Fig. 4, the results are not aligned very well, because points on the *Chinese character* shape are not clustered. The rightmost column of Fig. 4 shows the comparison of our results with the comparative methods. The difference between our method and other methods becomes larger as increasing the occlusion ratio. Most importantly, the errors of our method increase much slower than the others.

Outliers. The existence of outliers means many points in one point set that have no corresponding points (homologies) in the other and affects matching results significantly [4]. In this paper, five outlier to data ratios are used: 0, 0.5, 1.0, 1.5, 2.0, and the corresponding results are shown in the second and fourth columns of Fig. 5 respectively. Excitingly, correspondence points are aligned perfectly using our method even in the largest outlier ratio. The comparison of our results

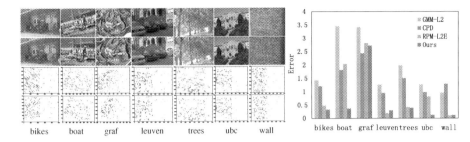

Fig. 6. Experiments on 2D real images. The third figure of each group denotes initial point sets (the *Model* set: blue crosses, the *Scene* set: red circles), and the last figure denotes the registration result of our method. The rightmost figure is a performance comparison of our results with GMM-L_2, CPD and RPM-L_2E methods. The height of each bar indicates the registration error means over 20 random trials (Color figure online).

with other methods, as shown in the rightmost column of Fig. 5, shows that our method outperforms GMM-L_2, CPD and RPM-L_2E significantly and is more robust than TPS-RPM.

4.2   Real Image Data

In this experiment, we select 7 image pairs from the Oxford affine covariant regions data set[1], as shown in the foremost two rows in Fig. 6. There are five different imaging conditions: image blur (bikes and trees), scale changes (boat), multi-viewpoint (graf and wall), JPEG compression (ubc), and illumination (leuven). We extract the SIFT [9] features of those image pairs, and construct initial correspondences using BBF (Best Bin First) method [9], the sparse initialization point sets as shown in the third row of Fig. 6. Note that the point sets do not satisfy arbitrary shapes. The TPS-RPM failed to match and register any point sets, so we did not draw its result in the rightmost figure of Fig. 6.

We repeated the process 20 times, and obtained standard deviations of the methods. GMM-L_2 and CPD are stable without deviations. The standard deviations of RPM-L_2E are 0.21, 0.39, 0.34, 0.03, 0.05, 0.04, 0.02, from left (bikes) to right (wall). However, the standard deviations of our method are almost zeros except the image pairs of graf (std: 0.52). The comparison of our results with other methods shows that our method outperforms GMM-L_2, CPD and RPM-L_2E significantly in most cases.

5   Conclusion

In this paper, we focus on the case of degradations in point matching problem. Under the previous work of literatures [3–7,10,14,21], we introduce a novel robust method for point matching. There are many registration methods based

---

[1] http://www.robots.ox.ac.uk/~vgg/data/.

the Gaussian model, while the asymmetric Gaussian model experimented more accurate than the former in this paper, such as comparing the proposed method with GMM-L_2 and RPM-L_2E which use Gaussian. Moreover, as pointed out in [8], asymmetric Gaussian can capture more accurate spatially asymmetric distributions than Gaussian. In addition, we choose L_2E [17], a robust estimator between two densities, to estimate the similarity between two input point sets. We use low-rank kernel matrix approximation to speed up our method. Note that our method is different with graph matching method [22], because the focus of our method is on the estimation robustness to noise, deformation, occlusion and outliers, while the latter one is mainly used to recover the correspondences accurately. Experimental results on synthetic and real image data illustrate that our proposed method outperforms the comparative methods. Future work includes validating our method on large number of data sets and applying it to many applications, *e.g.*, image retrieval, and 3D image registration.

Acknowledgement. This work was supported by National Natural Science Foundation of China (NSFC, No. 61103070).

References

1. Baldassarre, L., Rosasco, L., Barla, A., Verri, A.: Vector field learning via spectral filtering. In: Balcázar, J.L., Bonchi, F., Gionis, A., Sebag, M. (eds.) ECML PKDD 2010, Part I. LNCS, vol. 6321, pp. 56–71. Springer, Heidelberg (2010)
2. Belongie, S., Malik, J., Puzicha, J.: Shape matching and object recognition using shape contexts. IEEE Trans. Pattern Anal. Mach. Intell. **24**, 509–522 (2002)
3. Besl, P.J., McKay, N.D.: A method for registration of 3-D shapes. IEEE Trans. Pattern Anal. Mach. Intell. **14**, 239–256 (1992)
4. Chui, H., Rangarajan, A.: A new point matching algorithm for non-rigid registration. Comput. Vis. Image Underst. **89**, 114–141 (2003)
5. Granger, S., Pennec, X.: Multi-scale EM-ICP: a fast and robust approach for surface registration. In: Heyden, A., Sparr, G., Nielsen, M., Johansen, P. (eds.) ECCV 2002, Part IV. LNCS, vol. 2353, pp. 418–432. Springer, Heidelberg (2002)
6. Huang, X., Paragios, N., Metaxas, D.N.: Shape registration in implicit spaces using information theory and free form deformations. IEEE Trans. Pattern Anal. Mach. Intell. **28**, 1303–1318 (2006)
7. Jian, B., Vemuri, B.C.: Robust point set registration using gaussian mixture models. IEEE Trans. Pattern Anal. Mach. Intell. **33**, 1633–1645 (2011)
8. Kato, T., Omachi, S., Aso, H.: Asymmetric Gaussian and its application to pattern recognition. In: Caelli, T.M., Amin, A., Duin, R.P.W., Kamel, M.S., de Ridder, D. (eds.) SPR 2002 and SSPR 2002. LNCS, vol. 2396, pp. 405–413. Springer, Heidelberg (2002)
9. Lowe, D.G.: Distinctive image features from scale-invariant keypoints. Int. J. Comput. Vis. **60**, 91–110 (2004)
10. Ma, J., Zhao, J., Tian, J., Tu, Z., Yuille, A.L.: Robust estimation of nonrigid transformation for point set registration. In: IEEE Conference on Computer Vision and Pattern Recognition (CVPR), IEEE, pp. 2147–2154 (2013)
11. Markovsky, I., Usevich, K.: Low Rank Approximation. Springer, London (2012)

12. Micchelli, C.A., Pontil, M.: On learning vector-valued functions. Neural Comput. **17**, 177–204 (2005)
13. Myronenko, A., Song, X., Carreira-Perpinn, M.A.: Non-rigid point set registration: coherent point drift. Adv. Neural Inf. Process. Syst. **19**, 1009–1016 (2007)
14. Myronenko, A., Song, X.: Point set registration: coherent point drift. IEEE Trans. Pattern Anal. Mach. Intell. **32**, 2262–2275 (2010)
15. Nocedal, J., Wright, S.J.: Conjugate Gradient Methods. Springer, New York (2006)
16. Chui, H., Rangarajan, A.: Regularized least-squares classification. Nato Sci. Ser. Sub Ser. III Comput. Syst. Sci. **190**, 131–154 (2003)
17. Scott, D.W.: Parametric statistical modeling by minimum integrated square error. Technometrics **43**, 274–285 (2001)
18. Tikhonov, A.N., Arsenin, V.I., John, F.: Solutions of Ill-Posed Problems. Winston, Washington, DC (1977)
19. Tschumperle, D., Deriche, R.: Vector-valued image regularization with PDEs: a common framework for different applications. IEEE Trans. Pattern Anal. Mach. Intell. **27**, 506–517 (2005)
20. Tsin, Y., Kanade, T.: A correlation-based approach to robust point set registration. In: Pajdla, T., Matas, J.G. (eds.) ECCV 2004. LNCS, vol. 3023, pp. 558–569. Springer, Heidelberg (2004)
21. Zheng, Y., Doermann, D.: Robust point matching for nonrigid shapes by preserving local neighborhood structures. IEEE Trans. Pattern Anal. Mach. Intell. **28**, 643–649 (2006)
22. Scott, D.W.: Deformable graph matching. In: IEEE Conference on Computer Vision and Pattern Recognition (CVPR), IEEE, pp. 2922–2929 (2013)

Multiple Object Tracking
by Efficient Graph Partitioning

Ratnesh Kumar$^{(\boxtimes)}$, Guillaume Charpiat, and Monique Thonnat

STARS Team, INRIA, Sophia Antipolis, France
fnu.ratnesh_kumar@inria.fr

Abstract. In this paper, we view multiple object tracking as a graph partitioning problem. Given any object detector, we build the graph of all detections and aim to partition it into trajectories. To quantify the similarity of any two detections, we consider local cues such as point tracks and speed, global cues such as appearance, as well as intermediate ones such as trajectory straightness. These different clues are dealt jointly to make the approach robust to detection mistakes (missing or extra detections). We thus define a Conditional Random Field and optimize it using an efficient combination of message passing and move-making algorithms. Our approach is fast on video batch sizes of hundreds of frames. Competitive and stable results on varied videos demonstrate the robustness and efficiency of our approach.

1 Introduction

The tracking of objects, persons or animals is required for high-level vision inference systems, from action recognition to animal behavior analysis. Other applications of tracking include video editing, *e.g.* inpainting, wherein a good tracking system can help in reducing the manual effort to annotate the parts of the video to keep or to remove.

In this paper, we address the problem of multiple person tracking in videos obtained from a single camera. We suppose that we are already given person detections in each frame, from any pre-trained detector. This detector is not assumed to be perfect, but may produce false negatives (persons missed) and false positives (extraneous detections). Our objective is to group detections into consistent trajectories, as well as to eliminate false negatives and false positives.

Tracking algorithms can be broadly divided into two categories: online and batch-based. Online methods infer the object state using the current frame and the previous ones; this can be achieved for instance with particle filtering [1]. On the opposite, batch-based tracking considers the entire temporal sequence at once, or at least a significant part of it (hundreds of frames). Such methods are also referred to as global tracking. Our approach belongs to the latter class, hence we focus on related work in the realm of batch-based tracking.

Global tracking should be in principle less prone to identity switches (confusion of several different persons) than online approaches, and provide better occlusion management as they have both present and future frames available

© Springer International Publishing Switzerland 2015
D. Cremers et al. (Eds.): ACCV 2014, Part IV, LNCS 9006, pp. 445–460, 2015.
DOI: 10.1007/978-3-319-16817-3_29

to determine the state of objects. This extra information brought by the 2D+T volume has led to the development of many different approaches utilizing all kinds of color and motion clues, as well as many different optimization methods. We discuss below some of the recent notable ones [2–11].

Reference [4] computes cliques on a graph of detection responses to find object trajectories. False negatives and occlusions are handled using hypothetical nodes by assuming linear motion of the object. Reference [5] presents another data association approach, based on maximum weight independent sets, to merge tracklets of length 2 to compute full trajectories. Reference [6] uses a network flow based approach to obtain person trajectories and incorporates an explicit occlusion handling mechanism to provide information such as *object i is occluded by object j*. The work by [9] also uses a network flow based model similar to [6]. By greedily computing shortest path problems, they reach near-linear time complexity in computing the global minimum of successive sub-problems, which however doesn't guarantee a global optimum on the real global problem.

Most network flow models suffer from the disadvantage that possible occlusions or false negatives are not handled from the start, but in a post-processing step by introducing iteratively new nodes in the graph, which asks for re-iterating the optimization process until convergence. Importantly all network flow approaches and [5] do not incorporate acceleration information for computing trajectories. Acceleration knowledge is vital for ensuring smooth velocity in trajectories, and at least three nodes (*i.e.* detections) located at different time frames are required to compute acceleration. Recently a proof-of-concept work by [12] have shown that a network flow model can only deal with pairwise factors and hence cannot incorporate a third (or higher order) factor. Reference [13] extends a typical network flow model by adding higher order connections. However in doing so they have to resort to a relaxation (discrete to continuous) based optimization scheme, as the model can no longer be minimized by efficient network flow approaches. For time critical vision applications such as tracking, a discrete to continuous relaxation approach should be avoided, as these do not provide a usable solution at all instants during their run times, and stopping the optimizer to meet time requirements might return a non usable solution.

Works by [2,3] use a discrete-continuous optimization model to optimize detections and trajectories. They incorporate statistical data analysis to compute the parameters of the energy along with adding exclusion constraints at both trajectory and detection levels. However for this they use an already-performed tracking (from [9]) as input to their approach. Hence these works should rather be seen as trajectory-refinement process.

All of the above approaches including our proposed approach is categorized as *tracking using detections* in the literature. Instead of using detections, [8] uses *probabilistic occupancy maps* obtained from a background subtraction process. Subsequently the scene space is discretized into grid cells, and targets are forced to move along the grid. A global optimum for this model is computed using K-Shortest Paths. This scene discretization is possible only for situations wherein the camera calibration parameters are known, and hence cannot be applied to moving camera scenarios. This approach is computationally fast but is prone to identity switches. Global appearance constraints are added by [7] to provide robustness to identity switches.

Another relevant aspect of tracking algorithms is their computational cost in practice. Most approaches performing well [2–4,7] mention speeds of several seconds per frame. In contrast we will show an appreciable gain of speed (factor 10), with near real time performance in complicated videos. Also, [4,7] require a lot of memory and consequently cannot handle batches of many frames (typically 50), while we do not suffer from memory consumption and will consider blocks of several hundreds of frames.

With respect to the literature, our approach has the following advantages:

- A principled way of unifying natural constraints that arise in tracking.
- Thanks to an apt combination of optimizers (Sect. 3.1), a novel triplet search for trajectory-curvature penalization (Sect. 2.5), and graph reduction (Sect. 3.2), the proposed approach is computationally efficient (in terms of both memory and time), and can operate on hundreds of frames of HD videos on a simple machine.
- Last, but not least, the proposed tracker is self contained and unlike [2,3], we do not require beforehand trajectories from an external tracker.

Following sections introduce our proposed model and the optimizers used. Subsequently Sect. 4 elaborates on experimental results and processing times.

2 Model

A reliable tracking model should have the following criteria:

(C_1) **Uniqueness:** An object label (identity) should never appear more than once inside any frame over the whole sequence (*cf.* Sect. 2.2).

(C_2) **Smooth Trajectories:** The trajectory of each object should be as smooth as possible in time. In particular, there should not be jumps in an object location in consecutive frames (*cf.* Sects. 2.2 & 2.5).

(C_3) **Robustness to Occlusions and False Negatives:** The trajectories should not be lost or confused during occlusions or when several detections are missed (*cf.* Sects. 2.3 & 2.4).

(C_3) **No Ghost Objects:** False Positives from the detector should be removed and not form output trajectories (*cf.* Sect. 3.4).

The incorporation of these traits into our model will be discussed in the following sections.

2.1   Approach and Formalization

A person detector is used to obtain detection responses for all frames of a batch. We then build a graph $G = (V, E)$ whose nodes correspond to detection responses. Our aim is to find an optimal partition of G such that each part corresponds to the trajectory of one person. The notations used in the paper are presented below:

L: Number of possible labels (i.e. of graph parts).
$\mathcal{X}$: Set of all possible partitions $\subset L^{|V|}$.
i: A node of the graph, *i.e.* a person detection.
x_i: Label of the node i, to be found.
w_{ij}: Edge weight between nodes i and j (benefit for them to have same label).

For a set of L labels, each of the $|V|$ nodes can then take any of L states. A labeling $\mathbf{x} = (x_i)_{i \in V} \in \mathcal{X}$ then defines a partition of V into subsets T_l assigned to each class $l \in L$. The quality of such a labeling, to be maximized, is the sum of weighted edges connecting vertices with the same label:

$$\operatorname*{argmax}_{\mathbf{x} \in \mathcal{X}} \sum_{ij} w_{ij}\, \delta_{x_i = x_j} \quad = \quad \operatorname*{argmin}_{\mathbf{x} \in \mathcal{X}} \sum_{ij} w_{ij}\, \delta_{x_i \neq x_j}$$

In the following sections, we will define the quantities relevant to the problem of tracking, and show how to set the interaction terms w_{ij} to express them.

2.2 Repulsive Constraints

Adhering to the criterion C_1, it is imperative to have repulsive constraints in the model. The goal of these constraints is to prevent nodes in a same frame from being allocated the same label. To this end we set repulsive constraints by assigning huge negative weights w_{ij} between all pairs of detections (i, j) from the same frames. We refer to this as *intra-frame* repulsive constraint.

In regard to C_2, the tracker should also prevent objects from jumping from one location in a frame to a complete different location in the next frame. Otherwisely said, two nodes far apart in consecutive frames should not have the same label. To this end, we define a maximum object speed ($4\,\mathrm{m/s}$) and set highly negative weights w_{ij} between detections (i, j) in consecutive frames if the speed required for such a displacement is higher. The speed between two such detections is converted from pixels/frame into m/s by multiplying them with the factor $2f/\min(H_i, H_j)$, where f is the frame rate and where H_i is the height (in pixels) of the bounding box of detection i. Indeed, $H_i/2$ is a simple yet practical and sufficient approximation of the number of pixels per meter, and it has the advantage of adapting automatically to the depth in the video. We denote these no-jump constraints as *inter-frame* constraints (*cf.* Middle Inset in Fig. 1).

2.3 Temporal Neighborhoods and Point Tracks

Motion estimates for each detection provide vital information regarding its possible temporal neighbors. Without such estimates, temporal neighborhoods could become significantly big, which in turn would restrict the amount of frames processed in one batch due to a larger number of variables. Moreover, detections may be infrequent (false negatives) and may contain false positives, which prevents obtaining good motion estimates.

Owing to these reasons we do not rely only on the location of the detections, but instead we use point tracks, which provide motion estimates on a pixel

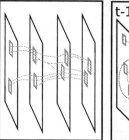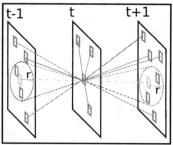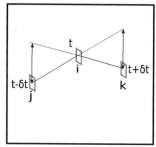

Fig. 1. Left: Point Tracks and detections. **Middle:** High repulsive exclusion constraints, shown for the central green bounding box in frame t, with **red** edges. Intra-frame repulsive constraints prevent this detection from having the same label as any other detection in the same frame t, while inter-frame repulsive constraints prevent it from having the same label as detections in previous and next frames $t-1$, $t+1$ that are too far. The maximum radius **r** is detection-dependent, in that it corresponds to the maximum physically-plausible displacement within a duration of one frame, and that speed estimation depends on object depth. **Right:** Computing the trajectory straightness for a triplet of detections j, i, k at the temporal scale δt (*cf.* sec 2.5) (Color figure online).

(or sub-pixellic) level. The proportion $F(i, j)$ of common point tracks between two nodes i and j, i.e. of points tracks which go through two given bounding boxes B_i and B_j from different times, defines a first similarity measure between these nodes. This similarity measure has the advantage of being robust to false detections (positive as negative) that occur between the two nodes. Also, in the case of partial occlusions, point tracks on the non-occluded part will still manage to follow the object and define a meaningful similarity, while overlapping detections make appearance-based affinities noisy in such partial occlusion cases.

2.4 Appearance Connections

In the previous sections, apart from defining repulsive constraints, we have added connections between the nodes which share common point tracks, as an incentive for them to choose the same label and consequently be part of the trajectory of the same object. But point tracks most often do not cover the full temporal span of the video and tracks may get lost or confused (aperture problem) after some time due to occlusion or pose changes. This calls for the need of *long temporal range connections* in the graph. To define such a similarity between detections from any frames, possibly far apart in time, we consider the appearance of objects. To cater this, we compute an appearance feature for each bounding box, and cluster these appearances into L groups using K-means. The appearance cluster of node i is denoted by A_i. The appearance similarity between any nodes belonging to a same cluster is then defined as a constant weight $\beta > 0$, while the one between nodes from different cluster is 0, which will lead to the quantity $\beta\, \delta_{A_i = A_j}$ in Eq. 3. For appearance clustering we do not need to know

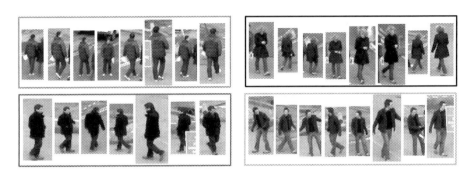

Fig. 2. Sample appearance clusters for PETS09 S2L1: Each box encloses a few samples belonging to the same cluster. Notice that the clustering is robust to scale changes.

the exact number of objects in the scene, as over-clustering is not an issue with our approach. In our experiments we set L to twice the maximum number of detections observed in a single frame of the current video batch.

The appearance feature for a detection is based on the histogram of colors inside the detection The distance between two appearances is computed by the L_2 norm between features. Figure 2 shows a few clusters from a PETS09 [14] video.

2.5   Favoring Smooth Trajectories

When the trajectories of people with a similar appearance cross each other, and that, in plus, full occlusion or detection mistakes (false positives or negatives) occur at this crossing, then the tracking based on the previous quantities may fail and induce small jumps in location or identity switches. This can be mitigated by *penalizing high curvature* of the trajectories. To this end we define an energy term which favors smooth trajectories, involving three detections j, i, k from different frames regularly spaced in time $(t - \delta t, t, t + \delta t)$, as shown in Right-most inset of Fig. 1. Given such detections, we compute a triplet factor $R(i, j, k)$ expressing the regularity of the associated trajectory. It is based on the Laplacian of the centroids p_i of the three bounding boxes:

$$\Delta_{ijk} = \frac{f}{H_i \, \delta t} \, \|p_j + p_k - 2p_i\| \tag{1}$$

and is expressed as:

$$R(i, j, k) = \frac{1}{\sqrt{\delta t}} \, \max(\tau - \Delta_{ijk}, \, 0) \tag{2}$$

Note that the Laplacian was normalized in order to be invariant to the video resolution and to the time interval, using the frame rate f, the frame interval δt

and the bounding box height H_i used as previously as a depth/resolution indicator. R denotes the benefit for the triplet j, i, k to belong to a same trajectory. The threshold τ indicates the maximum speed difference, or curvature, above which there is no gain. Note that $\tau = 1 \, \text{m/s}^2$ is video-invariant.

Considering all triplets in the graph is computationally prohibitive as there are $|V|^3$ possible triplets ($|V|^2$ symmetrical triplets). Furthermore searching only temporally successive triplets ($\delta t = 1$) would be sensitive to missed detections. Thus we compute $R(i, j, k)$ on various temporal scales, with $\delta t \in \{1, 2, 3, 4, 5, 10\}$. As object trajectory is more predictable at shorter temporal ranges, we decrease the importance of the smoothness assumption for longer time spans with the factor $1/\sqrt{\delta t}$.

Unlike [3], which requires the knowledge of trajectory proposals for curvature penalization, we model curvature penalization using an apt triplet search, thus making our model as unified and self contained as possible.

3 Optimization

Summing up all quantities defined in the previous section, we obtain the following similarity criterion to maximize over possible labellings $\mathbf{x}$:

$$S(\mathbf{x}) = \alpha \sum_{ij} F(i, j) \, \delta_{x_i = x_j} + \beta \sum_{ij} \delta_{A_i = A_j} \, \delta_{x_i = x_j}$$
$$+ \gamma \sum_{ijk} R(i, j, k) \, \delta^T_{x_i, x_j, x_k} - \Omega \sum_{(i,j) \in \mathcal{C}} \delta_{x_i = x_j} \tag{3}$$

where $\delta_{\text{true}} = 1$ and $\delta_{\text{false}} = 0$, where $\delta^T_{x_i, x_j, x_k} = \frac{1}{3} \left(\delta_{x_i = x_j} + \delta_{x_i = x_k} + \delta_{x_j = x_k} \right)$ is a good 2nd-order approximation of $\delta_{x_i = x_j = x_k}$. $\mathcal{C}$ denotes the set of all pairwise inter-frame or intra-frame constraints, and $\Omega > 0$ is sufficiently high to be dissuasive. Maximizing $S(\mathbf{x})$ in (3) is equivalent to minimizing $E(\mathbf{x}) = -S(\mathbf{x})$. Note that if one denotes by $\mathcal{X}$ the set of feasible labellings, i.e. satisfying all constraints, then solving $\text{argmin}_{\mathbf{x} \in L^V} E(\mathbf{x})$ with high Ω is equivalent to solving $\text{argmin}_{\mathbf{x} \in \mathcal{X}} E(\mathbf{x})$ with $\Omega = 0$, and that $E(\mathbf{x})$ in this latter formulation is submodular on $\mathcal{X}$, but to our knowledge there is no optimizer dedicated to the minimization of submodular functions over arbitrary sets.

3.1 Optimizers

The criterion (3) is a non-submodular Conditional Random Field, and a host of available optimization techniques can be employed. This section aims at providing a concise overview on selecting optimizers for $E(\mathbf{x})$.

Heuristic approaches such as Tabu Search (used by [4]) or Simulated Annealing can be used to optimize (3). However these suffer from at least two notable problems to applied to a tracking model. Firstly, they do not provide any indication certifying the vicinity of a solution from optimal. Secondly, in time critical applications it is often desirable to use techniques which can provide a usable solution (*i.e.* a solution satisfying all constraints) whenever required. These heuristic approaches along with relaxation techniques (*e.g.* Lagrangian relaxation), Polyhedral methods, do not provide a usable solution at all time instants of their operation. In a recent work by [15], the authors show that combinatorial methods (such as Integer Linear Programming, Max Cut using Reweighted Perfect Matching) based on branch-and-bound and cutting plane techniques do not scale well with the problem size.

Therefore we employ a fast message passing variant: Tree Re-Weighted Message Passing (**TRW-S**) [16]. TRW-S considers the full graph for labeling and provides good optima (along with the optimality bound). To make further improvements, we design local moves based on an Iterated Conditional Modes (ICM) that will satisfy the constraints and are likely to be useful.

ICM [17] is an iterative procedure, wherein an optimum labeling for a variable is chosen conditioned on all other variables. The process is repeated for all variables until convergence. Owing to this local nature of moves it is practically difficult for ICM to find a usable solution from scratch. However with a good initialization, ICM can find more meaningful solutions quickly. [18] proposed a variant of ICM: Lazy Flipper (**LF**). As opposed to ICM, a LF takes into account a large connected subset of variables up to a prescribed size. Upon convergence, the LF's labeling is guaranteed to be optimal within a Hamming distance equal to the subgraph size.

Inspired from LF, we search for flips of variables which reduce the energy, by considering a single variable or a subset of variables at a time. For a given subset size we repeat the above process until the energy cannot be reduced further. We also limit our search to only those subsets of variables which have a joint temporal distance of less than 20 frames, i.e. the maximum time scale in triplets. This structural information incorporation brings significant computational speed up on this part of the optimization process.

Notice that this flipper is different from the Block-ICM proposed by [12]. The authors in [12] sweep in a temporally forward manner, and check for flips *locally* in two frames. The flipper in our approach is more general as the nodes considered for flips have no time ordering restrictions. Furthermore as an ICM is susceptible to initialization [12], we provide a good usable solution satisfying all constraints to our flipper, obtained from TRW-S.

We experimented with recently proposed optimizers based on dual decomposition [19] and linear programming relaxations [20]. Both these techniques were excruciatingly slow on finding one usable solution.

3.2   Graph Reduction

Point tracks can be used to reduce the initial graph, and consequently speed up the optimization, by fusing nodes for which there is no tracking ambiguity. More precisely, two nodes are fused if *all* point tracks inside both bounding boxes move into one another. When fusing nodes i and j, their edge weights (towards any other node k) are accumulated, as in Fig. 3 : $w_{\{ij\},k} = w_{ik} + w_{jk}$. Thus the criterion optimized does not change.

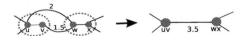

Fig. 3. Graph reduction by fusing nodes u,v and w,x.

The ratio of the fused graph size to the original size translates directly to the optimization speed, as we observe a reduction in the computational cost by the same ratio. Figure 4 shows a simple illustration for the speed gain due to this graph reduction step (*cf.* Fig. 4 caption for details).

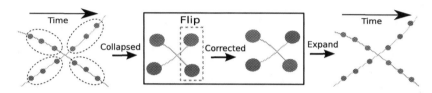

Fig. 4. Graph reduction and flipper speed gain. Leftmost drawing shows the labeling of 12 nodes. Node colors indicate a labeling (stuck at a local minima) and the colored lines (*green* and *yellow*) correspond to the groundtruth trajectories. Middle inset drawing shows the reduced graph by fusing nodes inside the *dotted* ellipse in the Leftmost drawing (*cf.* Sect. 3.2). Since the graph is reduced, we only need to search for flips of subgraphs of size = 2 (*i.e.* $O(|V|^2)$), instead of enumerating over all possible subgraphs of size = 6 (*i.e.* $O(|V|^6)$). The subgraph-flip required to correct the initial labeling is shown by *magenta* colored rectangular box in the middle inset. The Rightmost drawing correspond to the final correct output in the original graph (Color figure online).

3.3 Parameter Setting

We have three constant factors in CRF, namely α, β and γ (*cf.* Eq. (3)). These have to be set considering the relative importance of each term, and this setting should be as invariant to videos as possible. We set $\Omega = 1000000$, sufficiently high to enforce repulsive constraints. The rationale in setting these parameters is outlined below.

- The main contribution of point tracks is to obtain motion estimates which help in fusing the graph. On the fused graph, the nodes are either close to occlusion vicinity or false negatives. In both these situations, we need to look at appearance and trajectory curvature in time to decide about the labeling. Hence we set more weight on triplets and appearance clusters.
- Near occlusion vicinity, it is important to consider both motion difference and appearance. However trajectory curvature in short temporal scale should have higher weight than appearance due to following reasons: Firstly, trajectories are not supposed to change their path substantially in course of a few frames, and secondly, the appearance of persons can be similar either due to the presence of noise or persons having the same appearance. Hence $\beta = 0.5$ is set lower than $\gamma = 50$, with $\alpha = 0.01$. A small perturbation of these values while respecting the relative order does not change the results.

3.4   Graph Cleaning

After solving the optimization on a batch, any temporal gap along a trajectory due to false negatives is filled by assuming linear motion between the closest detected bounding boxes on either side of the temporal axis. False positives from detections usually form short trajectories and with long temporal gaps, and these tracks are removed.

Streaming Trajectory Computation is performed using a sliding window approach, with an overlap of 15 frames from the previous batch.

4   Experimental Results and Evaluation

Comparative quantitative evaluation is challenging due to the lack of benchmark datasets, such as [21] for optical flow evaluation purpose. For our evaluation purposes, we use the metrics proposed by [6][1]. Recently, [22] has thrown light on the ambiguities in evaluation due to dissimilarities in groundtruth annotations and evaluation codes used by different tracking approaches. Taking these ambiguities into account we provide other relevant information, *e.g.* type of detector, groundtruth and the code used for computing the metrics.

4.1   Evaluation Metrics

- **Recall:** % of correct detections w.r.t. total detections in groundtruth.
- **Precision:** % of correct detections w.r.t. total detections in tracking.
- **FAF:** False alarms per frame. **GT:** Number of trajectories in groundtruth.
- **MT:** Number of trajectories successfully tracked for >80 % of their groundtruth time span. **ML:** Number of trajectories successfully tracked for <20 % of their groundtruth time span.
- **IDS:** Number of times a tracked trajectory changes its matched id.

Other widely adopted metrics are Multiple Object Tracking Accuracy/Precision (MOTA and MOTP) [23]. MOTA takes into account the number of false positives, false negatives and IDS. MOTP quantifies the average distance between the groundtruth and the estimated target locations. MOTA is the preferred metric for us as we do not change the locations of input detections.

4.2   Results and Discussion

We consider videos from public datasets for evaluation. TRW-S is run for a fixed number of iterations (50), and the output is then optimized by the flipper. **All our results are obtained with the same unique set of parameters.**

PETS Dataset: We use the S2L1 view. This video is challenging due to non linear motion, and persons of similar appearances occluding each other[2]. With global

---

[1] We use the code provided by [2] to compute these metrics.
[2] Detections from http://iris.usc.edu/people/yangbo/downloads.html.

Table 1. Comparison with the recent proposed approaches on PETS S2L1 Video. The metrics on the first and last row are obtained using the same code, while middle ones are taken from the respective papers as their result files are unavailable.

Method	Rec	Prec	FAF	GT	MT	ML	IDS	MOTA(3D)	MOTA(2D)
Milan et al. [3]	96.9	94.1	0.36	19	18	0	22	90	83.6
Shitrit et al. [7]	-	-	-	-	-	-	19	-	82
Berclaz et al. [8]	-	-	-	-	-	-	28	-	80
Zamir et al. [4]	-	69.4	-	-	-	-	8	-	90.3
Ours	95.8	90.8	**0.28**	19	18	0	13	**90**	81.8

appearance features, we are able to keep the same ID for persons exiting and re-entering the scene (*cf.* Fig. 5).

We observe (Table 1) that our approach performs well and is on par or better with the best in the metrics. At the same time our approach is much faster (*cf.* Sect. 4.3) and **do not rely** on external tracker as [3] or camera calibration as [3,7,8]. Also the model of [3] has 11 parameters and requires an explicit parameter estimation step for a video. [4] uses Tabu Search on their model and hence guarantees of a stable output on multiple runs are minimal. Moreover [4] do not cater to a proper video streaming, as merging trajectories from batches is based on solving a clique problem by considering multiple batches. Typically better cliques can be found if more batches are considered for merging, which in turn adds to the latency time.

Usefulness of Triplets: Triplets are necessary to maintain consistent identities in time. Indeed without using *triplets*, our results for MOTA (3D) would decrease to 84.4 and the *identity switches* would increase to 35.

Towncenter Dataset: For the evaluation on HD videos with higher person density, we consider Towncenter video [11]. The groundtruth, result and detection files can be obtained from the webpage of [11]. We achieve competitive MOTA[3] (*cf.* Table 3, Fig. 7). [11] uses a head detector along with motion estimates to make precise the location of body and head bounding boxes, hence achieves higher MOTP. Also [11] requires camera calibration and a parameter estimation step which takes several hours.

Although [24] is a frame-by-frame method, we compare to this approach as the output files are available, and as it outperforms other previous approaches. While being competitive, we are 6 times faster on a single core implementation than the dual core implementation of [24].

Optimizer Scaling w.r.t. Problem Size: With this proposed combination of optimizers on a batch of 400 frames (with a high density of 15 persons/frame), we achieve competitive MOTA as shown in Table 2. The maximum memory consumed by our algorithm is under 6 GB, demonstrating the memory efficiency.

---

[3] MOTA code from https://github.com/glisanti/CLEAR-MOT.

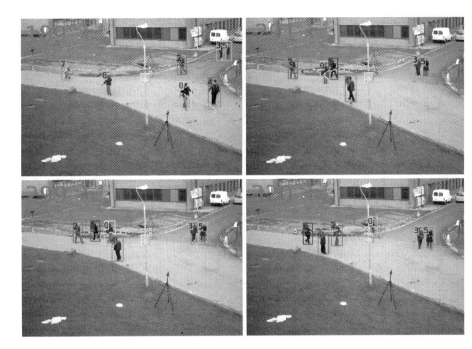

Fig. 5. Consistent tracks before and after occlusion: Frame numbers are shown on Top-Left of each image. The dotted points show the trajectories of bounding boxes in previous and successive frames. To reduce clutter in display, we show 3 trajectories and their *few* previous and future locations. Owing to the global appearance incorporation, **ID 4 is kept intact** for the person as he leaves and comes back in the view. This immaculate consistency in identities during crossing is obtained due to *triplet factors*.

Table 2. Results on a crowded batch of 400 frames. There are 6000 detections in this batch starting at the 450th frame.

Towncenter			
Method	MOTA	MOTP	Detector
Benfold et al. [11]	55.8	84.4	[11]
Zhang et al. [24]	66.4	75.2	[11]
Ours	66.5	75.8	[11]

Table 3. Results for first 1000 frames (50 frame batches). Competitive accuracy is obtained at **6x** faster speed.

Towncenter			
Method	MOTA	MOTP	Detector
[11]	55.9	84.7	[11]
[24]	64.9	76.4	[11]
Ours	64.6	75.0	[11]

Stable Output on Multiple Runs: We performed 5 trials on 50 frame batches for the first 1000 frames, and obtain a stable MOTA with a standard deviation of 0.7. In these trials we stop the optimizer to meet a requirement of **5–10 fps** (by stopping the flipper). Such stability guarantees can not be provided by heuristic (or stochastic) optimization approaches *e.g.* Tabu Search.

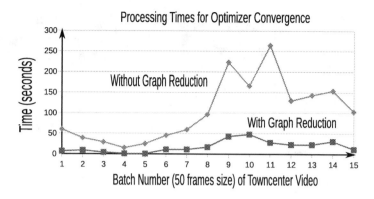

Fig. 6. Processing time improvement using graph reduction (similar MOTA in both cases), for the first 15 batches. High processing times from batch 8 to 12 are due to high detection rate/frame. In the above cases we let the optimizer run until convergence.

Usefulness of Point Tracks: Point tracks are an integral part of many vision systems. For our tracking system, point tracks help in reducing the graph and in-turn aid in swift convergence of our optimizer. On standard GPUs, optical flow based point-tracker such as [25] and the KLT based point-tracker from [26] provide dense point tracks at 25 fps and 200 fps, respectively for high resolution videos. Moreover as ours is a batch based tracker, a simple dual-threaded implementation with a dedicated thread for computation of point tracks for the successive batch can remove any probable latency. In order to demonstrate the advantage of graph reduction, we consider the complete batch of 794 frames of the PETS S2L1 video, with or without the graph reduction step (*cf.* Table 4). We observe a **4x** increase in efficiency with the graph reduction step. Similar comparative details on Towncenter video can be seen in Fig. 6.

Table 4. Usefulness of graph reduction: PETS S2L1 computation times (in **seconds**) for the cases when the graph reduction step is either chosen (*Row 1*) or discarded (*Row 2*). The column **App + k-means**, shows cumulative times for both appearance feature computation and clustering. The quantitative results for both rows are similar.

Batch Size (Number of Frames)	$App+k$-means	TRW-S	Flipper	Total	Memory
794 (With Graph Reduction)	35	95	370	**500**	2.5 GB
794 (Without Graph Reduction)	35	350	1500	**1885**	5 GB

4.3 Processing Time

Computational times are one of the major factors in choosing a tracking algorithm. Comparing exact running times is challenging, as peers often do not provide them (nor the code) or quote only average times over a set of varied videos. Our optimizer takes 0.01 s/frame on average for 50 frames batches

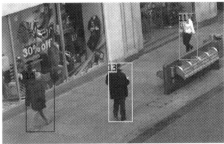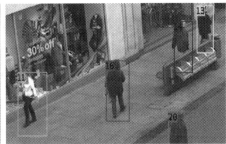

Fig. 7. Consistent people crossing over a span of **134** frames. The above images are cropped to show the crossing.

(8 persons/frame, PETS S2L1) on a **single 2.4 GHz core**, which is **100x** faster than the best case of [3] in 2013. The run time of optimizer from [3] is 1–2 s/frame. The average run time for [4] optimizer is 4.4 s/frame on **four** 2.4 GHz cores. On videos similar to PETS S2L1, [7] takes 4s/frame on 3 GHz CPU. Table 5 shows computational efficiency of our approach w.r.t. recent approaches.

We perform optimization at a speed of 5–11 fps (on 50 frames batches the Towncenter with 10–17 persons/frame), which is **20x–40x** faster than the 4-core implementation of [4], and **6x–10x** faster than the 2-core implementation of [24]. [11] achieves a real time performance on Towncenter using parallel CPU implementation, however the tracking accuracy is significantly lower than us.

Table 5. Approximate comparison of computation times for PETS S2L1, showing a significant positive gap between ours and state-of-the-art approaches in terms of speed *vs.* accuracy.

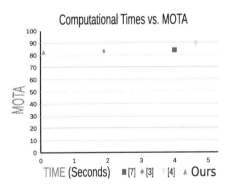

Table 6. State-of-the-art approaches and their incorporation of local and global clues. TOF stands for 3rd order factor (triplet). GAF denotes global appearance factor.

Method	Optimization	TOF	GAF
[9]	K-Shortest Paths	×	×
[4]	Tabu Search	×	✓
[3]	α-Expansion, TRW-S	✓	×
[11]	Markov Monte-Carlo	×	×
[7]	Integer Programming	×	✓
[13]	Lagrange Relaxation	✓	×
Ours	TRW-S, Flipper	✓	✓

5   Conclusion

We proposed a novel tracking algorithm which exploits local and global cues in the most unified manner as compared to the state-of-the-art (*cf.* Table 6). Furthermore an apt combination of optimizers and suitable graph reduction lends robustness, stability and efficiency (5–10 fps on HD video of busy town street, on a single core CPU) to the model. The results obtained are competitive or better than the state-of-the-art at this speed. The proposed model has two degrees of freedom, and hence would be highly amenable to parameter learning using scene context and other relevant inputs. Also the algorithm is easy to implement and reproduce. Future prospects include tracking object parts and providing feedback to the point-trackers about incorrect tracks.

Supplementary materials can be found at the project webpage.[4]

Acknowledgements. This work has received funding from the European Community's FP7/2007-2013 - under grant agreement n° 248907-VANAHEIM.

References

1. Breitenstein, M., Reichlin, F.: Robust tracking-by-detection using a detector confidence particle filter. In: ICCV (2009)
2. Andriyenko, A., Schindler, K., Roth, S.: Discrete-continuous optimization for multi-target tracking. In: CVPR (2012)
3. Milan, A., Schindler, K., Roth, S.: Detection-and trajectory-level exclusion in multiple object tracking. In: CVPR, June 2013
4. Roshan Zamir, A., Dehghan, A., Shah, M.: GMCP-tracker: global multi-object tracking using generalized minimum clique graphs. In: Fitzgibbon, A., Lazebnik, S., Perona, P., Sato, Y., Schmid, C. (eds.) ECCV 2012, Part II. LNCS, vol. 7573, pp. 343–356. Springer, Heidelberg (2012)
5. Brendel, W., Amer, M., Todorovic, S.: Multiobject tracking as maximum weight independent set. In: CVPR (2011)
6. Zhang, L., Li, Y., Nevatia, R.: Global data association for multi-object tracking using network flows. In: CVPR (2008)
7. Shitrit, H.B., Berclaz, J., et al.: Tracking multiple people under global appearance constraints. In: ICCV (2011)
8. Berclaz, J., Fleuret, F., Turetken, E., Fua, P.: Multiple object tracking using K-shortest paths optimization. TPAMI **33**, 1806–1819 (2011)
9. Pirsiavash, H., Ramanan, D., Fowlkes, C.C.: Globally-optimal greedy algorithms for tracking a variable number of objects. In: CVPR (2011)
10. Russell, C., Agapito, L., Setti, F.: Efficient second order multi-target tracking with exclusion constraints. In: BMVC (2011)
11. Benfold, B., Reid, I.: Stable multi-target tracking in real-time surveillance video. In: CVPR (2011)
12. Collins, R.T.: Multitarget data association with higher-order motion models. In: CVPR (2012)

---

[4] http://www-sop.inria.fr/stars/Documents/tracking/.

13. Butt, A., Collins, R.: Multi-target tracking by Lagrangian relaxation to min-cost network flow. In: CVPR (2013)
14. Ellis, A., Shahrokni, A., Ferryman, J.: PETS2009 and Winter-PETS 2009 results: A combined evaluation. In: PETS Workshop. IEEE (2009)
15. Kappes, J.H., Speth, M., Reinelt, G., Schnorr, C.: Towards efficient and exact MAP-inference for large scale discrete computer vision problems via combinatorial optimization. In: CVPR (2013)
16. Kolmogorov, V.: Convergent tree-reweighted message passing for energy minimization. TPAMI 28(10), 1568–1583 (2006)
17. Besag, J.: On the statistical analysis of dirty pictures. Stat. Mehodological Soc. 48(3), 259–302 (1986)
18. Andres, B., Kappes, J.H., Beier, T., Köthe, U., Hamprecht, F.A.: The lazy flipper: efficient depth-limited exhaustive search in discrete graphical models. In: Fitzgibbon, A., Lazebnik, S., Perona, P., Sato, Y., Schmid, C. (eds.) ECCV 2012, Part VII. LNCS, vol. 7578, pp. 154–166. Springer, Heidelberg (2012)
19. Martins, A.F.T., Figueiredo, M.A.T., Aguiar, P.M.Q., Smith, N.A., Xing, E.P.: An augmented Lagrangian approach to constrained MAP inference. In: ICML (2011)
20. Sontag, D., Choe, D., Li, Y.: Efficiently searching for frustrated cycles in MAP inference. In: Uncertainty in Artificial Intelligence (2012)
21. Butler, D.J., Wulff, J., Stanley, G.B., Black, M.J.: A naturalistic open source movie for optical flow evaluation. In: Fitzgibbon, A., Lazebnik, S., Perona, P., Sato, Y., Schmid, C. (eds.) ECCV 2012, Part VI. LNCS, vol. 7577, pp. 611–625. Springer, Heidelberg (2012)
22. Milan, A., Schindler, K., Roth, S.: Challenges of Ground Truth Evaluation of Multi-Target Tracking. In: CVPR Workshops (2013)
23. Bernardin, K., Stiefelhagen, R.: Evaluating multiple object tracking performance: the CLEAR MOT metrics. EURASIP JIVP 2008, 1:1–1:10 (2008). doi:10.1155/2008/246309
24. Zhang, J., Presti, L., Sclaroff, S.: Online multi-person tracking by tracker hierarchy. In: AVSS (2012)
25. Senst, T., Eiselein, V., Sikora, T.: Robust local optical flow for feature tracking. IEEE Trans. Circuits Syst. Video Technol. 22(9), 1377–1387 (2012)
26. Zach, C., Gallup, D., Frahm, J.: Fast gain-adaptive KLT tracking on the GPU. In: CVPR Workshops (2008)

Fast Approximate Nearest-Neighbor Field by Cascaded Spherical Hashing

Iban Torres-Xirau, Jordi Salvador$^{(\boxtimes)}$, and Eduardo Pérez-Pellitero

Technicolor R&I, Hannover, Germany
i.torres@nki.nl,
{jordi.salvador,eduardo.perezpellitero}@technicolor.com

Abstract. We present an efficient and fast algorithm for computing approximate nearest neighbor fields between two images. Our method builds on the concept of Coherency-Sensitive Hashing (CSH), but uses a recent hashing scheme, Spherical Hashing (SpH), which is known to be better adapted to the nearest-neighbor problem for natural images. Cascaded Spherical Hashing concatenates different configurations of SpH to build larger Hash Tables with less elements in each bin to achieve higher selectivity. Our method is able to amply outperform existing techniques like PatchMatch and CSH. The parallelizable scheme has been straightforwardly implemented in OpenCL, and the experimental results show that our algorithm is faster and more accurate than existing methods.

1 Introduction

Computing Approximate Nearest Neighbor Field (ANNF) between image patches has become a main building block for many computer vision and image processing algorithms, such as image re-targeting tools, image denoising or texture synthesis among others. Given two images A and B, the goal is to find for every patch in A a similar patch in B. The large size of images translates into millions of patches for each image A and B, and computing ANNF quickly becomes a challenge.

We propose the introduction of a recent hashing scheme, namely Spherical Hashing [1], in order to reduce the spatial and temporal complexity: we only require one set of hashing functions against the several sets of functions typically required when using planar function-based hashing (CSH [2]). In comparison to CSH and randomized search schemes like PatchMatch [3], we reduce the number of required iterations to just one to reach superior results.

To achieve this performance, we first introduce the general Spherical Hashing framework, and detail its applicability in ANNF estimation (Sect. 3). After observing its limitations, in Sect. 4 we propose a novel cascaded configuration for enhanced search without increasing testing time. Furthermore, we shed light on the implementation details of propagation strategies exploiting both local spatial coherence and similar appearance in both linear and hash space (using spherical Hamming distance).

We finally compare our proposed method to existing approaches in Sect. 5 and show the improvements achieved by our proposed contributions.

© Springer International Publishing Switzerland 2015
D. Cremers et al. (Eds.): ACCV 2014, Part IV, LNCS 9006, pp. 461–475, 2015.
DOI: 10.1007/978-3-319-16817-3_30

2   Related Work

Efros and Leung [4] proposed a simple non-parametric texture synthesis method based on sampling patches from a texture example and pasting them in the synthesized image. Various improvements for better structure preservation have been carried out by [5,6] and outperformed by [7] obtaining globally consistent completions of large missing regions by formulating the problem as a global optimization.

Ashikhmin [8] introduced for the first time the concept of coherency and spatial propagation, which lead to speed up many previous non-parametric texture synthesis works by limiting the search space for a patch to the neighboring area of the match in the source texture. An extension of this work was carried out by Tong et al. [9], where the propagation algorithm is combined with a precomputed set of k nearest neighbors and used to quickly search for ANN.

The principle proposed in Locality-Sensitive Hashing [10] is that given a set of points in a metric space, with high probability the hashing function families will distribute points that are close to each other to the same bin. The scheme proposed by Datar et al. [11] uses a particular family of LSH functions to determine regions in the space: $h_{a,b}(v) = \frac{a \cdot v + b}{r}$ where r is a predefined integer, b is a value drawn uniformly at random from $[0, r]$, and a is a d-dimensional vector with entries chosen independently at random from a Gaussian distribution.

The idiosyncrasy of PatchMatch (PM) [3] relies on the dependency among queries. It observes the spatial coherence of images and propagates good matches to their neighbors (coherence-based propagation). That is, for a pair of similar patches in two images, their neighbors are also likely to be similar. PM has a first stage of initialization to seed the nearest neighbor field, and an iterative process to improve the search by propagating good matches. Since initialization can be done by assigning random values, and because PatchMatch does not organize the data beforehand, after seeding most candidates are unlikely to be good matches.

Coherence Sensitive Hashing (CSH) [2] at its turn relies on LSH and on PM, and it is a state-of-the-art method for ANN search that exploits the idea of randomly partitioning the data space proposed by LSH, generating a family of hash functions to index the patches and store them in bins in a hash table. But alternatively to LSH, CSH uses a different set of functions (Walsh Hadamard kernels) to achieve the dispersion to be as large as possible when projecting the patches into the kernels, and also because of its low computational cost. CSH outperforms LSH by generating a larger number of (nearest neighbor) candidates since, according to PM, it also exploits coherence in images and furthermore combines it with appearance-based candidates.

Another method for ANNF is Propagation-Assisted KD-Trees (PAKT) [12], which improves PM and CSH in terms of accuracy and performance, and therefore becomes a current state-of-the-art algorithm. It merges contributions from kd-trees [13] and PM, so it is also based on (deterministically) partitioning the space, but its key insight is to exploit both the distribution of the candidates of patches in the source image as the dependency of the query patches. Tree-based methods such as kd-trees organize the candidates adaptively to their distribution in the search space, and a query can find its ANN by checking a small number of candidates. Indeed, PAKT introduces a propagation step after organizing the candidates in a traditional kd-tree, in which the tree nodes checked by each query are propagated from the nearby queries to its own leaf and to a nearby extra leaf. In contrast with general search schemes based on kd-trees, PAKT has no backtracking when descending the tree to a leaf, but it only checks a small number of candidates hence it becomes a fast method for computing ANNF. The principle of PAKT is similar to the one assumed at hashing: one bin has such a high likelihood to contain the NN patch that there is no need to check in other bins, but we must note that spherical hashing provides better partitioning than the tree scheme based on hyperplanes.

The Spherical Hashing (SpH) algorithm introduced by Heo et al. [1], uses a family of spherical hashing functions because it considers that the partitioning of the data space by means of hyperplanes can be improved by using hyperspheres: a higher number of closed regions can be constructed by using multiple hyperspheres, while the distances between points located in each region are bounded. The SpH algorithm has an initialization step to conveniently choose the spherical hashing functions in order to balance the amount of data falling in each bin. When trained with a large data set, the content in bins is likely to be uniformly distributed in the hash table. Although SpH does not focus on ANNF (it does so on data mining), its idea is still extrapolable for our purpose, and the improvement at partitioning the data space is a key insight for our method.

Our method builds on previous approaches like CSH and SpH, therefore it is able to quickly find similar patches with more accuracy and reducing the computational time over CSH, since the spherical hashing algorithm guarantees an increment of closed regions with less functions. The propagation step of our method is similar to the one adopted in CSH, which, based on PM, exploits query dependence. Our method additionally makes use of the Spherical Hamming Distance introduced by [1] and proposes a new class of candidates (spherical-neighbor propagation) to enlarge the list.

3   Spherical Hashing for ANNF

In this section we present the general idea behind our coherence-sensitive ANNF search method based on a spherical hashing scheme. We first discuss the training stage for an optimal choice of the hashing functions for image patches.

3.1   Training

At the training stage we use a large set of data patches from a wide range of images to create a family of data-dependent hashing functions that guarantees a good partitioning of the space, aiming to similar amount of data falling in each region (balance). Given a sufficiently large training set, the functions selection will remain valid for any new given data we may process.

We treat each patch as a D-dimensional vector in Euclidean space. These m vectors $X = \{x_1, x_2 \ldots x_m\}, x_i \in \mathbb{R}^D$ form an input manifold M of dimension D. Compared to previous hashing approaches, which used hyperplanes as splitting functions, spherical hashing considers the inclusion in hyperspheres. The algorithm models those hyperspheres by a pivot $p_k \in \mathbb{R}^D$ and a distance threshold (i.e. radius) $t_k \in \mathbb{R}^+$. Each data point x_i is then encoded with a binary number $b_k = \{-1, +1\}^c$ being c the number of hyperspheres and the length of the code, where the k-th bit is computed as follows:

$$
b_k(x) = \begin{cases} -1, & d(p_k, x) > t_k \\ 1, & d(p_k, x) \leqslant tk \end{cases}, \tag{1}
$$

where $d(\cdot, \cdot)$ denotes the Euclidean distance between two points in $\mathbb{R}^D$. The main benefit of using hyperspheres instead of hyperplanes is that defining closed regions in the spherical case is much more accurate, since these regions are bounded, and elements belonging to a region must be strictly closer; moreover, the number of spheres needed to define a closed region is minor than the number of hyperplanes, therefore the number of functions is also lower and the computational time decreases significantly.

Following the scheme proposed by SpH [1], the algorithm aims to minimize the search time in the bins of the hash table and improve the accuracy of the search, which can be achieved by reaching independence between hashing functions and a balanced partitioning of the data space. The two conditions to satisfy are the following:

$$
Pr[h_x(x) = 1] = \frac{1}{2}, \; x \in X, \; 1 \leq k \leq c \tag{2}
$$

$$
Pr[h_i(x) = 1, h_j(x) = 1] = Pr[h_i(x) = 1] \cdot Pr[h_j(x) = 1] = \tfrac{1}{2} \cdot \tfrac{1}{2} = \tfrac{1}{4}, \\ x \in X, \; 1 \leq i, j \leq c \tag{3}
$$

To fulfill these conditions, an iterative step for the selection of the functions has to be carried out, so that the centers of the hyperspheres p_k and their radii t_k (thresholds) are refined at every iteration. In order to accomplish Eqs. 2 and 3, the algorithm uses two variables to help these computations:

$$
o_i = |\{s_k \mid h_i(s_k) = 1, \; 1 \leq k \leq m\}|
$$

$$
o_{i,j} = |\{s_k \mid h_i(s_k) = 1, \; s_k \mid h_j(s_k) = 1, \; 1 \leq k \leq m\}|
$$

o_i denotes the number of data points which have 1 bit set for the i-th hashing function (number of data points falling inside the i-th hypersphere) and is used to satisfy balanced partitioning for each bit following Eq. (2), while $o_{i,j}$ counts the number of patches that are contained within both of two (i-th and j-th) spheres and is used to guarantee the independence between the i-th and j-th hashing functions following Eq. (3).

The iterative process for pivots refinement first adjusts the pivot centers of two hyperspheres in a way that $o_{i,j}$ becomes close to $\frac{m}{4}$, and then a threshold t_i is chosen such that o_i becomes $\frac{m}{2}$ to meet balanced partitioning. At each iteration the centers of the pivots are moved to new locations according to the forces computed regarding to each $o_{i,j}$. For each pair of spheres i and j, a repulsive or attractive force from p_j to p_i, $f_{i \leftarrow j}$ is computed as the following:

$$f_{i \leftarrow j} = \frac{1}{2} \frac{o_{i,j} - m/4}{m/4} (p_i - p_j),$$

and the accumulated force f_i is the average of all the computed forces from all the other pivots:

$$f_i = \frac{1}{c-1} \sum_{j \neq i} f_{i \leftarrow j} .$$

Convergence of the system is achieved when the ideal values for mean and the standard deviation of $o_{i,j}$ are $\frac{m}{4}$ and zero respectively (within $100\epsilon_m\%$ and $100\epsilon_s\%$ error tolerances).

3.2   Indexing and Building the Hash Table

A hash code of length c is computed for each patch of a new source image using Eq. (1) and is stored in a bin with all its similar patches, as shown in Fig. 1. At the indexing stage, a total of c patch-to-pivot squared L_2 distances are computed, which translates into a computational cost of $O(Dc)$ operations per patch. We build a hash table (HT) of 2^c entries of different sizes to store the entire image.

The building process is divided into two runs: we first compute all patch indices and determine the size of each bin in the hash table, and then we create the table according to the dimensions of each bin and we orderly store each patch in its position in the HT. However, we reduce the equivalent building time and search time compared to similar structures as PAKT [12], since the kd-tree scheme requires the decomposition in a suitable basis, while the hashing algorithm allows more flexible partitions in a native way. Furthermore, our algorithm is highly and easily parallelizable so the final build time is reduced to practically $O(Dc)$ in e.g. an OpenCL implementation.

3.3   Direct Search

For every patch in a given query image we compute its index, so that a list of similar candidates with the property of space similarity due to belonging to the same region can be found in the hashed bin. Since bins often contain several patches, various techniques can be carried out to select the ANNF, e.g. a re-ranking algorithm based on similarity between images (L_2), which increases the computational time in exchange for higher accuracy, or a random sampling within the HT entry that provides a fast approximate match.

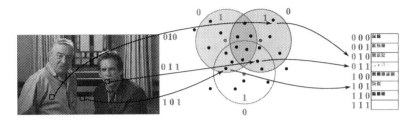

Fig. 1. Spherical hashing for ANNF places data points in a $\mathbb{R}^D$ space ($D = 2$ in the figure) and a set of c spheres (to be computed at the training phase) determine which region each point belongs to. The hash table on the right side stores in a bin every point falling in its correspondent region. The search stage hashes query points through the same system of spheres as the indexing phase. Patches of the query image point to bins of the hash table where the source data is stored creating a list of match candidates.

Even though the system is designed to achieve balance in the HT, when increasing the number of spheres up to a certain limit, this property becomes unstable, so a closed region in the $\mathbb{R}^D$ space is likely to contain no data points. This is the main reason why we cannot build a highly discriminative set of spheres and the motivation of our proposal in Sect. 4.

3.4   Drawbacks

For large values of c, a small number of patches in each bin is expected, and hence the re-ranking algorithm in the search is less expensive. However, this assumption is not always valid. Given the dimensionality of the $\mathbb{R}^D$ space determined for the size of the patches, a certain threshold value for c exists, at which convergence to guarantee the properties of Eqs. (2) and (3) is not achievable when we create the hash functions. Beyond this level, several bins result to be empty after building the HT and some others are overpopulated. We propose an extension of the given scheme to scalably increase the number of filled bins making them less populated and increase accuracy without introducing any cost during testing.

4   Cascaded Spherical Hashing for ANNF

We propose a novel approach to exploit the space partitioning with special influence in the densest areas. Despite the fact that spherical hashing guarantees a good equability in the HT, given the dimensionality D of the $\mathbb{R}^D$ space it turns into a nearly impossible task to unlimitedly increase the number of hyperspheres and still ensure balancing. Concatenating multiple dependent systems of hyperspheres and building a novel multi-dimensional hash table based on this cascading concept results to be a more accurate method, since, although it does not guarantee perfect balance in the final HT, we reduce the overfilling and simultaneously enlarge the number of filled bins, which translates into better performance in terms of accuracy at no additional processing cost during the testing time.

Points falling in a certain region in one system are then distributed according to the region they belong to in the next dimension and so on, hence our method provides more similarity between patches belonging to the intersection of closed regions between cascaded systems of spheres.

A total of 2^c bins are created for a chosen number of spheres c in the original SpH. For a large set of m random data distributed in the space, each bin is likely to store $\frac{m}{2^c}$ patches, but when trained with real data, we observe that the distribution of the source patches in the space is not uniform and therefore some bins happen to end up empty while others are overpopulated, especially for large c. Our approach concatenates various hashing systems of different numbers of spheres $c_1, c_2, \ldots, c_N$, and builds a final hash table of $2^{c_1} \cdot 2^{c_2} \cdot \ldots \cdot 2^{c_N}$ bins, achieving high discrimination at indexing.

4.1   Cascade Training

The offline training is an iterative algorithm where each iteration consists of two phases carried out to concatenate N dependent hash systems, in order to make every system more discriminative to the regions presenting more data (Fig. 2).

4.1.1   Spheres Training

In this phase a data set is trained following the scheme detailed in Sect. 3.1 to obtain a system of c_i hyperspheres.

4.1.2   Data Set Refinement

The HT deduced from the previous system(s) is filled by the whole data set, and observing the density of data falling in each entry we determine whether a region is overpopulated. We generate a subset of all vectors/patches lying in overpopulated bins and train a specialized sphere system as in Sect. 4.1.1.

4.2   Indexing and Building the Hash Table

Actually, the way we create the resulting hash table can be seen as a multi-dimensional Spherical Hashing, where every dimension (or spheres set) contributes to higher accuracy. For a given source patch, its index is created by a combination of the N hash codes generated using the function of Eq. 1 for each system. The source data is stored in the resulting HT which owns a large number of bins and, since the different spherical hashing systems are built in cascade, no bin contains a large amount of data and it yields a higher number of filled ones.

Building the cascaded-HT requires the same computational cost than the building time of the method proposed in Sect. 3 when we compare both approaches with the same total amount of hyperspheres. Besides, this interpretation comes handy to introduce the spherical propagation introduced in Sect. 4.4.2.

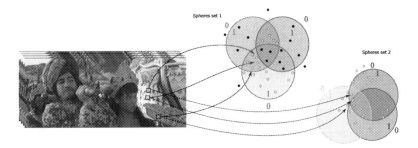

Fig. 2. Cascaded training: the data set is trained to obtain the first set of spheres (top) using the hashing scheme of Sect. 3.1 until convergence is achieved. When the Hash Table is filled by the data set, our training stage observes the density of data in space regions, and uses the subset of data contained in the most populated regions (highlighted data points) to train the next system of spheres (bottom). This is similar to the procedure in other cascaded methods, such as AdaBoost [14].

4.3   Direct Search

For a given query image every patch is hashed to an entry of the cascaded-HT in order to find a list of patches of the source image simultaneously belonging to the same regions in the N sets of spheres. It is interesting to note that, if $c_1 \leq c_2 \leq \ldots \leq c_N$, the sets of hashing systems ensure more stability for the firsts systems, so that if a query patch is hashed to an intersection of regions where no source data is stored, the algorithm can fall back to the other (lower) dimensions to find plausible matches (Fig. 3). All patches belonging to the hashed bin are likely to be a good match and, again for the ANNF search, a re-ranking or an in-bin random sampling are the main alternatives to adopt. However, since we manage to have more non-empty bins and containing less data at the same time, the re-ranking technique results to be faster and the random search is more accurate compared to the original method. In our experiments we avoid re-ranking thanks to the accurate partition obtained with the cascaded setup (we just perform random sampling within the selected bin).

4.4   Propagation

We improve the search by exploiting both local spatial coherence and hashing appearance in both linear and hash space.

4.4.1   Spatial Propagation

To enlarge the candidates list provided by the Hashing scheme and following the idea proposed by PM, we also adopt the concept of image coherence to propagate good matches to their spatial neighbors. We do so in a similar way to the extended mechanism introduced by PAKT [12], a bin-propagation to find better matches. Suppose a query patch $p_A(x - 1, y)$ has found a similar patch $p_B(x' - 1, y')$, we improve the result of $p_A(x, y)$ trying patches belonging to the

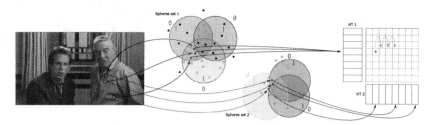

Fig. 3. Cascaded Hash Table search: Patches are hashed to bins in the corresponding HT for each set of spheres ($N = 2$), and by combining them we obtain a cascaded-HT capable of distributing data with high discrimination based on the closed region defined by the intersection of the systems where data falls. When the cascaded-HT of the figure is filled with real data from an image, not all bins happen to store data, but significantly more than in a single HT (and also less populated). Indeed, we still observe empty bins due to physical impossibility of belonging to regions which never intersect, although with the procedure we follow to create the HT it does not represent a cost in memory nor time. When a query patch is hashed to a bin that contains no source data (red point), the naive process of our method relies in the lower dimensions (or hyperspheres systems) by a linear search until a filled bin is found to find matches (Color figure online).

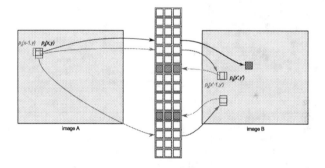

Fig. 4. Bin-Propagation in Spherical Hashing Scheme: If the spatial neighbor of $p_A(x, y)$ (black patch), $p_A(x - 1, y)$ (red), has a good match $p_B(x' - 1, y')$ (red), the spatial neighbor of the match, $p_B(x', y')$ (black) belongs to a bin in the Hash Table where all the patches are plausible candidates (shaded) (Color figure online).

same bin as $p_B(x', y')$, and so on with the other directions (Fig. 4). By proceeding this way, we obtain $x4$ times candidates for every query patch.

We analyze the benefits of the propagation step, adopted from the spatial coherence concept proposed by PM, to find out the impact of the accuracy gain over the cost in time. In the same scenario we reconstruct 2500 independent images using the single and the cascaded algorithm both with and without propagation, and the results are shown in Fig. 5. Note that propagation has notable influence but also implies a computational cost penalty avoided by the proposed cascaded approach.

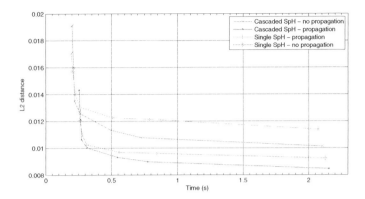

Fig. 5. Error/Time tradeoffs of Cascaded and Single Spherical Hashing, both with and without propagation.

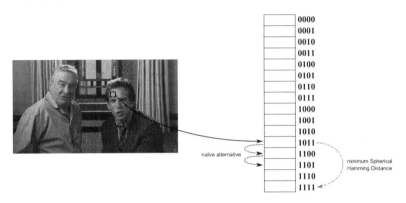

Fig. 6. Spherical Hamming Distance in the Hash Table: a patch hashed to an empty bin is likely to have better matches using the SHD to compute the spherical-neighboring cell instead of looking into the consecutive bins until a filled one is found.

4.4.2   Spherical Propagation

We make use of the concept of Spherical Hamming Distance (SHD) introduced by [1], which computes the distance between codes of two bounded regions (in one dimension of our multi-SpH) as follows:

$$d_{shd}(b_i, b_j) = \frac{\mid b_i \oplus b_j \mid}{\mid b_i \wedge b_j \mid}, \tag{4}$$

where b_i, b_j are the hash codes of patches i, j, and $\mid b_i \oplus b_j \mid$ measures the number of different bits (belonging to different spheres) and the term $\mid b_i \wedge b_j \mid$ denotes the number of common +1 bit (belonging to same spheres). This distance is useful when a given query patch hashes to a bin where no source data is stored. When searching in a bin that happens to be empty, a straightforward implementation could initially rely on looking into the following bins until one contains data (Fig. 3). Since this situation does not happen often ($\sim 0,005\,\%$ of patches in our experiments), empirical results show that this is often a good assumption. Nevertheless, an improvement in accuracy/speed-up versus the naive approach is achieved by using the Spherical Hamming distance to look in spherical-neighboring cells at minimum distance, as Fig. 6 shows.

5   Results

All algorithms were run on a PC with an Intel Xeon CPU 2.67 GHz CPU and 12 GB RAM. Note that all the methods use the same CPU platform, even for the parallelized OpenCL code. We test the search algorithms on a subset of the public data set VidPairs [15] and the training of our method is carried out using the publicly available Kodak data set.

5.1   Validation

In order to validate the proposed approach, we test different hypersphere configurations. Figure 7 shows that the best performance is achieved when using our proposed cascaded approach. We also train and test independent systems of hyperspheres and combin them, obtaining worse performance results than with single SpH. This proves that there is no benefit in training independent system without focusing on the overpopulated bins.

Finally, we validate that our Cascaded SpH method is more accurate than the single SpH at no additional testing computational cost, obtaining results up to 0.7 dB higher in PSNR.

Note how the progressive improvements by adding more cascading levels outperform the other alternavies, e.g. our method with 21 bits and 3 cascades outperforms both alternatives with 25 bits. The small margins reflect the already excellent performance of spherical hashing in the basic configuration with a relatively high number of bits, but the interesting aspect is that the gain of the cascaded configuration comes at literally no computational cost.

5.2   Comparison to State-of-the-Art

We compare our algorithm with PM [3] and CSH [2]. Our algorithm is implemented in OpenCL and exploits its parallel-friendly nature, yielding important speed-ups. We obtained the CSH code from the authors website [15], which is mainly implemented in C++. The PM algorithm is an OpenCL self-implemented code, which at its turn, outperforms the original PM in processing time.

Even though an open implementation of PAKT is not available, by the comparison against CSH published in the original paper [12], we can extrapolate that our algorithm is qualitatively competitive in terms of time and accuracy.

Figure 8 shows time-accuracy results for 4-by-4 patches and 2 Mp images. Accuracy is measured as the squared L_2 distance between the query patch and its nearest neighbor match found by PM, CSH, our single SpH and our cascaded SpH

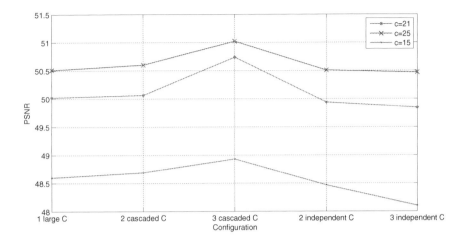

Fig. 7. Time-PSNR tradeoffs averaged on 225 reconstructions of independent images. The image size is 2 Mp and the patch size is 3-by-3. *1 large C* refers to a single spherical hashing system with large C, *2/3 independent C* refers to configurations of independent hyperspheres systems with multiple tables, and *2/3 cascaded C* refers to the proposed method. In the experiments, configurations for 2 and 3 stages with equal number of spheres as for *1 large C* are: $c_{15} = \{6,9\}, \{4,5,6\}$, $c_{21} = \{8,13\}, \{6,7,8\}$ and $c_{25} = \{11,14\}, \{7,8,10\}$.

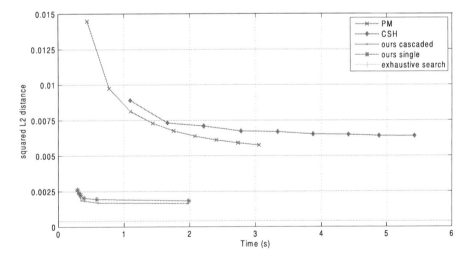

Fig. 8. Time vs accuracy averaged over 225 reconstructions of independent images. The image size is 2 Mp and the patch size is 4-by-4. Each marker on PM's and CSH's curves represents the performance for each iteration. Each marker on our method represents the performance for increasing total number of hyperspheres c_i $\{12, 15, 18, 21, 24, 27\}$. Exhaustive search is included to determine the lower bound error, but we avoid to show the long computation time to keep a proper scaling for the more efficient approaches.

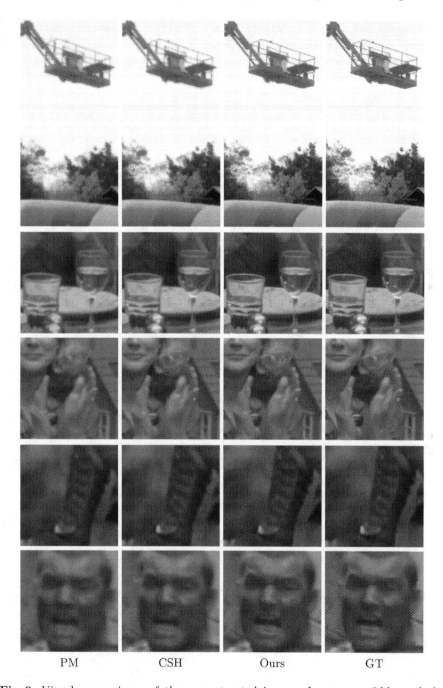

PM	CSH	Ours	GT

Fig. 9. Visual comparisons of the reconstructed images. Images are 2 Mp and the patches are 4-by-4. All methods are run in 1 iteration, and $N = 3$ in our method for a total number of hyperspheres equal to 18 ($c_1 = 5$, $c_2 = 6$, $c_3 = 7$). The running times are: 0.47s, 1.22s, and 0.35s, with PSNR values are: 39.08 dB, 41.44 dB and 48.23 dB for PM, CSH and ours, respectively.

(in the experiments $N = 3$). We also present results obtained by an exhaustive search to compare the measures to the maximum possible accuracy.

As Fig. 9 shows, our results at reconstruction are visually better than PM/CSH. When compared to the fastest method we achive speed-ups of ×1.3 with a quality difference of 9 dB in PSNR. When compared to the most accurate method, we still improve by 7 dB considering also that our method is ×3.5 faster.

It is interesting to note that reconstructed images obtained using PM are not able to accurately reconstruct some flat areas (especially noticeable in the first column of images in Fig. 9). This effect appears due to the search algorithm in PM, which considers the entire patch, while CSH and our method carry out the search by subtracting the mean value.

6   Conclusions

We propose a new algorithm for computing ANNF. We build on the Spherical Hashing algorithm of Heo et al. [1], originally presented in the context of data mining, which we adapt to the specific problem of ANNF estimation. We improve the baseline method by adding a propagation mechanism based on both local and visual coherence, inspired by the scheme proposed by PAKT [12], which in turn already extends the original PM local coherence concept [3].

We observed practical limitations in spherical hashing for ANNF when trained with large numbers of hyperspheres, and we overcome them by introducing a cascaded training approach. This cascaded scheme aims to improve the partitioning of the overpopulated regions without introducing any additional cost in testing time. In order to do so, we add complexity to the offline training stage to guarantee a better balance within the hash table.

We also introduce the usage of the spherical Hamming distance as an alternative hash selection for the rare situations in which a patch is hashed to an empty bin. Our algorithm, which allows straight-forward parallelization, has been compared to well-known state-of-the-art methods, obtaining the best-scoring results both in speed and quality.

We encourage to investigate further the benefits of our ANNF algorithm in other computer vision applications due to the applicability and feasibility of the method shown in the experimental results.

Acknowledgment. We thank the anonymous reviewers for their constructive feedback, which resulted in an improved manuscript.

References

1. Heo, J.P., Lee, Y., He, J., Chang, S.F., Yoon, S.: Spherical hashing. In: IEEE International Conference on Computer Vision and Pattern Recognition (CVPR) (2012)
2. Korman, S., Avidan, S.: Coherency sensitive hashing. In: Proceedings of the 2011 International Conference on Computer Vision, ICCV 2011, pp. 1607–1614. IEEE Computer Society, Washington, DC (2011)

3. Barnes, C., Shechtman, E., Finkelstein, A., Goldman, D.B.: PatchMatch: a randomized correspondence algorithm for structural image editing. ACM Trans. Graph. (Proc. SIGGRAPH) **28**, 24:1–24:11 (2009)
4. Efros, A.A., Leung, T.K.: Texture synthesis by non-parametric sampling. In: Proceedings of the International Conference on Computer Vision, ICCV 1999, vol. 2, pp. 1033–1038. IEEE Computer Society, Washington, DC (1999)
5. Efros, A.A., Freeman, W.T.: Image quilting for texture synthesis and transfer. In: Proceedings of the 28th Annual Conference on Computer Graphics and Interactive Techniques, SIGGRAPH 2001, pp. 341–346. ACM, New York (2001)
6. Kwatra, V., Schödl, A., Essa, I., Turk, G., Bobick, A.: Graphcut textures: image and video synthesis using graph cuts. In: ACM SIGGRAPH 2003 Papers, SIGGRAPH 2003, pp. 277–286. ACM, New York (2003)
7. Wexler, Y., Shechtman, E., Irani, M.: Space-time completion of video. IEEE Trans. Pattern Anal. Mach. Intell. **29**, 463–476 (2007)
8. Ashikhmin, M.: Synthesizing natural textures. In: Proceedings of the 2001 Symposium on Interactive 3D Graphics, I3D 2001, pp. 217–226. ACM, New York (2001)
9. Tong, X., Zhang, J., Liu, L., Wang, X., Guo, B., Shum, H.Y.: Synthesis of bidirectional texture functions on arbitrary surfaces. ACM Trans. Graph. **21**, 665–672 (2002)
10. Slaney, M., Casey, M.: Locality-sensitive hashing for finding nearest neighbors [lecture notes]. IEEE Sig. Process. Mag. **25**, 128–131 (2008)
11. Datar, M., Immorlica, N., Indyk, P., Mirrokni, V.S.: Locality-sensitive hashing scheme based on p-stable distributions. In: Proceedings of the Twentieth Annual Symposium on Computational Geometry, SCG 2004, pp. 253–262. ACM, New York (2004)
12. Sun, J.: Computing nearest-neighbor fields via propagation-assisted kd-trees. In: Proceedings of the 2012 IEEE Conference on Computer Vision and Pattern Recognition, CVPR 2012, pp. 111–118. IEEE Computer Society, Washington, DC (2012)
13. Friedman, J.H., Bentley, J.L., Finkel, R.A.: An algorithm for finding best matches in logarithmic expected time. ACM Trans. Math. Softw. **3**, 209–226 (1977)
14. Freund, Y., Schapire, R.E.: A decision-theoretic generalization of on-line learning and an application to boosting. J. Comput. Syst. Sci. **55**, 119–139 (1997)
15. Korman, S., Avidan, S.: Csh website.@ONLINE (2011)

Coupling Semi-supervised Learning and Example Selection for Online Object Tracking

Min Yang[(✉)], Yuwei Wu, Mingtao Pei, Bo Ma, and Yunde Jia

Beijing Laboratory of Intelligent Information Technology,
School of Computer Science, Beijing Institute of Technology, Beijing 100081, China
yangminbit@bit.edu.cn

Abstract. Training example collection is of great importance for discriminative trackers. Most existing algorithms use a sampling-and-labeling strategy, and treat the training example collection as a task that is independent of classifier learning. However, the examples collected directly by sampling are not intended to be useful for classifier learning. Updating the classifier with these examples might introduce ambiguity to the tracker. In this paper, we introduce an active example selection stage between sampling and labeling, and propose a novel online object tracking algorithm which explicitly couples the objectives of semi-supervised learning and example selection. Our method uses Laplacian Regularized Least Squares (LapRLS) to learn a robust classifier that can sufficiently exploit unlabeled data and preserve the local geometrical structure of feature space. To ensure the high classification confidence of the classifier, we propose an active example selection approach to automatically select the most informative examples for LapRLS. Part of the selected examples that satisfy strict constraints are labeled to enhance the adaptivity of our tracker, which actually provides robust supervisory information to guide semi-supervised learning. With active example selection, we are able to avoid the ambiguity introduced by an independent example collection strategy, and to alleviate the drift problem caused by misaligned examples. Comparison with the state-of-the-art trackers on the comprehensive benchmark demonstrates that our tracking algorithm is more effective and accurate.

1   Introduction

Object tracking aims to estimate the trajectory of an object automatically in a video sequence. Although the task is easily fulfilled by human vision system, designing a robust online tracker remains a very challenging problem due to significant appearance variations caused by factors such as object deformation, illumination change, occlusion, and background clutters.

Electronic supplementary material The online version of this chapter (doi:10.1007/978-3-319-16817-3_31) contains supplementary material, which is available to authorized users.

© Springer International Publishing Switzerland 2015
D. Cremers et al. (Eds.): ACCV 2014, Part IV, LNCS 9006, pp. 476–491, 2015.
DOI: 10.1007/978-3-319-16817-3_31

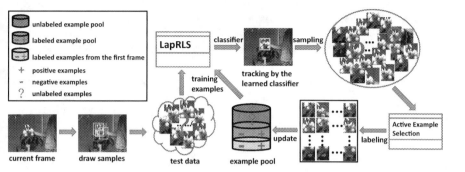

Fig. 1. Overview of our tracker. LapRLS is used to learn a robust classifier which is able to exploit both labeled and unlabeled data during tracking. An active example selection stage is introduced between sampling and labeling, which couples the objectives of semi-supervised learning and example selection. The figure is best viewed in color (Color figure online).

Numerous tracking algorithms have been proposed to address appearance variations, and most of them fall into two categories: generative methods and discriminative methods. Generative methods represent an object in a particular feature space, and then find the best candidate with maximal matching score. Some popular generative trackers include incremental visual tracking [1], visual tracking decomposition [2], sparse representation based tracking [3–7], and least soft-threshold squares tracking [8]. Discriminative methods cast tracking as a binary classification problem that distinguishes the object from the background [9–13]. Benefiting from the explicit consideration of background information, discriminative trackers usually are more robust against appearance variations under complex environments. In this paper, we focus on learning an online classifier which is able to capture appearance changes adaptively for object tracking.

The performance of discriminative trackers largely depends on the training examples used for classifier learning. Existing algorithms often collect training examples via a two-stage strategy [9]: sampling and labeling. The sampling process generates a set of examples around the current tracking result, and the labeling process estimates the labels of these examples using heuristic approach that depends on the current tracking result (*e.g.*, examples with small distance to the current track are labeled as positive, and examples far away from the current track are negative).

This widely used example collection strategy raises several issues. Firstly, the objective of the sampling process may not be consistent with the objective for the classifier, which makes the example collection strategy independent of classifier learning. The examples collected directly by sampling are neither necessarily informative nor intended to be useful for the classifier learning, and might introduce ambiguity to the tracker. Secondly, assigning labels estimated by the current tracking result to unlabeled examples may easily cause drift [9,14,15]. Slight inaccuracy of tracking results can lead to incorrectly labeled examples, and consequently degrades the classifier. State-of-the-art discriminative trackers mainly focus on learning a classifier that is robust to poorly labeled examples (*e.g.*, semi-supervised learning [14,16–18], P-N learning [19], multiple instance learning [15] and self-paced learning [20]). However, the first issue is rarely mentioned in the literature of object tracking.

In this paper, we propose an online object tracking algorithm which explicitly couples the objectives of semi-supervised learning and example selection. The overview of our tracker is shown in Fig. 1. We use a manifold regularized semi-supervised learning method, *i.e.*, Laplacian Regularized Least Squares (LapRLS) [21], to learn a robust classifier for object tracking. We show that it is crucial to exploit the abundant unlabeled data which can be easily collected during tracking to improve the classifier and alleviate the drift problem caused by label noisy. To avoid the ambiguity introduced by an independent example collection strategy, an *active example selection* stage is introduced between sampling and labeling to select the examples that are useful for LapRLS. The active example selection approach is designed to maximize the classification confidence of the classifier using the formalism of active learning [22,23], thus guarantees the consistency between classifier learning and example selection in a principled manner. Our experiments suggest that coupling semi-supervised learning and example selection leads to significant improvement on tracking performance. To make the classifier more adaptive to appearance changes, part of the selected examples that satisfy strict constraints are labeled, and the rest are considered as unlabeled data. According to the stability-plasticity dilemma [24], the additional labels provide reliable supervisory information to guide semi-supervised learning during tracking, and hence increases the plasticity of the tracker, which is validated in our experiments.

Semi-supervised tracking: Semi-supervised approaches have been previously used in tracking. Grabner *et al.* [14] proposed an online semi-supervised boosting tracker to avoid self-learning as only the examples in the first frame are considered as labeled. Saffari *et al.* [16] proposed a multi-view boosting algorithm which considers the given priors as a regularization component over the unlabeled data, and validate its robustness for object tracking. Kalal *et al.* [19] presented a P-N learning algorithm to bootstrap a prior classifier by iteratively labeling unlabeled examples via structural constraints. Gao *et al.* [18] employed the cluster assumption to exploit unlabeled data to encode most of the discriminant information of their tensor representation, and showed great improvement on tracking performance.

The methods mentioned above actually determine the "pseudo-label" of the unlabeled data, and do not discover the intrinsic geometrical structure of the feature space. In contrast, the LapRLS algorithm employed in our algorithm learns a classifier that predicts similar labels for similar data points by constructing a data adjacency graph. We show that it is crucial to consider the similarity in terms of label prediction during tracking. Bai and Tang [17] introduced a similar algorithm, *i.e.*, Laplacian ranking SVM, for object tracking. However, they adopt a handcrafted example collection strategy to obtain the labeled and unlabeled data, which limits the performance of their tracking method.

Active learning: Active learning, also referred to as experimental design in statistics, aims to determine which unlabeled examples would be the most informative (*i.e.*, improve the classifier the most if they were labeled and used as training data) [22,23], and has been well applied in text categorization [25] and image retrieval [26,27]. In this work, we propose an active example selection approach to couple semi-supervised learning and example selection by using the framework of active learning, in which the task is to select the examples that improve the prediction accuracy of LapRLS the most.

We show that the active example selection introduces several advantages for object tracking over existing methods. Firstly, it guarantees the consistency between classifier learning and example collection in a principled way. That is, the selected examples are meaningful for LapRLS, which can improve the classification performance. Secondly, the active example selection tends to choose the representative examples, which reduces the amount of training data without performance loss. Thirdly, assigning labels to the selected examples alleviates the drift problem caused by label noise. According to the theory of active learning, the examples, that minimize the predictive variance when they are used for training, will be selected. Thus misaligned examples are intended to be rejected by the active example selection.

2   The Proposed Tracking Algorithm

Our tracker operates by alternately performing two stages: classifier learning with LapRLS, and training example collection with active example selection. After describing these two stages in Sect. 2.1 and Sect. 2.2, respectively, we formulate object tracking in a Bayesian inference framework and summarize our tracking algorithm in Sect. 2.3.

2.1   Classifier Learning with LapRLS

Given a set of l labeled examples $\{(x_i, y_i)\}_{i=1}^{l}$, and a set of u unlabeled examples $\{x_i\}_{i=l+1}^{l+u}$, the LapRLS algorithm seeks for a real valued function $f : \mathcal{X} \to \mathbb{R}$ by solving the following optimization problem [21]:

$$f^* = \arg\min_{f \in \mathcal{H}_K} \sum_{i=1}^{l} (y_i - f(x_i))^2 + \lambda_1 \|f\|_K^2 + \frac{\lambda_2}{2} \sum_{i,j=1}^{l+u} (f(x_i) - f(x_j))^2 W_{ij}, \quad (1)$$

where $\mathcal{H}_K$ is a Reproducing Kernel Hilbert Space (RKHS) which is associated with a positive definite Mercer kernel $K : \mathcal{X} \times \mathcal{X} \to \mathbb{R}$, $\|\cdot\|_K$ is the norm defined in $\mathcal{H}_K$, and W is a $(l+u) \times (l+u)$ similarity matrix with entries W_{ij} indicating the adjacency weights between data points x_i and x_j. The last term in Eq. (1) is an approximated manifold regularizer that preserves the local geometrical structure represented by a weighted adjacency graph with similarity matrix W. It actually respects a smoothness assumption, that is, data points which are closed to each other in a high-density region should share similar measurements (or labels) given by trained function. According to the spectral graph theory, this regularized term can be rewritten as

$$\frac{1}{2} \sum_{i,j=1}^{l+u} (f(x_i) - f(x_j))^2 W_{ij} = \boldsymbol{f}^\top L \boldsymbol{f}, \tag{2}$$

where $\boldsymbol{f} = [f(x_1), f(x_2), \ldots, f(x_{l+u})]^\top$, and L is the graph Laplacian given by $L = D - W$. Here, D is a diagonal matrix defined as $D_{ii} = \sum_{j=1}^{l+u} W_{ij}$. We adopt the local scaling method [28] to define the similarity matrix,

$$W_{ij} = \begin{cases} \exp\left(-\frac{\|x_i - x_j\|_2^2}{\sigma_i \sigma_j}\right), & \text{if } i \in N_k^j \text{ or } j \in N_k^i, \\ 0, & \text{otherwise,} \end{cases} \tag{3}$$

where N_k^i indicates the index set of the k nearest neighbors of x_i in $\{x_i\}_{i=l}^{l+u}$, $\sigma_i = \|x_i - x_i^{(k)}\|_2$, and $x_i^{(k)}$ is the k-th nearest neighbor of x_i in $\{x_i\}_{i=l}^{l+u}$.

The Representer Theorem (see details in [21]) shows that the solution of Eq. (1) is an expansion of kernel functions over both labeled and unlabeled data,

$$f^*(x) = \sum_{i=1}^{l+u} \omega_i^* K(x, x_i). \tag{4}$$

By substituting this form into Eq. (1), we get a convex differentiable objective function of the $(l + u)$-dimensional vector $\boldsymbol{\omega} = [\omega_1, \ldots, \omega_{l+u}]^\top$,

$$\boldsymbol{\omega}^* = \arg\min_{\boldsymbol{\omega} \in \mathbb{R}^{l+u}} \|\tilde{\boldsymbol{y}} - \Lambda K \boldsymbol{\omega}\|^2 + \lambda_1 \boldsymbol{\omega}^\top K \boldsymbol{\omega} + \lambda_2 \boldsymbol{\omega}^\top K L K \boldsymbol{\omega}, \tag{5}$$

where K is the $(l + u) \times (l + u)$ Gram matrix with entries $K_{ij} = K(x_i, x_j)$, $\tilde{\boldsymbol{y}}$ is the augmented label vector given by $\tilde{\boldsymbol{y}} = [y_1, \ldots, y_l, 0, \ldots, 0]^\top$, and Λ is an $(l + u) \times (l + u)$ diagonal matrix with the first l diagonal entries being 1 and the rest 0, i.e., $\Lambda = diag(1, \ldots, 1, 0, \ldots, 0)$.

The solution of Eq. (5) can be acquired by setting the gradient $w.r.t$ $\boldsymbol{\omega}$ to zero,

$$\boldsymbol{\omega}^* = (\Lambda K + \lambda_1 I + \lambda_2 L K)^{-1} \tilde{\boldsymbol{y}}, \tag{6}$$

where I is an $(l+u) \times (l+u)$ identity matrix. Obviously, the prediction function can be efficiently obtained by solving a single system of linear equations described in Eq. (6), and then the predicted label of a test data x is given by Eq. (4).

2.2 Training Example Collection with Active Example Selection

Given the object location at the current frame, a large set of unlabeled examples is generated by random sampling around the object location, denoted as $P = \{p_i\}_{i=1}^{N_p}$, where N_p is the number of examples. Existing tracking algorithms directly employ a labeling process on this example set, and ignore the correlation between example collection and classifier learning. In this work, we propose an active example selection approach using the formulism of active learning to automatically select the most informative examples among P for LapRLS.

Now we consider the example selection problem from the perspective of active learning. Given the candidate set $V = \{v_i\}_{i=1}^n$, the task is to find a set of examples $Z = \{z_i\}_{i=1}^m$ that together are maximally informative [22]. Suppose that we can observe the labels of z_i by a measurement process $c_i = f(z_i) + \epsilon_i$, where c_i is the observed label of example z_i, f is the underlying label prediction function and $\epsilon_i \sim \mathcal{N}(0, \sigma^2)$ is measurement noise. Using Z as labeled data and the rest in V as unlabeled data, the estimate of f, denoted as $\hat{f}$, can be obtained by using LapRLS,

$$\hat{f}(x) = K_{x,V}\hat{\omega}, \tag{7}$$

$$\hat{\omega} = (K_{VZ}K_{ZV} + \lambda_1 K + \lambda_2 KLK)^{-1}K_{VZ}c, \tag{8}$$

where $(K_{x,V})_{1j} = K(x, v_j)$, $(K_{VZ})_{ij} = K(v_i, z_j)$, $(K_{ZV})_{ij} = K(z_i, v_j)$, $(K)_{ij} = K(v_i, v_j)$, and $c = [c_1, \ldots, c_m]^\top$. Note that Eq. (7) and Eq. (8) can be easily derived from Eq. (4) and Eq. (6), respectively.

Denote $H = K_{VZ}K_{ZV} + \lambda_1 K + \lambda_2 KLK$ and $\Delta = \lambda_1 K + \lambda_2 KLK$, the covariance matrix of $\hat{\omega}$ can be expressed as

$$\begin{aligned} Cov(\hat{\omega}) &= Cov(H^{-1}K_{VZ}c) \\ &= H^{-1}K_{VZ}Cov(c)K_{ZV}H^{-1} \\ &= \sigma^2(H^{-1} - H^{-1}\Delta H^{-1}), \end{aligned} \tag{9}$$

where the third equation uses the assumption $Cov(c) = \sigma^2 I$. The covariance matrix $Cov(\hat{\omega})$ characterizes the confidence of the estimation, or the informativeness of the selected examples [23]. Different criteria can be applied to the covariance matrix to obtain different active learning algorithms for LapRLS. He [27] used the D-optimality criterion that minimizes the determinant of $Cov(\hat{\omega})$ to design an active learning method for image retrieval. However, the criteria does not directly consider the quality of predictions on test data.

Inspired by the work in [25], we design the objective of our active example selection approach in a transductive setting. Let $\mathbf{f}_V = [f(v_1), \ldots, f(v_n)]^\top$ be the true labels of all examples in V given by the underlying label prediction function f, and $\hat{\mathbf{f}}_V = [\hat{f}(v_1), \ldots, \hat{f}(v_n)]^\top$ be the predictions on V given by the estimator $\hat{f}$, then the covariance matrix of the predictive error $\mathbf{f}_V - \hat{\mathbf{f}}_V$ is given by

$$\begin{aligned} Cov(\mathbf{f}_V - \hat{\mathbf{f}}_V) &= KCov(\hat{\omega})K \\ &= \sigma^2 K(H^{-1} - H^{-1}\Delta H^{-1})K. \end{aligned} \tag{10}$$

We aim to select m examples Z from V such that the average predictive variance $\frac{1}{n}\mathrm{Tr}(Cov(\mathbf{f}_V - \hat{\mathbf{f}}_V))$ is minimized, i.e., a high confidence of predictions on V is ensured. Since the regularization parameters (i.e., λ_1 and λ_2) are usually very small, we have

$$\mathrm{Tr}(K(H^{-1} - H^{-1}\Delta H^{-1})K) \approx \mathrm{Tr}(KH^{-1}K). \tag{11}$$

Algorithm 1. Sequential Active Example Selection

1: **Initialize:** $M = K(\lambda_1 K + \lambda_2 KLK)^{-1}K$; Z'; $Z = \emptyset$
2: $M \leftarrow M - M_{VZ'}(M_{Z'Z'} + I)^{-1}M_{Z'V}$
3: **while** $|Z| < m$ **do**
4:     select z according to Eq. (15);
5:     $Z' = Z' \cup \{z\}$, $Z = Z \cup \{z\}$;
6:     $M \leftarrow M - M_{V,z}M_{z,V}/(1 + M_{z,z})$;
7: **end while**
8: **return** Z

Therefore, the formulation of our active example selection approach can be expressed as

$$\max_{Z} \ \mathrm{Tr}\big(K(K_{VZ}K_{ZV} + \lambda_1 K + \lambda_2 KLK)^{-1}K\big)$$
$$s.t. \quad Z \subset V, \ |Z| = m. \tag{12}$$

Note that the example selection itself is independent of the observed labels **c**.

Let Δ^{-1} be the Moore-Penrose inverse of Δ, we can get the following equations by applying Woodbury matrix identity,

$$KH^{-1}K = K(K_{VZ}K_{ZV} + \Delta)^{-1}K$$
$$= K\Delta^{-1}K - K\Delta^{-1}K_{VZ}(K_{ZV}\Delta^{-1}K_{VZ} + I)^{-1}K_{ZV}\Delta^{-1}K, \tag{13}$$

where I is an $m \times m$ identity matrix. We define a new kernel matrix $M = K\Delta^{-1}K$, and rewrite Eq. (12) into a much simple form,

$$\max_{Z} \ \mathrm{Tr}\big(M_{VZ}(M_{ZZ} + I)^{-1}M_{ZV}\big)$$
$$s.t. \quad Z \subset V, \ |Z| = m \tag{14}$$

The problem of Eq. (14) is actually a combinatorial optimization problem which is NP-hard. We present a sequential greedy optimization approach to solve Eq. (14). The rational is two-fold. First, a sequential assumption greatly simplifies the problem and ensures the efficiency of our tracker. Second, it is straightforward to incorporate the current set of labeled examples in an incremental way. Considering the current set of labeled examples during example selection ensures the representativeness of the selected examples.

The sequential approach selects just one example in each iteration until m examples have been selected. Denote the selected examples in the previous iterations as Z', the task of each iteration is to seek for a new example $z \in V - Z'$ by solving Eq. (14). Denote $\tilde{\Delta} = K_{VZ'}K_{Z'V} + \Delta$, Eq. (14) can be rewritten into a canonical form,

$$\max_{z} \ \|\tilde{M}_{V,z}\|^2/(1 + \tilde{M}_{z,z})$$
$$s.t. \quad z \in V - Z' \tag{15}$$

where $\tilde{M} = K\tilde{\Delta}^{-1}K = M - M_{VZ'}(M_{Z'Z'} + I)^{-1}M_{Z'V}$, $\tilde{M}_{V,z}$ and $\tilde{M}_{z,z}$ are z's column and diagonal entry in $\tilde{M}$, respectively. Equation (15) can be easily solved by directly selecting $z \in V - Z'$ with the highest $\|\tilde{M}_{V,z}\|^2/(1 + \tilde{M}_{z,z})$.

Starting from a set Z' and $M = K(\lambda_1 K + \lambda_2 KLK)^{-1}K$, m most informative examples can be selected sequentially. We summarize our active example selection approach in Algorithm 1. Note that there is no need for matrix inverse at each iterative step.

Recall that we employ active example selection to automatically select informative examples from the set P generated by sampling. In addition, we intend to incorporate the current set of labeled examples into the example selection problem to ensures the representativeness of the selected examples. Hence, we set Z' as the current set of labeled examples and construct the candidate set as $V = Z' \cup P$ before we perform Algorithm 1 to select useful examples.

2.3   Bayesian Inference Framework

In this paper, we cast object tracking as a Bayesian inference task with a hidden Markov model. Given the observed image set $\mathcal{O}_{1:t} = \{o_1, \cdots, o_t\}$ up to time t, the optimal state s_t of an object can be estimated by Bayesian theorem,

$$p(s_t|\mathcal{O}_{1:t}) \propto p(o_t|s_t) \int p(s_t|s_{t-1})p(s_{t-1}|\mathcal{O}_{1:t-1}) \, ds_{t-1}, \qquad (16)$$

where $p(s_t|s_{t-1})$ is the motion model that predicts the next state s_t from the previous state s_{t-1}, and $p(o_t|s_t)$ is the observation model that estimates the likelihood of the observation o_t at the state s_t belonging to the object class. In practice, a particle filter [29] is used to approximate the posterior $p(s_t|\mathcal{O}_{1:t})$ by a finite set of N_s samples $\{s_t^i\}_{i=1}^{N_s}$ with importance weights $\{\pi_t^i\}_{i=1}^{N_s}$. The samples s_t^i are drawn from the motion model and the corresponding weights are given by the observation likelihood $p(o_t|s_t^i)$.

Motion model: We apply the affine transformation with six parameters to model the object motion. Formally, $s_t = (x_t, y_t, \sigma_t, \alpha_t, \theta_t, \phi_t)$ where (x_t, y_t) denote translation, $\sigma_t, \alpha_t, \theta_t, \phi_t$ are scale, aspect ratio, rotation angle, and skew direction at time t, respectively. The motion model is formulated as Brownian motion, i.e., $p(s_t|s_{t-1}) = \mathcal{N}(s_t; s_{t-1}, \Sigma)$, where Σ is a diagonal covariance matrix which indicates the variances of affine parameters.

Observation model: For the tracking at time t, we first generate N_s samples $\{s_t^i\}_{i=1}^{N_s}$ from the previous state s_{t-1}. Then the corresponding image regions can be cropped from the observed image o_t by applying affine transformations using s_t^i as parameters. After feature extraction, we can obtain a set of test data, denoted as $\{b_t^i\}_{i=1}^{N_s}$. Integrating this newly test data into the current set of unlabeled examples, denoted as U, together with the current set of labeled examples, denoted as L, an adaptive prediction function f_t can be learned with LapRLS. The observation likelihood of the sample s_t^i is given by

$$p(o_t|s_t^i) \propto exp\big(-\|1 - f_t(b_t^i)\|^2\big). \qquad (17)$$

Here we assume that positive examples are labeled with 1, and negative examples are labeled with 0. At each time stamp, the sample with the maximum observation likelihood is chosen as the tracking result.

Model update: Once the object is located, we sample a large set of unlabeled examples P, and employ active example selection to select a set of informative examples Z. To make the trained classifier more adaptive to appearance changes, we assign labels to part of the set Z according to the following constraints: the distances between positive examples and the current track should be smaller than a threshold τ, and negative examples should not overlap the current track. The rest examples that do not satisfy the constraints are considered as unlabeled data. Then the informative examples Z are used to update the current set of labeled examples L and the current set of unlabeled examples U, where random replacement happens once the number of examples in L or U reaches the maximum values $|L|$ or $|U|$.

3   Experimental Results

We evaluate our tracker with 10 state-of-the-art methods on a recent benchmark [30], where each tracker is tested on 51 challenging videos. The state-of-the-art trackers include TLD [19], MIL [15], VTD [2], Struck [9], SCM [4], CT [10], SPT [12], LSST [8], RET [13] and ONNDL [6]. We use the source codes publicly available on the benchmark (except that the source codes of SPT, LSST, RET and ONNDL are provided by the authors) with the same initialization and their default parameters. Since the trackers involve randomness, we run them 5 times and report the average result for each sequence.

3.1   Implementation Details

We normalize the object region to 32×32 pixels, and extract 9 overlapped 18×18 local patches within the region by sliding windows with 7 pixels as step length. Each patch is represented as a 32-dimensional HOG feature [31], and these features are grouped into a 288-dimensional feature vector. For LapRLS and active example selection, we apply linear kernel and empirically set the regularization parameters λ_1 and λ_2 to be 0.001 and 0.1, respectively. The parameter k in Eq. (4) is empirically chosen as 7 according to [28]. In the first frame, 20 positive examples, 80 negative examples and 300 unlabeled examples are used to initialize the classifier. The example set capacity $|L| = 200$ and $|U| = 600$. Given the object location at the current frame, $N_p = 1200$ unlabeled examples are generated by random sampling and 20 informative examples are selected by active example selection. We set the labeling constraint parameters τ to be 3 pixels. For particle filter, the number of samples $N_s = 600$, and the state transition matrix $\Sigma = diag(8, 8, 0.01, 0, 0, 0)$. Note that the parameters are fixed throughout the experiments in this section. Our tracker is implemented in MATLAB, which runs at 2 fps on an Intel Core i7 3.5 GHz PC with 16 GB memory.

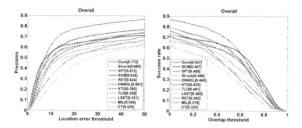

Fig. 2. Overall performance of the competing trackers on 51 video sequences. The precision plot and the success plot are used, and the performance score for each tracker is shown in the legend.

3.2 Quantitative Evaluation

We use the center location error as well as the overlap rate for quantitative evaluations. Center location error is the per frame distance (in pixels) between the center of the tracking result and that of ground truth. Overlap rate is defined as $\frac{area(R_T \cap R_G)}{area(R_T \cup R_G)}$, where R_T is the bounding box of tracking result and R_G denotes the ground truth. We employ precision plot and success plot [30] to evaluate the robustness of trackers, rather than directly using the average center location error and the average overlap rate over all frames of one video sequence to indicate the overall performance. The precision plot indicates the percentage of frames whose estimated location is within the given threshold distance of the ground truth, and the success plot shows the ratios of successful frames whose overlap rate is larger than the given threshold.

The overall performance of the competing trackers on the 51 sequences is illustrated by the precision plot and the success plot as shown in Fig. 2. For the precision plot, the results at error threshold of 20 pixels are used for ranking, while for the success plot we use area under curve (AUC) scores to summarize and rank the trackers.

We can observe from Fig. 2 that both our tracker and the SCM, SPT and Struck methods achieve good tracking performance. In the precision plot, our tracker performs 8.3 % better than the Struck, 10 % better than the SPT, and 13.6 % better than the SCM. In the success plot, our tracker performs 5 % better than the SCM, 5.8 % better than the SPT, and 6.1 % better than the Struck. We also observe that the SCM method provides higher precision and success rate when the error threshold is relatively small (*e.g.*, 5 pixels in the precision plot, and 80 % in the success rate). It owes to the fact that the SCM method exploits both holistic and local representation approaches based on sparse coding to handle appearance variations.

We also utilize the attribute based performance analysis approach [30] to demonstrate the robustness of our tracker. The video sequences used in the benchmark are annotated with 11 attributes which can be considered as different factors that may affect the tracking performance. One sequence can be annotated with several attributes. By putting the sequences that share a common attribute

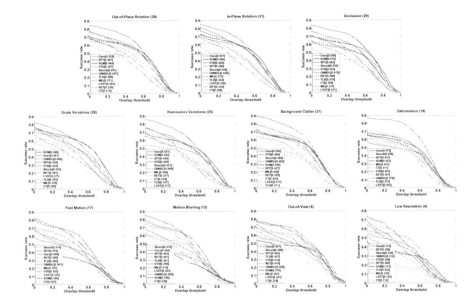

Fig. 3. Attribute based performance analysis using success plot. The number of video sequences in each subset is shown in the title. Best viewed on high-resolution display.

into a subset, we can analyze the performance of trackers to handle a specific challenging condition. Figure 3 illustrates the success plots of the competing trackers for these 11 attributes (arranged in ascending order of the number of video sequences in each subset), and the precision plots can be found in the *supplementary material*. As indicated in Fig. 3, our method provides the best tracking performance in 7 of the 11 video subsets and also performs well in the other 4 subsets, which demonstrates that the proposed algorithm is robust to appearance variations caused by a set of factors.

Overall, our tracker performs favorably against the state-of-the-art algorithms in terms of location accuracy and robustness. It can be attribute to the facts that LapRLS is effective for learning a robust classifier for object tracking, and that the proposed training example collection strategy which includes active example selection and the conservative labeling stage makes the classifier robust and adaptive to appearance changes. Our experimental results validate these claims in the following sections.

3.3 Diagnostic Analysis

As previously mentioned, our tracking method chooses the most informative examples for classifier learning via active example selection, leading to a significant improvement on tracking performance. In addition, we assign labels to part of the selected examples that satisfy strict constraints, which can increase the adaptivity of the classifier. To demonstrate the effectiveness of the active example

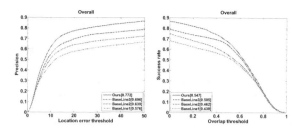

Fig. 4. Diagnostic Analysis. The overall performance of three baseline algorithms and our method on the 51 video sequences is presented for comparison in terms of precision and success rate.

selection approach and the conservative labeling strategy, we build three baseline algorithms to do validation and analyze various aspects of our method.

We begin with a "naive" tracker based on a classifier learned with LapRLS, denoted as BaseLine1. The BaseLine1 only exploits the labeled examples from the first frame, and collects unlabeled examples using random sampling. We add the active example selection stage after the sampling process to select informative examples for LapRLS, resulting in another baseline, denoted as BaseLine2. Both the BaseLine1 and the BaseLine2 are stable versions, since no supervisory information is added during tracking, *i.e.*, the training examples are collected without the labeling stage. We get the last baseline by allowing the BaseLine1 to assign labels to part of the unlabeled examples that satisfy the strict constraints described in Sect. 2.3, denoted as BaseLine3. Note that adding supervisory information to the BaseLine2 leads to the proposed method.

The overall tracking performance of these baseline algorithms and our method is presented in Fig. 4. Surprisingly, even without additional example selection and labeling process, the BaseLine1 produces good performance in terms of precision and robustness, outperforming the CT, MIL, LSST and TLD trackers and being comparable to the VTD. It demonstrates the effectiveness of LapRLS which can sufficiently exploit unlabeled data and preserve the local geometrical structure of feature space. The performance of our method and the Baseline3 is obviously better than the BaseLine1 and the BaseLine2, which demonstrates that the additional supervisory information is significant for object tracking. The conservative labeling strategy used in our tracking method achieves a suitable trade-off between stability and plasticity in terms of capturing appearance variations. The performance of our method is significantly better than BaseLine3, and the BaseLine2 outperforms the BaseLine1. It validates the effectiveness of selecting informative examples for classifier learning. The active example selection guarantees the consistency between example collection and classifier learning, and thus improves the tracking performance. Furthermore, assigning labels to examples selected by active example selection alleviates the drift problem caused by label noise, since misaligned examples will be rejected to ensure the high prediction confidence of the classifier.

3.4 Qualitative Evaluation

We present a qualitative evaluation of the tracking results in this section. 12 representative sequences are chose from the subsets of four dominant attributes, *i.e.*, occlusion, illumination variations, background clutter and deformation. Several screenshots of the tracking results on these 12 sequences are illustrated in Fig. 5. We mainly discuss the four dominant challenges in the following.

Occlusion is one of the most general yet crucial problems in object tracking, as shown in Fig. 5(a). In the *David3* sequence, the person suffers from partial occlusion as well as drastic pose variations (*e.g.*, #249). Only the LSST, RET, ONNDL and our method success in this sequence. In the *Jogging2* sequence, there is a short-term complete occlusion for the tracked object (*e.g.*, #60). The TLD, SCM, ONNDL and our method are able to reacquire the object and provide satisfactory tracks. Note that the TLD method employs a detector to reacquire the object and the SCM and ONNDL trackers involve occlusion resolving scheme based on sparse representation. In the *Woman* sequence, only the Struck, SPT and our method are able to track the object when the long-term occlusion happens (*e.g.*, #134). Most of the trackers lock onto a wrong object with similar appearances after occlusion. Our method selects informative examples for classifier learning via active example selection, and thus alleviates the drift problem caused by misaligned examples in handling occlusions.

The tracked objects in the *David1*, *Singer2* and *Trellis* sequences undergo significant illumination changes and pose variations, as shown in Fig. 5(b). Most of the trackers can not handle the appearance variations caused by illumination changes together with pose variations (*e.g.*, *David1* #161, *Singer2* #185 and *Trellis* #355), whereas the VTD and SCM methods perform better. In contrast, our method achieve stable performance in the entire sequences. In the *Singer2* sequence, the contrast between the foreground and the background is very low. Our method tracks the object accurately, but most trackers drift away at the beginning of the sequence (*e.g.*, #41). The robustness of our tracker against illumination variations comes from the fact that the adopted HOG feature has been proved to be invariant to illumination changes.

In the *Football*, *Lemming* and *Subway* sequences, the objects appear in background clutters, as shown in Fig. 5(c). Most trackers drift away from the objects as there exists the interference of similar appearances in the background (*e.g.*, *Football* #312, *Lemming* #545, *Subway* #46). Our method learns an online classifier that takes the background information into account, and thus can achieve robust performance under complex environments.

In the *Basketball*, *Bolt* and *Skating1* sequences, the object appearances change drastically due to significant non-rigid object deformation, such as viewpoint changes and pose variations, as shown in Fig. 5(d). We can see that only our method tracks the objects successfully in all these three sequences. In the *Basketball* sequence, the person changes his pose frequently and often partially occluded by other players. Only the VTD and our method can keep track all the time. In the *Bolt* sequences, there exist significant pose variations of the person, together with the viewpoint change. The trackers except the ONNDL and our method

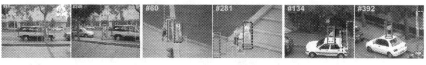

(a) Tracking results on sequence *David3*, *Jogging2* and *Woman* with occlusions.

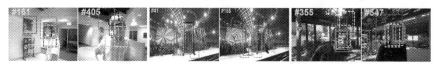

(b) Tracking results on sequence *David*, *Singer2* and *Trellis* with illumination changes.

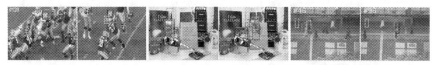

(c) Tracking results on sequence *Football*, *Lemming* and *Subway* with clustered background.

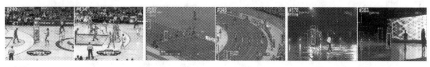

(d) Tracking results on sequence *Basketball*, *Bolt* and *Skating1* with object deformation.

| Ours | ONNDL | SPT | VTD | Struck | SCM | LSST | MIL | RET | CT | TLD |

Fig. 5. Sample tracking results of the competing trackers on 12 representative video sequences.

fail when the viewpoint start to change (*e.g.*, #107). In the *Skating1* sequence, all of the methods except our tracker gradually drift away when there is severe occlusion and large scale change of the object (*e.g.*, #178). We show that our method adaptively copes with appearance variations through online update with the selected informative examples, thus provides more accurate and consistent tracking results.

4   Conclusion

In this paper, we have presented a novel online object tracking algorithm that explicitly couples the objectives of semi-supervised learning and example selection in a principled manner. We have shown that selecting informative examples for classifier learning results in more robust tracking, and have proposed an active example selection approach using the formulism of active learning. We have also shown that assigning labels to part of the selected examples achieves a suitable trade-off between stability and plasticity in terms of capturing appearance variations. Both quantitative and qualitative evaluations compared with state-of-the-art trackers on a comprehensive benchmark demonstrate the effectiveness and robustness of our tracker.

Acknowledgement. This work was supported in part by the Natural Science Foundation of China (NSFC) under grant NO. 61203291, the 973 Program of China under grant NO. 2012CB720000, the Specialized Research Fund for the Doctoral Program of Higher Education of China (20121101120029), and the Specialized Fund for Joint Building Program of Beijing Municipal Education Commission.

References

1. Ross, D., Lim, J., Lin, R., Yang, M.H.: Incremental learning for robust visual tracking. Int. J. Comput. Vis. **77**, 125–141 (2008)
2. Kwon, J., Lee, K.: Visual tracking decomposition. In: CVPR, pp. 1269–1276 (2010)
3. Mei, X., Ling, H.: Robust visual tracking using ℓ1 minimization. In: ICCV, pp. 1–8 (2009)
4. Zhong, W., Lu, H., Yang, M.H.: Robust object tracking via sparsity-based collaborative model. In: CVPR, pp. 1838–1845 (2012)
5. Jia, X., Lu, H., Yang, M.H.: Visual tracking via adaptive structural local sparse appearance model. In: CVPR, pp. 1822–1829 (2012)
6. Wang, N., Wang, J., Yeung, D.Y.: Online robust non-negative dictionary learning for visual tracking. In: ICCV, pp. 657–664 (2013)
7. Wu, Y., Ma, B., Yang, M., Zhang, J., Jia, Y.: Metric learning based structural appearance model for robust visual tracking. IEEE Trans. Circuits Syst. Video Technol. **24**, 865–877 (2014)
8. Wang, D., Lu, H., Yang, M.H.: Least soft-thresold squares tracking. In: CVPR, pp. 2371–2378 (2013)
9. Hare, S., Saffari, A., Torr, P.H.: Struck: structured output tracking with kernels. In: ICCV, pp. 263–270 (2011)
10. Zhang, K., Zhang, L., Yang, M.-H.: Real-time compressive tracking. In: Fitzgibbon, A., Lazebnik, S., Perona, P., Sato, Y., Schmid, C. (eds.) ECCV 2012, Part III. LNCS, vol. 7574, pp. 864–877. Springer, Heidelberg (2012)
11. Li, X., Shen, C., Dick, A.R., van den Hengel, A.: Learning compact binary codes for visual tracking. In: CVPR, pp. 2419–2426 (2013)
12. Yao, R., Shi, Q., Shen, C., Zhang, Y., van den Hengel, A.: Part-based visual tracking with online latent structural learning. In: CVPR, pp. 2363–2370 (2013)
13. Bai, Q., Wu, Z., Sclaroff, S., Betke, M., Monnier, C.: Randomized ensemble tracking. In: ICCV, pp. 2040–2047 (2013)
14. Grabner, H., Leistner, C., Bischof, H.: Semi-supervised on-line boosting for robust tracking. In: Forsyth, D., Torr, P., Zisserman, A. (eds.) ECCV 2008, Part I. LNCS, vol. 5302, pp. 234–247. Springer, Heidelberg (2008)
15. Babenko, B., Yang, M.H., Belongie, S.: Robust object tracking with online multiple instance learning. IEEE Trans. Pattern Anal. Mach. Intell. **33**, 1619–1632 (2011)
16. Saffari, A., Leistner, C., Godec, M., Bischof, H.: Robust multi-view boosting with priors. In: Saffari, A., Leistner, C., Godec, M., Bischof, H. (eds.) ECCV 2010, Part III. LNCS, vol. 6313, pp. 776–789. Springer, Heidelberg (2010)
17. Bai, Y., Tang, M.: Robust tracking via weakly supervised ranking SVM. In: CVPR, pp. 1854–1861 (2012)
18. Gao, J., Xing, J., Hu, W., Maybank, S.: Discriminant tracking using tensor representation with semi-supervised improvement. In: ICCV (2013)
19. Kalal, Z., Matas, J., Mikolajczyk, K.: P-N learning: bootstrapping binary classifiers by structural constraints. In: CVPR, pp. 49–56 (2010)

20. Supancic III, J.S., Ramanan, D.: Self-paced learning for long-term tracking. In: CVPR, pp. 2379–2386 (2013)
21. Belkin, M., Niyogi, P., Sindhwani, V.: Manifold regularization: a geometric framework for learning from labeled and unlabeled examples. J. Mach. Learn. Res. **7**, 2399–2434 (2006)
22. Cohn, D.A., Ghahramani, Z., Jordan, M.I.: Active learning with statistical models. J. Artif. Intell. Res. **4**, 129–145 (1996)
23. Atkinson, A.C., Donev, A.N.: Optimum Experimental Designs. Oxford University Press, New York (2002)
24. Santner, J., Leistner, C., Saffari, A., Pock, T., Bischof, H.: PROST: parallel robust online simple tracking. In: CVPR, pp. 723–730 (2010)
25. Yu, K., Bi, J., Tresp, V.: Active learning via transductive experimental design. In: ICML, pp. 1081–1088 (2006)
26. He, X., Min, W., Cai, D., Zhou, K.: Laplacian optimal design for image retrieval. In: ACM SIGIR, pp. 119–126 (2007)
27. He, X.: Laplacian regularized d-optimal design for active learning and its application to image retrieval. IEEE Trans. Image Process. **19**, 254–263 (2010)
28. Zelnik-Manor, L., Perona, P.: Self-tuning spectral clustering. In: NIPS, pp. 1601–1608 (2004)
29. Isard, M., Blake, A.: Condensation - conditional density propagation for visual tracking. Int. J. Comput. Vis. **29**, 5–28 (1998)
30. Wu, Y., Lim, J., Yang, M.H.: Online object tracking: a benchmark. In: CVPR, pp. 2411–2418 (2013)
31. Dalal, N., Triggs, B.: Histograms of oriented gradients for human detection. In: CVPR, pp. 886–893 (2005)

Reconstructing Shape and Appearance of Thin Film Objects with Hyper Spectral Sensor

Yoshie Kobayashi[1(✉)], Tetsuro Morimoto[2], Imari Sato[3],
Yasuhiro Mukaigawa[4], and Katsushi Ikeuchi[1]

[1] The University of Tokyo, Tokyo, Japan
yoshie@cvl.iis.u-tokyo.ac.jp
[2] Toppan Printing Co. Ltd., Tokyo, Japan
[3] National Institute of Informatics, Tokyo, Japan
[4] Nara Institute of Science and Technology, Nara, Japan

Abstract. Modeling the shape and appearance of a thin film object has promising applications such as heritage-modeling and industrial inspections. In the same time, such modeling is a frontier of computer vision and contains various challenging issues to be solved. In particular, thin film colors show iridescence along the view and lighting directions and how to acquire and formalize the spectral iridescence for shape estimation. This paper aims to model the shapes and appearances of thin film objects from measured reflectance spectra. Thin film reflectance is represented by the incident angle on the object surface, the refractive index and the film thickness. First, we estimate the incident angle of a surface patch on a thin film based on monotonically increasing peak intensities. Then, we apply a characteristics strip expansion method to the peak intensity for estimating the surface normal of the patch. Based on this shape estimation, we estimate refractive index and film thickness from iridescence variance. We experimentally evaluate the accuracy of the estimated shape and estimated parameters. We also demonstrate to reconstruct appearances based on the shape and parameters.

1 Introduction

Modeling the shape and appearance of real world objects is one of the important research in computer graphics and computer vision fields. Such modeling results are widely used to games, movies and cultural heritage digitization to name a few. Appearances of many objects include several complex reflectance properties such as scattering, absorption, diffraction, refraction and interference. These properties make it difficult to model the shapes and appearances of such objects.

Various objects have interference optical properties, such as laminated materials, soap bubbles and oil films. Interference is one of the most intractable effects since its color varies iridescence along the viewing and lighting directions. Yet, modeling shapes and appearances of these objects with interference effects would be useful for diverse applications in industry, biology, archeology and medicine. For example, realizing the digitization of thin film objects, we can obtain more

© Springer International Publishing Switzerland 2015
D. Cremers et al. (Eds.): ACCV 2014, Part IV, LNCS 9006, pp. 492–506, 2015.
DOI: 10.1007/978-3-319-16817-3_32

realistic appearance of new coating products in digital space. Several Japanese art crafts such as Tamamushi Shrine were made of wings of green buprestids with interference.

Considering the iridescence of thin film objects, Iwasaki *et al.* [1] proposed a rendering method based on physical model. This method manually sets optical parameters such as the refractive index and film thickness. In the optics field, there are several methods for estimating the optical parameters of thin film. Interference spectroscopy [2] and ellipsometry [3] are suitable methods for estimating film thickness, but the refractive index and surface must be known and they handle only a spot measurement. Kitagawa [4,5] proposed an image-based method. Kitagawa used RGB values which change along the film thickness. However, this method needs to know the refractive index. Kobayashi *et al.* [6] proposed a method for estimating the unknown refractive indexes and film thicknesses by using hyper-spectral images. This method can only be applied to flat surfaces in order to control the incident angle.

This paper proposes a novel method for estimating the shape and appearance of thin film objects by using hyper-spectral images. The color variance of thin film is related to the shape and optical parameters. First, we estimate the incident angles of light on the surface. We focus on the monotonically increasing of the local maximum intensity in the hyper-spectral space, which is caused by interference of reflected light. This local maximum intensity depends on the refractive index of the bottom layer. From the known refractive index and the maximum intensity, we can estimate the incident angles. Second, we estimate the normal from the estimated incident angle by using the characteristic strip expansion method. Finally, we can estimate the optical parameters of thin film such as the refractive index and film thickness by least square minimization between measured reflectance and model reflectance. In our experiments, we confirm that our method theoretically works well. Furthermore, we synthesize the appearance of a thin film object by using estimated parameters and evaluate the accuracy.

We assume that a thin film object consists of the top layer, thin film layer and bottom layer as shown in Fig. 1. We also assume that the top layer is air, the target object is convex, and that the captured image is an orthographic projection of the object; hence, the distance between the object and camera is sufficiently far, and the refractive index of the bottom layer is known. In addition to these, we assume the refractive index is constant along wavelengths.

The rest of this paper is organized as follows. In Sect. 2, we introduce the methods for acquiring and estimating the shape and BRDF and structural color rendering. In Sect. 3, we introduce a reflectance model of thin film interference. In Sect. 4, we describe the method used to estimate the shape and BRDF parameters. In Sect. 5, we evaluate the proposed method on the basis of simulations and real data and discuss the estimation error in the experiment. In Sect. 6, we discuss experimental errors. In Sect. 7, we summarize results.

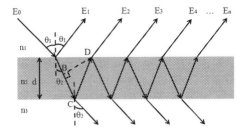

Fig. 1. Schematic diagram of thin film interference when considering multiple reflections. n_1, n_2 and n_3 are refractive indexes of top layer, thin film and bottom layer respectively. d is film thickness. θ_1 is incident angle. θ_2 is refracting angle. θ_3 is outgoing angle.

2   Related Work

In computer vision fields, many methods are proposed for estimating shape, for example the stereo method [7], photometric method [8]. All these methods work well for Lambertian, isotropic, and anisotropic reflectance properties. For more a complicated reflectance property, Morris et al. [9] estimate the shape of translucent objects. In an outdoor scene, Oxholm et al. [10] estimate the BRDF and shape from a single image under natural illumination. These methods do not consider the iridescence of thin film along the light and view directions. For the optical parameters of reflectance property, Morimoto et al. [11] estimated the optical thickness and opacity of layered surfaces, and represented the appearance of layered surfaces of arbitrary thickness. However, this method cannot handle the interference effect of the thin film.

In computer graphics fields, several methods are available for rendering multi-layer interference, diffraction gratings, and refraction. Hirayama et al. [12,13] used a multi-layered interference model based on physics and rendered both eyeglass lens and a mother-of-pearl. Modeling the micro-structure of CDs precisely, Sun et al. [14,15] were able to render them more realistically. Sadeghi et al. [16] calculated refracted ray in vapor by ray tracing and represented an accurate rainbow image that was close to the real one. Cuypers et al. [17] showed that the Wigner distribution function can represent the BRDF of diffraction grating as accurately as can a physical model. All these methods are based on physical models and represent the color changes well, but the optical parameters of models must be set manually. Therefore, it is difficult to represent the appearance of a real object without parameters information.

3   Thin-Film Interference Reflectance Model

In the optics fields, a reflectance model of thin film interference [18] was proposed. As shown in Fig. 1, the reflection of thin film consists of only specular reflection. Considering the multi-path reflection in Fig. 1, the observed light E can be represented by using Eq. (1).

$$
\begin{aligned}
E &= E_1 + E_2 + E_3 + E_4 + \cdots \\
&= E_0(r_{12} + t_{12}t_{21}r_{23}e^{i\Delta} + t_{12}t_{21}r_{23}^2 r_{21} e^{2i\Delta} \\
&\quad + t_{12}t_{21}r_{23}^3 r_{21}^2 e^{3i\Delta} + \cdots \\
&= E_0(r_{12} + t_{12}t_{21}r_{23}e^{i\Delta}(1 + r_{23}r_{21}e^{i\Delta} \\
&\quad + r_{23}^2 r_{21}^2 e^{2i\Delta} + \cdots)) \\
&= E_0(r_{12} + t_{12}t_{21}r_{23}e^{i\Delta}\frac{1}{1 - r_{23}r_{21}e^{i\Delta}}),
\end{aligned}
\tag{1}
$$

where r_{12}, r_{23} and r_{21} are the Fresnel reflection coefficients, and t_{12} and t_{21} are the Fresnel transmittance coefficients. Δ is the phase difference, and represented by Eq. (2). φ is the optical path difference which is the path distance of $BC + CD$ as shown in Fig. 1.

$$
\Delta = \frac{2\pi\varphi}{\lambda}
\tag{2}
$$

$$
\varphi = 2dn_2 \cos\theta_2
\tag{3}
$$

By setting $r_{21} = -r_{12}$ and $t_{21}t_{12} + r_{12}^2 = 1$, the amplitude of the reflection coefficients is defined as Eq. (4).

$$
\begin{aligned}
r &\equiv \frac{E}{E_0} \\
&= r_{12} + t_{12}t_{21}r_{23}e^{i\Delta}\frac{1}{1 - r_{23}r_{21}e^{i\Delta}} \\
&= \frac{r_{12} - r_{12}r_{23}r_{21}e^{i\Delta} + (1 - r_{12}^2)r_{23}e^{i\Delta}}{1 - r_{23}r_{21}e^{i\Delta}} \\
&= \frac{r_{12} + r_{23}e^{i\Delta}}{1 + r_{23}r_{12}e^{i\Delta}}
\end{aligned}
\tag{4}
$$

The reflectance is given by the square of the absolute value of Eq. (4).

$$
R = \left| \frac{r_{12} + r_{23}e^{i\Delta}}{1 + r_{23}r_{12}e^{i\Delta}} \right|^2
\tag{5}
$$

Fresnel reflection coefficients in Eq. (4) are defined for the perpendicular (S-wave) and parallel (P-wave) polarizations. r_{12} is defined as Eqs. (6) and (7). r_{23} is defined as Eqs. (8) and (9).

$$
r_{12}^s = \frac{n_1 \cos\theta_1 - n_2 \cos\theta_2}{n_1 \cos\theta_1 + n_2 \cos\theta_2}
\tag{6}
$$

$$
r_{12}^p = \frac{n_2 \cos\theta_1 - n_1 \cos\theta_2}{n_2 \cos\theta_1 + n_1 \cos\theta_2}
\tag{7}
$$

$$
r_{23}^s = \frac{n_2 \cos\theta_2 - n_3 \cos\theta_3}{n_2 \cos\theta_2 + n_3 \cos\theta_3}
\tag{8}
$$

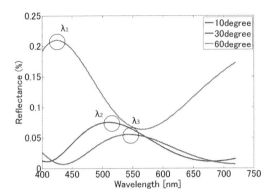

Fig. 2. Reflectance of thin film at 10, 30 and 60 degrees shown as blue, green and red lines respectively. The refractive index of these reflectance is 1.37 and the film thickness is 400 nm.

$$r_{23}^p = \frac{n_3 \cos\theta_2 - n_2 \cos\theta_3}{n_3 \cos\theta_2 + n_2 \cos\theta_3},\tag{9}$$

where n_1, n_2 and n_3 are the refractive index of the top layer, thin film and bottom layer respectively. θ_1 is the incident angle. θ_2 is the refracting angle. θ_3 is an angle of outgoing light transmitting the thin film and absorbed by the bottom layer.

With these above equations, Eq. (5) is represented by the incident angle, the refractive index and the film thickness. Equation (5) describes the reflectance along the incident angle. We use this equation for the BRDF model of the thin film interference.

4 Shape and BRDF Estimation

In this section, we describe a step by step algorithm for estimating the shape and reflectance parameters. First, we estimate the incident angle. Second, we estimate the surface normal from the estimated incident angle by using the characteristic strip expansion method. Finally, we estimate the BRDF parameters, such as refractive index and film thickness, from measured reflectance spectra.

4.1 Incident Angle Estimation

We propose an incident angle estimation method, focusing on the monotonically increasing of the "peak intensity" along the incident angle. Figure 2 shows an example of the peak intensity and peak wavelength enclosed by circles. The local maximum of the reflectance is caused by the full constructive interference. We call this local maximum reflectance "peak intensity" and the wavelength of this local maximum reflectance "peak wavelength".

We find the peak intensity is only dependent on the refractive index of the ground layer, when it becomes higher than the refractive index of the thin film.

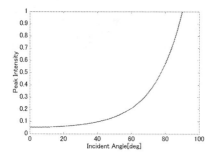

Fig. 3. Peak intensity along incident angle. We calculate intensity with refractive index of the bottom layer of 1.6.

Figure 3 shows the peak intensity along the incident angle. Using this monotonically increasing intensity, we can estimate the incident angle.

The phase difference (Eq. (2)) becomes 2π at the peak wavelength when the refractive index of the ground layer is higher than that of the thin film [19]. Therefore, $e^{i\Delta}$ becomes 1 at this wavelength, so the reflectance intensity at this wavelength $R(\lambda_t)$ can be determined by Eq. (10).

$$R(\lambda_t) = \left| \frac{r_{12} + r_{23}}{1 + r_{23} r_{12}} \right|^2 , \tag{10}$$

where λ_t is the peak wavelength.

Substituting Eqs. (6) and (8) with Eq. (10), the peak intensity of the perpendicular polarization is defined as Eq. (12).

$$R(\lambda_t) = \left| \frac{\cos\theta_1 - n_3 \cos\theta_3}{\cos\theta_1 + n_3 \cos\theta_3} \right|^2 = \left| \frac{\cos\theta_1 - n_3 \sqrt{1 - \sin\theta_3^2}}{\cos\theta_1 + n_3 \sqrt{1 - \sin\theta_3^2}} \right|^2 \tag{11}$$

By Snell's law, $n_1 \sin\theta_1 = n_2 \sin\theta_2 = n_3 \sin\theta_3$ and $n_1 = 1.0$, Eq. (11) becomes as follows.

$$R(\lambda_t) = \left| \frac{\cos\theta_1 - n_3 \sqrt{1 - \frac{1}{n_3^2} \sin\theta_1^2}}{\cos\theta_1 + n_3 \sqrt{1 - \frac{1}{n_3^2} \sin\theta_1^2}} \right|^2 = \left| \frac{\cos\theta_1 - \sqrt{n_3^2 - \sin^2\theta_1}}{\cos\theta_1 + \sqrt{n_3^2 - \sin^2\theta_1}} \right|^2 \tag{12}$$

The equation shows that the peak intensity of the perpendicular polarization depends on the incident angle and refractive index of the ground layer. In our method, we assume the refractive index of the ground layer is known. We also verified the integral intensity in the whole visible wavelength and found that it becomes monotonic increasing. However, this intensity depends not only on the refractive index of the ground layer but also on the refractive index of the thin film.

We determine the incident angle domain by minimizing the least square error between the peak intensity Eq. (12) and that of the measured reflectance.

$$\text{Arg} \min_{\theta_1} |R_o(\lambda_t) - R_m(\lambda_t)|^2 \tag{13}$$

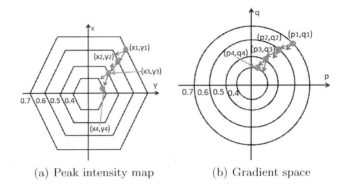

(a) Peak intensity map   (b) Gradient space

Fig. 4. Example of estimation using the characteristic expansion method. (a) the image which is mapped peak intensity to each pixel. (b) shows contour line in the gradient space.

$R_o(\lambda_t)$ is the measured reflectance at the peak wavelength. $R_m(\lambda_t)$ is calculated by using the known refractive index of the bottom layer.

4.2   Surface Normal Estimation

We estimate the surface normal of the thin film by using the characteristic strip expansion method proposed by Horn [20]. This method uses the monotonically increasing intensity and steepest ascent in the gradient space. As mentioned in previous section, the peak intensity monotonically increases. We find that the peak intensity corresponds to the gradient. We explain about the correspondence below.

In the image coordinate, an object point (x, y, z) is mapped to a pixel (u, v), for which $u = x$ and $v = y$ under the orthographic projection. If the object surface z is represented as follows,

$$z = f(x, y), \tag{14}$$

then the surface normal vector is defined by Eq. (15).

$$(p, q, -1) = \left[\frac{\delta f(x, y)}{\delta x}, \frac{\delta f(x, y)}{\delta y}, -1 \right], \tag{15}$$

where p and q are the parameters of the surface normal. The quantity (p, q) is the gradient of (x, y) and is called the "gradient space".

Normalizing Eq. (15) as 1, the z component of the surface normal becomes

$$z = \frac{1}{\sqrt{p^2 + q^2 + 1}} \tag{16}$$

This component is also equal to the cosine of the incident angle. Setting $x^2 + y^2 + z^2 = 1$, the existence domain of f (p, q) is on the circumference defined as Eq. (17).

$$p^2 + q^2 = \frac{1}{\cos^2 \theta_1} - 1 \tag{17}$$

By Eq. (17), the existence domein of gradients corresponds to the peak intensity. The peak intensity is determined uniquely by the incident angle. Also the existence domain is defined uniquely by the incident angle as shown in Eq. (17). This correspondence make it able to apply the characteristics strip expansion method to the thin film objects.

We describe the estimation procedure with Fig. 4. Red arrows are steepest ascents in the peak intensity map. Purple arrows are steepest ascent in the gradient space.

1. Drawing contour lines by sampling the peak intensity per 0.1.
2. Start from the pixel (x_1, y_1) in captured image which gradient $(p_1, q1)$ is known.
3. Moving to the steepest ascent direction of (p_1, q_1) in captured image and determining (x_2, y_2) as the next pixel where intersect with contour line of the peak intensity.
4. Moving to the steepest ascent direction of (x_1, y_1) in gradient space and determining (p_2, q_2) as the next gradient where intersect with contour line of the gradient.
5. Repeating steps 3 and 4 until the whole surface normal is estimated.

4.3   Refractive Index and Film Thickness Estimation

The refractive index and the film thickness are important optical parameters for reconstructing the appearance of thin film. We developed a more effective method for estimating these parameters.

By Snell's law, the optical path difference of Eq. (3) is rewritten as

$$\varphi = 2d\sqrt{n_2^2 - \sin^2 \theta_1} \tag{18}$$

The optical path difference becomes an integral multiple of the peak wavelength.

$$m\lambda_t = 2d\sqrt{n_2^2 - \sin^2 \theta_1}, \tag{19}$$

where m is a natural number. Using Eq. (19), the film thickness is defined as

$$d = \frac{m\lambda_t}{2\sqrt{n_2^2 - \sin^2 \theta_1}} \tag{20}$$

Therefore, we only need to check the combinations of the refractive index and the film thickness that fit the integral multiples of the peak wavelength. This enables us to reduce the computational time considerably, comparing with that required for the full search.

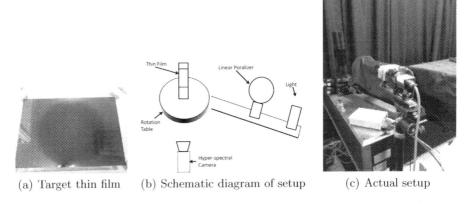

(a) Target thin film   (b) Schematic diagram of setup   (c) Actual setup

Fig. 5. Experimental setup for measuring thin film reflectance. (a) shows target thin film. (b) shows schematic diagram of setup. (c) shows actual setup. Distance between light source and the thin film was 0.8 m. Distance between the camera and the thin film was 0.6 m.

We determine the refractive index and film thickness by minimizing the square error between the reflectance model and the measured reflectance. The uniqueness of this minimization is guaranteed experimentally. Equation (21) has some local minima, but it only has global minimum around ground truth.

$$\text{Arg} \min_{n_2,m} | \sum_{\lambda} R_o(\lambda) - R_m(\lambda) |^2 \qquad (21)$$

$R_o(\lambda)$ is measured reflectance spectra. $R_m(\lambda)$ is calculated by using the reflectance model in Sect. 3.

As mentioned in the previous section, the refractive index n_2 is lower than that of the bottom layer. Also, it is higher than 1.0 which is the refractive index in a vacuum. Kobayashi et al. [6] showed that when the refractive index error is approximately 0.01, the color difference of the BRDF becomes sufficiently small. We change the refractive index n_2 by 0.01 from 1.0 to the refractive index of the bottom layer. We then increased the natural number m until the film thickness is less than 1000 nm.

5   Evaluation

We evaluate the accuracy of our method by simulation and real data. For the simulation, we used hemispherical and cylindrical objects. We set the refractive index of thin film to 1.37 and that of the bottom layer to 1.6 which was the same as that of the real object. We set the film thickness to 400 nm for the hemispherical object and 420 nm to 560 nm along the x-axis for the cylindrical object.

Figure 5 shows the setup for the thin film reflectance measurement to acquire the real data. A light source was attached to the rotation table to adjust the

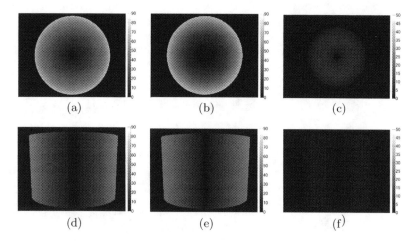

Fig. 6. Incident angle estimation results by simulation. (a) and (d) are ground truths. (b) and (e) are estimated results. (c) and (f) are estimation errors.

incident angle. The target thin film was MgF_2 which refractive index is 1.37. The film thickness was 400 nm. The refractive index of the bottom layer was 1.6, made of polyethylene terephthalate. We varied the incident angle from 10 to 42.5 degrees by 2.5 degrees.

The measurement device was a hyper-spectral camera, which consists of a liquid crystal tunable filter (Vari Spec CRI) and a monochrome camera. The liquid crystal tunable filter (LCTF) can change its transmitted wavelengths electrically. The viewing angle of the camera is approximately 30 degrees. The band width in this experiment was 4 nm. We putted a linear polarizer, which transmits S-wave. LCTF also transmits linearly polarized light, so we can capture S-wave reflectance. The transmittance of LCTF is only 4 % around 400 nm. The brightness of S-wave is stronger than that of P-wave, therefore we measure S-wave.

5.1   Incident Angle

Figure 6 shows the incident angle estimation results of the simulation. Figure 6(b) and (e) show the estimated incident angles. Figure 6(c) and (f) show the estimation errors. The error increased around 0 to 20 degrees. The error of the spherical object is about 10 degree in this area. In other area, it becomes less than 3 degree. The error of the cylindrical object is about 5 degree in this area. In other are, it becomes less than 3 degree.

Figure 7 shows the captured reflectance and the estimated result of the real data. The error also increased around 0 to 20 degrees. The error was approximately 9 degrees in this area. At other incident angles, the error was less than 5 degrees.

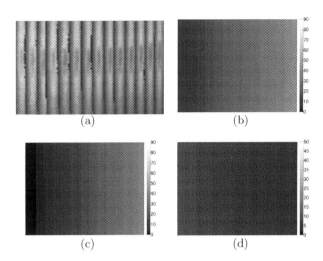

Fig. 7. Incident angle estimation results of real data. (a) shows input reflectance image. (b) shows ground truth incident angle. (c) shows estimated incident angle. (d) shows estimation error.

5.2   Surface Normal

By delimiting the estimated incident angle in Sect. 5.1 by 3 degrees, we estimated the surface normal by the characteristic strip expansion method. Figure 8(b) and (e) show the estimated results.

Figure 8(c) and (f) show the estimation errors. The estimation error was calculated as the angle between the ground truth normal and the estimated normal. The maximum error for the hemispherical object was approximately 10 degrees, and that of the cylinder was about 4 degrees. These errors include incident angle errors, then the error of surface normal estimation is about 1 degree. Therefore, the areas in which these errors occurred were the same as the areas where the incident angle errors were large.

5.3   Refractive Index and Film Thickness

We estimated the refractive index and film thickness, by using the estimated incident angle in Sect. 5.1. For the simulation, the estimated refractive index of the hemispherical and cylindrical objects was 1.37. Figure 9(b) and (e) show the estimated film thicknesses. Figure 9(c) and (f) show the estimation errors. The error of the hemispherical object was approximately 10 nm in the area where the error of the incident angle became larger. The error of cylindrical object was about 7 nm in the same area. For the real data, the estimated refractive index was 1.41. Figure 10(b) shows the estimated thickness. Figure 10(c) shows the estimation error. The average error was 45 nm.

We calculated the average color difference and root mean square error (RMSE) between the measured reflectance and the reflectance with estimated parameters.

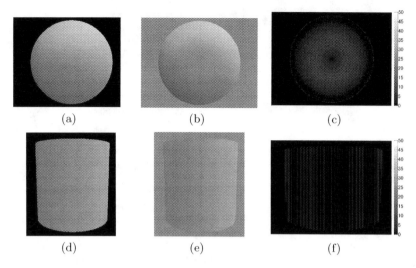

Fig. 8. Surface normal estimation results by simulation. (a) and (d) are ground truth. (b) and (e) are estimated normals. (c) and (f) are estimation errors.

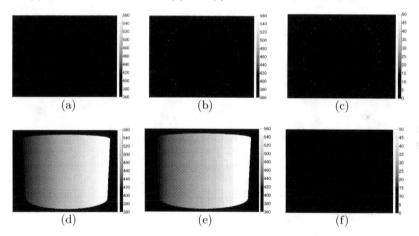

Fig. 9. Fim thickness estimation results by simulation. (a) and (d) are ground truths. (b) and (e) are estimated results. (c) and (f) are estimation errors.

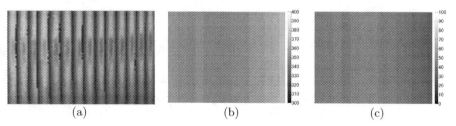

Fig. 10. Film thickness estimation result of real data. (a) shows input reflectance image. (b) shows estimated film thickness. (c) shows estimation error.

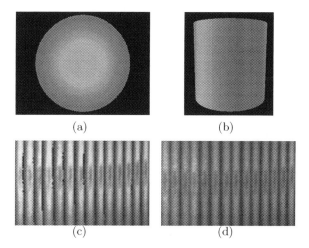

Fig. 11. Image synthesized with estimated surface normal, refractive index, and film thickness. (a) and (b) are results for simulation data. (c) is reflectance image by captured with the hyper-spectral camera. (d) is synthesized reflectance image for real data.

The color difference was calculated using Eq. (22).

$$\Delta E^* ab = \sqrt{(\Delta L^*)^2 + (\Delta a^*)^2 + (\Delta b^*)^2} \qquad (22)$$

The RMSE is defined as Eq. (23).

$$RMSE = \sqrt{(R_o(\lambda) - R_e(\lambda))^2 / N} \qquad (23)$$

$R_o(\lambda)$ is the measured reflectance. $R_e(\lambda)$ is reflectance calculated by using the estimated parameters. The color difference was approximately 3.33, which can be perceived as a slight difference from the levels given in Table 1. The RMSE was about 2 % for each wavelength intensity.

Figure 11 shows the rendering results with the estimated surface normal, refractive index and film thickness. Figure 11(a) and (b) are the reconstructed appearance of simulation data. Figure 11(c) is the image captured by using the hyper-spectral camera and (d) is the synthesized image.

6   Discussion

In this section, we discuss estimation results of the incident angle, surface normal, and optical parameters. The error of the incident angle became larger around 0 to 20 degrees. In these areas, the peak wavelengths were close to each other. This is very close to the sampling interval of the simulation data and the band width of the hyper-spectral camera, so intensity detection became difficult. The error of the surface normal and optical parameters became large in the same area where the error of the incident angle became large. This error occurred because

Table 1. Level of difference or distance between two Colors

Level of color difference	$\Delta E^* ab$
Trace	$0 \sim 0.5$
Slight	$0.5 \sim 1.5$
Noticable	$1.5 \sim 3.0$
Appreciable	$3.0 \sim 6.0$
Great	$6.0 \sim 12.0$
Very great	over 12.0

of the incident angle estimation error. The error of the optical parameters error of the real data becomes large outside these areas. The measured reflectance included noise which make the detection accuracy of the peak wavelength lower. Therefore, we can avoid these errors by using a high wavelength resolution and hyper-spectral camera with less noise.

Comparing the synthesized image Fig. 11(d) and real image Fig, 11(c), we can perceive the difference. The color difference occurs by the error of the incident angle and rounding error of captured reflectance spectra around 430 nm. Over 40 degree, the sample MgF_2 has the peak intensity around 430 nm, but hyper-spectral camera could not capture it with enough brightness because of its low transmittance. The low transmittance cause the rounding error which effects as noise, so we have the difference. The wavelength dependency of the refractive index is also considerable. However, we experimentally verified it does not effect to the estimated appearance for this sample.

We could estimate the incident angle and optical parameters even in darker areas in Fig. 11(c). In darker areas, just the intensity of the measured reflectance is small, and we could measure reflectance spectra correctly. Therefore, estimated results of Figs. 7(c) and 10(b) had parameters in darker areas in Fig. 11(c).

7   Conclusion

We proposed a novel method for estimating the shape and appearance of a thin film. We found that the peak intensity increased monotonically along incident angle, so we could use the characteristic strip expansion method to estimate the thin film surface normal. We also developed a more efficient method for estimating the refractive index and the film thickness by using the peak wavelength, where the optical path difference becomes an integral multiple of the peak wavelength. We conducted an experiment by simulation and real data and showed the effectiveness of our method. Our future work is to estimate more complicated shapes.

References

1. IWasaki, K., Matsuzawa, K., Nishita, T.: Real-time rendering of soap bubbles taking into account light interference. In: Proceedings of the Computer Graphics

International, CGI 2004, pp. 344–348. IEEE Computer Society, Washington, DC, USA (2004)

2. Meinster, K.W.: Interference spectroscopy. Part I. J. Opt. Soc. Am. **31**, 405–426 (1941)
3. Azzam, R., Bashara, N.: Ellipsometry and Polarized Light. North-Holland Personal Library. North-Holland Pub, Co, Amsterdam (1977)
4. Kitagawa, K.: Thin-film thickness profile measurement by three-wavelength interference color analysis. Appl. Opt. **52**, 1998–2007 (2013)
5. Kitagawa, K.: Transparent film thickness measurement by three-wavelength interference method: an extended application of global model fitting algorithm. In: 2012 13th Int'l Workshop on Mechatronics (MECATRONICS), 2012 9th France-Japan 7th Europe-Asia Congress on and Research and Education in Mechatronics (REM), pp. 94–100 (2012)
6. Kobayashi, Y., Morimoto, T., Sato, I., Mukaigawa, Y., Ikeuchi, K.: BRDF estimation of structural color object by using hyper spectral image. In: IEEE International Conference on Computer Vision Workshops (ICCVW), pp. 915–922 (2013)
7. Scharstein, D., Szeliski, R.: A taxonomy and evaluation of dense two-frame stereo correspondence algorithms. Int. J. Comput. Vis. **47**, 7–42 (2002)
8. Herbort, S., WUhler, C.: An introduction to image-based 3d surface reconstruction and a survey of photometric stereo methods. 3D Res. **2**, 40:1–40:17 (2011)
9. Morris, N.J.W., et al.: Reconstructing the surface of inhomogeneous transparent scenes by scatter-trace photography (2007)
10. Oxholm, G., Nishino, K.: Shape and reflectance from natural illumination. In: Fitzgibbon, A., Lazebnik, S., Perona, P., Sato, Y., Schmid, C. (eds.) ECCV 2012, Part I. LNCS, vol. 7572, pp. 528–541. Springer, Heidelberg (2012)
11. Morimoto, T., Tan, R., Kawakami, R., Ikeuchi, K.: Estimating optical properties of layered surfaces using the spider model. In: 2010 IEEE Conference on Computer Vision and Pattern Recognition (CVPR), pp. 207–214 (2010)
12. Hirayama, H., Kaneda, K., Yamashita, H., Monden, Y.: An accurate illumination model for objects coated with multilayer films. Comput. Graph. **25**, 391–400 (2001)
13. Hirayama, H., Yamaji, Y., Kaneda, K., Yamashita, H., Monden, Y.: Rendering iridescent colors appearing on natural objects. In: Proceedings of the Eighth Pacific Conference on Computer Graphics and Applications, pp. 15–433 (2000)
14. Sun, Y., David Fracchia, F., Drew, M.S., Calvert, T.W.: Rendering iridescent colors of optical disks. In: Péroche, B., Rushmeier, H. (eds.) Rendering Techniques 2000. Eurographics, pp. 341–352. Springer, Heidelberg (2000)
15. Sun, Y., Fracchia, F.D., Calvert, T.W., Drew, M.S.: Deriving spectra from colors and rendering light interference. IEEE Comput. Graph. Appl. **19**, 61–67 (1999)
16. Sadeghi, I., Muñoz, A., Laven, P., Jarosz, W., Seron, F., Gutierrez, D., Jensen, H.W.: Physically-based simulation of rainbows. ACM Trans. Graph. **31**, 3:1–3:12 (2012). (Presented at SIGGRAPH)
17. Cuypers, T., Haber, T., Bekaert, P., Oh, S.B., Raskar, R.: Reflectance model for diffraction. ACM Trans. Graph. **31**, 122:1–122:11 (2012)
18. Kinoshita, S.: Structural Colors in the Realm of Nature. World Scientific, Singapore (2008)
19. Pedrotti, L.S.: Basic Physical Optics. SPIE Press Book, Bellingham (2008)
20. Horn, B.K.: A problem in computer vision: orienting silicon integrated circuit chips for lead bonding. Comput. Graph. Image Process. **4**, 294–303 (1975)

A Two-Stage Approach for Bag Detection in Pedestrian Images

Yuning Du[1]([✉]), Haizhou Ai[1], and Shihong Lao[2]

[1] Computer Science and Technology Department,
Tsinghua University, Beijing, China
dyn10@mails.tsinghua.edu.cn
[2] OMRON Social Solutions Co., LTD, Tokyo, Japan

Abstract. Bag detection in pedestrian images is a very practical visual surveillance problem. It is challenging because bag appearance may vary greatly. In this paper, we propose a novel two-stage approach for bag detection in pedestrian images. Firstly, we utilize two stripe vocabulary forests to check whether a pedestrian is with a bag. Secondly, we locate the bag location by ranking the generated bottom-up region proposals. The ranker is learned with a convolutional neural network (CNN). Experiments are performed on a subset of CUHK person re-identification dataset that show the effectiveness of our approach for bag detection in pedestrian images. Although developed for a specific problem, our approach could be applied to detect other carrying objects in pedestrian images.

1 Introduction

In visual surveillance, people are interested in automatically searching persons from a huge amount of video data [1–11]. Because bag is a very common target appeared in surveillance video from public areas such as streets, subways, tourist attractions, airports and supermarkets, mining bag information is conducive to criminals monitoring, lost person search, video index and criminal investigation, and so on.

Bag detection plays an important role in bag information extraction. Firstly, it can greatly reduce the number of candidates for person searching when we only concern whether a person is with a bag. Secondly, it can also be used for the abnormal event detection, such as losing bag and stealing bag. Moreover, it provides prior knowledge for high level bag information extraction, such as bag color and type recognition, and so on. For convenience, in this paper, pedestrian images with bag will be called as bag images and those without bag as non-bag images. Some bag images and non-bag ones are shown in Fig. 1. When the bag area is too small, as seen in Fig. 1(c), although those pedestrians are with bags, they contain less bag information and it is hard to utilize. Besides, a person usually carries with one bag. Therefore, we mainly focus on the bag images where there is only one bag and more than 50 % the bag area is visible. Because bag appearance changes due to variations in bag type, illumination, pedestrian pose and background clutter, bag detection is a challenging problem.

© Springer International Publishing Switzerland 2015
D. Cremers et al. (Eds.): ACCV 2014, Part IV, LNCS 9006, pp. 507–521, 2015.
DOI: 10.1007/978-3-319-16817-3_33

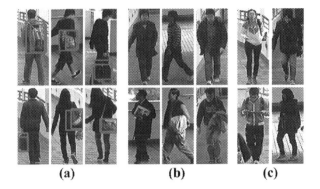

Fig. 1. (a) Some bag images. (b) Some non-bag images. (c) Some bag images where bag area is too small. The red boxes are ground truth of bag locations and the green ones are the detection results of our approach. All images in this paper are from CUHK person re-identification dataset [4] (Colour figure online).

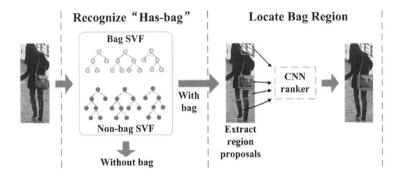

Fig. 2. Illustration of the framework of our approach.

Although there are some previous works [12–15, 29–31] on bag detection in short video sequences, to the best of our knowledge, no pervious work studies on this problem in a pedestrian image. It is also a valuable problem and more challenging than bag detection in short video sequences due to the less available information. Firstly, to extract pedestrian bag information (such as bag color, bag type) to retrieve a certain person from his tracklets, one effective way is by extracting bag information from some key pedestrian images of the tracklets. Then extracting bag information in the images is important. Secondly, bag detection in images is an important ingredient for tracking-by-detection approaches. Thirdly, bag detection in images is a specific problem, it provides insights on feature design and learning approaches.

In this paper, we propose a novel two-stage approach for bag detection in pedestrian images, as seen in Fig. 2. Firstly, we check whether a pedestrian is with a bag, i.e. recognize pedestrian attribute "has-bag". Secondly, we locate the bag region when there is a bag around the pedestrian, i.e. locate bag region.

To recognize "has-bag", we utilize the particular structure of pedestrian and construct two different stripe vocabulary forests (SVFs) from bag images and non-bag ones. Stripes are rectangle regions whose width are the same as that of the pedestrian image and they are widely used in person re-identification [5,8,9,11]. We estimate the likelihood of each stripe of the test image containing bag regions by SVFs. Then, combine those likelihoods of the above stripes to recognize "has-bag". When a pedestrian is with a bag, a small number of bottom-up region proposals will be extracted by selective search algorithm [16]. Those region proposals give high quality locations of bag. Then, we rank those region proposals with a convolutional neural network and regard the top 1 region proposal as the location of bag. Our main contribution is a novel two-stage approach for bag detection in pedestrian images and we show the effectiveness of our approach on a subset of CUHK person re-identification dataset. Although our approach is developed for bag detection in pedestrian images, it can be also applied to detect other carrying objects.

The rest of the paper is organized as follows. In Sect. 2, we present the related work of our approach. In Sect. 3, we show how to recognize "has-bag" with the stripe vocabulary forests. In Sect. 4, we show how to locate the bag region with selective search and CNN. In Sect. 5, we give and discuss experimental results. In Sect. 6, we conclude this paper.

2   Related Work

There are some previous works [10,11,17–19] on other pedestrian attributes recognition in a person image for "is-male", "has-hat", "has-shorts", "has-vnecks", "pedestrian orientation", etc. The approaches for pedestrian attributes recognition can be broadly categorized in two directions. In one direction, some works train discriminative models using Support Vector Machine (SVM) [11], Adaboost [19] and Random Forest [18] to recognize pedestrian attributes with a feature vector extracted from full body images. However, they neglect that bag regions exist in bag images. Those bag regions have stronger capacity for distinguishing bag images and non-bag ones than other regions. In another direction, some works utilize body segmentation and pose estimation [10,17] to recognize person attributes. But it is hard to take advantage of them to recognize "has-bag". There are two main reasons. Firstly, "has-bag" is different from other pedestrian attributes such as "has-hat". Human usually wears a hat on the head, but the location of the bag in images varies dramatically and bag may appear anywhere in bag images, as seen in Fig. 1(a). Secondly, bag may not appear in human body regions.

A sliding window approach for object detection is common. However, because there are large number of candidate windows to be distinguished, the sliding window approach is hard to use for bag detection. Recently, many works [16,20,21] attempt to generate a small set of high quality windows. Since bag regions in pedestrian images are always compact, it is easier to recall the bag regions by those bottom-up region proposal generation approaches. Nevertheless, this is

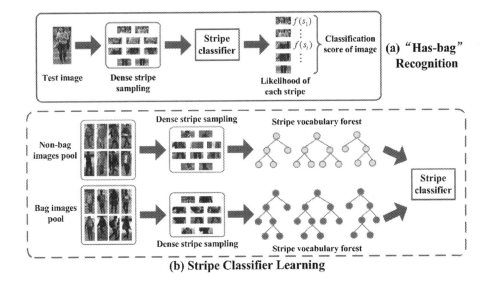

Fig. 3. (a) The framework of "has-bag" recognition in our approach. (b) The flowchart of the stripe classifier learning with two stripe vocabulary forests.

merely a preprocessing step and lots of non-bag regions need to be filtered out. Krizhevsky et al. [22] show that deep convolutional neural network achieved better results on the 2012 ImageNet Large Scale Visual Recognition Challenge (ILSVRC) using purely supervised learning. Inspired from their work, in this paper we learn a ranker with a convolutional neural network to rank the region proposals and locate the bag region.

3   Recognize "has-bag" with Stripe Vocabulary Forests

Figure 3 shows the framework of "has-bag" recognition in our approach with two stripe vocabulary forests. Given a test image p, at first, we densely sample stripes from the image, denoted as $S^p = \{s_1^p, s_2^p, \cdots, s_{n_s}^p\}$. Then we estimate the likelihood of each stripe in S^p containing bag regions with a stripe classifier and combine those likelihoods to recognize "has-bag". To learn the stripe classifier, we densely sample stripes from non-bag images to form the negative stripe set, denoted as Θ^N. Similarly the positive stripe set is from bag images, denoted as Θ^P. Then, we build two stripe vocabulary forests from Θ^P and Θ^N separately and learn the stripe classifier with the above two stripe vocabulary forests.

3.1   Stripe Vocabulary Forest Construction

Given a stripe set Θ, we apply the hierarchical k-means algorithm presented in [24,25] to build a stripe vocabulary tree T from Θ and estimate the similarity $sim(s, \Theta)$ between one stripe s and the stripe set Θ. The hierarchical k-means

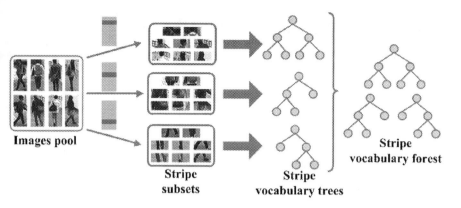

Fig. 4. Illustration of the stripe vocabulary forest construction.

algorithm is scalable and to achieve good performance in other image retrieval problems. Send the stripes in Θ to the stripe vocabulary tree, the stripes reach the same leaf node will form a stripe set. Then, each leaf node will associate with a stripe set, denoted as $\{\tilde{S}_1^T, \tilde{S}_2^T, \cdots, \tilde{S}_m^T\}$, where m is the number of the leaf node in the stripe vocabulary tree T.

Estimating $sim(s, \Theta)$ only with the stripe vocabulary tree constructed from all stripes in Θ ignores the particular structure of pedestrian. Intuitively, although the pose of pedestrian may vary dramatically, vertical misalignment of two pedestrian images is slight. For example, the vertical range of head, upper body and lower body are similar between two different pedestrian images. Thus we build a stripe vocabulary forest instead of above stripe vocabulary tree by utilizing the particular structure of pedestrian, as seen in Fig. 4. When we densely sample stripes from an image, assume h_i is the center position of the ith stripe in vertical. At first, we generate stripe subsets $\{\Theta_1, \Theta_2, \ldots, \Theta_n\}$ from the stripe set Θ according to the center position of the stripe in vertical, where n is the number of stripes of one image and all of the stripes in Θ_i have the same center position in vertical as h_i. Considering the slight vertical misalignment, we relax the above strict constraint to a larger space. Then,

$$\Theta_i = \{s_j | s_j \in \Theta, |h(s_j) - h_i| \le h_\theta\}, \tag{1}$$

where $h(s)$ is the center position of the stripe s in vertical, h_θ is the size of relaxed space. In our setting, h_θ is equal to the stride for stripe sampling. When the stripe subsets are generated, we build stripe vocabulary trees for each stripe subset with the hierarchical k-means algorithm, denoted as $\{T_1, T_2, \ldots, T_n\}$. Then, those stripe vocabulary trees form a stripe vocabulary forest $F = \{T_1, T_2, \ldots, T_n\}$ and $sim(s, \Theta)$ can be estimated with it. Given a stripe s, when $h(s) = h_i$, then send s to T_i and s reaches the rth leaf node of T_i,

$$sim(s, \Theta) = \min_{s_j \in \tilde{S}_r^{T_i}} (d(s, s_j)), \tag{2}$$

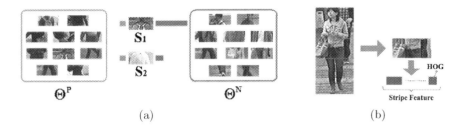

(a)   (b)

Fig. 5. (a) Illustration of the distance between different kinds of stripes and the stripe sets Θ^{P} and Θ^{N}. The distance is represented with the bar and the longer bar means the larger distance. S_1 is the stripe containing bag regions. S_2 is the stripe without bag regions. (b) Illustration of stripe feature extraction.

where $\tilde{S}_r^{T_i}$ is the stripe set associated with the rth leaf node of T_i and $d(s, s_j) = \left\| \mathbf{v}_s - \mathbf{v}_{s_j} \right\|_2$, $\mathbf{v}_x$ is the feature vector of the stripe x.

There are two advantages of adopting the stripe vocabulary forest. (1) $sim(s, \Theta)$ estimation is more accurate since it considers the particular structure of pedestrian and doesn't match the stripes in upper body to the ones in lower body. (2) It reduces the time consumption for estimating $sim(s, \Theta)$ due to $\Theta_i \subset \Theta$.

3.2   Classification Score Estimation

To recognize "has-bag", we firstly build two stripe vocabulary forests F^{P} and F^{N} with the stripe set Θ^{P} and Θ^{N}. Then learn a stripe classifier and estimate the likelihood of one stripe containing bag regions. The likelihood of stripe s_i can be represented as follows:

$$f(s_i) = \frac{sim(s_i, \Theta^{\mathrm{P}})}{sim(s_i, \Theta^{\mathrm{N}})} \tag{3}$$

As seen in Fig. 5(a), when the stripe s_i contains bag regions, $sim(s_i, \Theta^{\mathrm{P}})$ will be small and $sim(s_i, \Theta^{\mathrm{N}})$ will be large, then $f(s_i)$ will be small. On the contrary, when the stripe s_i is without bag regions, because not all the stripes in bag images contain bag regions, both $sim(s_i, \Theta^{\mathrm{P}})$ and $sim(s_i, \Theta^{\mathrm{N}})$ will be small, then $f(s_i)$ will be large.

With the stripe classifier, we introduce a function $score(p)$ to check whether or not a pedestrian p is with a bag. This function can be represented as follows:

$$score(p) = \sum_{s_i \in S^p} f(s_i), \tag{4}$$

The final decision is made by assigning a confidence threshold.

3.3   Stripe Feature Extraction

A stripe is always represented by color and texture histogram features in person re-identification [5, 8, 9, 11], but those features ignore the spatial distribution and

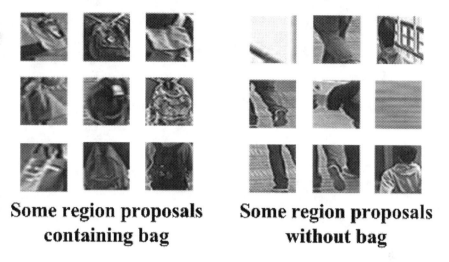

Some region proposals containing bag

Some region proposals without bag

Fig. 6. Some warped region proposals generated with selective search.

the neighborhood context of object. In our approach, we utilize contour features to describe a stripe. Figure 5(b) shows the procedure of stripe feature extraction. Given a stripe, we densely sample a set of 16 × 16 patches from this stripe and set the shift stride to 4 pixels both on vertical and horizontal direction. For each patch, we extract HOG feature [26] that is widely used to describe the contour information of object and of which gradient is voted into 9 orientation bins in $0° - 180°$. Then this stripe is depicted by concatenating HOG features of all patches.

4   Locate Bag Region

In this section, at first, we will show how to generate the region proposals. Then, we will present how to learn a region proposal ranker with a convolutional neural network.

4.1   Region Proposals Generation

In our approach, we use selective search [16] to generate the region proposals. Selective search exploits the structure of the image and generates object locations from super pixels. It uses a variety of complementary grouping criteria to diversify the sampling techniques and account for as many image conditions as possible. To be considered as a correct region proposal, the area of overlap a_o between the predicted bounding box B_p and the ground truth bounding box B_{gt} must exceed 50 % by the formula:

$$a_o = \frac{area(B_p \cap B_{gt})}{area(B_p \cup B_{gt})},$$

(5)

Input

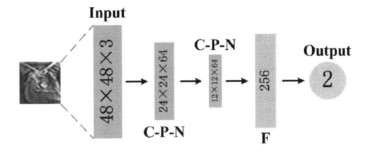

Fig. 7. Schematic view of the CNN model for ranking the region proposals. We visualize the network layers with their corresponding output dimensions.

We observe that selective search will yield 96.04 % recall and the average number of region proposals is only 463 for each pedestrian image containing bag in CUHK dataset (the size of the images is 160 × 60). Thus, selective search is fit for generating the region proposals for bag detection in pedestrian images. To facilitate the following convolutional neural network design, we warp all region proposals in a fixed 48 × 48 pixel size. Figure 6 shows some warpped bag region proposals and some non-bag ones.

4.2   Region Proposal Ranking

To rank the region proposals, inspired from the classification on CIFAR-10 dataset with cuda-convnet [23], we consider the bag region proposals and the non-bag ones as two different classes and redesign a simple convolutional neural network. Figure 7 gives the schematic view of our CNN model. Denote by C a convolutional layer, by N a local response normalization one, by P a max pooling layer and by F a fully connected one. The network can be described concisely as follows: C (48 × 48 × 64)-P(24 × 24 × 64)-N(24 × 24 × 64)-C(24 × 24 × 64)-P(12 × 12 × 64)-N(12 × 12 × 64)-F(256). For C, P and N layers, the size is defined as width × height × depth, where the first two dimensions have a spatial meaning while the depth defines the number of filters. The input to the net is a 48 × 48 warped region proposal. The output layer of the net is a softmax layer with 2 output values that are the probabilities of a region proposal belonging to bag or not. The total number of parameters of the above CNN is about 2.5 million. For further details, we refer the reader to [23]. To train the above CNN model, we use only purely supervised learning approach as same as the procedure for training the traditional neural network.

5   Experiments

We utilize the pedestrian images from the public available dataset CUHK Person Re-identification Dataset [4] to evaluate our approach. The pedestrian images in this dataset are collected from the campus where the bag appearance and

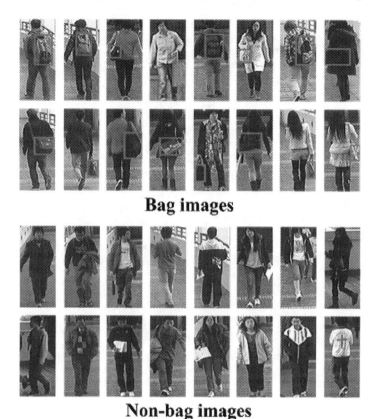

Bag images

Non-bag images

Fig. 8. Some bag images and some non-bag ones in CUHK dataset. The green boxes are ground truth of bag locations (Color figure online).

location change greatly, as seen in Fig. 8. The size of these pedestrian images is 160×60 pixels and the type of bag includes handbag, backpack, briefcase, laptop bag, satchel, sling bag and hip bag.

To evaluate the performance of "has-bag" recognition, we manually label 1363 bag images and 1534 non-bag ones. Half of them are selected randomly for training and the other half for testing. To densely sample stripes from an image, the height of a stripe is set to be 32 pixels and the shift stride is set to be 4 pixels. Then the number of stripes of one image is 33. We use a branch factor $k = 5$ to train the stripe vocabulary forest. All experiments related to "has-bag" recognition were carried out with C++ implementation on a CPU.

To evaluate the performance of bag location, we manually label the ground truth bounding box of the above 1363 bag images. Half of them are selected randomly for training and the other half for testing. Because the number of bag region proposals is far less than non-bag ones, we adapt the following strategy to augment the amount of the bag region proposals. At first, we extend the 48×48 warped region proposals into 56×56 according to the original image. Then, we

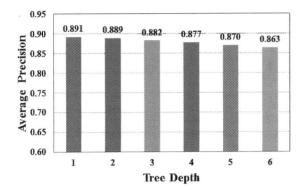

(a) The average precision of precision-recall curve.

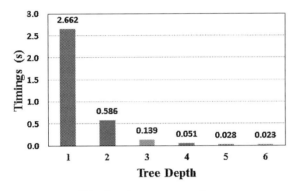

(b) The time consumption.

Fig. 9. Comparison of different tree depths for "has-bag" recognition.

densely sample a set of 48×48 region proposals from a 56×56 region proposal and set the shift stride to 1 pixels both at vertical and horizontal direction. Therefore, for training the CNN model, the number of the bag region proposals is about 3×10^5 and the non-bag ones are also about 3×10^5. All experiments related to bag location were carried out with Matlab and Python implementation on a GPU.

5.1 Evaluation on "has-bag" Recognition

The Tree Depth Exploration: The depth of the hierarchical k-means tree is a key parameter of our approach for "has-bag" recognition. Figure 9 compare the performance of different tree depths. When the tree depth is 1, it means that the similarity $sim(s, \Theta)$ between a stripe s and a stripe set Θ is estimated by 1-NN search and without the stripe vocabulary forests in our approach. When the tree depth is increased, although the average precision will be decreased, the time consumption will be reduced too. It is easy to observe that the average

Table 1. Comparisons of the stripe vocabulary forest (SVF) and the stripe vocabulary tree (SVT) for "has-bag" recognition.

Method	Average Precision	Timings (s)
SVF	**0.882**	**0.139**
SVT	0.871	1.237

precisions are comparable when the tree depth is changed from 1 to 3, but the time consumption is reduced obviously. When the tree depth is 3, it is about **20** times faster than the tree depth is 1. Although the time consumption is reduced further when the tree depth changes from 4 to 6, the average precisions are worse than the tree depth is 1. In the following sections, we will evaluate our approach for "has-bag" recognition under the tree depth is 3.

Forest Vs. Tree: To estimate the similarity between a stripe and a stripe set, we utilize the stripe vocabulary forest instead of the stripe vocabulary tree constructed from all stripes in the stripe set. Table 1 compares the performance of our approach with the stripe vocabulary forest (SVF) and the stripe vocabulary tree (SVT). The average precision of SVF is about 1.1 % higher than SVT and the time consumption of SVF is around 10 times faster than SVT for testing an image. SVF is superior to SVT.

Comparison with Other Approaches: To demonstrate the effectiveness of our approach for "has-bag" recognition, we will compare some other approaches that use features extracted from full body image. In those approaches, two kinds of feature vector are taken into account: histogram of oriented gradients (HOG) and histogram of color and texture (HCT). The HOG feature vector is similar as our stripe feature and is densely sampled a set of patches from an image. Then concatenate the HOG features of all patches to form the feature vector. The HCT feature vector is the same as [9,11]. A pedestrian image is divided into six stripes equally. For each stripe, 8 color channels (RGB, YCbCr and HSV) and 21 texture filters (Schmid, Gabor) are used and each channel is described by a 16 dimensional histogram. Then, concatenate all histograms to form the feature vector. In order to recognize "has-bag", we train binary classifiers with KNN and SVM for each feature type separately. Learning KNN classifier is similar as our stripe classifier. Because the dimensionality of HOG feature vector is 15984 for a 160×60 image and it is large, the nonlinear mapping does not improve the performance [27], we train the SVM classifier by LibLinear [28]. For HCT feature vector, the dimensionality is 2784 for a 160×60 image and not large, we train the SVM classifier by LibSVM [27] and select RBF as the kernel function.

Figure 10 compares our approach with the other approaches for "has-bag" recognition. The average precision of our approach is about 2.9 % higher than HOG-KNN, 4.6 % higher than HOG-SVM, 23.7 % higher than HCT-KNN and 15.1 % higher than HCT-SVM. Our approach outperforms all the comparison approaches. Moreover, since concatenated HOG feature takes into account the

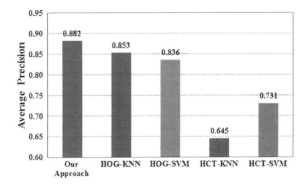

Fig. 10. Comparisons of our approach and the other approaches for " has-bag" recognition.

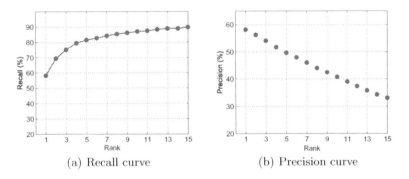

(a) Recall curve   (b) Precision curve

Fig. 11. Recall and precision of the ranked region proposals. "Rank = r" denotes the region proposals of each image in top r are regarded as the location results.

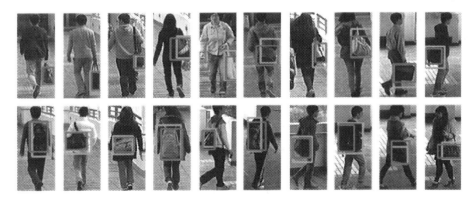

Fig. 12. Some bag location results of our approach. The red boxes are ground truth of bag locations and the green ones are the detection results of our approach (Color figure online).

spatial distribution and the neighborhood context of object, the performance of HOG feature is better than HCT feature.

5.2 Evaluation on Bag Location

Figure 11 shows the performance of our approach for bag location. When we regard the region proposals of each image in top 1 as the location results, both the precision and recall of our approach for bag location is 58.1 %. Our approach can locate the bag regions effectively. Two points are worth highlighting concerning our bag location approach. (1) When we consider the region proposals in top 15, the recall is 89.7 %. Our approach can also yield a high quality locations with a small number of the region proposals. (2) Assume that "Rank $= r$" denotes the region proposals of each image in top r are regarded as the location results. When Rank $= 3$, although the precision is 54.1 % that is lower than Rank $= 1$, the recall is 75.2 % that is much higher than Rank $= 1$. This indicates that we can utilize context information of the region proposals to further improve the bag location performance. Figure 12 shows some bag location results of our approach.

6 Conclusion

In this paper, we investigate bag information extraction in pedestrian images and attempt to tackle a practical visual surveillance problem of bag detection in pedestrian images. We propose a novel two-stage approach for this problem. At first, we check whether a pedestrian is with a bag using two stripe vocabulary forests. Then, we combine selective search and convolutional neural network to locate the bag region in the bag images. Experiments show that our approach is effective for bag detection in pedestrian images. In the future, we will utilize more bag images and non-bag ones and mine the context information of the region proposals to improve bag detection performance.

Acknowledgement. This work is supported in part by National Basic Research Program of China under Grant No.2011CB302203, and it is also supported by a grant from OMRON Corporation.

References

1. Zhao, R., Ouyang, W., Wang, X.: Unsupervised salience learning for person re-identification. In: CVPR (2013)
2. Li, W., Wang, X.: Locally aligned feature transforms across views. In: CVPR (2013)
3. Ma, B., Su, Y., Jurie, F.: BiCov: a novel image representation for person re-identification and face verification. In: BMVC (2012)
4. Li, W., Zhao, R., Wang, X.: Human reidentification with transferred metric learning. In: Lee, K.M., Matsushita, Y., Rehg, J.M., Hu, Z. (eds.) ACCV 2012, Part I. LNCS, vol. 7724, pp. 31–44. Springer, Heidelberg (2013)

5. Zheng, W., Gong, S., Xiang, T.: Transfer re-identification: from person to set-based verification. In: CVPR (2012)
6. Hirzer, M., Roth, P.M., Köstinger, M., Bischof, H.: Relaxed pairwise learned metric for person re-identification. In: Fitzgibbon, A., Lazebnik, S., Perona, P., Sato, Y., Schmid, C. (eds.) ECCV 2012, Part VI. LNCS, vol. 7577, pp. 780–793. Springer, Heidelberg (2012)
7. Wu, Y., Minoh, M., Mukunoki, M., Lao, S.: Set based discriminative ranking for recognition. In: Fitzgibbon, A., Lazebnik, S., Perona, P., Sato, Y., Schmid, C. (eds.) ECCV 2012, Part III. LNCS, vol. 7574, pp. 497–510. Springer, Heidelberg (2012)
8. Gray, D., Tao, H.: Viewpoint invariant pedestrian recognition with an ensemble of localized features. In: Forsyth, D., Torr, P., Zisserman, A. (eds.) ECCV 2008, Part I. LNCS, vol. 5302, pp. 262–275. Springer, Heidelberg (2008)
9. Zheng, W., Gong, S., Xiang, T.: Person re-identification by probabilistic relative distance comparison. In: CVPR (2011)
10. Satta, R., Fumera, G., Roli, F.: A general method for appearance-based people search based on textual queries. In: Fusiello, A., Murino, V., Cucchiara, R. (eds.) ECCV 2012. LNCS, pp. 453–461. Springer, Heidelberg (2012)
11. Layne, R., Hospedales, T.M., Gong, S.: Towards person identification and re-identification with attributes. In: Fusiello, A., Murino, V., Cucchiara, R. (eds.) ECCV 2012. LNCS, vol. 7583, pp. 402–412. Springer, Heidelberg (2012)
12. Damen, D., Hogg, D.: Detecting carried objects from sequences of walking pedestrians. IEEE Trans. PAMI **34**, 1056–1067 (2012)
13. Damen, D., Hogg, D.C.: Detecting carried objects in short video sequences. In: Forsyth, D., Torr, P., Zisserman, A. (eds.) ECCV 2008, Part III. LNCS, vol. 5304, pp. 154–167. Springer, Heidelberg (2008)
14. BenAbdelkader, C., Davis, L.: Detection of people carrying objects: a motion-based recognition approach. In: FG (2002)
15. Haritaoglu, I., Cutler, R., Harwood, D., Davis, L.: Backpack: detection of people carrying objects using silhouettes. In: ICCV (1999)
16. Uijlings, J., Sande, K., Gevers, T., Smeulders, A.: Selective search for object recognition. Int. J. Comput. Vis. **104**, 154–171 (2013)
17. Bourdev, L., Maji, S., Malik, J.: Describing people: a poselet-based approach to attribute classification. In: ICCV (2011)
18. Baltieri, D., Vezzani, R., Cucchiara, R.: People orientation recognition by mixtures of wrapped distributions on random trees. In: Fitzgibbon, A., Lazebnik, S., Perona, P., Sato, Y., Schmid, C. (eds.) ECCV 2012, Part V. LNCS, vol. 7576, pp. 270–283. Springer, Heidelberg (2012)
19. Cao, L., Dikmen, M., Fu, Y., Huang, T.: Gender recognition from body. In: ACM MM (2008)
20. Alexe, B., Deselaers, T., Ferrari, V.: Measuring the objectness of image windows. IEEE Trans. PAMI **34**, 2189–2202 (2012)
21. Endres, I., Hoiem, D.: Category independent object proposals. In: Daniilidis, K., Maragos, P., Paragios, N. (eds.) ECCV 2010, Part V. LNCS, vol. 6315, pp. 575–588. Springer, Heidelberg (2010)
22. Alex, K., Ilya, S., Geoffrey, H.: Imagenet classification with deep convolutional neural networks. In: NIPS (2012)
23. Alex, K.: Cuda-convnet. (https://code.google.com/p/cuda-convnet/)
24. Wang, X., Hua, G., Han, T.: Detection by detections: non-parametric detector adaptation for a video. In: CVPR (2012)
25. Nister, D., Stewenius, H.: Scalable recognition with a vocabulary tree. In: CVPR (2006)

26. Dalal, N., Triggs, B.: Histograms of oriented gradients for human detection. In: CVPR (2005)
27. Hsu, C., Chang, C., Lin, C.: A practical guide to support vector classification. Technical report, Department of Computer Science, National Taiwan University (2003)
28. Fan, R., Chang, K., Hsieh, C., Wang, X., Lin, C.: LIBLINEAR: a library for large linear classification. JMLR **9**, 1871–1874 (2008)
29. Amer, M.R., Xie, D., Zhao, M., Todorovic, S., Zhu, S.-C.: Cost-sensitive top-down/bottom-up inference for multiscale activity recognition. In: Fitzgibbon, A., Lazebnik, S., Perona, P., Sato, Y., Schmid, C. (eds.) ECCV 2012, Part IV. LNCS, vol. 7575, pp. 187–200. Springer, Heidelberg (2012)
30. Zhu, Y., Nayak, N., Roy-Chowdhury, A.: Context-aware modeling and recognition of activities in video. In: CVPR (2013)
31. Bhargava, M., Chen, C., Ryoo, M., Aggarwal, J.: Detection of object abandonment using temporal logic. Mach. Vis. Appl. **20**, 271–281 (2009)

Recognizing Daily Activities from First-Person Videos with Multi-task Clustering

Yan Yan[1]([✉]), Elisa Ricci[2,3], Gaowen Liu[1], and Nicu Sebe[1]

[1] Department of Information Engineering and Computer Science,
University of Trento, Trento, Italy
yan@disi.unitn.it
[2] Fondazione Bruno Kessler, Trento, Italy
[3] Department of Engineering, University of Perugia, Perugia, Italy

Abstract. The widespread adoption of low-cost wearable devices requires novel paradigms for analysing human behaviour. In particular, when focusing on first-person cameras continuously recording several hours of the users life, the task of activity recognition is especially challenging. As a huge amount of unlabeled data is automatically generated in this scenario, despite recent notable attempts, more scalable algorithms and more effective feature representations are required. In this paper, we address the problem of *everyday activity recognition* from visual data gathered from a *wearable camera* proposing a novel *multi-task learning* framework. We argue that, even if label information is not provided, we can take advantage of the fact that the tasks of recognizing activities of daily life of multiple individuals are related, *i.e.* typically people tend to perform the same actions in the same environment (*e.g.* people at home in the morning typically have breakfast and brush their teeth). To exploit this information we propose a novel multi-task clustering approach. With our method, rather than clustering data from different users separately, we look for data partitions which are similar among related tasks. Thorough experiments on two publicly available first-person vision datasets demonstrate that the proposed approach consistently and significantly outperforms several state-of-the-art methods.

1 Introduction

Human behaviour analysis is an important research area in computer vision. Automatically understanding *what people do* by analyzing visual streams recorded from surveillance cameras is a challenging task and implies recognizing the activities of the people of interest, the environment where they operate, the other people with whom they interact, the objects they manipulate and even their future intentions. While many progresses have been made in this area, recent works [1] have demonstrated as the traditional "third-person" view perspective (*i.e.* employing fixed cameras mounted all around in the user's environment) may be insufficient for understanding people activities and intentions and that wearable cameras can provide an alternative or complementary source of information. Wearable cameras can be employed in many different applications, such

© Springer International Publishing Switzerland 2015
D. Cremers et al. (Eds.): ACCV 2014, Part IV, LNCS 9006, pp. 522–537, 2015.
DOI: 10.1007/978-3-319-16817-3_34

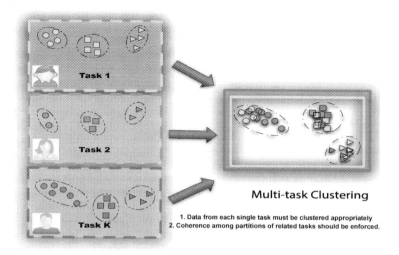

Fig. 1. Overview of our proposed multi-task clustering approach for First Person Vision activity recognition (Figure is best viewed in color and zoom) (Color figure online).

as in driver's assistance systems, for monitoring assembly operations in manufacturing, in ambient assisted living and, more recently, in the context of the so called "life-logging" [2,3] (*i.e.* where a first-person camera continuously records a whole day of its wearer life).

In this paper, we focus specifically on everyday activity recognition from a "first-person" vision (FPV) perspective. This problem poses several challenges. With wearable cameras typically several hours of videos are recorded. This generates a large amount of data for which labels are not available as the annotation would require a massive human effort. Thus, for accurate recognition, algorithms which are both scalable and able to operate in an unsupervised setting are required. Moreover, designing effective visual features representations in this unconstrained FPV scenario is much more challenging than in the case of fixed cameras. In this paper, we propose to address the problem of everyday activity recognition from unlabeled visual data within a multi-task learning framework. When considering the tasks of recognizing activities of daily living of many individuals, it is natural to assume that these tasks are related. For example, people working in an office environment tend to perform the same kind of activities (*e.g.* typing on keyboard in front of a personal computer, reading and writing documents). Similarly, most people when they wake up in the morning use to drink coffee and brush their teeth. Thus, it is intuitive that, when performing activity recognition, learning from data of all the individuals simultaneously is advantageous with respect to considering each person separately. However, the data distributions of single tasks can be different, since visual data corresponding to different people may exhibit different features. In particular if there are limited data for a single person, typical clustering methods may fail to discover the correct clusters. In this case, using data from other people as an auxiliary source of information can improve clustering results. However, simply combining data from different people together and applying traditional clustering approach does not necessarily increase accuracy, because the data distributions of single tasks can be different, violating *i.i.d.* assumptions. To address this problem, we propose to invoke the novel paradigm of multi-task clustering (MTC). Specifically, we introduce two novel methods, derived by a common framework based on the minimization of an objective function balancing two terms, one which ensures the data of each single task to be clustered appropriately, the other which enforces some coherence between the clustering results of related tasks. We demonstrate the effectiveness of our approaches on two recent FPV datasets, the FPV activity of daily living dataset [3] and the coupled ego-motion and eye-motion dataset introduced in [4], comparing them with several single task and multi-task learning methods. Figure 1 depicts an overview of the proposed method.

The main contributions of this work are the following: (i) To our knowledge, this paper is the first to address the problem of everyday activity recognition within a MTC framework. While our framework can be used to analyze visual streams recorded from fixed cameras, we tackle the more challenging scenario of egocentric vision. (ii) The two proposed multi-task clustering approaches are novel and two efficient algorithms are derived for solving the associated optimization problems. (iii) Our experimental evaluation demonstrates that, independently of the adopted feature representations, a multi-task learning framework is greatly advantageous for FPV activity recognition with respect to traditional single task approaches. (iv) The proposed MTC algorithms are general and can be applied to many other computer vision and pattern recognition problems.

2 Related Works

Activity Recognition in Egocentric Videos. Analysing human behaviors from data collected from wearable devices has received considerable attention recently, not only in computer vision but also in other related research areas, *e.g.* ubiquitous computing [5,6]. While many recent works are based on the use of RFID tags or inertial sensors, systems based on first-person cameras still play an important role being generally cheap and easy to deploy. Aghazadeh *et al.* [7] considered the problem of discovering anomalous events analysing the video stream captured from a small video camera attached to a person's chest. In [2] a summarization approach targeted to egocentric videos is presented. Fathi *et al.* [8] introduced a method for individuating social interactions in first-person videos collected during social events. Some recent works have faced the multiple challenges of recognizing complex activities of everyday life from an egocentric perspective in different scenarios (*e.g.* kitchen, office, home) [3,4,9,10]. In [3] the authors demonstrated the importance of using features based on object detectors' output in the challenging unconstrained scenario of everyday at home activity recognition. In [9] RGB-D sensors are employed for fine-grained recognition of kitchen activities. In [4] the task of recognizing egocentric activities in an office environment is considered and motion descriptors extracted from an outside looking camera are used jointly with features modeling the eye movements of the wearer captured by an inside looking camera. In [10] activity recognition in a kitchen scenario (multiple subjects preparing different recipes) is considered. A codebook learning framework is proposed in order to alleviate the problem of the large within-class data variability due to the different execution styles and speed among different subjects.

In this paper, we address the problem of analysing activities of daily living under the perspective of multi-task learning. Multi-task learning methods have been previously investigated in the context of visual-based activity recognition from fixed cameras and in a supervised setting [11–13]. In this paper, we consider the more challenging scenario where no annotated data are provided, which is typical when analyzing visual streams from wearable cameras.

Multi-task Learning. Recently multi-task learning (MTL) approaches [14] have demonstrated their effectiveness in several applications in computer vision, such as object detection [15], indoor localization [16], face verification [17] or head pose estimation [18]. The idea of multi-task learning is simple: learning from data of multiple related tasks simultaneously produces more accurate classification and regression models with respect to learning on every single task independently. While many works have introduced supervised MTL approaches, only few have considered an unsupervised setting [19–21], *i.e.* the scenario where all the data are unlabeled and the aim is to predict the cluster labels in each single task. Gu *et al.* [19] proposed to learn a subspace shared by all the tasks, through which the knowledge of one task can be transferred to all the others. Zhang *et al.* [21] introduced a MTC approach based on a pairwise agreement term which encourages coherence among clustering results of multiple tasks. In [20] the k-means algorithm is revised from a Bayesian nonparametric viewpoint and extended to MTL.

In this paper, we propose two novel approaches for multi-task clustering. The first one is inspired by the work in [21] but it is based on another objective function and thus on a radically different optimization algorithm. Furthermore, in the considered application, it provides superior accuracy with respect to [21]. Our second approach instead permits to easily integrate prior knowledge about the tasks and the data of each task (*e.g.* temporal consistency among subsequent video clips). Moreover, it relies on a convex optimization problem, thus avoids the issues related to local minima of previous methods [19–21].

3   Multi-task Clustering for FPV Activity Recognition

In this paper, we focus on the problem of everyday activity recognition from wearable cameras. More specifically, we consider several video clips collected by a certain number of people involved in activities of daily living. No labeled data are provided. We only assume that people perform about the same tasks, a very reasonable assumption in the context of everyday activity analysis. Considering each individual's data as a specific task, we propose a MTC approach. To stress

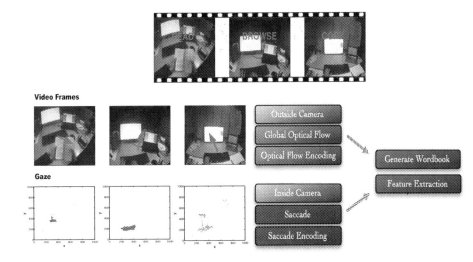

Fig. 2. Feature extraction pipeline on the FPV office dataset. Some frames correspond-ing to the actions *read*, *browse* and *copy* are shown together with the corresponding optical flow features (top) and eye-gaze patterns depicted on the 2-D plane (bottom). It is interesting to observe the different gaze patterns among these activities.

the generality of our method, we apply it in two different scenarios: an office environment where people are involved in typical activities such as browsing the web or writing documents and a home environment where a chest mounted camera records users' activities such as opening a fridge or preparing tea. To perform experiments we use two publicly available datasets, corresponding to the scenarios described above: the FPV office dataset introduced in [4] and the FPV activity of daily living dataset described in [3]. Both datasets contains visual streams recorded from an outside-looking wearable camera while the office dataset also has informations about eye movements acquired by an inside-looking camera. Further details about the datasets are provided in the experimental section. In the following we describe the adopted feature descriptors and the proposed MTC framework.

3.1   Features Extraction in Egocentric Videos

Due to the large variability of visual data collected from wearable cameras there exist no typical feature descriptors but different representations are adopted dependently on the context. While in some situations extracting motion infor-mation by computing optical flow vectors may suffice [4], in other cases motion patterns may be too noisy and other kind of informations (*e.g.* presence/absence of objects) must be exploited. In this paper we demonstrate that, independently from the employed feature descriptors, MTC is an effective strategy for recog-nizing everyday activities. We now describe the adopted feature representations respectively for the considered office and home scenarios.

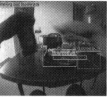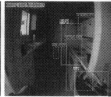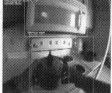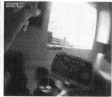

Fig. 3. FPV home dataset: frames depicting examples of the activities *making cold food/snack* and *making tea* and the detected objects.

FPV office dataset. We follow [4] and extract features describing both the eye motion (obtained by the inside-looking camera) and the head and body motion (computed processing the outside camera's stream). To calculate the eye motion features, we consider the gaze coordinates provided in the dataset and smooth them applying a median filter. Then the continuous wavelet transform is adopted for saccade detection separately on the x and y motion components [22]. The resulting signals are quantized according to magnitude and direction and are coded with a sequence of discrete symbols. To analyze the streams of the output camera, for each frame the global optical flow is computed by tracking corner points over consecutive frames and taking the mean flow in the x and y directions. Then, the optical flow vectors are quantized according to magnitude and direction with the same procedure adopted in the eye motion case. The obtained sequences of symbols are then processed to get the final video clip descriptors. We use a temporal sliding window approach to build a n-gram dictionary over all the dataset. Then each video is divided into segments corresponding to 15 s, each of them representing a video clip. For each sequence of symbols associated to a video clip, a histogram over the dictionary is computed. The final feature descriptor $\mathbf{x}_i$ is calculated by considering some statistics over the clip histogram and specifically computing the maximum, the average, the variance, the number of unique n-grams, and the difference between maximum and minimum count. Figure 2 shows the feature extraction pipeline.

FPV home dataset. We adopt the same object-centric approach proposed in [3], *i.e.* to compute features for each video clip, we consider the output of several object detectors. More specifically, we use the pre-segmented video clips and the active object models in [3]. Active object models are introduced to exploit the fact that objects look different when being interacted with (*e.g.* open and close fridge). Therefore in [3] additional detectors are trained using a subset of training images depicting object appearance when objects are used by people. Figure 3 shows some frames associated to the activities *making cold food/snack* and *making tea*: the output of the object detectors are depicted. To obtain object-centric features for each frame a score for each object model and each location is computed. Then the maximum scores of all the object models are used as frame features. To compute the final clip descriptors $\mathbf{x}_i$, two approaches are adopted: one based on "bag of features" (accumulating frame features over time) and the other based on temporal pyramids. The temporal pyramid features are obtained concatenating several histograms constructed with accumulation: the first is a histogram over the full temporal extent of a video clip, the next is the concatenation of two histograms obtained by temporally segmenting the video into two parts, and so on.

3.2   Multi-task Clustering

We consider T related tasks corresponding to T different people. For each task t, a set of data samples $X^t = \{\mathbf{x}_1^t, \mathbf{x}_2^t, ..., \mathbf{x}_{N_t}^t\}$ is available, where $\mathbf{x}_j^t \in I\!\!R^d$ is the d-dimensional feature vector describing the j-th video clip and N_t is the total number of samples associated to the t-th task. In the following we denote with $(\cdot)'$ the transpose operator, $N = \sum_{t=1}^T N_t$ is the total number of datapoints, while $\mathbf{X} \in I\!\!R^{N \times d}$, $\mathbf{X} = [\mathbf{X}^{1'}\ \mathbf{X}^{2'}\ ...\ \mathbf{X}^{T'}]'$ is the data matrix obtained by concatenating the task specific matrices $\mathbf{X}^t = [\mathbf{x}_1^t\ \mathbf{x}_2^t\ ...\ \mathbf{x}_{N_t}^t]' \in I\!\!R^{N_t \times d}$. To discover people activities, we want to segment the entire video clip into parts, *i.e.* we want the data in the set X^t to be grouped into K_t clusters, where the number of required partitions can be different in different tasks. This is reasonable in the context of everyday activity recognition where people perform about the same activities. Furthermore, as we assume the tasks to be related, we also require that the resulting partitions are consistent with each other. This can be obtained by defining the following optimization problem:

$$\min_{\Theta_t}\ \sum_{t=1}^T \Lambda(\mathbf{X}^t, \Theta^t) + \sum_{t=1}^T \sum_{s=t+1}^T R(\Theta^t, \Theta^s) \tag{1}$$

The problem (1) corresponds to the general problem of multi-task clustering, where the term $\Lambda(\cdot)$ represents a reconstruction error which must be minimized by learning the optimal task-specific model parameters Θ^t (*i.e.* typically the cluster centroids and the associated assignment matrix), while $R(\cdot)$ is an "agreement" term imposing that, since the multiple tasks are related, also the associated model parameters should be similar. Under this framework, in this paper we propose two different approaches for MTC which mainly differ for the definition of the "agreement term". In the following subsections we present them in detail.

Notation. In the following $\mathbf{A}_{i\cdot}$, $\mathbf{A}_{\cdot j}$ denote respectively the i-th row and the j-th column of the matrix $\mathbf{A}$.

3.3   Earth Mover's Distance Multi-task Clustering

Given the task data matrices $\mathbf{X}^t$, we are interested in finding the centroid matrices $\mathbf{C}^t \in I\!\!R^{K_t \times d}$, and the cluster indicators matrices $\mathbf{W}^t \in I\!\!R^{N_t \times K_t}$ by solving the following optimization problem:

$$\min_{\mathbf{C}^t,\mathbf{W}^t,f_{ij}^{st}\geq 0} \sum_{t=1}^{T}\left\|\mathbf{X}^t - \mathbf{W}^t\mathbf{C}^t\right\|_F^2 + \lambda\sum_{t=1}^{T}\sum_{s=t+1}^{T}\sum_{i=1}^{K_t}\sum_{j=1}^{K_s}f_{ij}^{st}(\mathbf{C}_{i\cdot}^t - \mathbf{C}_{j\cdot}^s)'(\mathbf{C}_{i\cdot}^t - \mathbf{C}_{j\cdot}^s) \quad (2)$$

$$\text{s.t.} \quad \sum_{j=1}^{K_s}f_{ij}^{st} = \sum_{n=1}^{N_t}\mathbf{W}_{ni}^t \;\; \forall t,i \qquad \sum_{i=1}^{K_t}f_{ij}^{st} = \sum_{n=1}^{N_s}\mathbf{W}_{nj}^s \;\; \forall s,j$$

$$\sum_{i=1}^{K_t}\sum_{j=1}^{K_s}f_{ij}^{st} = 1 \;\; \forall s,t$$

The first term in the objective function is a relaxation of the traditional k-means objective function for T separated data sources. The second term, *i.e.* the agreement term, is added to explore the relationships between clusters of different data sources. It consists in the popular Earth Mover's Distance (EMD) [23] computed considering the signatures $\mathcal{T}$ and $\mathcal{S}$ obtained by clustering the data associated to task t and s separately, *i.e.* $\mathcal{T} = \{(\mathbf{C}_{1\cdot}^t, w_t^1), \ldots, (\mathbf{C}_{K_t\cdot}^t, w_t^{K_t})\}$, $w_t^i = \sum_{n=1}^{N_t}\mathbf{W}_{ni}^t$, and $\mathcal{S} = \{(\mathbf{C}_{1\cdot}^s, w_s^1), \ldots, (\mathbf{C}_{K_s\cdot}^s, w_s^{K_s})\}$, $w_s^i = \sum_{n=1}^{N_s}\mathbf{W}_{ni}^s$. In practice $\mathbf{C}_{i\cdot}^t$ and $\mathbf{C}_{j\cdot}^s$ are the cluster centroids and w_i^s, w_i^t denote the weights associated to each cluster (reflecting somehow the number of datapoints in each cluster). In practice the second term represents a sum of distances between two distributions and minimizing it we impose the found partitions between pairs of related tasks to be consistent. The variables f_{ij}^{st} are flow variables as follows from the definition of EMD as a transportation problem [23].

In (2) there are no constraints on the $\mathbf{C}_t$ values. In this paper we define the matrix $\mathbf{C} \in \mathbb{R}^{K\times d}$, $\mathbf{C} = [\mathbf{C}^{1'} \ldots \mathbf{C}^{T'}]'$, $K = \sum_{t=1}^{T}K_t$, and we impose that the columns of $\mathbf{C}$ are a weighted sum of certain data points, *i.e.* $\mathbf{C} = \mathbf{PX}$ where $\mathbf{P} = \text{blkdiag}(\mathbf{P}^1,\ldots,\mathbf{P}^T)$, $\mathbf{P} \in \mathbb{R}^{K\times N}$. In the following, for sake of simplicity and easy interpretation, we consider only a two tasks problem. The extension to T tasks is straightforward. Defining $\mathbf{F} = \text{diag}(f_{11}\ldots f_{K_1K_2})$, $\mathbf{F} \in \mathbb{R}^{K_1K_2\times K_1K_2}$ and the block diagonal matrix $\mathbf{W} = \text{blkdiag}(\mathbf{W}^1,\mathbf{W}^2)$, $\mathbf{W} \in \mathbb{R}^{N\times K}$, the optimization problem (2) becomes:

$$\Delta(\mathbf{P},\mathbf{W},\mathbf{F}) = \min_{\mathbf{P},\mathbf{W},\mathbf{F}\geq 0}\|\mathbf{X} - \mathbf{WPX}\|_F^2 + \lambda\text{tr}(\mathbf{MPXX}'\mathbf{P}'\mathbf{M}'\mathbf{F}) \quad (3)$$

$$\text{s.t.} \quad \|\mathbf{P}_{i\cdot}^t\|_1 = 1, \;\; \forall i = 1,\ldots,K \;\; \forall\, t = 1,2$$

$$\text{tr}(\mathbf{I}_j\mathbf{F}) = \sum_{i=1}^{N}\mathbf{W}_{ij}, \;\; \forall j = 1,\ldots,K \quad (4)$$

$$\text{tr}(\mathbf{F}) = 1$$

where $\mathbf{I}_j \in \mathbb{R}^{K_1K_2\times K_1K_2}$ and $\mathbf{M} \in \mathbb{R}^{K_1K_2\times K}$ are appropriately defined selection matrices as $\mathbf{I}_j = \begin{bmatrix} 1 & 0 & \cdots & 0 \\ 0 & 1 & \cdots & 0 \\ & & \ddots & \\ 0 & 0 & \ddots & 0 \\ \vdots & \vdots & & \vdots \\ 0 & 0 & \cdots & 0 \end{bmatrix}$, $\mathbf{M} = \begin{bmatrix} 1 & 0 & 0 & \cdots & -1 & 0 & \cdots \\ 1 & 0 & 0 & \cdots & 0 & -1 & \cdots \\ 1 & 0 & 0 & \cdots & 0 & \cdots & -1 \\ 0 & 1 & 0 & \cdots & -1 & 0 & \cdots \\ \vdots & \vdots & \vdots & & \vdots & \vdots & \\ 0 & 0 & 1 & \cdots & 0 & \cdots & -1 \end{bmatrix}$.

$$\underbrace{}_{1:K_1}\quad\underbrace{}_{K_1+1:K_1+K_2}$$

Algorithm 1. Algorithm for solving (3).

Input: the data matrices $\mathbf{X}^1, \mathbf{X}^2$, the numbers of clusters K_1, K_2, the parameter λ.
1. Initialize $\mathbf{F}$ as an identity matrix.
2. Initialize $\mathbf{W} > 0$ with l_1 normalized columns and $\mathbf{P} > 0$ with l_1 normalized rows.
3. **repeat**

> Given $\mathbf{W}^k, \mathbf{P}^k$, compute $\mathbf{F}^{k+1}$ using a linear programming solver.
> Given $\mathbf{F}^{k+1}, \mathbf{P}^k$, compute $\mathbf{W}^{k+1}$ using a projected gradient method:
> $$\mathbf{W}^{k+1} = \max(0, \mathbf{W}^k - \alpha_k \nabla_{\mathbf{W}} \Delta(\mathbf{P}^k, \mathbf{W}^k, \mathbf{F}^{k+1})).$$
> Given $\mathbf{F}^{k+1}, \mathbf{W}^{k+1}$, compute $\mathbf{P}^{k+1}$ using a projected gradient method:
> $$\mathbf{P}^{k+1} = \max(0, \mathbf{P}^k - \alpha_k \nabla_{\mathbf{P}} \Delta(\mathbf{P}^k, \mathbf{W}^{k+1}, \mathbf{F}^{k+1})).$$
> Normalize $\mathbf{P}$ by $\mathbf{P}^{k+1}_{ij} \leftarrow \dfrac{\mathbf{P}^{k+1}_{ij}}{\sum_j \mathbf{P}^{k+1}_{ij}}.$

until *convergence*;
Output: the optimized matrices $\mathbf{W}, \mathbf{P}$.

Optimization. To solve the proposed problem (3), we first note that the optimal solution of (3) can be found adopting an alternating optimization scheme, *i.e.* optimizing separately (3) first with respect to $\mathbf{P}$ and then with respect to $\mathbf{W}$ and $\mathbf{F}$ jointly. In both cases, a non-negative least square problem with constraints arises, for which standard solvers can be employed. However, due to computational efficiency, in this paper we consider an approximation of (3), replacing the constraints (4) with $\text{tr}(\mathbf{I}_j \mathbf{F}) = \mathbf{e}$, where $\mathbf{e} \in I\!\!R^{K_1 K_2}$, $\mathbf{e}_i = \frac{1}{K_1}$, if $i \leq K_1$, $\mathbf{e}_i = \frac{1}{K_2}$ otherwise. This approximation implies that for each task the same number of datapoints is assigned to all the clusters. In this way a more efficient solver can be devised. Specifically, we adopt an alternating optimization strategy, *i.e.* we optimize (3) separately with respect to $\mathbf{F}$, $\mathbf{W}$ and $\mathbf{P}$ until convergence. The algorithm for solving (3) is summarized in Algorithm 1.

Kernelization. Finally, to kernelize the proposed method we consider a feature mapping $\phi(\cdot)$ and the associated kernel matrix $\mathbf{K_X} = \phi(\mathbf{X})\phi(\mathbf{X})'$. The objective function of (3) is:

$$\|\phi(\mathbf{X}) - \mathbf{W}\mathbf{P}\ \phi(\mathbf{X})\|^2_F + \lambda \text{tr}(\mathbf{M}\mathbf{P}\phi(\mathbf{X})\phi(\mathbf{X})'\mathbf{P}'\mathbf{M}'\mathbf{F}) =$$
$$\text{tr}(\mathbf{K_X} - 2\mathbf{K_X}\mathbf{P}'\mathbf{W}' + \mathbf{W}\mathbf{P}\mathbf{K_X}\mathbf{P}'\mathbf{W}' + \lambda \mathbf{M}\mathbf{P}\mathbf{K_X}\mathbf{P}'\mathbf{M}'\mathbf{F})$$

The update rules of the kernelized version of our method can be easily derived similarly to the linear case using $\mathbf{K_X}$ instead of $\mathbf{X}'\mathbf{X}$.

3.4 Convex Multi-task Clustering

Given the task specific training sets X^t, we propose to learn the sets of cluster centroids $\Pi^t = \{\boldsymbol{\pi}^t_1, \boldsymbol{\pi}^t_2, ..., \boldsymbol{\pi}^t_{N_t}\}$, $\boldsymbol{\pi}^t_i \in I\!\!R^d$, by solving the following optimization problem:

$$\min_{\boldsymbol{\pi}^t_i} \sum_{t=1}^{T}\left(\sum_{i=1}^{N_t} \|\mathbf{x}^t_i - \boldsymbol{\pi}^t_i\|^2_2 + \lambda_t \sum_{\substack{i,j=1 \\ j>i}}^{N_t} w^t_{ij}\|\boldsymbol{\pi}^t_i - \boldsymbol{\pi}^t_j\|_1\right) + \lambda_2 \sum_{\substack{t,s=1 \\ s>t}}^{T} \gamma_{st} \sum_{i=1}^{N_t}\sum_{j=1}^{N_s} \|\boldsymbol{\pi}^t_i - \boldsymbol{\pi}^s_j\|^2_2 \quad (5)$$

Algorithm 2. Algorithm for solving (5).

Input: The data matrix $\mathbf{X}, \mathbf{E}, \mathbf{B}$, the parameter λ_2.
1. Set $\mathbf{Q} = \rho\mathbf{E}'\mathbf{E} + 2\mathbf{I} + 2\lambda_2\mathbf{B}$.
2. Compute Cholesky factorization of the matrix $\mathbf{Q}$.
3. **for** $j=1{:}d$ **do**
> **repeat**
>> Set $\mathbf{b}^k = \rho\mathbf{E}'\mathbf{q}^k - \mathbf{E}'\mathbf{p}^k + 2\mathbf{X}_{\cdot j}$
>> *Update* $\mathbf{\Pi}_{\cdot j}$
>>> Solve $\mathbf{Q}[\mathbf{\Pi}_{\cdot j}]^{k+1} = \mathbf{b}^k$
>> *Update* $\mathbf{q}$ *using the operator* $ST_\lambda(x) = sign(x)\max(|x| - \lambda, 0)$
>>> $\mathbf{q}^{k+1} = ST_{1/\rho}(\mathbf{E}[\mathbf{\Pi}_{\cdot j}]^{k+1} + \frac{1}{\rho}\mathbf{p}^k)$
>> *Update* $\mathbf{p}$
>>> $\mathbf{p}^{k+1} = \mathbf{p}^k + \rho(\mathbf{E}[\mathbf{\Pi}_{\cdot j}]^{k+1} - \mathbf{q}^{k+1})$
> **until** *convergence*;

Output: The final centroid matrix $\mathbf{\Pi}$.

In (5) the first two terms guarantees that the data of each task are clustered: specifically with $\lambda_t = 0$ the found centroids are equal to the datapoints while as λ_t increases the number of different centroids π_i^t reduces. The last term in (5) instead imposes the found centroids to be similar if the tasks are related. The relatedness between tasks is modeled by the parameter γ_{st} which can be set using an appropriate measure between distributions. We consider the Maximum Mean Discrepancy $\mathcal{D}(X^t, X^s) = \|\frac{1}{N_t}\sum_{i=1}^{N_t} \phi(\mathbf{x}_i^t) - \frac{1}{N_s}\sum_{i=1}^{N_s} \phi(\mathbf{x}_i^s)\|^2$ [24], we computed it using a linear kernel and we set $\gamma_{st} = e^{-\beta\mathcal{D}(X^t, X^s)}$ with β being a user-defined parameter ($\beta = 0.1$ in our experiments). The parameters w_{ij}^t are used to enforce datapoints in the same task to be assigned to the same cluster and can be set according to some *a-priori* knowledge or in a way such that the found partitions structure reflects the density of the original data distributions.

Optimization. To solve (5) we propose an algorithm based on the alternating direction method of multipliers (ADMM) [25]. We consider the matrix $\mathbf{\Pi} = [\mathbf{\Pi}^{1'} \ \mathbf{\Pi}^{2'} \ \dots \ \mathbf{\Pi}^{T'}]'$, $\mathbf{\Pi} \in I\!R^{N \times d}$, obtained concatenating the task-specific matrices $\mathbf{\Pi}^t = [\pi_1^t \ \pi_2^t \ \dots \ \pi_{N_t}^t]'$. The problem (5) can be solved considering d separate minimization subproblems (one for each column of $\mathbf{X}$) as follows:

$$\min_{\mathbf{q}, \ \mathbf{\Pi}_{\cdot j}} \|\mathbf{X}_{\cdot j} - \mathbf{\Pi}_{\cdot j}\|_2^2 + \|\mathbf{q}\|_1 + \lambda_2\|\mathbf{B}\mathbf{\Pi}_{\cdot j}\|_2^2$$
$$\text{s.t.} \quad \mathbf{E}\mathbf{\Pi}_{\cdot j} - \mathbf{q} = 0 \tag{6}$$

where $\mathbf{E}$ is a block diagonal matrix defined as $\mathbf{E} = \text{blkdiag}(\mathbf{E}^1, \mathbf{E}^2, \dots, \mathbf{E}^T)$ and $\mathbf{E}^t \in I\!R^{|\mathcal{E}_t| \times N_t}$ is a matrix with $|\mathcal{E}_t| = \frac{N_t(N_t-1)}{2}$ rows. Each row is a vector of all zeros except in the position i where it has the value $\lambda_t w_{ij}^t$ and in the position j where it has the value $-\lambda_t w_{ij}^t$. Similarly the matrix $\mathbf{B} \in I\!R^{|\mathcal{B}| \times N}$, where $|\mathcal{B}| = \frac{T(T-1)}{2}$, imposes smoothness between the parameters of related tasks. A row of the matrix $\mathbf{B}$ is a vector with all zeros except in the terms

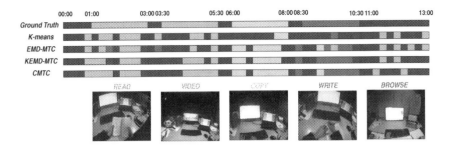

Fig. 4. FPV Office dataset. Temporal video segmentation on the second sequence of subject-3 (13 min): comparison of different methods. (Best viewed in color) (Color figure online).

corresponding to datapoints of the t-th task which are set to γ_{st} and to the terms corresponding to datapoints of the s-th task which are all set to $-\gamma_{st}$. To solve (6) we consider the associated lagrangian $L_\rho(\mathbf{\Pi}_{\cdot j}, \mathbf{q}, \mathbf{p})$:

$$\|\mathbf{X}_{\cdot j} - \mathbf{\Pi}_{\cdot j}\|_2^2 + \|\mathbf{q}\|_1 + \lambda_2\|\mathbf{B}\mathbf{\Pi}_{\cdot j}\|_2^2 + \mathbf{p}'(\mathbf{E}\mathbf{\Pi}_{\cdot j} - \mathbf{q}) + \frac{\rho}{2}\|\mathbf{E}\mathbf{\Pi}_{\cdot j} - \mathbf{q}\|_2^2$$

with $\mathbf{p}$ being the vector of augmented Lagrangian multipliers and ρ being the dual update step length. We devise an algorithm based on the ADMM where three steps, corresponding to the update of the three variables $\mathbf{\Pi}_{\cdot j}, \mathbf{q}, \mathbf{p}$, are performed. We summarize our approach in Algorithm 2.

4   Experimental Results

4.1   Datasets and Experimental Setup

The growing interest in the vision community towards novel approaches for FPV analysis has led to the creation of several publicly available datasets [2–4,8]. In this paper we consider two of them, the FPV office dataset [4] and the FPV home dataset [3].

FPV office dataset [4]. This dataset consists of five activities which frequently occur in an office environment (*reading a book, watching a video, copying text from screen to screen, writing sentences on paper* and *browsing the internet*). Each action was performed by five subjects, who were instructed to execute each task for about two minutes, while 30 s intervals of void class were placed between target tasks. To provide a natural experimental setting, the void class contains a wide variety of actions such as conversing, singing and random head motions. The sequence of five actions was repeated twice to induce interclass variance. The dataset consists of over two hours of data, where the video from each subject is a continuous 25–30 min. video.

FPV home dataset [3]. This dataset contains videos recorded from chest-mounted cameras by 20 different users. The users perform 18 non scripted daily activities in the house, like *brushing teeth, washing dishes,* or *making tea.* The length of the videos is in the range of 20–60 min. The annotations about the presence of 42 relevant objects (*e.g.* kettle, mugs, fridge) and about temporal segmentation are also provided.

Setup. In the experiments, we compare our methods (EMD Multi-task Clustering with linear and rbf kernel and Convex Multi-task Clustering denoted as EMD-MTC, KEMD-MTC, CMTC respectively) with single task clustering approaches, *i.e.* k-means (KM), kernel k-means (KKM), convex (CNMF) and semi (SemiNMF) nonnegative matrix factorization [26]. We also consider recent multi-task clustering algorithms such as the SemiEMD-MTC proposed in [21], its kernel version KSemiEMD-MTC and the LS-MTC method in [19]. To evaluate the clustering results, we adopt two metrics widely used in the literature: the clustering accuracy (Acc) and the normalized mutual information (NMI). For all the methods, except than for CMTC, 10 runs are performed corresponding to different initializations conditions. The average results are shown. In CMTC the parameters λ_t are varied in order to obtain the desired number of clusters. The value of the regularization parameters of our approaches (λ for the methods based on EMD regularization and λ_2 for CMTC) are set in the range $\{0.01, 0.1, 1, 10, 100\}$.

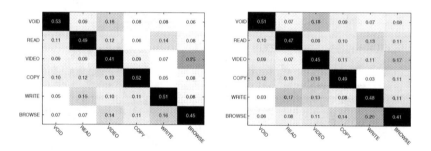

Fig. 5. FPV Office dataset. Confusion matrices using saccade+motion features obtained with (left) KEMD-MTC and (right) CMTC methods.

4.2   Results

FPV office dataset [4]. To conduct experiments on this dataset, we consider $T = 5$ tasks, as the dataset contains videos corresponding to five people. As each datapoint corresponds to a video clip in this dataset, we set the parameters w_{ij}^t in CMTC in order to enforce temporal consistency, *i.e.* for each task t, $w_{ij}^t = 1$ if the features vectors $\mathbf{x}_i^t$ and $\mathbf{x}_j^t$ correspond to temporal adjacent video clips, otherwise $w_{ij}^t = 0$. Table 1 shows a comparison of the results associated to different clustering methods based on different types of features (*i.e.* only saccade, only motion and saccade+motion features). The last three rows correspond to methods which employ a non-linear kernel. From Table 1, several observations can be made. First, independently on the adopted features representation, multi-task

Table 1. Clustering results on FPV office dataset: comparison of different methods using saccade (S), motion (M) and saccade+motion (S+M) features.

	Avg. Acc			Avg. NMI		
	S	M	S+M	S	M	S+M
KM	0.230	0.216	0.257	0.029	0.021	0.045
SemiNMF [26]	0.320	0.303	0.358	0.149	0.131	0.166
SemiEMD-MTC [21]	0.371	0.349	0.415	0.229	0.209	0.259
LSMTC [19]	0.286	0.261	0.335	0.043	0.031	0.071
CNMF [26]	0.328	0.301	0.357	0.152	0.139	0.170
EMD-MTC	0.389	0.363	0.442	0.239	0.221	0.273
CMTC ($\lambda_2 = 0$)	0.367	0.346	0.413	0.224	0.209	0.244
CMTC	0.425	0.401	0.468	0.259	0.238	0.305
KKM	0.345	0.316	0.377	0.159	0.152	0.185
KSemiEMD-MTC [21]	0.387	0.359	0.432	0.241	0.228	0.287
KEMD-MTC	0.436	0.419	0.485	0.268	0.244	0.311

clustering approaches always perform better than single task clustering methods (*e.g.* SemiEMD-MTC outperforms SemiNMF, EMD-MTC provide higher accuracy than CNMF, a value of λ_2 greater than 0 leads to an improvement in accuracy and NMI in CMTC). Confirming the findings reported in [4], we also observe that combining motion and saccade features is advantageous with respect to considering each single feature representation separately. Noticeably, our methods are among the best performers, with KEMD-MTC reaching the highest values of accuracy and NMI. This is somehow expected probably due to both the use of kernels and the adoption of the multi-task learning paradigm. Moreover, CMTC outperforms EMD-MTC by up to 4 % which means that incorporating information about temporal consistency in the learning process is beneficial. Furthermore, in this case the use of Maximum Mean Discrepancy may capture better the relationship among tasks with respect to EMD. Figure 4 shows some qualitative temporal segmentation results on the second sequence of subject-3. In this case for example the CMTC methods outperforms all the other approaches and the effect of enforcing temporal consistency among clips is evident.

Finally, Fig. 5 shows the confusion matrices associated to our methods KEMD-MTC and CMTC. Examining the matrix associated to KEMD-MTC, we observe that the *void, copy* and *write* actions achieve relative high recognition accuracies compared with the *video* and *browse* actions. It is also interesting to note that 25 % and 17 % of the *video* actions are recognized as *browse* actions for KEMD-MTC and CMTC respectively, because of the similarity among motion and eye-gaze patterns.

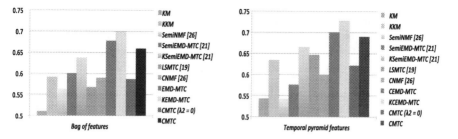

Fig. 6. Comparison of different methods using (left) bag of features and (right) temporal pyramid features on FPV home dataset. (Figure is best viewed in color) (Color figure online).

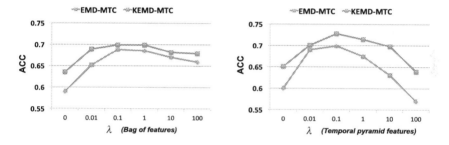

Fig. 7. FPV home dataset: performance variations of EMD-MTC and KEMD-MTC at different values of λ using (left) bag of features and (right) temporal pyramid features.

FPV home dataset [3]. In this dataset there are 18 different non scripted activities. Since each person typically performs a small subset of the 18 activities, in our experiments we consider a series of three tasks problems, selecting videos associated to three randomly chosen users but imposing the condition that videos corresponding to the three users should have at least three activities in common. We perform 10 different runs. Figure 6 shows the results (average accuracy) obtained with different clustering methods for both the bag-of-words and the temporal pyramid features representation. In this series of experiments, we did not cluster video clips of fixed size as in the office dataset, but we consider the pre-segmented clips as provided with the dataset. In this scenario, it does not make sense to set w_{ij}^t in CMTC to model temporal consistency. Therefore, we set $w_{ij}^t = e^{-\|\mathbf{x}_i^t - \mathbf{x}_j^t\|^2}$ if $e^{-\|\mathbf{x}_i^t - \mathbf{x}_j^t\|^2} \leq \theta$ and $w_{ij}^t = 0$ otherwise. This is meant to enforce that the found partitions structure reflects the density of the original data distributions. Analyzing the results in Fig. 6, it is evident that the MTC approaches outperforms their single task version (*e.g.* CMTC outperforms CMTC with $\lambda_2 = 0$, EMD-MTC outperforms CNMF, SemiEMD-MTC outperforms SemiNMF). On the other hand, our algorithms based on EMD regularization and CMTC achieve a considerably higher accuracy with respect to all the other methods. Finally, we also investigate the effect of different values of the regularization parameter λ in (3) on clustering performance. As shown in Fig. 7, independently from the adopted feature representation, the accuracy values are sensitive to varying λ. Figure 7 shows that choosing a value of $\lambda = 0.1$ always lead to similar or superior performance with respect to adopting a single-task clustering approach ($\lambda = 0$). The value $\lambda = 0.1$ correspond to the results reported in Fig. 6. This clearly confirms the advantage of using a MTC approach for FPV analysis.

5 Conclusions

In this paper, we consider the problem of egocentric activity recognition from unlabeled data within a multi-task clustering framework. Two novel MTC algorithms have been proposed and evaluated extensively on two FPV datasets. Our experimental results clearly demonstrate the advantage of sharing informations among tasks over single tasks algorithms. Among our methods the approach based on EMD regularization achieves the best performance when used in its kernel version. On the other hand, our second algorithm is also effective as it is based on a convex optimization problem and it is particularly useful when one needs to incorporate some *a-priori* knowledge. In this paper we consider embedding information about temporal consistency but the CMTC method also permits to integrate *a-priori* knowledge about task dependencies if available (*e.g.* people performing the same activities in the same rooms correspond to more related tasks with respect to people operating in different rooms). This can be easily done by defining an appropriate matrix $\mathbf{B}$. Future works include exploiting the suitability of the proposed algorithms for other vision applications, as well as investigating how to improve our MTC methods (*e.g.* by detecting outlier tasks).

Acknowledgement. This work has been supported by the project Cluster Active Ageing at Home.

References

1. Kanade, T., Hebert, M.: First-person vision. Proc. IEEE **100**, 2442–2453 (2012)
2. Lu, Z., Grauman, K.: Story-driven summarization for egocentric video. In: CVPR (2013)
3. Pirsiavash, H., Ramanan, D.: Detecting activities of daily living in first-person camera views. In: CVPR (2012)
4. Ogaki, K., Kitani, K.M., Sugano, Y., Sato, Y.: Coupling eye-motion and ego-motion features for first-person activity recognition. In: CVPR Workshop on Egocentric Vision (2012)
5. Tapia, E.M., Intille, S.S., Larson, K.: Activity recognition in the home using simple and ubiquitous sensors. In: Ferscha, A., Mattern, F. (eds.) PERVASIVE 2004. LNCS, vol. 3001, pp. 158–175. Springer, Heidelberg (2004)
6. Casale, P., Pujol, O., Radeva, P.: Human activity recognition from accelerometer data using a wearable device. In: Vitrià, J., Sanches, J.M., Hernández, M. (eds.) IbPRIA 2011. LNCS, vol. 6669, pp. 289–296. Springer, Heidelberg (2011)

7. Omid, A., Josephine, S., Stefan, C.: Novelty detection from an egocentric perspective. In: CVPR (2011)
8. Fathi, A., Rehg, J.M.: Social interactions: a first-person perspective. In: CVPR (2012)
9. Lei, J., Ren, X., Fox, D.: Fine-grained kitchen activity recognition using rgb-d. In: UBICOMP (2012)
10. Taralova, E., De la Torre, F., Hebert, M.: Source constrained clustering. In: ICCV (2011)
11. Mahasseni, B., Todorovic, S.: Latent multitask learning for view-invariant action recognition. In: ICCV (2013)
12. Yan, Y., Liu, G., Ricci, E., Sebe., N.: Multi-task linear discriminant analysis for multi-view action recognition. In: ICIP (2013)
13. Yuan, C., Hu, W., Tian, G., Yang, S., Wang, H.: Multi-task sparse learning with beta process prior for action recognition. In: CVPR (2013)
14. Caruana, R.: Multitask learning. Mach. Learn. **28**, 41–75 (1997)
15. Salakhutdinov, R., Torralba, A., Tenenbaum, J.: Learning to share visual appearance for multiclass object detection. In: CVPR (2011)
16. Lu, G., Yan, Y., Sebe, N., Kambhamettu, C.: Knowing where i am: exploiting multi-task learning for multi-view indoor image-based localization. In: BMVC (2014)
17. Wang, X., Zhang, C., Zhang, Z.: Boosted multi-task learning for face verification with applications to web image and video search. In: CVPR (2009)
18. Yan, Y., Ricci, E., Subramanian, R., Lanz, O., Sebe, N.: No matter where you are: flexible graph-guided multi-task learning for multi-view head pose classification under target motion. In: ICCV (2013)
19. Gu, Q., Zhou, J.: Learning the shared subspace for multi-task clustering and transductive transfer classification. In: ICDM (2009)
20. Kulis, B., Jordan, M.I.: Revisiting k-means: new algorithms via bayesian nonparametrics. In: ICML (2012)
21. Zhang, J., Zhang, C.: Multitask bregman clustering. Neurocomput. **74**, 1720–1734 (2011)
22. Bulling, A., Ward, J.A., Gellersen, H., Troster, G.: Eye movement analysis for activity recognition using electrooculography. TPAMI **33**, 741–753 (2011)
23. Rubner, Y., Tomasi, C., Guibas, L.J.: A metric for distributions with applications to image databases. In: ICCV (1998)
24. Borgwardt, K., Gretton, A., Rasch, M., Kriegel, H.P., Schoelkopf, B., Smola, A.: Integrating structured biological data by kernel maximum mean discrepancy. Bioinformatics **22**, 1–9 (2006)
25. Boyd, S., Parikh, N., Chu, E., Peleato, B., Eckstein, J.: Distributed optimization and statistical learning via the alternating direction method of multipliers. Found. Trends Mach. Learn. **3**, 1–122 (2011)
26. Ding, C., Li, T., Jordan, M.I.: Convex and semi-nonnegative matrix factorizations. TPAMI **32**, 45–55 (2010)

Multi-view Recognition Using Weighted View Selection

Scott Spurlock[✉], Hui Wu, and Richard Souvenir

University of North Carolina at Charlotte, Charlotte, NC 28223, USA
{sspurloc,hwu13,souvenir}@uncc.edu

Abstract. In this paper, we present an algorithm for multi-view recognition in a distributed camera setting that learns which viewpoints are most discriminative for particular instances of ambiguity. Our method is built on top of 2D recognition algorithms and casts view selection as the problem of optimizing kernel weights in multiple kernel learning. The main contribution is a locality-sensitive meta-training step to learn a disambiguation function to select the relative weighting of available viewpoints needed to classify a 2D input example. Our method outperforms related approaches on benchmark multi-view action recognition data sets.

1 Introduction

Multi-view human action recognition is an active area of research with applications to surveillance, robotics, and human-computer interaction. Figure 1 shows a scene captured from multiple cameras with two tracked people, where the goal is to recognize the actions of each tracked person. In general, there are two main approaches to recognition from multiple viewpoints: integrate data from all the views to build a 3D model and solve a 3D recognition problem, or consider some combination of multiple 2D views. In general, 3D approaches tend to perform well, but require unobstructed views and, usually, a high computational cost for 3D model construction or finding correspondences. For the 2D case, a major challenge is caused by the unknown relative viewpoint or pose of the object, whereby instances from the same class may appear different from different viewpoints, while, from other viewpoints, instances from different classes may appear similar.

Our approach is applicable to distributed camera networks for human activity understanding (e.g., Fig. 1). In particular, we consider architectures with peer camera nodes, where for a given target, there is a *primary* camera and the rest of the camera nodes are *secondary*. This designation can be fixed, where a particular camera is primary for targets in a specified region, or dynamic, e.g., the primary camera is selected to track a target [1]. In either case, secondary views are represented by their *relative offset* from the primary camera.

Our focus is to only incorporate secondary views when necessary by learning a model that recognizes potentially confusing poses and determines the relative value of secondary viewpoints for disambiguation. That is, we not only determine

© Springer International Publishing Switzerland 2015
D. Cremers et al. (Eds.): ACCV 2014, Part IV, LNCS 9006, pp. 538–552, 2015.
DOI: 10.1007/978-3-319-16817-3_35

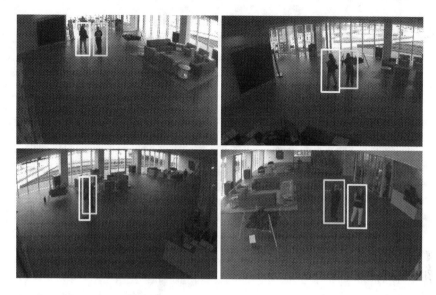

Fig. 1. In distributed camera networks, some viewpoints are more discriminative for action recognition. Our method learns *which* viewpoints are most discriminative for *particular instances* of ambiguity.

if information from additional viewpoints is needed, but *which* viewpoints would provide the most discriminative power. Our two-stage learning algorithm casts the problem of combining views as that of learning weights for multiple kernel learning (MKL), and we build off the efficient algorithms that have been developed for MKL.

2   Related Work

The idea of using information from one view to inform view selection is often framed as active vision [2], usually in the context of a mobile agent. For example, in [3], agents perform object recognition using entropy maps, which model the predicted suitability of potential viewpoints to help determine the object. This differs from the distributed camera setting, in that active vision approaches are typically carried out in a sequential fashion (during, for example, robot navigation), while all the views are available simultaneously in multi-camera networks. For multi-view action recognition [4], there are two broad categories of methods: (1) 3D methods, which explicitly build a 3D model, and (2) 2D methods, like ours, which may incorporate multiple 2D views, but do not build 3D models.

3D action descriptors include motion history volumes [5,6], a compact representation of the animated visual hull of a person performing an action. While complex 3D models often achieve high recognition rates, they also tend to be computationally expensive. A recent hybrid 2D/3D approach determines the best viewpoint of an action in isolation after constructing a 3D model [7]. This approach differs from ours in that it is focused on finding the single best view from the perspective of a human observer, while our method learns how to combine views to improve recognition. Other hybrid approaches that include strong 3D correspondences during the training phase include methods designed for cross-view recognition (e.g., [8,9]), which is a version of multi-view recognition where synchronized views from all views are not available for both training and testing.

For 2D multi-view recognition, there are a variety of approaches. One method models 2D feature descriptors as a function of viewpoint [10]. Farhadi et al. distinguish between geometric and discriminative aspect, where geometric aspect corresponds to canonical views (front, side), while discriminative aspect encodes the ways in which different things look similar or different [11]. Their method learns the parameters governing these latent variables and weights features accordingly to improve classification. These approaches of specifically learning a viewpoint manifold or discriminative aspect model are very different from ours in that we do not learn to distinguish viewpoints, but instead seek to recognize when additional viewpoints are needed and their relative utility. A number of approaches seek to identify view-invariant features (e.g., [12]) or extract features that exhibit low intra-class, but high inter-class variation (e.g., [13]). Our method is agnostic to the base feature; rather than relying on view-invariance, our method learns cases where disambiguation is needed.

In Sect. 3, we describe our classification approach and how we cast the view combination problem as kernel weight learning. By applying a kernel-based approach, our method is applicable to a variety of feature transforms used in action recognition, and in Sect. 4, we show high recognition rates on benchmark datasets for multi-view action recognition.

3 Approach

Figure 2 presents an overview of our approach to example disambiguation.[1] Each example, $\mathbf{X}_i = \langle \mathbf{x}_{i,0}, \ldots, \mathbf{x}_{i,V-1} \rangle$ represents V videos of a particular action instance captured by a primary camera, $\mathbf{x}_{i,0}$, and $V - 1$ secondary cameras, ordered by their offset to the primary camera (as shown in Fig. 3). As illustrated in Fig. 3, each instance of an action could represent up to V different training examples corresponding to each of the V cameras serving as the primary camera. Each example $\mathbf{X}_i$ has class label y_i. In this section, we describe our approach to identifying ambiguous examples, learning to disambiguate, and training the combined classifier. Finally we describe the complete algorithm in Sect. 3.3.

---

[1] For illustration, Fig. 2 depicts a 2-dimensional feature space, but each step of our procedure can be kernelized, so a direct feature vector representation of the data is not necessary.

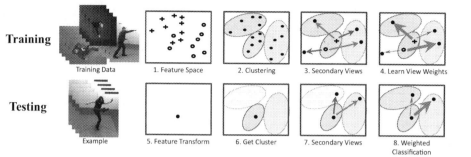

Fig. 2. The recognition procedure. For training, (1,2) the videos from all views are clustered. Some clusters (e.g., blue and orange) are homogeneous, while others (e.g., gray) contain examples from multiple classes. (3) In non-homogeneous clusters, secondary views are identified for each instance (green and purple arrows). (4) A classifier is trained that simultaneously learns the relative weights of each view for each cluster (represented by arrow thickness). For testing, (5,6) the input is assigned to a cluster. (7) If the cluster is non-homogeneous, secondary views are obtained, and (8) the input is classified using the weighted model learned for the cluster (color figure online).

3.1 Identifying Ambiguous Examples

The first step toward estimating view utility is identifying examples that are similar in appearance, but may represent different classes. Let $\kappa(\mathbf{x}, \mathbf{x}')$ be a kernel function, which we refer to as the *base kernel* that can be applied to the video feature representation. Using κ, we perform kernel k-means (KKM) [14] to partition the training data into C clusters, where each primary video, $\mathbf{x}_{i,0}$, receives cluster label $c_i \in [1, C]$. Even though KKM is unsupervised, with modern feature transforms designed for discriminative action recognition, a significant fraction of the clusters are *homogeneous*, containing only examples from a single class. These clusters demarcate regions of the feature space where input from a single, primary camera is sufficient for classification. However, the remaining *heterogeneous* clusters contain examples from multiple classes nearby in feature space, representing border cases that would typically be misclassified using standard classification methods. In each cluster, we will learn the relative utility of the secondary views for disambiguating the input (Sect. 3.2).

To disambiguate test examples, an efficient method to assign new examples to clusters is needed. Using the training examples, corresponding cluster labels $\{c_i\}$, and base kernel, κ, a support vector machine (SVM) is trained for *cluster assignment classification*. Methods exist for unsupervised support vector clustering that return support vectors suitable for cluster assignment classification. However, these methods tend to return large numbers of support vectors [15], so this two-stage (cluster-then-classification) approach can be more efficient for evaluating the SVM at run-time.

A common approach to handling multiple representations of the same object is feature vector concatenation. For multi-view recognition, this corresponds to

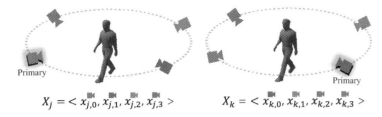

$$X_j = < x_{j,0}, x_{j,1}, x_{j,2}, x_{j,3} >$$ $$X_k = < x_{k,0}, x_{k,1}, x_{k,2}, x_{k,3} >$$

Fig. 3. For a given primary view, the offsets to other cameras are *relative*. The same instance of an action leads to different feature representations depending on which camera is selected as primary. On the left, selecting the red camera to be primary leads to X_j, while, on the right, selecting the purple camera as primary leads to X_k. With recorded data, during the training phase, each instance of an action could represent up to V different examples. For testing, the primary camera is determined as part of distributed network sensing. (Figure best viewed in color.) (color figure online)

concatenating the feature representations of the same action from different viewpoints. One drawback to using this combined representation directly in a standard supervised learning scheme is that multiple viewpoints are incorporated even if one of the viewpoints is highly discriminative, and, worse, the addition of a difficult, ambiguous feature vector to the joint representation can result in misclassification in some cases. Our approach, for a given ambiguity, is to learn the relative utility of secondary viewpoints for discrimination. The rest of this section explains how we cast the problem of estimating view offset utility as kernel weight learning.

3.2   Learning Discriminative View Combinations

For kernel-based methods, such as support vector machines (SVM), selecting an appropriate kernel function is a key step. There are a number of common choices (e.g., linear, RBF) and custom kernels (e.g., spatial pyramid kernel [16] for sets of local image features). Multiple kernel learning (MKL) has emerged as an alternative to simply selecting a single kernel function, with multiple approaches to learning weighted combinations of kernels [17]. MKL is often used to fuse different types of features, and has been used in this way for action recognition (e.g., [18]). By contrast, we propose to use multiple kernel learning for weighted view selection, rather than feature weighting.

Kernel functions can be combined; for example, a linear combination of kernels is itself a kernel. That is, $\kappa_\beta(\cdot) = \sum_{i=1}^{M} \beta_i \kappa_i(\cdot)$, where β is a vector of weights for M kernels, $\{\kappa_i\}$. In the case of convex β (i.e., $\beta \in \mathbb{R}_+^M$ and $\sum \beta_i = 1$), the weights represent the importance of each kernel and the combined kernel represents the similarity in a feature space defined by the concatenation of the individual feature vectors. While most of the focus in MKL has been on linear combinations of kernels, recent work [19] with nonlinear kernel combinations has shown they can be more effective. For our approach, we use the quadratic kernel:

$$\kappa_\beta(\mathbf{X}_i, \mathbf{X}_j) = \sum_{m=0}^{V-1} \sum_{l=0}^{V-1} \beta_m \beta_l \kappa(\mathbf{x}_{i,m}, \mathbf{x}_{j,m}) \kappa(\mathbf{x}_{i,l}, \mathbf{x}_{j,l}) \tag{1}$$

where each kernel represents one of the viewpoints in the system.

Many approaches to multiple kernel learning incorporate the problem of learning kernel weights with the optimization of the classification margin. However, as the complexity of the kernel combination increases, so does the complexity of the resulting optimization problem. For example, incorporating Eq. 1 into the usual SVM optimization leads to a difficult non-convex optimization. We apply an iterative approach [20], modified for SVM [17], to this MKL optimization:

$$\min_{\beta \in \mathcal{M}} \max_{\alpha \in \mathbb{R}^N} \sum_i \alpha_i - \frac{1}{2} \sum_{i,j} \alpha_i \alpha_j y_i y_j \kappa_\beta(\mathbf{X}_i, \mathbf{X}_j) \tag{2}$$

where $\mathcal{M}$ is the norm-1 bounded set which constrains β to be convex. This optimization can be solved iteratively, alternately finding α by solving the inner SVM problem with the current combined kernel, κ_β, and then finding the weights, β, using projection-based gradient descent.

3.3   Algorithm

Training Consider a set of N actions, each captured from V different viewpoints. This gives a training set of $N \times V$ labeled examples, where example $\mathbf{X}_i$ has class label y_i. Let $\kappa(\mathbf{x}, \mathbf{x}')$ be the *base kernel*, which can be applied to the video feature representation. The two-stage training procedure is as follows:

1. Cluster the training videos to learn cluster labels $\{c_i\}$.
   (a) Using the base kernel, κ, and cluster labels, train cluster assignment SVM, $\mathcal{C}_{cluster}$.
   (b) For homogeneous clusters, no further work is needed.
2. For each non-homogeneous cluster, c_i, train multi-class SVM classifier (Eq. 2), $\mathcal{C}_{c_i}$, and learn cluster weights, β_{c_i}, with the classes represented in cluster c_i.

Classification. Given a new query example (action captured from V different views), $\mathbf{X}_q$, the classification procedure follows an analogous two-stage approach.

1. Using SVM, $\mathcal{C}_{cluster}$, get cluster, c_q, for $\mathbf{x}_{q,0}$.
2. Classify $\mathbf{x}_{q,0}$:
   (a) If c_q is homogeneous, $\mathbf{X}_q$ is classified immediately.
   (b) Otherwise, $\mathbf{X}_q$ is classified using SVM $\mathcal{C}_{c_q}$, and cluster-specific weights, β_{c_q}.

Using this locality-sensitive approach, similar to [21], kernel combinations can be applied in a data-dependent fashion rather than learning a global combination across the whole input space.

4   Results

We evaluated our method on three publicly-available multi-view recognition datasets. Our algorithm was implemented in Matlab on a standard PC, using libsvm [22] for support vector classification. For multi-class classification, we use the one-versus-all (OVA) approach. The SVM cost parameter, C_{SVM}, was selected using cross-validation for each experiment. For clustering, we initialized kernel k-means 25 times and selected the cluster assignment with minimum energy, as measured by average intra-class similarity.

4.1   Action Recognition

Our approach is neither specific to particular camera configurations nor video feature representations. We evaluated our algorithm using two widely-used multi-view human action datasets with two different feature representations.

Data Sets. For these experiments, we used the i3DPost multi-view human action data set [23] and the INRIA Xmas Motion Acquisition Sequences (IXMAS) data set [5]. i3DPost includes 10 actions performed by 8 actors recorded by 8 synchronized cameras. IXMAS, which is commonly used as a benchmark for multi-view action recognition, contains multiple actors performing various actions, captured by five synchronized cameras. Compared with i3DPost, IXMAS is more challenging, containing fewer cameras, more easily confused actions, and more instances of self occlusion. Figure 4 shows sample frames from both datasets.

Features. To demonstrate the ability of our method to handle different underlying motion features, we used the Motion Context (MC) transform [24] and the $\mathcal{R}$ Transform Surface (RT) video descriptor [10]. MC computes frame-based histograms of the localized optic flow and silhouette occupancy. The base kernel for an image sequence is the histogram intersection kernel on quantized

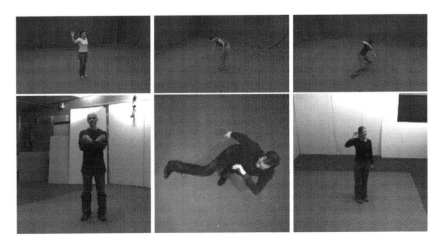

Fig. 4. Example frames from the i3Dpost (top) and IXMAS (bottom) data sets.

features, with a dictionary size, $|D| = 800$. RT is a silhouette-based descriptor that extends the Radon transform. The base kernel is the Gaussian radial basis function of the diffusion distance [25] between the base features.

Methods. Using the same features, base kernel, and free parameters, we compare the performance of our multi-view learning (mvl) approach to several other kernel-based schemes for multi-view classification:

View-Insensitive SVM (svm). The basic classifier where the SVM is trained with the base kernel without respect to viewpoint.

SVM Voting (vote). An example is classified from each viewpoint and the majority decision serves as the final classification.

Weighted SVM Voting (wvote). Similar to vote, but SVM posterior probabilities [26] are used to weight each vote.

Winner Take All (wta). Using SVM posterior probabilities as a proxy for classifier confidence, the most confident classifier provides the final classification.

Uniform-Weighting SVM (uwsvm). Each example is represented as the concatenation of all the views. This is equivalent to using the uniformly-weighted convex combination of base kernels for each view representation.

Table 1. Multi-view classification rates on the i3DPost and IXMAS data sets. (Top) Rates for our approach, mvl, and kernel-based variants using two different feature representations (RT & MC). (Bottom) Representative recognition rates reported in the literature on IXMAS using the same experimental protocol.

Method	i3Dpost		IXMAS	
	RT	MC	RT	MC
mvl	**73.75%**	**96.25%**	**90.91%**	**93.58%**
uwsvm	72.50%	95.00%	87.27%	92.42%
vote	66.56%	93.75%	81.82%	89.15%
wvote	66.25%	92.50%	75.09%	82.79%
wta	**73.75%**	93.75%	74.18%	79.39%
svm	63.75%	91.25%	71.88%	77.15%
Wu et al. [18]	-		88.2%	
Zhu et al. [27]	-		88.0%	
Parrigan and Souvenir [28]	-		84.0%	

Results. Table 1 shows the multi-view classification rates for both data sets with both feature representations. In general, our method, mvl, outperformed competing approaches, except for an unusual case where an otherwise underperforming method, wta, matched our performance for a particular feature-dataset combination.

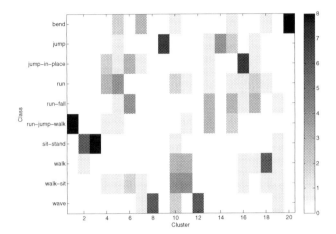

Fig. 5. Distribution of class labels in clusters for i3DPost. In most cases, clusters were either homogeneous (e.g., clusters 8 and 12 contain only wave actions) or represented specific instances of ambiguity (e.g., run and run-fall tend to co-cluster).

For i3DPost, we employed 2-fold cross-validation, with half the actors in each set, and included 4 views and 10 actions. For both features, `mvl` returned the highest classification rates (except as noted above), improving on the baseline kernel classification by up to 10 %. Figure 5 shows an example from an experiment with 20 clusters and the MC features. Several of the clusters are homogeneous. For example, cluster 1 contains only run-jump-walk actions, while clusters 8 and 12 contain only wave actions. Overall in this experiment, 34 % of test examples fell into homogeneous clusters, which results in immediate (single-camera) classification and computational savings compared to the other aggregation approaches that always incorporate each viewpoint.

There does not appear to be a commonly-used experimental protocol in the literature for i3Dpost. To our knowledge, the best reported accuracy is 97.50 % using a full 3D (not 2D multi-view) approach [29]. In addition to the inherent complexity of 3D reconstruction, this method uses leave-one-actor-out (LOAO) cross-validation, where for each fold, a single actor is used for testing, while the remainder are used for training. With LOAO on i3DPost, our `mvl` method also resulted in 97.50 % accuracy. However, the other multi-view methods also performed well, so this may be a function of the complexity of the dataset rather than the effectiveness of the classification approaches.

Compared to i3Dpost, IXMAS contains more self-occlusion and similar-looking actions. For IXMAS, we followed the LOAO protocol, which is the experimental setup most commonly found in the literature (see, e.g., [30]). The experiment uses 10 actors, each performing one of 11 actions three times. As shown in Table 1, `mvl` far outperforms the baseline `svm` and voting approaches. While the MC feature outperformed RT on each test, our method boosted the performance of both feature descriptors. The 93.58 % classification accuracy

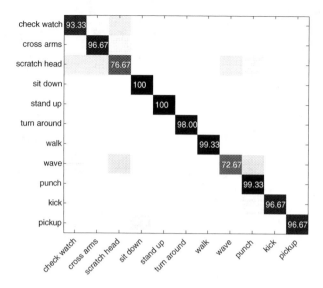

Fig. 6. Confusion matrix for `mvl` classification on IXMAS data. Each row represents the actual class and each column represents the predicted class. Our method achieved 93.58 % accuracy.

achieved by our `mvl` approach not only out-performs other recent 2D methods, it approaches the performance of 3D approaches, but without the computational expense of building 3D models.

For `mvl`, Fig. 6 shows the confusion matrix for the classification experiment on IXMAS with the MC feature, where each row represents the actual class and each column represents the predicted class. For many actions (e.g., sit, stand, turn, walk, pickup), accuracy was above 95 %. The most challenging cases involved confusions between waving, punching, and scratching head. These results are expected as the base descriptors are primarily silhouette-based, and these motions include self-occlusion from most viewpoints. Additionally, by comparing the per-class accuracies between `mvl` and the best-performing 2D method from the literature [18], we find that the achieved per-class accuracy for eight of the actions is similar (and relatively high). However, for three actions (check watch, cross arms, scratch head), our method shows noticeable gains: from 78 % to 93 % for check watch, 83 % to 97 % for cross arms, and 72 % to 77 % for scratch head. This suggests that the superior performance of `mvl` is mainly due to correctly classifying the most challenging cases of confusion, which, for our approach, tend to fall in heterogeneous clusters.

As the same base kernel was used for both clustering and classification, the clustering step provides an initial partition of the data into groups that are either mostly homogeneous with regards to the class of the examples or require disambiguation. For the IXMAS data with $C = 50$ clusters and RT feature, Fig. 7 shows the distribution of class labels in each cluster. It can be seen that

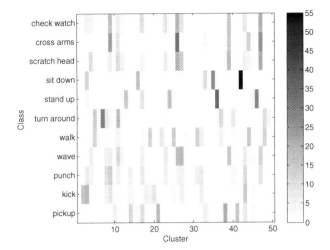

Fig. 7. Distribution of class labels in clusters for IXMAS. In most cases, clusters were either homogeneous (e.g., clusters 35 and 42 contain only sit actions) or represented specific instances of ambiguity (e.g., check watch, cross arms, wave, and scratch head tend to co-cluster).

the classes that resulted in the highest recognition rates (e.g., sit, stand, turn) tend to lie in homogeneous clusters. For example, clusters 35 and 42 contain only sit actions, while cluster 7 contains only turn. By contrast, classes that were more likely to be confused by our method tend to lie in more heterogeneous clusters. The most frequently confused action, punch, is present in 28 of the 50 clusters in this experiment.

Figure 8 shows examples views of actions that were co-clustered during an experiment. The top row contains examples from a cluster containing primarily kick and walk motions. From the given viewpoint, these actions are visually similar and indistinguishable for most feature transforms. The bottom row shows examples from a cluster containing punches and kicks from a viewpoint directly overhead. In this case, the silhouette-based descriptors are similar for these semantically different actions. However, incorporating almost any of the other viewpoints would serve to disambiguate this confusion and correctly classify these actions. Figure 9 shows two examples of the weighting learned by our method for secondary views. For each row, the left image is a frame from an action that was not immediately classified. The next three images show frames from secondary viewpoints, sorted in order of weights learned by our method. The highest weighted viewpoint often corresponds to views that are highly discriminative, with minimal self-occlusion.

4.2   Object Recognition

While our method was originally intended for action recognition from video, we also applied it to object recognition from images. The 3D object data set

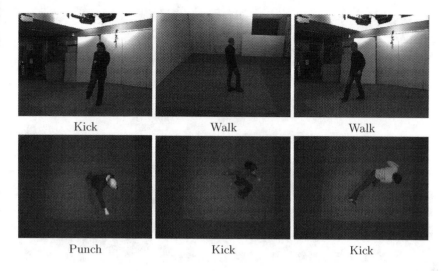

Fig. 8. Each row shows a set of three example frames from viewpoints that were co-clustered by our algorithm. The label indicates the action represented.

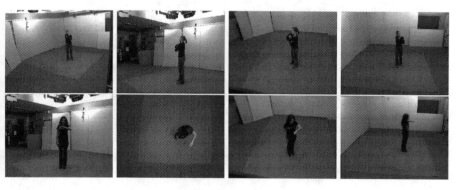

Fig. 9. For each row, the left image is a frame from an action that was not immediately classified. The following images show frames from secondary viewpoints, sorted in order of weights learned by our method.

(3DO) [31] consists of examples of 10 object categories from several different views, elevations, and scales. Figure 10 shows some example images from the data set. We selected a subset of seven categories for which 10 examples were available with four different views at the same elevation and scale (bicycle, car, cellphone, head, iron, monitor, and mouse). For each image, we calculated SIFT descriptors for 16×16 patches on a regular grid, with a spacing of 8, and used the Spatial Pyramid [16] (number of levels, $L = 3$, and the vocabulary size, $M = 200$) as the base kernel. For evaluation, we divided the data in half and performed 2-fold testing. The basic svm approach achieved 81.43 % accuracy.

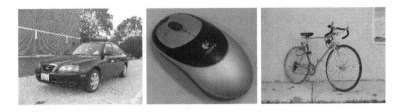

Fig. 10. Example images from the 3DO data set.

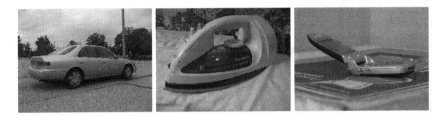

Fig. 11. Example images that were co-clustered by our method.

Integrating multiple views was beneficial as vote achieved 87.50 % accuracy. Our approach, mvl, achieved 90.71 % accuracy.[2] Like the action recognition data, classification ambiguity in this data set appears to be tied to ambiguous viewpoints. Figure 11 shows an example of co-clustered object views. Unlike the examples for action recognition, for this data set, it is not always apparent that co-clustered images should share similar feature representations. Nonetheless, the results demonstrate that incorporating weighted view aggregation provides additional discriminative power.

5   Conclusions and Future Work

In this paper, we presented a multi-view recognition method for identifying when input is ambiguous and learning the relative utility of secondary views as a function of the particular ambiguity. We cast the problem of viewpoint weighting as kernel weight optimization for multiple kernel learning, localized in feature space, and took advantage of efficient solutions in the MKL domain. A significant amount of research effort in the action recognition domain focuses on devising new, more discriminative, feature representations. However, by applying a strategy to account for the inherent ambiguity in certain poses from certain viewpoints, our method boosted the performance of existing features and achieved high recognition accuracy on a benchmark action recognition data set, outperforming other recent 2D multi-camera methods, and similar to 3D approaches,

---

[2] We were unable to directly compare these results with those previously reported. Unlike with the IXMAS set, there is little agreement in the literature on an experimental protocol for 3DO.

with reduced computational effort. For future work, we plan to investigate early identification of potentially ambiguous actions and learn the *single* view shift that would best disambiguate the input to allow for dynamic camera switching in distributed camera networks on untrimmed video.

References

1. Wang, X.: Intelligent multi-camera video surveillance: A review. Pattern Recogn. Lett. **34**(1), 3–19 (2012)
2. Dutta Roy, S., Chaudhury, S., Banerjee, S.: Active recognition through next view planning: a survey. Pattern Recogn. **37**, 429–446 (2004)
3. Arbel, T., Ferrie, F.: Viewpoint selection by navigation through entropy maps. In: Proceedings of the International Conference on Computer Vision, vol. 1, pp. 248–254 (1999)
4. Weinland, D., Ronfard, R., Boyer, E.: A survey of vision-based methods for action representation, segmentation and recognition. Comput. Vis. Image Underst. **115**, 224–241 (2011)
5. Weinland, D., Ronfard, R., Boyer, E.: Free viewpoint action recognition using motion history volumes. Comput. Vis. Image Underst. **104**, 249–257 (2006)
6. Turaga, P., Veeraraghavan, A., Chellappa, R.: Statistical analysis on stiefel and grassmann manifolds with applications in computer vision. In: Proceedings of the IEEE Conference on Computer Vision and Pattern Recognition, pp. 1–8 (2008)
7. Rudoy, D., Zelnik-Manor, L.: Viewpoint selection for human actions. Int. J. Comput. Vis. **97**, 243–254 (2012)
8. Li, R., Zickler, T.: Discriminative virtual views for cross-view action recognition. In: IEEE Conference on Computer Vision and Pattern Recognition, pp. 2855–2862 (2012)
9. Zhang, Z., Wang, C., Xiao, B., Zhou, W., Liu, S., Shi, C.: Cross-view action recognition via a continuous virtual path. In: IEEE Conference on Computer Vision and Pattern Recognition, pp. 2690–2697 (2013)
10. Souvenir, R., Babbs, J.: Learning the viewpoint manifold for action recognition. In: Proceedings of the IEEE Conference on Computer Vision and Pattern Recognition, pp. 1–7 (2008)
11. Farhadi, A., Tabrizi, M., Endres, I., Forsyth, D.: A latent model of discriminative aspect. In: Proceedings of the International Conference on Computer Vision, pp. 948–955 (2009)
12. Ali, S., Shah, M.: Human action recognition in videos using kinematic features and multiple instance learning. IEEE Trans. Pattern Anal. Mach. Intell. **32**, 288–303 (2010)
13. Sharma, A., Kumar, A., Daume, H., Jacobs, D.: Generalized multiview analysis: A discriminative latent space. In: Proceedings of the IEEE Conference on Computer Vision and Pattern Recognition, pp. 2160–2167 (2012)
14. Dhillon, I., Guan, Y., Kulis, B.: Kernel k-means: spectral clustering and normalized cuts. In: Proceedings of the ACM SIGKDD International Conference on Knowledge Discovery and Data Mining, pp. 551–556. ACM (2004)
15. Zhang, K., Tsang, I., Kwok, J.: Maximum margin clustering made practical. IEEE Trans. Neural Netw. **20**, 583–596 (2009)

16. Lazebnik, S., Schmid, C., Ponce, J.: Beyond bags of features: Spatial pyramid matching for recognizing natural scene categories. In: Proceedings of the IEEE Conference on Computer Vision and Pattern Recognition, vol. 2, pp. 2169–2178. IEEE (2006)

17. Gönen, M., Alpaydın, E.: Multiple kernel learning algorithms. J. Mach. Learn. Res. 12, 2211–2268 (2011)

18. Wu, X., Xu, D., Duan, L., Luo, J.: Action recognition using context and appearance distribution features. In: Proceedings of the IEEE Conference on Computer Vision and Pattern Recognition, pp. 489–496 (2011)

19. Levinboim, T., Sha, F.: Learning the kernel matrix with low-rank multiplicative shaping. In: Proceedings of the National Conference on Artificial Intelligence (2012)

20. Cortes, C., Mohri, M., Rostamizadeh, A.: Learning non-linear combinations of kernels. In: Advances in Neural Information Processing Systems 22, pp. 396–404 (2009)

21. Yang, J., Li, Y., Tian, Y., Duan, L., Gao, W.: Group-sensitive multiple kernel learning for object categorization. In: Proceedings of the International Conference on Computer Vision, pp. 436–443 (2009)

22. Chang, C.C., Lin, C.J.: LIBSVM: A library for support vector machines. ACM Trans. Intell. Syst. Technol. 2, 27:1–27:27 (2011)

23. Gkalelis, N., Kim, H., Hilton, A., Nikolaidis, N., Pitas, I.: The i3dpost multi-view and 3d human action/interaction database. In: Conference for Visual Media Production, pp. 159–168. IEEE (2009)

24. Tran, D., Sorokin, A.: Human activity recognition with metric learning. In: Forsyth, D., Torr, P., Zisserman, A. (eds.) ECCV 2008, Part I. LNCS, vol. 5302, pp. 548–561. Springer, Heidelberg (2008)

25. Ling, H., Okada, K.: Diffusion distance for histogram comparison. In: Proceedings of the IEEE Conference on Computer Vision and Pattern Recognition, pp. 246–253. IEEE Computer Society, Washington, DC (2006)

26. Lin, H.T., Lin, C.J., Weng, R.C.: A note on platts probabilistic outputs for support vector machines. Mach. Learn. 68, 267–276 (2007)

27. Zhu, F., Shao, L., Lin, M.: Multi-view action recognition using local similarity random forests and sensor fusion. Pattern Recogn. Lett. 24, 20–24 (2012)

28. Parrigan, K., Souvenir, R.: Aggregating low-level features for human action recognition. In: Bebis, G., Boyle, R., Parvin, B., Koracin, D., Chung, R., Hammoud, R., Hussain, M., Kar-Han, T., Crawfis, R., Thalmann, D., Kao, D., Avila, L. (eds.) ISVC 2010, Part I. LNCS, vol. 6453, pp. 143–152. Springer, Heidelberg (2010)

29. Holte, M.B., Chakraborty, B., Gonzalez, J., Moeslund, T.B.: A local 3-d motion descriptor for multi-view human action recognition from 4-d spatio-temporal inter-est points. IEEE J. Sel. Top. Sig. Process. 6, 553–565 (2012)

30. Weinland, D., Boyer, E., Ronfard, R.: Action recognition from arbitrary views using 3d exemplars. In: Proceedings of the International Conference on Computer Vision, pp. 1–7 (2007)

31. Savarese, S., Fei-Fei, L.: 3d generic object categorization, localization and pose estimation. In: Proceedings of the International Conference on Computer Vision, pp. 1–8 (2007)

Graph Transduction Learning of Object Proposals for Video Object Segmentation

Tinghuai Wang$^{(\boxtimes)}$ and Huiling Wang

Nokia Technologies, Tampere, Finland
tinghuai.wang@nokia.com

Abstract. We propose an unsupervised video object segmentation algorithm that detects recurring objects and learns cohort object proposals over space-time. Our core contribution is a graph transduction process that learns object proposals densely over space-time, exploiting both appearance models learned from rudimentary detections of sparse object-like regions, and their intrinsic structures. Our approach exploits the fact that rudimentary detections of recurring objects in video, despite appearance variation and sporadity of detection, collectively describe the primary object. By learning a holistic model given a small set of object-like regions, we propagate this prior knowledge of the recurring primary object to the rest of the video to generate a diverse set of object proposals in all frames, incorporating both spatial and temporal cues. This set of rich descriptions underpins a robust object segmentation method against the changes in appearance, shape and occlusion in natural videos.

1 Introduction

Video segmentation remains an open challenge for Computer Vision, with recent advances relying upon prior knowledge supplied via interactive initialization or correction [1–6]. Yet fully unsupervised video segmentation [7–11] remains useful in Big Data scenarios such as video summarization or ingest pre-processing for video indexing or recognition, where the human in the loop is impractical. This is a very challenging task due to the lack of prior knowledge about object appearance, shape or position. Furthermore, variance in illumination and occlusion relationships introduce ambiguities that in turn induce instability in boundaries and the potential for localized under- or over-segmentation (Fig. 1).

This paper proposes a novel automatic video object segmentation algorithm in which the segmentation of each frame is driven by set of rich object models learned from *spatio-temporally dense and coherent object proposals*. The core novel contribution is our *graph transduction* approach to the efficient learning of the dense video object proposals which enables the detection and segmentation of objects in complex dynamic scenes without suffering from appearance variation or object occlusion over time. In contrast to previous techniques, our algorithm learns and extracts object proposals from scratch to account for the evolution of

---

T. Wang and H. Wang—Indicates equal contribution.

© Springer International Publishing Switzerland 2015
D. Cremers et al. (Eds.): ACCV 2014, Part IV, LNCS 9006, pp. 553–568, 2015.
DOI: 10.1007/978-3-319-16817-3_36

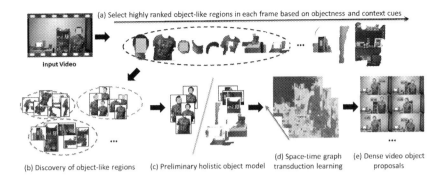

Fig. 1. Generation of dense video object proposals.

object's appearance, shape and location with time, as opposed to selecting from existing per-frame detections of object-like regions [9–12].

The key idea is to create feature-based rudimentary detections of regions for the primary object by discriminative learning from labelled examples of sparse object-like regions. These detections serve as informative indicators of the appearance and location of the object. We propagate this labeled data on an undirected space-time graph consisting of regions, solving the graph transduction learning efficiently with a fast convergence technique [13]. Inference at the region level further makes our dense video object proposal extraction approach a practical solution for unsupervised object segmentation on natural video sequences (Fig. 1).

2   Related Work

Video object segmentation methods requiring user to provide an initial annotation of the first frame have been proposed, which either propagate the annotation to drive the segmentation in successive frames [1–6] or perform spatio-temporal grouping [14,15]. The former group of methods heavily rely on motion estimates and may fail in segmenting videos with complex motions or varying object appearance. Although stability is achieved in the latter methods, they usually become computationally infeasible for pixel counts in even moderate size videos, and often fail in dealing with fast moving objects.

Automatic or unsupervised methods have also been proposed as a consequence of the prohibitive cost of user intervention in processing large amounts of video data in most computer vision applications. Methods like [16–21] achieve segmentation in a bottom-up approach based on spatio-temporal appearance and motion constraints. Motion segmentation methods cluster pixels or superpixels in video employing long-term motion trajectories analysis, which require the motion of the primary object to be neither too similar with the background nor too fast. Methods which generate over-segmentations for later processing analog to still-image superpixels [22] have also been proposed [23,24], by applying spatio-temporal clustering based on low level features. However, without any top-down explicit notion of object, all of these automatic methods produce segmentations without corresponding to any particular object with semantic meaning.

Several recent methods [9–12] are proposed based on exploring recurring object-like regions from still images by measuring generic object appearance [25]. Lee *et al.* [9] proposed to extract 'key-segments' of the primary object by performing clustering in a pool of object proposals from each frame of the video. The weakness of this approach is that the object proposal pool combines regions across all frames and discards the spatial and temporal information of each region. Ma and Latecki [10] proposed to leverage the temporal information by utilizing binary appearance relation between regions in different frames and model the object region selection as a constrained Maximum Weight Cliques problem. Zhang *et al.* [11] improved this approach by introducing optical flow to track the evolution of object shape and appearance and solving the primary object proposal selection problem as the longest path problem for Directed Acyclic Graph (DAG). There are mainly two limitations with these later two approaches [10,11]. First, both approaches propose to select or merge per-frame extracted object-like regions based on the objectness score which is computed locally in each frame, regardless of the prior knowledge of the corresponding object learned from other frames; their performance heavily relies on the quality of the initial rudimentary detection of object-like regions which is highly unreliable in practice. The initial object proposals generated using [25] normally contain a large amount of erroneous regions. Second, both approaches assume all object-like regions within each frame are independent and do not explicitly consider spatial affinity. This substantially limits the size of the object proposal especially when the primary object is comprised of multiple regions with distinct appearances. An additional limitation of [11] is that it employs optical flow warped region overlap to merge object-like regions into a new region which may introduce further spurious proposals due to inherent motion estimate error. Li *et al.* [12] proposed to track a pool of figure-ground segments in each frame and incrementally to learn a long-term object appearance model. However the incrementally built appearance model heavily relies on greedy matching and also suffers from the cumulative motion estimation error. All the above methods do not build an explicit holistic appearance model but relies on local heuristics and motion for selecting the object proposals.

To address the limitations of the above approaches [9–12], we propose to learn a holistic appearance model from the rudimentary detection of object-like regions across the whole video to drive the generation of dense object proposals. We propagate the prior knowledge from rudimentary detections on an undirected space-time graph consisting of regions by performing transduction learning, with respect to both low level cues collectively revealed by the appearance model and the intrinsic structure within video data. The transduction learning is guided by the initially detected evidence by collectively learning the initial sparse object-like regions, rather than directly using the local static 'objectness' score. Spatio-temporally coherent and dense object proposals are generated to facilitate robust object segmentation in challenging natural videos.

Our approach advances the state-of-the-art mainly in three aspects: (1) it explores the holistic patterns of primary object which are collectively revealed by a small set of object-like regions, and thus it prunes the spurious regions due to the independent rudimentary detection from a particular frame without considering the object-like regions generated in adjacent frames (2) it employs an efficient graph transduction learning approach to generating object proposals evenly and consistently distributed spanning the whole video, by exploiting both the local evidence and the intrinsic structure within video data (3) this set of object proposals provides sufficient and diverse appearance, shape, and location prior information to drive object segmentation while preserving spatio-temporal coherence.

3   Video Object Proposals

Our approach to generating video object proposals is comprised of three main steps: (1) object-like regions are extracted from each frame and a small set of the most likely object regions associated with the primary object in the video are identified (2) a holistic appearance model is learned from the object-like regions to describe the primary object spanning the whole video (3) in a top-down approach, transduction learning is performed on a space-time graph of regions to efficiently *generate* object proposals in each frame integrating the shared object models, temporal correlation and intrinsic structure within video data.

3.1   Initial Detection of Object-Like Regions

Since we assume no prior knowledge on the size, shape, appearance or location of the primary object, our algorithm operates by producing a diverse set of object proposals in each frames using [25] which is a category independent method to identify object-like regions in still image. To find the object-like regions among the proposals, we compute the 'objectness' of each region r as

$$S(r) = A(r) + M(r)$$

where $A(r)$ is the appearance score and $M(r)$ is the motion score. The static intra-frame appearance score $A(r)$ is computed using [25]. Motion score $M(r)$ reflects the disparity of motions between primary object and background. We compute optical flow [26] histograms for region r and $\bar{r}$ which is formed by merging all the closest surrounding regions of r. Using surrounding regions is more informative than using pixels in a loosely fit bounding box around r in [9]. We compute $M(r)$ as $M(r) = 1 - \exp(-\chi^2_{flow}(r, \bar{r}))$, where $\chi^2_{flow}(r, \bar{r})$ is the χ^2 distance between L_1-normalized optical flow histograms for regions r and $\bar{r}$.

Following [9], we firstly form a candidate pool $\mathcal{C}$ by taking the top N ($N = 10$) highest-scoring regions from each frame, and then identify groups of object-like regions that may represent a foreground object by performing spectral clustering in $\mathcal{C}$. All clusters are ranked based on the average score $S(r)$ of its comprising regions. The clusters among the highest ranks correspond to the most object-like regions but there may also be noisy regions, which is denoted as $\mathcal{H}$.

3.2   Holistic Appearance Model

Each object-like region from the rudimentary detection may correspond to different part of the primary object from particular frames, whereas they collectively describe the primary object. We could devise a discriminative model to learn the appearance of those most likely object regions. The initial set of object-like regions $\mathcal{H}$ form the set of all instances with a positive label (denoted as $\mathcal{P}$), while negative regions ($\mathcal{N}$) are randomly sampled outside the bounding box of the positive example. We use this labeled training set to learn linear SVM classifier for two categories. The classifier provides a confidence of class membership taking the features of a region which combines texture and color features, as input. This classifier is then applied to all the unlabeled regions across the whole video. After this classification process, each unlabelled region i is assigned with a weight Y_i from SVM, i.e. the signed distance to the decision boundary. All weights are normalized between -1 and 1, by the sum of unsigned distances to the decision boundary.

3.3   Graph Transduction Learning of Object Proposals

The holistic appearance model provides an informative yet independent and incoherent prediction on each of the unlabelled regions regardless the inherent structure revealed by both labeled and unlabeled regions. To generate robust dense video object proposals, we adopt a graph transduction learning approach, exploiting both the *intrinsic structure* within data and the *initial local evidence* from the holistic appearance model.

Space-Time Graph of Regions. To perform transduction learning, we define a weighted space-time graph $\mathcal{G}_s = (\mathcal{V}, \mathcal{E})$ spanning the whole video with each node corresponding to a region, and each edge connecting two regions based on spatial and temporal adjacencies. Temporal adjacency is coarsely determined based on motion estimates. Each region r_i^k in frame i is warped by the forward optical flow to frame $i + 1$ and the overlap ratio between the warped region r_i^k and the overlapped regions r_{i+1}^j in frame $i + 1$ are computed as $S_{\text{overlap}}(k, j) = \frac{|\tilde{r}_i^k \cap r_{i+1}^j|}{|\tilde{r}_i^k|}$, where $\tilde{r}_i^k$ is the warped region of r_i^k by optical flow to frame $i + 1$, and $|r|$ is the cardinality of region r. If $S_{\text{overlap}}(k, j)$ is greater than 0.5 for a pair of regions, i.e. r_i^k and r_{i+1}^j, in two successive frames, they are deemed temporally adjacent. Note that accurate motion estimation is neither assumed nor required to construct this graph.

We compute the affinity matrix W of the graph using the feature histogram representation h_{r_i} of each region r_i as $W_{ij} = \exp(-\frac{\chi^2(h_{r_i}, h_{r_j})}{2\beta})$, where β is the average χ^2 distance between all adjacent regions. Since sparsity is important to remove label noise and semi-supervised learning algorithms are more robust on sparse graphs [27], we set all W_{ij} are set to zero if r_i and r_j are not adjacent.

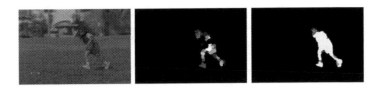

Fig. 2. Positive predictions of each region and the brightness indicates probability of being an object: (a) source image (b) independent SVM predictions (c) predictions from graph transduction capturing the coherent intrinsic structure within visual data, using SVM predictions as input.

Graph Transduction Learning. Graph transduction learning propagates label information from labeled nodes to unlabeled nodes. Let the node degree matrix $D = \text{diag}[d_1, \ldots, d_N]$ be defined as $D_i = \sum_{j=1}^{N} W_{ij}$, where $N = |\mathcal{V}|$. We follow a similar formulation with [13] to minimize an energy function $E(F)$ with respect to all region labels F ($F \in [-1, 1]$):

$$E(F) = \sum_{i,j=1}^{N} W_{ij} |\frac{F_i}{\sqrt{D_i}} - \frac{F_j}{\sqrt{D_j}}|^2 + \mu \sum_{i=1}^{N} |F_i - Y_i|^2, \qquad (1)$$

where $\mu > 0$ is the regularization parameter, and Y are the desirable labels of nodes which are normally imposed by prior knowledge. The first term in (1) is the *smoothness constraint*, which encourages the coherence of labelling among adjacent nodes, whilst the second term is the *fitting constraint* which enforces the labelling to be similar with the initial label assignment.

The optimization problem in (1) is solved by an iteration algorithm in [13]. Alternatively we solve it as a linear system of equations. Differentiating $E(F)$ with respect to F we have

$$\nabla E(F)|_{F=F^*} = F^* - SF^* + \mu(F^* - Y) = 0 \qquad (2)$$

where $S = D^{-1/2} W D^{-1/2}$. It can be transformed as

$$F^* - \frac{1}{1+\mu} SF^* - \frac{\mu}{1+\mu} Y = 0 \qquad (3)$$

Denoting $\gamma = \frac{\mu}{1+\mu}$, we have $(I - (1 - \gamma)S)F^* = \gamma Y$. An optimal solution for F can be solved using the Conjugate Gradient method with very fast convergence.

We use the predictions from SVM classifier to assign the values of Y. The diffusion process can be performed for positive and negative labels separately, with initial labels Y in (1) substituted as Y_+ and Y_- respectively:

$$Y_+ = \begin{cases} Y & \text{if } Y > 0 \\ 0 & \text{otherwise} \end{cases} \qquad (4)$$

and

$$Y_- = \begin{cases} -Y & \text{if } Y < 0 \\ 0 & \text{otherwise.} \end{cases} \qquad (5)$$

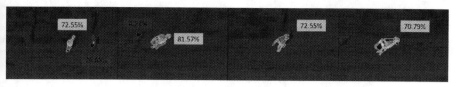

Fig. 3. Exemplar video object proposals from CHEETAH sequence. Colors of contour indicate different proposals. The transparency of each region indicates the objectness (F) from graph transduction learning. The objectness of each final object proposal is computed by averaging the constituent region-wise objectness F weighted by area (color figure online).

Combining the diffusion processes of both the object-like regions and background can produce more efficient and coherent labelling, taking advantage of their complementary properties. We perform the optimization for two diffusion processes simultaneously as follows:

$$F^* = \gamma(I - (1 - \gamma)S)^{-1}(Y_+ - Y_-). \tag{6}$$

This enables a faster and stable optimization avoiding separate optimizations while giving equivalent results to the individual positive and negative label diffusion. Figure 2 shows the positive predictions of each region, from SVM predictions and graph transduction learning respectively. The prediction from SVM exhibits unappealing incoherence, nonetheless, using it as initial input, graph transduction gives smooth predictions exploiting the inherent structure of data.

Finally, the regions which are assigned with label $F > 0$ from each frame are grouped. Specifically, we use the final label F to indicate the level of objectness of each region. The final proposals are generated by grouping the spatially adjacent regions ($F > 0$), and assigned by an objectness value by averaging the constituent region-wise objectness F weighted by area. The grouped regions with the highest objectness per frame are added to the set of object proposals $\mathcal{P}$. Exemplar video object proposals are shown in Fig. 3.

4   Video Object Segmentation

We formulate video object segmentation as a pixel-labelling problem of assigning each pixel with a binary value which represents background or foreground (object) respectively. We define a space-time graph by connecting frames temporally with optical flow displacement. In contrast to the previous space-time graph during transduction learning, each of the nodes in this graph is a pixel as opposed to a region, and edges are set to be the 4 spatial neighbors within the same frame and the 2 temporal neighbors in adjacent frames. We define the energy function that minimizes to achieve the optimal labeling:

$$E(x) = \sum_{i \in \mathcal{V}} \psi_i(x_i) + \lambda \sum_{i \in \mathcal{V}, j \in N_i} \psi_{i,j}(x_i, x_j)$$

where N_i is the set of pixels adjacent to pixel i in the graph and λ is a parameter. The pairwise term $\psi_{i,j}(x_i, x_j)$ penalizes different labels assigned to adjacent pixels:

$$\psi_{i,j}(x_i, x_j) = [x_i \neq x_j]\exp(-d(x_i, x_j))$$

where $[\cdot]$ denotes the indicator function. The function $d(x_i, x_j)$ computes the color and edge distance between neighboring pixels:

$$d(x_i, x_j) = \beta(1 + |SE(x_i) - SE(x_j)|) \cdot ||c_i - c_j||^2$$

where $SE(x_i)$ ($SE(x_i) \in [0, 1]$) returns the edge probability provided by the Structured Edge (SE) detector [28], $||c_i - c_j||^2$ is the squared Euclidean distance between two adjacent pixels in CIE Lab colorspace, and $\beta = (2 < ||c_i - c_j||^2 >)^{-1}$ with $< \cdot >$ denoting the expectation.

The unary term $\psi_i(x_i)$ defines the cost of assigning label $x_i \in \{0, 1\}$ to pixel i, which is defined based on the per-pixel probability map by combining color distribution and region objectness:

$$\psi_i(x_i) = \begin{cases} -\log(w \cdot U_i^c(x_i) + (1 - w) \cdot U_i^o(x_i)) & \text{if } x_i \in \mathcal{P} \\ -\log U_i^c(x_i) & \text{otherwise} \end{cases} \tag{7}$$

where $U_i^c(\cdot)$ is the color likelihood and $U_i^o(\cdot)$ is the objectness cue. The definitions of these two terms are explained in detail next.

4.1 Color Likelihood

To model the appearance of the object and background, we estimate two Gaussian Mixture Models (GMM) in CIE Lab colorspace. Pixels belonging to the set of object proposals are used to train the GMM representing the primary object, whilst randomly sampled pixels in the complement of object proposals are adopted to train the GMM for the background. Given these GMM color models, per-pixel probability $U_i^c(\cdot)$ is defined as the likelihood observing each pixel as object or background respectively can be computed.

4.2 Objectness Cue

Extracted object proposals provide explicit information of how likely a region belongs to the primary object (objectness) which can be directly used to drive the final segmentation. Per-pixel likelihood $U_i^o(\cdot)$ is set to be the objectness value (F in (6)) of the region it belongs to.

4.3 Optimization

We adopt the binary graph cut [29] to minimize (7) and the resulting label assignment gives the foreground object segmentation of the video.

5   Implementation Details

We start by computing feature descriptors for all the regions in video. Two types of bag-of-features histograms are used: Texton Histograms (TH) and Color Histograms (CH). For TH, a filter bank with 18 bar and edge filters (6 orientations and 3 scales for each), 1 Gaussian and 1 Laplacian-of-Gaussian filters, is used. 400 textons are quantized via k-means. For CH, we use CIE Lab color space with 20 bins per channel (60 bins in total). All histograms are concatenated to form a single feature vector for each region. We learn 5 components per GMM to model the color distribution.

We empirically set $\mu = 3.0$ to balance the impact of the prior labelling and the local labelling smoothness. For graph cut optimization, we set $\lambda = 5$ and $w = 0.35$ by optimizing segmentation against ground truth over a training set of 5 videos which proved to be a versatile setting for a wide variety of videos. These parameters are fixed for the evaluation.

For efficiency and scalability, our region graph transduction learning is sequentially performed on clips of 20 frames by dividing the source video. The efficient transduction learning normally takes ~ 18 s on a clip of 20 frames with an unoptimized MATLAB implementation. The final graph cut based pixel labelling is sequentially performed in each frame in turn, using a space-time graph of three consecutive frames.

6   Experimental Results

We evaluate our method on two datasets: SegTrack [4] and a new dataset consisting of five videos. Two videos (*waterski, yunakim*) of this new dataset are from GaTech video segmentation dataset [19], two (*jump, gymnastic*) from the challenging VOT2013 [30] dataset, and one (*monkeybar*) from video tooning [14]. The SegTrack dataset comes with pixel-level ground truth for the task of video object segmentation. We manually labelled the ground-truth segmentation of all the frames in the new dataset for evaluation. We measure the segmentation performance as the average number of per-frame pixel error compared to the ground-truth, which is defined as [4] error $= \frac{XOR(S,GT)}{NF}$, where S denotes the label for every pixel in the video, GT is the ground-truth, and NF is the total number of frames in the video.

6.1   SegTrack Dataset

There are totally six videos (*birdfall, cheetah, girl, monekeydog, parachute, penguin*) in SegTrack dataset. We follow the setup in previous works [9–12,21] and discard the *penguin* video, since only a single penguin is labelled in the ground-truth amidst a group of penguins. Those videos exhibit a variety of challenges, including objects of similar color to the background, fast motion, non-rigid deformations, and fast camera motion.

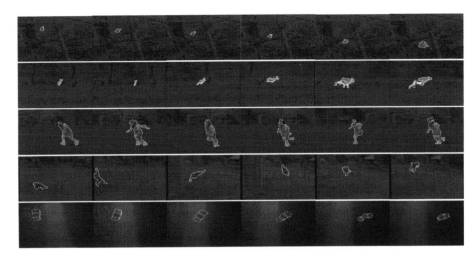

Fig. 4. Primary object proposals generated by the proposed graph transduction learning method.

Table 1. Quantitative results on SegTrack. The proposed video object proposals are compared with the per-frame top-scoring object proposal from [25], and also the lowest/highest error rates of all existing video object segmentation methods.

Video (No. frames)	Our proposal	[25]	Lowest error	Highest error
Birdfall (30)	264	22167	151	454
Cheetah (29)	869	20649	633	1217
Girl (21)	1683	8176	1121	1785
Monkeydog (71)	839	29058	284	3859
Parachute (51)	450	82934	201	855

Evaluation of Video Object Proposals. To evaluate our method's capability to detect and generate spatio-temporal coherent and dense video object proposals, we firstly compare with [25], one of the state-of-the-art segment based object proposal methods on still images, as the baseline. Table 1 compares the per-pixel error rate of our object proposals, per-frame best scoring object proposal generated from [25], and also the lowest/highest error rates of all existing methods on SegTrack dataset. We observe that [25] returns inconsistent and sporadic object proposals independently in each frame, whilst our object proposal captures the coherent essence of primary object, despite appearance variation and sporadity of detection. The comparison against the existing lowest/highest error rates of video object segmentation methods shows that the object regions generated by efficient graph transduction learning alone can be regarded as coarse segmentation, even without the pixel-based object segmentation described in Sect. 4. The

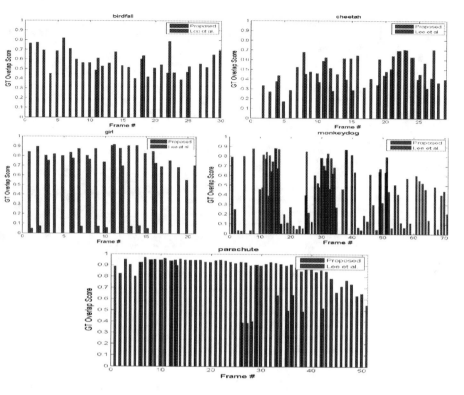

Fig. 5. Ground-truth overlap score of our object proposals and the 'key-segments' from Lee et al. [9].

qualitative evaluation of primary object proposals in Fig. 4 further confirms the advantages of the proposed method in SegTrack dataset.

We also compare the object proposals generated from our graph transduction learning with the 'key-segments' generated by Lee et al. [9]. Figure 5 shows the per-frame ground-truth overlap score of those generated object proposals from both methods on SegTrack dataset. The results clearly demonstrate that our method can generate object proposals which are not only temporally dense in each frame, but also break the lower-bound posed by the accuracy of the region candidates produced by [25] by learning a holistic appearance model (note that most of the blue bars are taller than the corresponding red bars in Fig. 5).

Evaluation of Video Object Segmentation. We compare our video object segmentation method with five state-of-the-art unsupervised methods [9–12,21] and two supervised methods [1,4]. Following [10,11], we also compute the average number of incorrect pixels over all frames in the five videos as they are roughly of the same frame size. Our method achieves the lowest average number of per-frame pixel error along with superior performance on two out of five videos compared with all 7 state-of-the-art methods with or without supervision

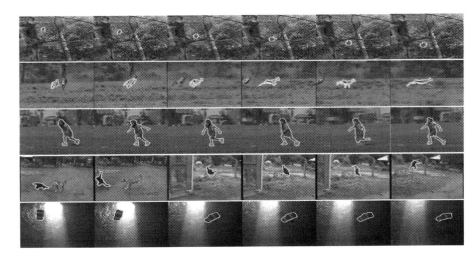

Fig. 6. Segmentation results on SegTrack dataset. The contour of segmented primary object is shown in green (color figure online).

(Table 2). It produces second best results on the rest three videos. Note that our method consistently segments all the videos with low error rate which reflects its robustness on various challenging situations (Fig. 6). As a contrast, previous 'object proposal' based methods are limited to the existing region candidates which contain a large amount of label noise (Fig. 6).

Table 2. Quantitative segmentation results on SegTrack. Segmentation error as measured by the average number of incorrect pixels per frame. Lower values are better. The best result is shown in red and second best in blue

Video (No. frames)	Ours	[12]	[21]	[11]	[10]	[9]	[4]	[1]
birdfall (30)	151	188	217	155	189	288	252	454
cheetah (29)	672	983	890	633	806	905	1142	1217
girl (21)	1121	1573	3859	1488	1698	1785	1304	1755
monkeydog (71)	359	558	284	365	472	521	563	683
parachute (51)	204	339	855	220	221	201	235	502
Average	413	614	876	452	542	592	594	791
Supervision	N	N	N	N	N	N	Y	Y

Table 3. Quantitative segmentation results on Sports dataset

Video (No. frames)	Ours	Lee *et al.* [9]	Zhang *et al.* [11]
gymnastic (100)	523	1595	1951
jump (105)	364	1261	3456
monkeybar (200)	833	1496	2108
waterski (48)	1582	2107	3084
yunakim (200)	319	907	4038

6.2   Sports Dataset

We have manually generated ground-truth for a new dataset collecting videos from other datasets for video object segmentation. The dataset is challenging: those videos are generally longer than SegTrack dataset; person's varying poses cause frequent self-occlusions and consequently appearance variations; some persons move fast so causing blur whilst some are slow which is very hard to perform motion segmentation. We find that the results on longer and complex videos can better demonstrate the strength of our approach, especially in dealing with fast appearance variation, cluttered scene and complex motions (Table 2).

We firstly compare the proposed approach with Lee et al. [9] which is one of the state-of-the-art 'object proposal' approach, both quantitatively and qualitatively[1]. Table 3 shows the segmentation error on five videos of Sports dataset, comparing our method with [9]. Our method substantially outperforms [9] with low segmentation error across all videos. The qualitative comparison in Fig. 7 further confirms the advantages of the proposed method over [9]. In *gymnastic* (first video), the appearance of the athlete varies quickly due to the fast motion and pose variation. The sparse and noisy 'key-segments' generated by [9] can no longer deal with this complex situation. As a contrast, our approach robustly segments the athlete based on rich descriptions of the primary object regardless of the video length and appearance variation. Similar situations are also present in *monkeybar* (third video), *waterski* (fourth video) and *yunakim* (fifth video) where, in meanwhile, self-occlusion aggravates the failure of [9], due to the lack of prior knowledge in the corresponding frames. The result on *jump* (second video) demonstrates that our method can stably segment small object while preserving temporal coherence (see the missegmentations in the background from [9]).

We also quantitatively and qualitatively compare with Zhang et al. [11] on Sports dataset[2]. The quantitative and qualitative comparisons are shown in Table 3 and Fig. 7 respectively. Using local motion-warped overlapping to form new object regions from the region candidates produced by [25], [11] tends to produce either under- or over-segmentations (e.g. the *gymnastic, jump* and *yunakim* sequences) due to the spurious object regions and heavy reliance on accurate motion estimation. Zhang et al. [11] further assume all object-like regions within each frame are independent and do not explicitly consider spatial affinity, which substantially limits the size of the object region especially when the primary object is comprised of multiple regions with distinct appearances (e.g. the *monkeybar* sequence). Distinctively, our method learns a holistic appearance model to diffuse the prior knowledge from the initial region candidates using graph transduction learning and thus can cope with more complex scenes in natural videos.

---

[1] We used the publicly available source code from: http://vision.cs.utexas.edu/projects/keysegments/code/.

[2] We used the publicly available source code from: http://dromston.com/projects/video_object_segmentation.php.

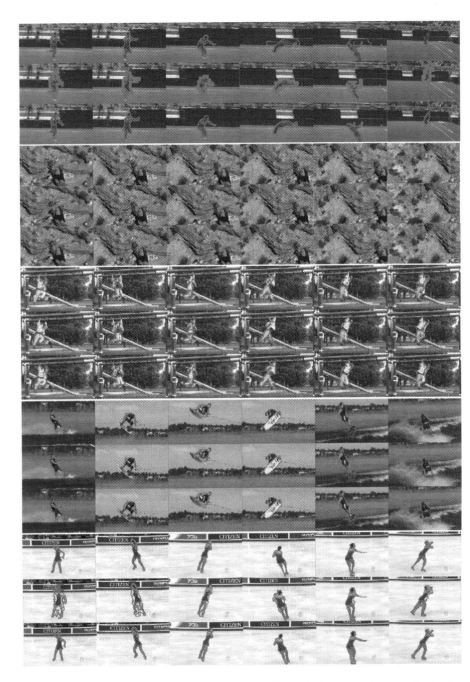

Fig. 7. Segmentation results on Sports dataset. Row 1: Segmentation results by Lee *et al.* [9]. Row 2: Segmentation results by Zhang *et al.* [11]. Row 3: Segmentation by the proposed method.

7 Conclusion

We have proposed a novel unsupervised video object segmentation method by generating a diverse set of video object proposals in a bottom-up approach. This set of rich descriptions underpin robust segmentations against the large variations of appearance, shape and occlusion in natural videos. The generation of dense video object proposals is cast as performing efficient graph transduction learning based on a holistic appearance model to describe the object-like regions, incorporating both spatial and temporal cues. The proposed approach exhibits superior performance in comparison with the state of the art on the SegTrack dataset and additional challenging data sets posing different challenges.

References

1. Chockalingam, P., Pradeep, S.N., Birchfield, S.: Adaptive fragments-based tracking of non-rigid objects using level sets. In: ICCV, pp. 1530–1537 (2009)
2. Bai, X., Wang, J., Simons, D., Sapiro, G.: Video snapcut: robust video object cutout using localized classifiers. ACM Trans. Graph. **28**, 70:1–70:11 (2009)
3. Price, B.L., Morse, B.S., Cohen, S.: Livecut: Learning-based interactive video segmentation by evaluation of multiple propagated cues. In: ICCV, pp. 779–786 (2009)
4. Tsai, D., Flagg, M., Nakazawa, A., Rehg, J.M.: Motion coherent tracking using multi-label mrf optimization. Int. J. Comput. Vision **100**, 190–202 (2012)
5. Wang, T., Collomosse, J.P.: Probabilistic motion diffusion of labeling priors for coherent video segmentation. IEEE Trans. Multimedia **14**, 389–400 (2012)
6. Wang, T., Han, B., Collomosse, J.P.: Touchcut: Fast image and video segmentation using single-touch interaction. Comput. Vis. Image Underst. **120**, 14–30 (2014)
7. Sheikh, Y., Javed, O., Kanade, T.: Background subtraction for freely moving cameras. In: ICCV, pp. 1219–1225 (2009)
8. Brox, T., Malik, J.: Object segmentation by long term analysis of point trajectories. In: Daniilidis, K., Maragos, P., Paragios, N. (eds.) ECCV 2010, Part V. LNCS, vol. 6315, pp. 282–295. Springer, Heidelberg (2010)
9. Lee, Y.J., Kim, J., Grauman, K.: Key-segments for video object segmentation. In: ICCV, pp. 1995–2002 (2011)
10. Ma, T., Latecki, L.J.: Maximum weight cliques with mutex constraints for video object segmentation. In: CVPR, pp. 670–677 (2012)
11. Zhang, D., Javed, O., Shah, M.: Video object segmentation through spatially accurate and temporally dense extraction of primary object regions. In: CVPR, pp. 628–635 (2013)
12. Li, F., Kim, T., Humayun, A., Tsai, D., Rehg, J.M.: Video segmentation by tracking many figure-ground segments. In: ICCV (2013)
13. Zhou, D., Bousquet, O., Lal, T.N., Weston, J., Sch, B.: Learning with local and global consistency. In: NIPS, vol. 1 (2004)
14. Wang, J., Xu, Y., Shum, H.Y., Cohen, M.F.: Video tooning. ACM Trans. Graph. **23**, 574–583 (2004)
15. Collomosse, J.P., Rowntree, D., Hall, P.M.: Stroke surfaces: Temporally coherent artistic animations from video. IEEE Trans. Vis. Comput. Graph. **11**, 540–549 (2005)
16. Brendel, W., Todorovic, S.: Video object segmentation by tracking regions. In: ICCV, pp. 833–840 (2009)

17. Huang, Y., Liu, Q., Metaxas, D.N.: Video object segmentation by hypergraph cut. In: CVPR, pp. 1738–1745 (2009)
18. Vazquez-Reina, A., Avidan, S., Pfister, H., Miller, E.: Multiple hypothesis video segmentation from superpixel flows. In: Daniilidis, K., Maragos, P., Paragios, N. (eds.) ECCV 2010, Part V. LNCS, vol. 6315, pp. 268–281. Springer, Heidelberg (2010)
19. Grundmann, M., Kwatra, V., Han, M., Essa, I.A.: Efficient hierarchical graph-based video segmentation. In: CVPR, pp. 2141–2148 (2010)
20. Xu, C., Xiong, C., Corso, J.J.: Streaming hierarchical video segmentation. In: Fitzgibbon, A., Lazebnik, S., Perona, P., Sato, Y., Schmid, C. (eds.) ECCV 2012, Part VI. LNCS, vol. 7577, pp. 626–639. Springer, Heidelberg (2012)
21. Papazoglou, A., Ferrari, V.: Fast object segmentation in unconstrained video. In: ICCV (2013)
22. Achanta, R., Shaji, A., Smith, K., Lucchi, A., Fua, P., Süsstrunk, S.: Slic superpixels compared to state-of-the-art superpixel methods. IEEE Trans. Pattern Anal. Mach. Intell. 34, 2274–2282 (2012)
23. Greenspan, H., Goldberger, J., Mayer, A.: A probabilistic framework for spatio-temporal video representation & indexing. In: Heyden, A., Sparr, G., Nielsen, M., Johansen, P. (eds.) ECCV 2002, Part IV. LNCS, vol. 2353, pp. 461–475. Springer, Heidelberg (2002)
24. Wang, J., Thiesson, B., Xu, Y., Cohen, M.: Image and video segmentation by anisotropic kernel mean shift. In: Pajdla, T., Matas, J.G. (eds.) ECCV 2004. LNCS, vol. 3022, pp. 238–249. Springer, Heidelberg (2004)
25. Endres, I., Hoiem, D.: Category independent object proposals. In: Daniilidis, K., Maragos, P., Paragios, N. (eds.) ECCV 2010, Part V. LNCS, vol. 6315, pp. 575–588. Springer, Heidelberg (2010)
26. Brox, T., Bruhn, A., Papenberg, N., Weickert, J.: High accuracy optical flow estimation based on a theory for warping. In: Pajdla, T., Matas, J.G. (eds.) ECCV 2004. LNCS, vol. 3024, pp. 25–36. Springer, Heidelberg (2004)
27. Jebara, T., Wang, J., Chang, S.F.: Graph construction and b-matching for semi-supervised learning. In: ICML, p. 56 (2009)
28. Dollar, P., Zitnick, C.L.: Structured forests for fast edge detection. In: ICCV (2013)
29. Boykov, Y., Veksler, O., Zabih, R.: Fast approximate energy minimization via graph cuts. IEEE Trans. Pattern Anal. Mach. Intell. 23, 1222–1239 (2001)
30. VOT2013: The vot2013 challenge dataset (2013). http://www.votchallenge.net

Forecasting Events Using an Augmented Hidden Conditional Random Field

Xinyu Wei[1,2]([✉]), Patrick Lucey[2], Stephen Vidas[1,3], Stuart Morgan[4], and Sridha Sridharan[1]

[1] Queensland University of Technology, Brisbane, Australia
s.sridharan@qut.edu.au
[2] Disney Research Pittsburgh, Pittsburgh, USA
{felix.wei,patrick.lucey}@disneyresearch.com
[3] Nanyang Technological University, Singapore, Singapore
svidas@ntu.edu.sg
[4] Australian Institute of Sport, Canberra, Australia
stuart.morgan@ausport.gov.au

Abstract. In highly dynamic and adversarial domains such as sports, short-term predictions are made by incorporating both local immediate as well global situational information. For forecasting complex events, higher-order models such as Hidden Conditional Random Field (HCRF) have been used to good effect as capture the long-term, high-level semantics of the signal. However, as the prediction is based solely on the hidden layer, fine-grained local information is not incorporated which reduces its predictive capability. In this paper, we propose an "augmented-Hidden Conditional Random Field" (a-HCRF) which incorporates the local observation within the HCRF which boosts it forecasting performance. Given an enormous amount of tracking data from vision-based systems, we show that our approach outperforms current state-of-the-art methods in forecasting short-term events in both soccer and tennis. Additionally, as the tracking data is long-term and continuous, we show our model can be adapted to recent data which improves performance.

1 Introduction

With the recent deployment of vision-based player and ball tracking systems in professional sports, researchers are looking at leveraging this data to forecast future events [1–3]. Application wise, this is useful as knowing the location of a future event would allow a camera to be intelligently positioned for automatic broadcasting [4]. An additional by-product is that higher-level analysis such as tactics and strategy can be gleaned from such systems which can aid in decision-making and story-telling aspects for coaches, broadcasters and viewers alike [5,6]. Beyond sport, intelligent systems that can predict situations that can cause disruptions before they occur could be useful for logistics and surveillance and security domains.

© Springer International Publishing Switzerland 2015
D. Cremers et al. (Eds.): ACCV 2014, Part IV, LNCS 9006, pp. 569–582, 2015.
DOI: 10.1007/978-3-319-16817-3_37

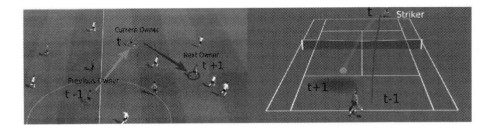

Fig. 1. In this paper, we use our a-HCRF method to: (left) predict the next pass in soccer, and (right) predict the location of the next shot in tennis.

An example of the problem we investigate in this paper is depicted in Fig. 1, where given observations from the past n seconds, we wish to forecast/predict a future event. The event can vary from predicting the next ball owner in soccer (a), or predicting the location of the next shot in tennis (b). Even though the variance in decisions that can be made is extremely high, the number of feasible decisions can be greatly truncated by using recent contextual cues. For example in tennis, when the opponent is out of position, we can predict with high confidence that a player will hit the ball to the open side of the court in order to win the point. Our goal of this paper is to incorporate these factors into a statistical model to accurately predict these events.

Popular methods such as hidden Markov models (HMMs), dynamic Bayesian networks (DBNs), linear-chain Conditional Random Field (LCRF) obey the Markov assumption where the future state depends only upon the present state. However for complex systems where more temporal information is required, higher order models such as the HCRF (Hidden Conditional Random Field) [7] have been used to good effect. These models are effective as they decompose the input signal into a series of semantically meaningful sub-states which are hidden. However, the issue with such approaches is that the final prediction is based solely on the hidden-layer, meaning that no features directly influence the prediction.

In this paper, we propose an augmentation to HCRF which we call an *augmented-Hidden Conditional Random Field* (a-HCRF). By making the final prediction contingent on directly the hidden-layer as well as the observation, we show that we can improve prediction performance. This modification allows our model to not only capture a coarse summarization of what has happen so far through the hidden layer but also include fine-grained information of the current situation via the features. The advantages of using this configuration rather than the original HCRF or other models (e.g., DBNs, LCRF) are demonstrated by the model learning and evaluation. Additionally, as sports are adversarial and long-term, we show that our model can be adapted to match the prediction outputs. Experimental results show that our approach outperforms current state-of-the-art method in forecasting events short-term events both in soccer and tennis.

1.1 Related Work

In the computer vision literature, there has been recent work focussing both on early-event detection and event forecasting. Early event detection has the aim of detecting an event as soon as possible given that we know it has started (i.e., after it starts but before it ends) [8,9]. Event forecasting is more complicated, as the goal is to predict what and when the event/action occurred and for how long. In terms of early-event detection, Hoai et al. [9] used a structured-output SVM to detect the length of emotions directly from faces. Ryoo [8], used a dynamic bag-of-words and maximum a posteriori (MAP) classifier to recognize human actions. In terms of event forecasting, Pellegrini et al. [10] and Mehran et al. [11] both modeled the social factors between pedestrians (i.e., avoid collisions) to improve their tracking performance. While Kitani et al., [12], utilized other factors such as nearby objects to improve the prediction of the most likely trajectory path using a partial observable Markov decision process (POMDP). In terms of predicting future crowd behavior, Zhou et al., [13] learned a mixture model of dynamic pedestrian-agents to estimate and simulate the flow of people at the Grand Central Station in New York.

In terms of adversarial behaviors, Kim et al. [1] used motion fields to predict where the play will evolve in soccer based on a region of convergence. In the subsequent work, they then used stochastic fields for predicting important future regions of interest as the scene evolves dynamically for a variety of team sports [14]. In [2,3], a Dynamic Bayesian Network (DBN) to predict the type and location of the future shot in tennis was used. To circumvent the issue of prediction, Carr et al. [4] used an alternative approach by using virtual camera on a one-second delay and an L_1 filter to predict future behaviors.

2   Augmented Hidden Conditional Random Field

Given a period of past observations of an event, the goal of this paper is to forecast or predict what is going to happen in the short-term future (i.e., in the next 1 to 10 s). We do not assume past states of an event are given and only observations are available. Before we describe the method, we will first compare and contrast various models to explain the motivation of our approach.

2.1   Modeling Approaches

Linear-Chain Models: A popular way to perform prediction is to employ a HMMs or DBNs. In these models, a label of the future is dependent on its previous state as well as its observation. However, two assumptions are made here. First, it assumes each state y_i is independent of all its ancestors $y_1, y_2, ..., y_{i-2}$ given its previous state y_{i-1} which is the Markov assumption. Secondly, to ensure the computational tractability, Bayesian models assumes features are independent. A linear conditional random field (LCRF) [15] relaxes this assumption by directly modeling the conditional distributions. However, for more complex tasks like predicting future behaviors in sport the Markovian assumption maybe limiting.

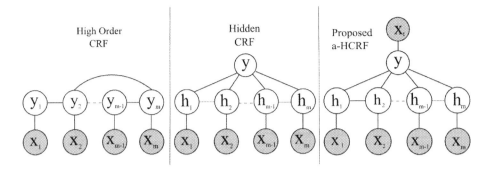

Fig. 2. (Left) Example of a higher order CRF. Output is a sequence. (Middle) Depiction of a hidden CRF (HCRF) where the sequence label y only depends on hidden states. (Right) Our proposed a-HCRF, where x_i is a past observation from $t_i - w$ to t_i, w is a feature window, h_i is a historical state at t_i, y is our prediction in the future. $\mathbf{x}$ is a global feature describes current game/player status. x_i is used for providing evidence for h_i. $\mathbf{x}$ is used for predicting the future event.

Higher-Order Models: Higher-order models, as the name suggest incorporates more than one previous state which means that the future label, y_i can depend on any number of its ancestors $y_1, y_2, ..., y_{i-1}$. A popular example of a higher-order model is a higher-order CRF. Such models predict a *sequence* of labels - instead of making a single prediction (e.g., Fig. 2 (Left)). A hidden Conditional Random Field (HCRF) can circumvent this problem by making past states hidden. It only optimizes one label and it is a high order CRF. The idea is that it summarizes a temporal signal into a sequence of hidden sub-states and use these sub-states to predict the sequence label. The drawback, however, is that the prediction of y is solely based on the hidden layer. No features can directly influence y (Fig. 2 (Middle)).

Augmented-Hidden Conditional Random Field (a-HCRF): We modified the original HCRF by directly connecting the observation to y (Fig. 2 (Right)). This way, our model can not only capture fine grained information of the current situation via the top feature layer $\mathbf{x}$, but also incorporate a coarse summarization of what has happen so far (the context of the game) through the hidden layer $\mathbf{h}$. This modification is important since present information could be a strong cue for a future event. Here x_i is a feature extracted from $t_i - w$ to t_i to provide evidence for past state h_i. w is the feature window. $\mathbf{x}$ are features for predicting y. For example, $\mathbf{x}$ can be features which indicate the current game phase, player positions, player fatigue factor or any features which are predictive of the future event.

2.2   Formulation

The formulation of our a-HCRF is similar to the HCRF [7] with the key difference being the potential function. Given a set of observations $\mathcal{X} = \{\mathbf{x}_0, \mathbf{x}_1, \ldots, \mathbf{x}_m\}$, we wish to learn a mapping to class labels $y \in \mathcal{Y}$. Each local observation $\mathbf{x}_j$ is represented by a feature vector $\phi(\mathbf{x}_j) \in \Re^d$. The posterior of a-HCRF is given by the following form,

$$P(y|\mathbf{x}, \theta) = \sum_{\mathbf{h}} P(y, \mathbf{h}|\mathbf{x}, \theta) = \frac{\sum_{\mathbf{h}} e^{\Psi(y, \mathbf{h}, \mathbf{x}; \theta)}}{\sum_{y' \in \mathcal{Y}, \mathbf{h} \in \mathcal{H}^m} e^{\Psi(y', \mathbf{h}, \mathbf{x}; \theta)}}. \tag{1}$$

Each y is a member of a set $\mathcal{Y}$ of possible labels. For prediction, y refers to the label of a future event. The layer $\mathbf{h} = \{h_1, h_2, ..., h_m\}$, where each $h_i \in \mathcal{H}$ is a historical state of an event at time t_i. The term, θ is a set of parameters describing the feature functions. If the historical states are observed, then $\mathbf{x}$ will not influence $\mathbf{h}$. Therefore, this model can be simplified to just the top layer.

The potential function, $\Psi(y, \mathbf{h}, \mathbf{x}; \theta)$ measures the compatibility between a label, a set of observations and a configuration of the historical states,

$$\begin{aligned}
\Psi(y, \mathbf{h}, \mathbf{x}; \theta) = &\sum_{j=1}^{n} \varphi(\mathbf{x}, j, \omega) \cdot \theta_h[h_j] + \sum_{j=1}^{n} \theta_y[y, h_j] \\
&+ \sum_{(j,k) \in \mathcal{E}} \theta_e[y, h_j, h_k] \\
&+ \frac{\varphi(\mathbf{x}, \omega) \cdot \theta_p[y]}{k},
\end{aligned} \tag{2}$$

where n is the total number of historical states in the model, $\varphi(\mathbf{x}, j, \omega)$ is a vector that can include any feature of the observation sequence for a specific time window ω, (i.e., each historical state can include features from $t - \omega$ to t).

The parameter vector, θ can be represented as $\theta = [\theta_{\mathbf{h}} \ \theta_y \ \theta_e \ \theta_p]$. In our work we use the same notation as [7] where $\theta_{\mathbf{h}}[h_j]$ is the parameters that correspond to state $h_j \in \mathcal{H}$. The function $\theta_y[y, h_j]$ indicates the parameters that correspond to class y and state h_j and $\theta_e[y, h_j, h_k]$ refers to parameters that between each edge h_j and h_i. Additionally, $\theta_p[y]$ defines the parameters for y given the features over the past.

The dot product $\varphi(\mathbf{x}, j, \omega) \cdot \theta_h[h_j]$ measures the compatibility between the observation and the state at time j, while the dot product between $\varphi(\mathbf{x}, \omega) \cdot \theta_p[y]$ measures the compatibility between the observation and the future event y. The total number of possible combinations of $\mathbf{h}$ is k and dividing by k avoids adding this term multiple times. This last term is added to capture the influence of features to a future event. Without it, a future event will only depend on past states.

2.3   Learning and Inference

Parameters can be learnt in many ways and use different objective functions. A common objective is to maximize the likelihood from labelled training data. Using the same definition in previous CRF work [16], the likelihood function is defined as follows

$$L(\theta) = \sum_{i=1}^{n} \log P(y_i|\mathbf{x_i}, \theta) - \frac{1}{2\sigma^2} ||\theta||^2, \tag{3}$$

where n is the total number of training examples. The first term is the log-likelihood and the second term refers to a Gaussian prior. Given a new input test sequence $\mathbf{x}$, and trained parameter θ^* we can obtain the estimated label y^* as

$$y^* = \arg\max_{y \in \mathcal{Y}} P(y|\mathbf{x}, \omega, \theta^*). \tag{4}$$

In some situations, optimizing the likelihood on the training set may not generalize well to the test set. Alternatively, one can utilize a max margin criterion [17] or diverse M-best solutions [18] to learn these parameters. Other objective functions may also be used depending on the specific application (e.g., minimizing the distance between predicted location and estimated location). We used the maximum likelihood as the objective function in both of our experiments in sports.

Since the edge E in our model is a chain, exact methods for inference and parameter estimation are available. Gradient Ascent is used for each step of the tempered maximum likelihood learning. For labeling in test sequences, Maximum a Posteriori (MAP) inference is carried out using Belief Propagation.

3 Predicting Future Ball Location in Soccer

Given player tracking data over the past n seconds, our goal is to predict the owner of the ball in the future. Having the ability to predict the future ball owner has many foreseeable benefits across automatic sports broadcasting as well as improving real time ball tracking performance. This is a relatively unexplored area due to the lack of available data. Most current works are still centered on ball tracking. Recently, Wang et al. [19] formulated the ball tracking task in terms of deciding which player, if any, owns the ball at any given time. Our work extends this work, where instead of finding the ball owner at the present time, we are interested in predicting where the ball will be based in the short-term future.

3.1 Data

Spatiotemporal data has been used extensively in the visualization and officiating of sports action [20–22], but considerably fewer works [23–25] have used these large datasets to perform predictive analysis. In this experiment, we utilized the (x, y) positions of both players and the ball across 9 complete matches (over 13 h) from a top-tier soccer league. Meta data such as the team label for each player, owner of the ball and event labels are also included. The granularity of the data is at the centimeter level, and was sampled at 10 fps. In each of these 9 matches, the team of interest was flipped to left in order to normalize team features.

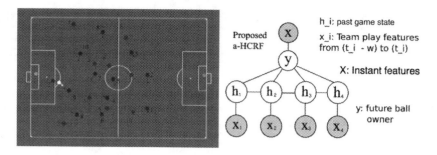

Fig. 3. (Left) In each frame, we extract speed, position and moving direction for each player. (Right) Model Representation for future ball owner prediction.

3.2   Model Representation

For this experiment, h_i is a past state of the game at t_i which is hidden, y is the owner in the future, x_i is the observation of h_i. In each frame, we compute speed, position and moving direction for each player. The top x include features of current game phase (i.e. defence, attack, counter attack, corners, free kick), number of opponents currently near each player and team formation. The pairwise potential between h_i and h_{i+1} measures the transition of the game states. The unary potential between h_i and x_i measures the compatibility between a particular player and a set of features. Both potentials are automatically learned from data. A future owner is influenced by game states over the past as well as features of the current situation. Features extracted from each frame are illustrated in Fig. 3 (Left).

3.3   Experimental Setup

Given 9 matches of soccer data, we first segment it into continuous plays and stoppages. In this research, we are only interested in predicting a future ball owner when the game is in the continuous state. For training, we have the event label which indicates the current state of the game. For testing, we employed a random forest to perform the segmentation. The idea is to break a continuous match into small chunks and assign labels to these chunks based on player features (i.e., player speed, location, etc.). This task can be achieved at an average rate of 92.25 % correct.

Once the segmentation is completed, the remaining frames are divided equally for training and testing. We extract data for the team of interest and its oppositions and train two models respectively. We use four nodes for the bottom chain structured CRF. Each node is 2 s later than the previous one. The historical state h_i can take one of 11 discrete values (i.e. 11 players of this team). The future state y can take one of 12 values (representing the 11 players of the team + one for a turn over event). We only make a prediction if the same team keeps the ball in the past 8 s. If there is a lot of turn over in the past 8 s, the prediction will be unreliable therefore it is not considered in this work. When testing, since

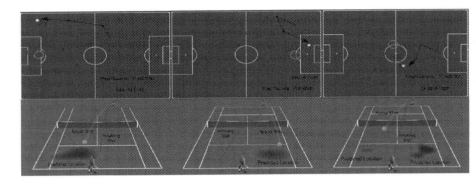

Fig. 4. Examples of our prediction results. Top: Examples of ball owner prediction in soccer. Black trajectories indicate the past passing patterns over the last four time steps, yellow circle shows the predicted ball owner while blue circle shows the ground truth. Bottom: Examples of shot prediction in tennis, yellow is the true shot trajectory while red area indicates the probability of the next shot location.

our data provides the team label for each player, we can easily find out which team has the ball over the past 8 s and therefore apply the correct model. If the team label is not given (raw videos), one can use color features of player's jersey or optical flow combined with the ball evidence to find out which team has the ball over the last 8 s (Fig. 4).

To the best of our knowledge, this is the first work on ball ownership prediction using spatiotemporal data. No existing work is available for comparison. In order to demonstrate the advantage of a-HCRF, we compare our result with other models, namely a Dynamic Bayesian Networks (DBNs), a linear chain CRF (CRF), and a Hidden CRF (HCRF). Each model has four past nodes and a future node. The last node (right most node) in DBNs or CRF is the future node and we only give past observations to that node. In HCRF, the sequence label is the future node while hidden nodes are past states. We also create two versions of our proposed model, a-HCRF-1 and a-HCRF-2. In a-HCRF-1, we set feature window ω as 1. That is, each past state can take features from the previous 2 s. In a-HCRF-2, feature window ω is set as 2. Thus, each state can take features from the last 4 s. We conduct experiments to answer three questions: (i) Which model is the best? (ii) How far in the future can we predict? (iii) How many past features do we need?

3.4   Experimental Result and Discussion

In order to answer the above questions, we plot the prediction rate against the number of seconds in the future ranging from 1 s to 10 s (at 10 fps) which is shown in Fig. 5. If we look in the immediate future (i.e., 1 s), the same player is more likely to have the ball which makes sense as the player needs time to control the ball and then execute their next decision. The black triangle curve at the bottom in Fig. 5 illustrates the result if we always assign the previous owner as

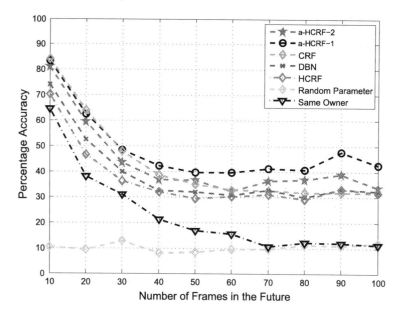

Fig. 5. Plot shows the ball owner prediction accuracy of different models at different time of the future. CRF and a-HCRF have similar performance within 2 s. After 2 s, proposed a-HCRF outperforms all other models. The black triangle curve at the bottom shows the result if we always assign the previous owner as the future owner.

the future owner. Since the output can take one of twelve values, the cyan curve at bottom indicates the result of random assignment which is approximately 9 %. When the future state is less than 2 s from the current time, the a-HCRF-1, a-HCRF-2 and CRF models have similar performance. However after 2 s, the a-HCRF-1 outperforms other methods. The a-HCRF-2 model is the second best method after 5 s. The HCRF model performs worse than DBNs, which we think is due to the model not utilizing any of the current features. Another thing to note is that at 9 s, there is a peak for all three CRF methods. We think this is a sweet-spot in soccer where it is more predictable.

3.5 Model Adaptation

In the previous section, our model is trained using all data from team of interest from all matches. This model assumes that a player/team will have the same behavior regardless of the opposition. This represents an area of improvement as the behavior or tactics of a player/team are heavily dependent on the opposition in adversarial activities (e.g., sports). However, to train a model between the exact two teams/players is problematic as obtaining enough data is difficult (players/teams may only play each other several times a year). A method to resolve this issue is to employ model adaptation. In this paper, we adapted a well trained generic behavior model (GBM) with a opposition-specific model

Table 1. Comparison of performance of generic behavior model (GBM), opposition specific model (OSM) and combine model (Comb).

	GBM	OSM	Comb
ω (soccer)	0.78	0.22	N/A
Prediction rate (soccer)	42.6	42.4	**45.1**

(OSM) for a team/player to improve the predictive capability. Use tennis as an example, we can first use a-HCRF to train an GBM for Djokovic using data from all his matches. Then we train another model (OSM) using data just between Djokovic and a specific opponent (e.g., Nadal). Finally, we adaptively combine these two models. We expect this combined model will achieve a better prediction performance for Djokovic when he is against Nadal. The fusion can be implemented on several levels (e.g., feature, parameter, or output level.) While these combination schemes can all be explored for this task, output-level combination is of particular interest due to its simplicity (models can easily have over 1000 parameters). To do this task, we linearly combine the probability output from GBM and OSM as: $P_{comb} = \omega_1 P_{GBM} + \omega_2 P_{OSM}$ with weight ω. Here, $\omega_i \geq 0, i = 1, 2$. and $\omega_1 + \omega_2 = 1$. The optimum ω is found by maximizing the prediction rate.

Result: We test the adaptation result on ball prediction in soccer in 4 s future. a-HCRF-1 is used to train both generic behavior model (GBM) and opposition specific model (OSM). The performance of adapted model is compared with each individual model in Table 1. The adaptive model achieves an improvement of 2.5 %.

4   Predicting Shot Location in Tennis

Given features of the past n shots in a rally in tennis, the goal here is to accurately predict the location of the next shot. This task is much more challenging than the previous work of Wei et al. [2], where they predicted "what" type of shot (i.e. winner, error or continuation) but not "where" which is a potentially infinitely larger output state space. This experiment has potential value in high performance sport coaching.

4.1   Data

Using multiple fixed cameras, we used Hawk-Eye data which captured the (x, y, z) positions of the ball over time t [22]. Player court positions are recorded as the (x, y) positions of players on the court at 20 frames per second. For this work, we used the data from the 2012 Australian Open Men's draw which consisted of more than 10,000 points. We specifically modeled the behavior of Novak Djokovic at the tournament as he had the most data (winner of the tournament).

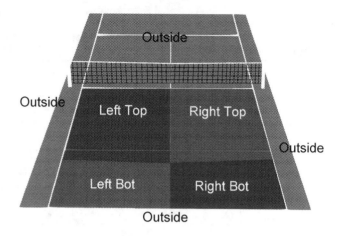

Fig. 6. An example of our court quantization scheme. Here quantization level is 2. There is 4 + 1 possible output locations for a future shot. (4 inner areas + outside).

4.2 Model Representation

Ideally, we want to predict the location of the shot at the most precise level (e.g., millimeter). However, as this essentially represents an infinite output state-space, we instead utilize a quantization scheme to make the problem more tractable. In order to find out the best quantization scheme, different levels of quantization are tested. The idea is we divide the receiving player's side of the court into d areas where $d = n^2 + 1$. Here n is the quantization level, $n \in \{1, 2, 3, 4, 5, 6\}$. d is the number of areas under a particular quantization level. 1 is added to n^2 because there is a catch-all area which captured all shots that fell outside these d areas (an outside shot). For example, if we are currently using quantization level 3, then there will be $(3^2 + 1 = 10)$ possible output locations for an incoming shot (see Fig. 6).

In this experiment, h_i is a past state of the game at t_i. y is the impact location of the next shot in the future. When $n = 3$, h_i can take 1 of 9 values representing the 9 inner areas of the court. (Previous shots can not be outside). y_i can take 1 of 10 values. The pairwise potential between h_i and h_{i+1} measures the transition of the game. Features used in this experiment can be found in Table 2.

4.3 Experimental Setup

We extract data for Novak Djokovic from an entire tournament of Australia Open 2012 Hawk-eye data. There are in total 1916 points played by him and 3410 shots. We divide this data equally for training and testing. We test our model with other models, namely DBNs, CRF and HCRF. Each model has four past nodes (the last four shots in this rally). We also create two versions of our model, a-HCRF-1 and a-HCRF-2 corresponds to different size of feature window ω. Conditional decoding is used for all models to find the optimum future

Table 2. Description of the shot variables used in this paper.

Feature	Description
Speed	Shot average speed
Angle	Angle between shot & center line
Feet Location	Player and opponent court position when shot starts
Shot-Start Loc.	Location where shot starts
Shot-End Loc.	Location where shot impacts the court
No. of shots	Total number of shots in the point
Opponent Movement	Local speed & direction of the opponent before the player strikes the ball

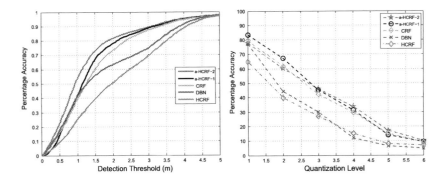

Fig. 7. (Left) Plot shows the prediction accuracy of each model against different detection threshold at quantization level 3. Proposed a-HCRF-2 (red curve) achieves the best result. (Right) Plot shows the prediction accuracy of each model at different quantization level. a-HCRF-1 achieves the best performance before level 3. a-HCRF-2 slightly outperforms other models after level 3 (Color figure online).

label. Experiments are conducted to answer three questions: (i) Which is the best model? (ii) How many quantization level can we achieve while maintaining a reasonable accuracy? (iii) How many history features are required?

4.4 Experimental Result

We first calculate the mean error (distance) between predicted location and actual location for each method at each quantization levels. We use the center of the predicted zone as the predicted location. Each method is tested 10 times and the average result is reported. Except DBN, all other models achieve the best result at quantization level 3. a-HCRF-2 gives the best result of 1.68 m mean error[1]. Next, we plot the prediction rate against detection threshold for

---

[1] Each side of the tennis court is 11 m wide and 11.9 m long.

each model at level 3 (See Fig. 7 Left). The red curve (a-HCRF-2) achieves the best result which indicates that features of two shots ago are still useful when predicting the next shot. Finally, we plot the prediction accuracy against different quantization levels (See Fig. 7 Right). At level 1 (only two zones), a-HCRF-1 can predict whether a shot is inside or outside at 83 % accuracy.

Table 3. Comparison of performance of generic behavior model (GBM), opposition specific model (OSM) and combine model (Comb).

	GBM	OSM	Comb
ω (tennis)	0.69	0.31	N/A
Prediction rate (tennis)	48.1	39.8	**53.9**

In addition, we apply the same adaptation method on tennis. We test its performance on shot prediction in tennis at quantization level 3. a-HCRF-1 is used to train both generic behavior model (GBM) and opposition specific model (OSM). The performance of adapted model is compared with each individual model in Table 3. The adaptive model achieves an improvement of 5.8 %.

5 Summary and Future Work

In this paper, we have proposed an augmented-Hidden Conditional Random Field (a-HCRF) which adds another feature layer to an HCRF to allow more effective prediction of a future event. The proposed model outperforms other models (CRF, HCRF, DBNs) across various spatiotemporal dataset for both ball ownership prediction in soccer and shot prediction in tennis. By adaptively combining a generic behavior model with an opposition-specific model of a team/player, we further improve its predictive capability. Future research will investigate other model training methods such as max-margin [17] or diverse M-best solutions. We will also explore the application of this modeling approach on other domains such as surveillance as well as trying it on datasets of larger magnitudes (e.g., seasons worth of sports data).

References

1. Kim, K., Grundmann, M., Shamir, A., Matthews, I., Hodgins, J., Essa, I.: Motion fields to predict play evolution in dynamic sport scenes. In: CVPR (2010)
2. Wei, X., Lucey, P., Morgan, S., Sridharan, S.: Sweet-spot: using spatiotemporal data to discover and predict shots in tennis. In: MIT Sloan Sports Analytics Conference (2013)
3. Wei, X., Lucey, P., Morgan, S., Sridharan, S.: Predicting shot locations in tennis using spatiotemporal data. In: DICTA (2013)
4. Carr, P., Mistry, M., Matthews, I.: Hybrid robotic/virtual pan-tilt-zoom cameras for autonomous event recording. In: ACM Multimedia (2013)

5. Bialkowski, A., Lucey, P., Carr, P., Yue, Y., Matthews, I.: "Win at home and draw away": automatic formation analysis highlighting the differences in home and away team behaviors. In: MIT Sloan Sports Analytics Conference (2014)
6. Lucey, P., Bialkowski, A., Carr, P., Yue, Y., Matthews, I.: "How to get an open shot": analyzing team movement in basketball using tracking data. In: MIT Sloan Sports Analytics Conference (2014)
7. Quattoni, A., Wang, L., Morency, L., Collins, M., Darrell, T.: Hidden-state conditional random fields. PAMI **29**, 1848–1852 (2007)
8. Ryoo, M.S.: Human activity prediction: early recognition of ongoing activities from streaming videos. In: ICCV (2011)
9. Hoai, M., Torre, F.: Max-margin early event detectors. In: CVPR (2012)
10. Pellegrini, S., Ess, A., Schindler, K., Van Gool, L.: You'll never walk alone: modeling social behavior for multi-target tracking. In: CVPR (2009)
11. Mehran, R., Oyama, A., Shah, M.: Abnormal crowd behavior detection using a social force model. In: CVPR (2009)
12. Kitani, K.M., Ziebart, B.D., Bagnell, J.A., Hebert, M.: Activity forecasting. In: Fitzgibbon, A., Lazebnik, S., Perona, P., Sato, Y., Schmid, C. (eds.) ECCV 2012, Part IV. LNCS, vol. 7575, pp. 201–214. Springer, Heidelberg (2012)
13. Zhou, B., Wang, X., Tang, X.: Understanding collective crowd behaviors: learning a mixture model of dynamic pedestrian-agents. In: CVPR (2012)
14. Kim, K., Lee, D., Essa, I.: Detecting regions of interest in dynamic scenes with camera motions. In: CVPR (2012)
15. Lafferty, J., McCallum, A., Pereira, F.: Conditional random fields: probabilistic models for segmenting and labeling sequence data. In: ICML (2001)
16. Wang, S., Quattoni, A., Morency, L., Demirdjian, D.: Hidden conditional random fields for gesture recognition. In: CVPR (2006)
17. Wang, Y., Mori, G.: Max-margin hidden conditional random fields for human action recognition. In: CVPR (2009)
18. Batra, D., Yadollahpour, P., Guzman-Rivera, A., Shakhnarovich, G.: Diverse M-best solutions in markov random fields. In: Fitzgibbon, A., Lazebnik, S., Perona, P., Sato, Y., Schmid, C. (eds.) ECCV 2012, Part V. LNCS, vol. 7576, pp. 1–16. Springer, Heidelberg (2012)
19. Wang, X., Ablavsky, V., Shitrit, H.B., Fua, P.: Take your eyes off the ball: improving ball-tracking by focusing on team play. In: CVIU (2013)
20. SportsVision. http://www.sportsvision.com.au
21. Stats. http://www.stats.com/
22. Hawk-Eye. http://www.hawkeyeinnovations.co.uk
23. Lucey, P., Bialkowski, A., Carr, P., Foote, E., Matthews, I.: Characterizing multi-agent team behavior from partial team tracings: evidence from the English premier league. In: AAAI (2012)
24. Lucey, P., Oliver, D., Carr, P., Roth, J., Matthews, I.: Assessing team strategy using spatiotemporal data. In: ACM SIGKDD Conference on Knowledge, Discovery and Data Mining (KDD) (2013)
25. Wei, X., Sha, L., Lucey, P., Morgan, S., Sridharan, S.: Large-scale analysis of formations in soccer. In: DICTA (2013)

Camera Motion and Surrounding Scene Appearance as Context for Action Recognition

Fabian Caba Heilbron[1,2], Ali Thabet[1], Juan Carlos Niebles[2],
and Bernard Ghanem[1]($\boxtimes$)

[1] King Abdullah University of Science and Technology (KAUST),
Thuwal, Saudi Arabia
bernard.ghanem@kaust.edu.sa
[2] Universidad del Norte, Barranquilla, Colombia

Abstract. This paper describes a framework for recognizing human actions in videos by incorporating a new set of visual cues that represent the *context* of the action. We develop a weak foreground-background segmentation approach in order to robustly extract not only foreground features that are focused on the actors, but also global camera motion and contextual scene information. Using dense point trajectories, our approach separates and describes the foreground motion from the background, represents the appearance of the extracted static background, and encodes the global camera motion that interestingly is shown to be discriminative for certain action classes. Our experiments on four challenging benchmarks (HMDB51, Hollywood2, Olympic Sports, and UCF50) show that our contextual features enable a significant performance improvement over state-of-the-art algorithms.

1 Introduction

Human action recognition is a challenging task for computer vision algorithms due to the large variabilities in video data caused by occlusions, camera motion, actor and scene appearances, among others. A popular current trend in action recognition methods relies on using local video descriptors to represent visual events in videos [4,12,22]. These features are usually aggregated into a compact representation, namely the bag-of-features (BoF) representation [13]. The advantage of this simple representation is that it avoids difficult pre-processing steps such as motion segmentation and tracking. In the BoF representation, local descriptors are quantized using a pre-computed codebook of visual patterns. This representation combined with discriminative classifiers such as support vector machines (SVM), has been quite successful in recognizing human actions in controlled scenarios [3,21]. Due to its simplicity, BoF requires the use of strong, robust and informative features, which can be obtained reliably in such simplified scenarios.

However, recent efforts have been made to collect more realistic video datasets (*e.g.* from movies and personal videos uploaded to video sharing websites [11,15]), which are useful for evaluating human action recognition methods in more natural settings. In fact, these datasets represent a challenge for existing

© Springer International Publishing Switzerland 2015
D. Cremers et al. (Eds.): ACCV 2014, Part IV, LNCS 9006, pp. 583–597, 2015.
DOI: 10.1007/978-3-319-16817-3_38

BoF-based methods due to dynamic backgrounds, variations in illumination and viewpoint, and camera motion among other visual nuisances that can severely affect recognition performance. To mitigate the effect of camera motion in describing the action of interest in a video, recent methods [22,23] have proposed using dense point trajectories in a video. In fact, these trajectories can separate background from foreground using a simple camera motion model (*i.e.* an affine or homography transform between consecutive frames). Such separation allows action recognition approaches to robustly extract and describe foreground motion, which is otherwise contaminated by camera motion and the background. Inspired by this work, our proposed method also makes use of these dense trajectories; however, we enlist a more general camera model (by estimating the fundamental matrix between video frames) that allows for a more reliable separation between foreground and background pixels, especially in non-planar cluttered scenes.

Unlike most other methods, we claim that the *context* of a human action, namely global camera motion and static background appearance, can also be used to discriminate between certain human actions. These cues are considered as contextual features for an action, which would allow classification algorithms to mine the relationship between the human action and both the background scene as well as the camera motion. The appearance of the scene in which an action occurs can be helpful in recognizing the action, as validated by previous work in [15]. For example, a 'cooking' action tends to occur indoors, while a 'jogging' action usually exists outdoors. Interestingly, the manner in which the *cameraman* records a particular action can also be indicative of the action. For example, camera zoom with minimal panning usually indicates an action that is spatially limited to a smaller physical space (*e.g.* juggling balls), while significant panning is indicative of actions that require a much larger spatial support (*e.g.* practicing long jump). Our proposed approach mines these two sources of contextual information, as well as, the separated foreground motion to describe and recognize an action. Figure 1 illustrates our claims.

Related work

A large body of work has studied the problem of human action recognition in video. For a survey of this work, we refer the reader to [1]. In this section, we give an overview of previous work that is most relevant to our proposed method.

Action Recognition Pipeline. The majority of action recognition methods rely on local descriptors to represent visual events in videos [4,12,22]. Traditionally, these features are usually aggregated into a compact representation using the bag-of-features (BoF) framework [5,13]. Moreover, recent studies show that using soft encoding techniques, such as Fisher Vectors [19] and Vectors of Locally Aggregated Descriptors (VLAD) [9], can lead to a boost in action recognition performance. These representations combined with discriminative classifiers such as support vector machines (SVM), have been quite successful in discriminating human action classes. However, as discussed in [24], there remain many details of the overall action recognition pipeline that can be extensively explored, including

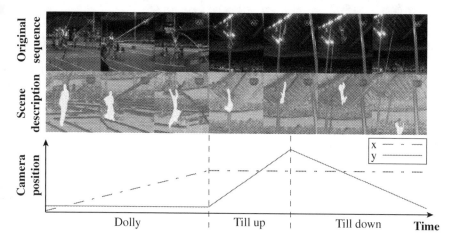

Fig. 1. Some human actions have important correlations with surrounding cues. As observed in the first row, there is a video sequence associated with the human action pole vault. It is also noticeable that the camera moves according to some specific patron for capturing the movement of the subject. Specifically, the camera moves within dolly panning tracking when the athlete is approaching the plant and take off. Then, camera slightly starts to tilling up and tilling down when the person is flying away and falling respectively. Additionally, a better description can be performed if visual appearance of the track field is captured.

feature extraction, feature pre-procesing, codebook generation, feature encoding and pooling and normalization. In this paper, we propose a new set of features that can be used to address some of the limitations of conventional feature extraction methods.

Feature Extraction. When applied to videos with substantial camera motion, traditional feature extraction approaches [4,12] tend to generate a large number of features, which are inherently dependent on the camera motion in a video, thus, limiting their discriminative power among action classes. In order to overcome this issue, Wu *et al.* [25] propose the use of Lagrangian point trajectories for action description in videos captured by moving cameras. Their method compensates for global camera motion by only extracting features that exhibit motion that is independent of the camera motion, thus, outperforming traditional feature extraction algorithms. In [2], these trajectories are used to recognize human actions using Fisher Kernel features for discrimination. Park *et al.* [18] use a weak video stabilization method based on extracting coarse optical flow to isolate limb motion while canceling pedestrian translation and camera motion. Wang *et al.* [22] present a method for action recognition using dense sampling of point trajectories. Their method handles large camera motions by limiting the maximum length of tracked trajectories. Despite their simplicity, these dense trajectory features have been shown to achieve a significant performance improvement as compared to conventional spatiotemporal point features [12].

More recent methods improve upon the aforementioned dense trajectory features. For example, Jain *et al.* [8] propose a method to estimate more reliable trajectory features for action recognition. This method lends additional reliability and robustness to trajectory extraction by decomposing optical flow into dominant and residual motions. Dominant motion is estimated using an affine frame-to-frame motion model and is subtracted from the computed optical flow to obtain the residual motion, which is attributed to the human action of interest. Similarly, 'improved trajectories' are proposed in [23] to stabilize features and compensate for simple camera motion. This is done by fitting a frame-to-frame homography (using RANSAC) to separate moving points of the human action from those of the background. By explicitly canceling out the camera motion, their framework improves the performance of several motion descriptors, including trajectory shape, histogram of optical flow (HOF), and motion boundary histograms (MBH). While these methods have been successful in separating background and residual motions, contextual cues of actions are usually discarded, thus, ignoring relevant information such as static scene appearance and distinctive camera motions correlated with some actions.

Moreover, a few approaches have investigated ways to involve background scene information in the action recognition pipeline. Marszalek *et al.* [15] incorporate context information from movie scripts by modeling the relationship between human actions and static scenes based on textual co-occurrence. While such textual co-occurrence helps recognition, they are restricted only to video sources where scripts are available. In [7], multiple feature channels are integrated from different sources of information including human motion, scene information, and objects in the scene. However, this approach makes use of all pixels (corresponding to both the human action and background scene) to generate a global descriptor of the static scene [17]. Rather than computing a holistic representation, our proposed method computes a static scene descriptor only from the extracted background, a motion descriptor from the extracted foreground trajectories, and a camera motion descriptor from the estimated transformations between consecutive frames.

In this paper, our goal is to reliably alleviate the effect of camera motion, as well as, incorporate features describing the surrounding of an action to build a richer representation for human actions. We are motivated by the fact that most videos are filmed with an intention and therefore there exists a correlation between the inherent camera motion in a video and the portrayed human action itself. We encode this intention with a weak camera motion model based on frame-to-frame fundamental matrices in a video. To the best of our knowledge, this is the first work to mine such a relationship between human actions and the filming process.

2   Proposed Methodology

This section gives a detailed description of our proposed approach for action recognition in video. The methodology in this paper follows the conventional

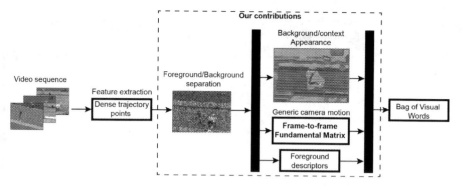

Fig. 2. Given a video sequence, a set of dense point trajectories are extracted. Then, a fundamental matrix is estimated and used to compensate for camera motion and to separate foreground from background trajectories. Each type of trajectories is encoded by a different descriptor. Specifically, frame-to-frame fundamental matrices are used to describe the camera motion. Moreover, surrounding scene appearance is explicitly computed on background trajectories. Traditional foreground descriptors (*e.g.* MBH, HOF, HOG and trajectory shape) are also aggregated in action description. Finally, this set of descriptors is encoded separately using the BoF framework.

action recognition pipeline. Given a set of labelled videos, a set of features is extracted from each video, represented using visual descriptors, and combined into a single video descriptor used to train a multi-class classifier for recognition.

In this paper, we use dense point trajectories (short tracks of a densely sampled set of pixels in a video [23]) as our primitive features. By estimating frame-to-frame camera motion (fundamental matrix), we separate foreground trajectories (corresponding to the action) from background ones. Each type of trajectory is represented using a different descriptor. Foreground trajectories are represented using conventional visual properties (*e.g.* MBH, HOF, HOG, and trajectory shape), while the surrounding scene appearance is described using SIFT. Foreground and background trajectories are then encoded separately using the BoF framework as illustrated in Fig. 2. Unlike other action recognition methods, we not only use the frame-to-frame camera motion to separate foreground from background, but we also use it to *describe* a video. This is done by encoding all frame-to-frame fundamental matrices in a video using the BoF framework. We use all three descriptors (foreground, surrounding scene appearance, and camera motion) to train a multi-class classifier for recognition. In this paper, we argue and show that combining a foreground-only description [23] with additional cues (background/context and camera motion) provides a richer and more discriminative description of actions.

2.1 Camera Motion

Since videos are normally filmed with the intention of maintaining the subject within the image frame, there exists a relationship between the estimated camera motion and the underlying action. In this paper, we argue and show that this relationship can be a useful cue for discriminating certain action classes. As observed in the three top rows of Fig. 3, there is a correlation between how the camera moves and the actor For example, in the second row, the cameraman performs a downward tilt to follow the diver's movement. Here, we do not claim that this cue is significant for all types of actions, since very similar camera motion can be shared among classes, as shown in Fig. 3 (last two rows). Instead of using a homography to encode camera motion, we estimate the more general fundamental matrix for each pair of frames in a video using the well-known 8-point algorithm [6]. As mentioned earlier, a homography is suitable when the camera is not translating or when the background is planar; however, it is not applicable in more complex or cluttered scenes.

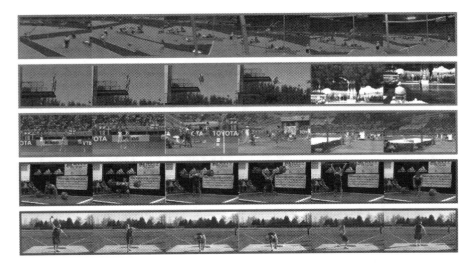

Fig. 3. A generic camera motion descriptor can be a useful cue for discriminating specific action classes. The first three rows contain a characteristic correlation between how the camera moves and the action itself. However, this cue is not significant for all action classes, as exemplified in the last two rows, where there is no camera motion.

In this paper, we compute the camera motion descriptor as follows. After estimating all pairwise fundamental matrices using RANSAC, we encode the camera motion of a video using the BoF framework. We call this descriptor CamMotion and it is complementary to other visual descriptors of the action. Unlike most existing work, we embrace camera motion and employ a low-level feature to represent it in a video.

2.2   Foreground/Background Separation

We use the global motion model introduced in Sect. 2.1 to compensate for camera motion in the extracted point trajectories. To separate background from

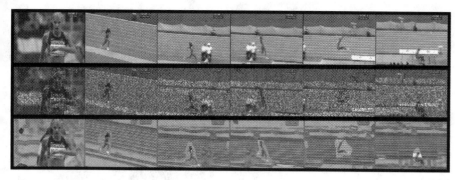

Fig. 4. Results from our foreground-background separation and illustration of the encoded information by the surrounding scene features. (*top*) Frame sequence sampled from a 'long jump' video. Note that the camera is panning to follow the actor. (*middle*) Camera compensation allows to perform a background-foreground separation. Noticeably, foreground feature points are mostly related with the actor. (*bottom*) Illustration of information captured by our surrounding appearance SIFT descriptor. In order to achieve a meaningful illustration, descriptor dimensionality is reduced to 3 dimensions to produce a color-coded image. Surrounding appearance is represented using background points only, thus, avoiding confusion with pixels of the actor him/herself.

foreground, we assume that a background trajectory produces a small frame-to-frame trajectory displacement, after camera motion compensation. In fact, we simply threshold the overall displacement, which is computed for the ith trajectory as

$$D(i) = \sum_{j=1}^{L-1} \left\| \mathbf{x}_{j+1}^i - \mathbf{x}_j^i \right\|_2^2. \tag{1}$$

Here, $\mathbf{x}_j^i$ represents the jth point in the ith trajectory. Trajectories are associated with the background if $D(i) \leq \alpha$; otherwise, they are labeled as foreground. Empirically, we set this threshold value to $\alpha = 3$ pixels. Figure 4 shows an example of our foreground-background separation in a video associated with the action *long jump*. Here, foreground and background trajectories are color-coded in red and blue respectively. Clearly, the foreground trajectories correspond to the underlying action itself, while background trajectories correspond to *static* background pixels undergoing camera motion only. Our proposed separation will allow each type of trajectory (foreground and background) to be represented independently and thus more reliably than other methods that encode context information using information from entire video frames [15].

In this paper, we represent foreground trajectories using a foreground descriptor, comprising of Trajectory Shape, HOG, HOF, and MBH as in [23]. In the following section, we detail how surrounding scene appearance is encoded.

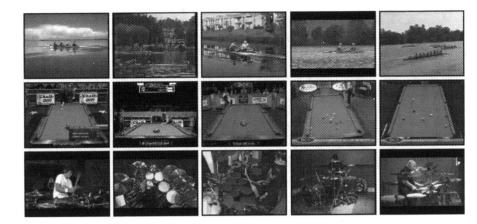

Fig. 5. Each row presents five different thumbnails taken from different videos of UCF50 dataset. (*top*) Visual examples of the 'rowing' action class. As observed all thumbnails share distinct background appearance *i.e.* in all water is present and also in the majority there is a common landmark. (*middle*) Visual examples of the 'billiard' action class. A billiard table and the indoor environment of the action, enable our surrounding appearance descriptor to capture critical information about that action. (*bottom*) Visual examples of the 'drumming' class. Note that these examples share visual cues that are largely ignored if only foreground features are encoded.

2.3   Background/Context Appearance

Many visual cues can be used to discriminate human actions. Beyond local motion and appearance properties, the surrounding in which an action is performed is a critical component to recognize actions. For example, a 'springboard' action can only be executed if there is a pool, which has distinctive appearance properties. This motivates us to encode the visual appearance of the static scene. Surrounding scene appearance is encoded using SIFT descriptors [14] around trajectory points associated with the background. We detect SIFT keypoints in a dense manner and then filter out those that fall within the union of foreground trajectories. Context appearance focuses more on the scene itself, as observed in Fig. 5, where it can be used to aggregate meaningful information about the action. For example, all the examples of the action 'rowing' contain a shared scene appearance and layout which can be exploited to model the background trajectories. Unlike other methods that encode scene context holistically (using both foreground and background) in a video [15], separating the background (or context) from the foreground produces a more reliable and robust context descriptor.

2.4   Implementation Details

Codebook Generation. We generate the visual codebook in two different ways: (a) using k-means clustering or (b) using a Gaussian Mixture Model (GMM),

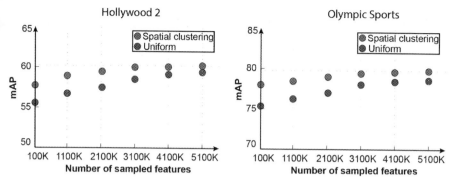

Fig. 6. Due to the large number of features extracted by the dense trajectory method, sub-sampling is required to generate a codebook. Here, we explore the effect of the number of sampled features on the overall performance. A comparison is done on two different datasets under the Bag-of-Features framework. Also, the performance of two different sampling strategies is reported: uniform and spatial clustering. As noticed, selecting more features to form the codebook and using the spatial clustering approach improve recognition performance in both datasets.

which captures a probability distribution for the feature space. In both cases, a codebook is computed for each descriptor (context appearance, foreground, and camera motion) separately. Since the trajectory extraction method produces a large number of features from the training videos resulting in intractable code-book computation, it is necessary to sub-sample these features. In order to estab-lish a trade-off between computation cost and recognition performance, we study the effect of the number of sampled features for computing a visual codebook, as observed in Fig. 6. This experiment includes results on two different datasets using k-means clustering to form the visual dictionary. Moreover, we investigate two types of sub-sampling strategies, namely uniform random sampling and ran-dom sampling based on spatially clustered (using simple distance thresholding) trajectories. Based on results in Fig. 6, the latter strategy outperforms the for-mer one, especially when a small number of features are sampled. Therefore, in our experiments, we generate the visual codebook from 5 million feature points (8 GB RAM required per descriptor) sampled by the spatial clustering strategy.

Representation and Classification. Feature encoding can be performed using one of two popular approaches: (a) traditional histogram quantization (VQ), or (b) Fisher vectors introduced in [19]. Different types of normalization are performed to provide robustness to feature vectors: (a) *l2* normalization (L2) [19], (b) power normalization (PW) [19], and (c) intra-normalization (IN) [24]. In our experi-ments, we focus on two classification frameworks that have been widely adopted in the action recognition literature. For simplicity, we summarize the details of each framework in Table 1. The first follows the Bag of Features (BoF) para-digm, using k-means for visual codebook generation, VQ for feature encoding,

L2 normalization, and a χ^2 kernel SVM within a multichannel approach (MCSVM) [26]. In this case, the kernel is defined as

$$K(\mathbf{x}_i, \mathbf{x}_j) = \exp\left(-\sum_c \frac{1}{2\Omega_c} D_c(\mathbf{x}_i, \mathbf{x}_j)\right), \qquad (2)$$

where $D_c(\mathbf{x}_i, \mathbf{x}_j)$ is the χ^2 distance for channel c and Ω_c is the average channel distance. For the second framework, we enlist a more robust feature encoding scheme (Fisher vectors) using a visual codebook generated by learning a GMM on the subsampled training data. Here, each action video is represented as a high dimensional Fisher vector that undergoes three normalization procedures, L2, PW and IN as in [24]. The three normalized features channels are concatenated and discriminative action models are learned using a linear SVM (LSVM).

Table 1. Comparison of adopted frameworks for action recognition.

Representation ↓	Codebook	Encoding	Normalization	Classifier
Bag of features	k-means	VQ	L2	MCSVM
Fisher vectors	GMM	Fisher vectors	L2+PW+IN	LSVM

3   Experimental Results

In this section, we present extensive experimental results that validate our contextual features within the action recognition pipeline. We compare the performance of both classifications frameworks mentioned in Sect. 2.4, as well as, state-of-the-art recognition methods on benchmark datasets, when possible.

3.1   Datasets and Evaluation Protocols

We use four public datasets [11,15,16,20] and their corresponding evaluation protocols. In this section, we briefly describe each dataset.

HMDB51 [11] includes a large collection of human activities categorized on 51 classes. It comprises 6766 videos from different media resources *i.e.* digitized movies, public databases and user generated web video data. Since many of the videos contain undesired camera motions, the authors provide a stabilized version of the dataset. However, since we look at the camera motion as an informative cue, the pre-stabilized version of the dataset is used. To evaluate classification performance, we adopt the same protocol proposed by the authors, namely the mean accuracy under three fixed train/test splits of the data.

Hollywood2 [15] contains a large number of videos retrieved from 69 different Hollywood movies. It is divided into 12 categories including short actions such as 'Kiss', 'Answer Phone' and 'Stand Up'. This dataset remains one of the most challenging despite the small number of action classes. Change of camera view, camera motion and unchoreographed execution introduces significant difficulty to the recognition task. To evaluate performance, we follow the authors' protocol, whereby videos are separated in two different sets: a training set of 823 videos and a testing set of 884 videos. We use training videos to learn our action models and then compute the mean average precision (mAP) over all action classes.

Olympic Sports [16] or Olympic comprises a set of 783 sport related YouTube videos. This set of videos are semi-automatically labeled using Amazon Mechanical Turk. This dataset establish new challenges for recognition because the underlying action classes range from simple actions (*e.g.* 'Kiss') to complex actions (*e.g.* 'Hammer Throw'). All of these complex actions are related to olympic sports including actions like 'Long Jump', 'Pole Vault' and 'Javelin Throw'. As proposed by the authors, we measure performance by computing the mAP over all action classes.

UCF50 [20] includes 6618 videos of 50 different human actions. This dataset presents several recognition challenges due to large variations in camera motion, cluttered background, viewpoint, etc. Action classes are grouped into 25 sets, where each set consists of more than 4 action clips. Recognition performance is measured by applying a leave-one-group-out cross-validation and average accuracy over all group splits is reported.

3.2   Impact of Contextual Features

In this section, we conduct experiments to evaluate the contribution of our proposed camera motion (CamMotion) and surrounding scene appearance descriptor (SIFT) to overall action recognition performance. Our baseline corresponds to using only Foreground features for describing actions. Using descriptors individually is compared to this baseline. Also, we investigate the effect of combining the proposed features with Foreground cues. As mentioned earlier, both action recognition frameworks (BoF and Fisher vectors) are explored. Below, we present an analysis of our obtained results.

Representation. As suggested in recent works [19,23,24], Fisher vectors register an improved performance over traditional BoF representations. We found in our experiments that Fisher vectors also boost the performance of using our contextual descriptors. These results are reported in Table 2. However, we note that using Fisher vectors is less important with our CamMotion descriptor due to its low dimensionality.

Surrounding Appearance. While the surrounding SIFT features achieves a discrete performance by itself, it also produces a notable improvement when combined with foreground descriptors. As Table 2 reports, performance is significantly improved over all datasets. Interestingly, we note that this features produces higher improvements in HMDB51 and UCF50 *i.e.* +2.7 % and +2.4 % re-spectively.

Table 2. Impact of our surrounding scene appearance and camera motion features on recognition performance. Bag-of-Features encoding generally performs worse than Fisher vectors. Both surrounding SIFT and CamMotion show important improvements in performance when they are combined with foreground descriptors.

Features			Datasets			
Foreground	SIFT	CamMotion	HMDB51	Hollywood2	Olympics	UCF50
Framework: Bag of features						
✓			51.2 %	60.1 %	79.8 %	85.9 %
	✓		19.5 %	28.7 %	36.4 %	45.7 %
		✓	13.5 %	21.8 %	26.9 %	19.3 %
✓	✓		53.8 %	60.9 %	81.1 %	87.2 %
✓		✓	50.9 %	60.4 %	80.6 %	86.8 %
	✓	✓	20.7 %	36.2 %	43.7 %	50.3 %
✓	✓	✓	51.7 %	61.6 %	81.7 %	87.6 %
Framework: Fisher vectors						
✓			56.5 %	62.4 %	90.4 %	90.9 %
	✓		20.1 %	28.5 %	39.6 %	49.8 %
		✓	14.1 %	22.1 %	27.2 %	19.5 %
✓	✓		**59.2 %**	**63.5 %**	**91.6 %**	**93.3 %**
✓		✓	55.9 %	62.9 %	91.3 %	93.1 %
	✓	✓	22.3 %	36.5 %	46.5 %	54.3 %
✓	✓	✓	**57.9 %**	**64.1 %**	**92.5 %**	**93.8 %**

Camera Motion. Our experiments provide evidence that action recognition performance can be improved when global camera motion is incorporated with Foreground features. Our CamMotion feature provides slightly lower contributions in performance than the surrounding SIFT feature, in general. We observe a contribution over all datasets except on HMDB51 where recognition performance decreases. This negative effect is attributed to the extensive shared shaky camera motion in most video sequences of this dataset. This prevents CamMotion from capturing discriminative cues across the action classes.

Foreground-Background Separation. As described in Sect. 2, we perform a weak separation between background and foreground feature trajectories. Here, we measure the effect on performance of this separation. We note that this separation provides a significant boost in performance, as observed in Table 3. When feature points are localized on the background, surrounding SIFT focuses on the scene appearance avoiding information of actors and foreground objects. Unlike other methods that extract context information from all the trajectories (both background and foreground) in the video, we see that extracting surrounding SIFT and CamMotion features from the background alone improves overall

Table 3. Effect of separating background feature points on the surrounding SIFT and CamMotion features. These features are extracted using foreground and/or background trajectories. Our results consistently show that our proposed contextual features are most discriminative when they are extracted from background trajectories only. This motivates our proposed weak separation step and validates why it should be used in the action recognition pipeline.

Feature ↓	Feature points		Datasets			
	Foreground	Background	HMDB51	Hollywood2	Olympics	UCF50
SIFT	✓		19.5 %	22.1 %	33.5 %	44.7 %
SIFT		✓	**20.1 %**	**28.5 %**	**39.6 %**	**49.8 %**
SIFT	✓	✓	19.8 %	24.3 %	34.4 %	45.9 %
CamMotion	✓		9.7 %	14.9 %	19.5 %	13.7 %
CamMotion		✓	**14.1 %**	**22.1 %**	**27.2 %**	**19.5 %**
CamMotion	✓	✓	12.9 %	18.7 %	21.8 %	17.2 %

Table 4. Comparison with the state-of-the-art on four benchmark datasets. Our method improves reported results in the state-of-the-art for three different datasets, HMDB51, Olympic Sports and UCF50 and obtains comparable performance on Hollywod2. Note that our proposed method does not require explicit human detection.

Approach ↓	HMDB51	Hollywood2	Olympics	UCF50
Jiang et al. [10]	40.7 %	59.5 %	80.6	-
Jain et al. [8]	52.1 %	62.5 %	83.2	-
Wang et al. [23] non-HD	55.9 %	63.0 %	90.2 %	90.5 %
Wang et al. [23] HD	57.2 %	**64.3 %**	91.1 %	91.2 %
Our methods with Fisher vectors				
Baseline (Foreground)	56.5 %	62.4 %	90.4 %	90.9 %
Foreground + SIFT	**59.2 %**	63.5 %	**91.6 %**	**93.3 %**
Foreground + SIFT + CamMotion	57.9 %	64.1 %	**92.5 %**	**93.8 %**

performance. These results motivate our weak separation step as a necessary strategy in the action recognition pipeline. For the surrounding SIFT features, this step improves performance by +0.3 % for HMDB51, +4.2 % for Hollywood2, +5.2 % for Olympics and +3.9 % for UCF50. The same behavior is observed with our CamMotion descriptor, where performance is boosted in all datasets when the Fundamental Matrix is computed using background trajectories.

3.3   Comparison with State-of-the-Art

Here, we compare our proposed method with recent and popular methods in the literature [8, 10, 23]. The results of this comparison are reported in Table 4.

We present results of our own implementation of [23], which corresponds to our baseline (Foreground). The performance gain over the method in [23], which reports the best performance in the literature, is as follows: $+2\,\%$ for HMDB51, $+1.4\,\%$ for Olympic Sports and $2.6\,\%$ for UCF50. We also achieve a comparable performance on the Hollywood2 dataset with only $0.2\,\%$ less in the mAP score. It is noteworthy to mention that the method in [23] requires a human detection (HD) step to perform recognition. Since human detection is not included in our trajectory extraction stage, a more direct comparison is done with the non-HD version of [23]. In this case, our method outperforms their improved trajectory approach by $3.3\,\%$ for HMDB51, $1.1\,\%$ for Hollywood2, $2.3\,\%$ for Olympic Sports and $3.3\,\%$ for UCF50.

4   Conclusion

In this paper, we propose a set of novel contextual features that can be incorporated into a trajectory-based action recognition pipeline for improved performance. By separating background from foreground trajectories in a video, these features encode the appearance of the surrounding as well as the global camera motion, which can be shown to be discriminative for a large number of action classes. When combined with foreground trajectories, we show that these features, can improve state-of-the-art recognition performance on popular and challenging action datasets, without resorting to any additional processing stages (e.g. human detection).

Acknowledgment. Research reported in this publication was supported by competitive research funding from King Abdullah University of Science and Technology (KAUST). F.C.H. was also supported by a COLCIENCIAS Young Scientist and Innovator Fellowship. J.C.N. is supported by a Microsoft Research Faculty Fellowship.

References

1. Aggarwal, J., Ryoo, M.S.: Human activity analysis: a review. ACM Comput. Surv. (CSUR) **43**, 1–43 (2011)
2. Atmosukarto, I., Ghanem, B., Ahuja, N.: Trajectory-based fisher kernel representation for action recognition in videos. In: International Conference on Pattern Recognition, pp. 3333–3336 (2012)
3. Blank, M., Gorelick, L., Shechtman, E., Irani, M., Basri, R.: Actions as space-time shapes. In: ICCV (2005)
4. Dollar, P., Rabaud, V., Cottrell, G., Belongie, S.: Behavior recognition via sparse spatio-temporal features. In: 2005 Visual Surveillance and Performance Evaluation of Tracking and Surveillance (2005)
5. Escorcia, V., Niebles, J.C.: Spatio-temporal human-object interactions for action recognition in videos. In: ICCV (2013)
6. Hartley, R.: In defense of the eight-point algorithm. TPAMI **19**, 580–593 (1997)

7. Ikizler-Cinbis, N., Sclaroff, S.: Object, scene and actions: combining multiple features for human action recognition. In: Daniilidis, K., Maragos, P., Paragios, N. (eds.) ECCV 2010, Part I. LNCS, vol. 6311, pp. 494–507. Springer, Heidelberg (2010)

8. Jain, M., Jégou, H., Bouthemy, P.: Better exploiting motion for better action recognition. In: CVPR (2013)

9. Jégou, H., Perronnin, F., Douze, M., Sánchez, J., Pérez, P., Schmid, C.: Aggregating local image descriptors into compact codes. PAMI **34**, 1704–1716 (2012)

10. Jiang, Y.-G., Dai, Q., Xue, X., Liu, W., Ngo, C.-W.: Trajectory-based modeling of human actions with motion reference points. In: Fitzgibbon, A., Lazebnik, S., Perona, P., Sato, Y., Schmid, C. (eds.) ECCV 2012, Part V. LNCS, vol. 7576, pp. 425–438. Springer, Heidelberg (2012)

11. Kuehne, H., Jhuang, H., Garrote, E., Poggio, T., Serre, T.: Hmdb: a large video database for human motion recognition. In: ICCV (2011)

12. Laptev, I.: On space-time interest points. IJCV **64**, 107–123 (2005)

13. Laptev, I., Marszalek, M., Schmid, C., Rozenfeld, B.: Learning realistic human actions from movies. In: CVPR (2008)

14. Lowe, D.G.: Distinctive image features from scale-invariant keypoints. IJCV **60**, 91–110 (2004)

15. Marszalek, M., Laptev, I., Schmid, C.: Actions in context. In: CVPR (2009)

16. Niebles, J.C., Chen, C.-W., Fei-Fei, L.: Modeling temporal structure of decomposable motion segments for activity classification. In: Daniilidis, K., Maragos, P., Paragios, N. (eds.) ECCV 2010, Part II. LNCS, vol. 6312, pp. 392–405. Springer, Heidelberg (2010)

17. Oliva, A., Torralba, A.: Modeling the shape of the scene: a holistic representation of the spatial envelope. IJCV **42**, 145–175 (2001)

18. Park, D., Zitnick, C.L., Ramanan, D., Dollár, P.: Exploring weak stabilization for motion feature extraction. In: CVPR (2013)

19. Perronnin, F., Sánchez, J., Mensink, T.: Improving the fisher kernel for large-scale image classification. In: Daniilidis, K., Maragos, P., Paragios, N. (eds.) ECCV 2010, Part IV. LNCS, vol. 6314, pp. 143–156. Springer, Heidelberg (2010)

20. Reddy, K.K., Shah, M.: Recognizing 50 human action categories of web videos. Mach. Vis. Appl. **24**, 971–981 (2013)

21. Schuldt, C., Laptev, I., Caputo, B.: Recognizing human actions: a local SVM approach. In: ICPR (2004)

22. Wang, H., Klaser, A., Schmid, C., Liu, C.L.: Action recognition by dense trajectories. In: CVPR (2011)

23. Wang, H., Schmid, C.: Action recognition with improved trajectories. In: ICCV (2013)

24. Wang, X., Wang, L.M., Qiao, Y.: A comparative study of encoding, pooling and normalization methods for action recognition. In: Lee, K.M., Matsushita, Y., Rehg, J.M., Hu, Z. (eds.) ACCV 2012, Part III. LNCS, vol. 7726, pp. 572–585. Springer, Heidelberg (2013)

25. Wu, S., Oreifej, O., Shah, M.: Action recognition in videos acquired by a moving camera using motion decomposition of lagrangian particle trajectories. In: ICCV (2011)

26. Zhang, J., Marszałek, M., Lazebnik, S., Schmid, C.: Local features and kernels for classification of texture and object categories: a comprehensive study. IJCV **73**, 213–238 (2007)

Semi-Supervised Ranking for Re-identification with Few Labeled Image Pairs

Andy Jinhua Ma$^{(\boxtimes)}$ and Ping Li

Department of Statistics, Department of Computer Science,
Rutgers University, Piscataway, NJ 08854, USA
jma@stat.rutgers.edu

Abstract. In many person re-identification applications, typically only a small number of labeled image pairs are available for training. To address this serious practical issue, we propose a novel semi-supervised ranking method which makes use of unlabeled data to improve the re-identification performance. It is shown that low density separation or graph propagation assumption is not valid under some conditions in person re-identification. Thus, we propose to iteratively select the most confident matched (positive) image pairs from the unlabeled data. Since the number of positive matches is greatly smaller than that of negative ones, we increase the positive prior by selecting positive data from the top-ranked matching subset among all unlabeled data. The optimal model is learnt by solving a regression based ranking problem. Experimental results show that our method significantly outperforms state-of-the-art distance learning algorithms on three publicly available datasets using only few labeled matched image pairs for training.

1 Introduction

Person re-identification under non-overlapping camera views has become an active research topic due to its important applications in video surveillance systems, such as criminal detection, human tracking and behavior understanding across camera views. This problem can be extremely challenging because variations of illumination condition, background, human pose, scale, etc., are usually significant among disjoint camera views. Many research works [1–12] have been developed to extract robust features invariant to deal with these variations. To take advantage of label information of persons, discriminative learning methods were employed in [13–20]. With person labels for training, matched (positive) and unmatched (negative) image pairs are generated to learn the discriminative models for the query image. Although the re-identification performance is improved by supervised learning, these methods require a large number of positive image pairs for training.

In large-scale camera networks containing (e.g.) hundreds of thousands of cameras, it is extremely time-consuming and expensive to collect the label information of numerous training subjects from every camera. In this context,

---

Electronic supplementary material The online version of this chapter (doi:10. 1007/978-3-319-16817-3_39) contains supplementary material, which is available to authorized users.

© Springer International Publishing Switzerland 2015
D. Cremers et al. (Eds.): ACCV 2014, Part IV, LNCS 9006, pp. 598–613, 2015.
DOI: 10.1007/978-3-319-16817-3_39

a domain transfer support vector ranking method was proposed in [21] by adapting the classifier learnt from the source domain with plenty of label information to the target domain without any labels. To align the distribution mismatch between the source and target domains, this domain transfer learning method assumes that the target positive (matched image pairs) distribution can be represented by the target positive mean. While this assumption can simplify the problem, it may degrade the performance when the assumption is not valid.

In this paper, we address the problem that only a small number of persons are labeled to generate few positive image pairs for training. Under this scenario, we develop a novel semi-supervised ranking algorithm which make use of the unlabeled data to boost the re-identification performance. By analyzing the data distribution of absolute difference vectors, we show that the widely used low density separation and graph propagation assumptions in many semi-supervised algorithms [22,23] are not valid under some conditions in person re-identification. Therefore, we follow the self training direction to iteratively label the most confident positive image pairs from the unlabeled data. Since the number of positive matches is much smaller than that of negative ones, it is difficult to correctly select the true positive image pairs with a small amount of positive data. Therefore, we take advantages of properties in person re-identification and increase the positive prior by selecting potential positive data from the rank-one matching subset in all the unlabeled data. The optimal classification model is learnt by solving a regression based ranking problem with the selected positive data. The contributions of this paper are two-fold.

• We propose a new method to select positive image pairs for semi-supervised learning in person re-identification under data imbalance problem. It is shown that the positive prior in the rank-one matching subset is much larger than that in all the unlabeled data due to properties in re-identification. Thus, we propose to select the most confident positive matches from the rank-one matching subset for higher positive prior, which gives higher precision in selecting positive image pairs. On the other hand, we define a more robust confidence measure using negative data generated under non-overlapping cameras to select the potential positive data more accurately.

• We develop a novel semi-supervised ranking algorithm for person re-identification using only a small number of positive image pairs for training. Based on the potential positive image pairs selected from the unlabeled data, we formulate the ranking problem by least-square regression and propose an efficient updating method to determine the optimal solution. Since the proposed method updates the classification model iteratively, the classification model becomes more discriminative with iteration to better select the potential positive data.

The rest of the paper is organized as follows. Section 2 provides a brief review on person re-identification and semi-supervised learning. Section 3 reports the proposed Semi-Supervised Ranking method with Increased Positive Prior (SSR-IPP). Experimental results are given in Sect. 4. Finally, Sect. 5 concludes the paper.

2   Related Works

2.1   Supervised and Semi-supervised Person Re-identification

To take advantages of person labels, many existing supervised re-identification algorithms [14,16–18,20] convert the multi-class person identification problem into a two-class matching problem by training a unified classification model for different individuals. In [14], the Ranked Support Vector Machines (RSVM) model was employed to assign higher confidence to the positive image pairs and vice versa. To exploit higher-order correlations among features, Zheng et al. [17] proposed a Relative Distance Comparison (RDC) method using second-order distance learning. For solving the computational complexity issue, a Relaxed Pairwise Metric Learning (RPML) method was proposed in [16] by relaxing the original hard constraints, which leads to a simpler problem that can be solved more efficiently. On the other hand, more recently, there have been some research works on semi-supervised learning for person identification or re-identification [24–26]. While these methods employed the concept of semi-supervised learning, they did not address the problem that only a small number of matched image pairs are available to train a discriminative re-identification model.

2.2   Semi-supervised Learning

Semi-supervised learning attempts to train a better classification model by incorporating a small amount of labeled data with a large amount of unlabeled data. Many semi-supervised learning algorithms were developed based on low density separation or graph propagation assumption [22,23]. Under low density separation assumption, it is believed that the classification boundary lies in the low density region within which there are few data points. For the graph propagation approach, a regularization term is added to the objective function for the smoothness of the classification model. Besides classification, semi-supervised learning has been employed for ranking in information retrieval. Semi-supervised ranking methods were proposed in [27] based on low density separation assumption and [28] based on graph propagation approach. However, they do not take full advantages of the available information and it is shown by our analysis that these assumptions are not valid under some conditions in person re-identification.

3   Proposed Method

For clear presentation, we consider the re-identification task for images from a pair of cameras a and b. For multiple cameras, multiple classification models can be trained for each camera pair. As indicated in [17], the absolute difference space shows some advantages over the common difference space, so we use the Absolute Difference Vector (ADV) as the feature representation method for both positive and negative image pairs. Given two feature vectors x_i^a and x_j^b

representing two images under cameras a and b, respectively, the ADV z_{ij} is defined by

$$z_{ij} = d(x_i^a - x_j^b) = (|x_i^a(1) - x_j^b(1)|, \cdots, |x_i^a(R) - x_j^b(R)|)^T \quad (1)$$

where $x(r)$ is the r-th element of feature vector x and R is the dimension of x.

Given a small number of labeled person images under both cameras a and b for training, positive image pairs can be constructed for $y_i^a = y_j^b$, where y_i^a and y_j^b are person labels of feature vectors x_i^a and x_j^b, respectively. Denote positive ADVs as z_{ij}^+. Similarly, negative ADVs z_{ik}^- can be obtained for $y_i^a \neq y_k^b$. On the other hand, we are given a large number of unlabeled person images under both cameras and their ADVs are denoted by z_{mn}^u. Since the same person cannot be presented at the same instant under different non-overlapping cameras a and b, negative image pairs can be obtained for each unlabeled feature vector x_m^a or x_n^b. This means we can easily get some negative ADVs from the unlabeled images and denote them as z_{mk}^- and z_{ln}^-. Therefore, the key problem is to determine the potential positive image pairs from the unlabeled ones.

3.1   Data Distribution Analysis in Person Re-identification

Let us consider the distance between a positive ADV z_{ij}^+ and an unlabeled one z_{mn}^u. According to the definition given by (1), we have

$$\|z_{ij}^+ - z_{mn}^u\|_p = \left(\sum_{r=1}^{R} \left| |x_i^a(r) - x_j^b(r)| - |x_m^a(r) - x_n^b(r)| \right|^p \right)^{\frac{1}{p}} \quad (2)$$

where $\| \cdot \|_p$ denotes l_p norm. To show that the low density assumption may not be valid, we consider the unlabeled ADV z_{mn}^u for $y_m^a \neq y_n^b$. In this case, z_{mn}^u is negative. And, the difference between the r-th elements of feature vectors x_m^a and x_n^b could be large, i.e., $|x_m^a(r) - x_n^b(r)|$ is a large number. If the difference between $x_i^a(r)$ and $x_j^b(r)$ is small for positive image pair, we have the conclusion that the distance between z_{ij}^+ and z_{mn}^u is large by (2) for $y_m^a \neq y_n^b$. However, it cannot be guaranteed that $|x_i^a(r) - x_j^b(r)|$ for $y_i^a = y_j^b$ is significantly smaller than $|x_m^a(r) - x_n^b(r)|$ for $y_m^a \neq y_n^b$, since feature vectors x_i^a and x_j^b are extracted from images under non-overlapping camera views. Thus, $|x_i^a(r) - x_j^b(r)|$ could be large. Due to the large amount of negative image pairs, it is likely that there exists z_{mn}^u for $y_m^a \neq y_n^b$ such that the distance between z_{ij}^+ and z_{mn}^u is small, i.e.,

$$\exists z_{mn}^u, \text{s.t.} \ \|z_{ij}^+ - z_{mn}^u\|_p \leq \varepsilon, y_m^a \neq y_n^b \quad (3)$$

where ε is a small positive number. This equation means that for each positive ADV z_{ij}^+ there are probably some negative ones around them. Therefore, the low density region separating the positive and negative data does not exist. This means the low density separation assumption in many semi-supervised learning methods is not valid under this condition in person re-identification.

On the other hand, for the positive ADVs from the unlabeled data, i.e., $y_m^a = y_n^b$, we expand the element-wise difference in (2) as follows,

$$
\begin{aligned}
&\left| |x_i^a(r) - x_j^b(r)| - |x_m^a(r) - x_n^b(r)| \right| \\
&= \begin{cases} |(x_i^a(r) - x_m^a(r)) + (x_n^b(r) - x_j^b(r))|, (x_i^a(r) - x_j^b(r))(x_m^a(r) - x_n^b(r)) \geq 0 \\ |(x_i^a(r) - x_n^b(r)) + (x_m^a(r) - x_j^b(r))|, (x_i^a(r) - x_j^b(r))(x_m^a(r) - x_n^b(r)) < 0 \end{cases}
\end{aligned}
\tag{4}
$$

Let us consider the first case in (4), i.e., $(x_i^a(r) - x_j^b(r))(x_m^a(r) - x_n^b(r)) \geq 0$. If there exists r_0 such that the signs of $x_i^a(r_0) - x_m^a(r_0)$ and $x_n^b(r_0) - x_j^b(r_0)$ are the same, i.e., $(x_i^a(r_0) - x_m^a(r_0))(x_n^b(r_0)) - x_j^b(r_0)) \geq 0$, we have

$$
\begin{aligned}
&|(x_i^a(r_0) - x_m^a(r_0)) + (x_n^b(r_0) - x_j^b(r_0))| \\
&= |x_i^a(r_0) - x_m^a(r_0)| + |x_n^b(r_0) - x_j^b(r_0))|
\end{aligned}
\tag{5}
$$

Denote the value of (5) as λ. Since persons in the unlabeled set are likely to be different from the ones in the labeled set using few labeled image pairs, the absolute differences $|x_i^a(r_0) - x_m^a(r_0)|$ and $|x_n^b(r_0) - x_j^b(r_0)|$ could be large due to different identities (though the differences are calculated for feature vectors from the same camera). Therefore, the element-wise difference λ of (5) is a large number, which implies the distance between z_{ij}^+ and z_{mn}^u for $y_m^a = y_n^b$ is large by (2). Similarly, for the second case that $(x_i^a(r) - x_j^b(r))(x_m^a(r) - x_n^b(r)) < 0$, the norm $\|z_{ij}^+ - z_{mn}^u\|_p$ is large, if there exists r_0 such that $(x_i^a(r_0) - x_n^b(r_0))(x_m^a(r_0) - x_j^b(r_0)) \geq 0$. Under this condition, the distances between z_{ij}^+ and z_{mn}^u are large for any $y_i^a = y_j^b$ in the labeled set and $y_m^a = y_n^b$ in the unlabeled set, i.e.,

$$
\|z_{ij}^+ - z_{mn}^u\|_p \geq \lambda, \forall y_i^a = y_j^b, y_m^a = y_n^b, y_i^a \neq y_m^a
\tag{6}
$$

In this case, the positive information from the labeled data cannot be propagated to the unlabeled data. As a results, the graph propagation assumption cannot be employed under this condition in person re-identification.

Based on the above analysis, we follow the self training approach to iteratively label the most confident positive image pairs from the unlabeled data which will be discussed in the following sections.

3.2   Selecting Potential Positive Data by Increasing Positive Prior

Given a classification model f on the ADVs, one way to determine the positive data is to label the potential positive image pairs with very high scores, i.e.,

$$
\hat{E}^+ = \{z_{mn}^u | f(z_{mn}^u) \geq \theta\}
\tag{7}
$$

where $\hat{E}^+$ denotes the set of potential positive ADVs selected from the unlabeled data and θ is a threshold for the selection. However, according to (3), the region with high confidence may contain both positive and negative image pairs. On the other hand, according to (6), the scores of positive image pairs do not change continuously. This means not all the positive ADVs give very high confidence scores. Consequently, it may not be a good strategy to label positive image pairs from the unlabeled data using (7).

To deal with this problem, we propose to take advantages of properties in person re-identification and define a better confidence measure ρ by both the classification function f and negative data z_{mk}^- and z_{ln}^- generated under non-overlapping camera views. If the score difference between z_{mn}^u and the negative data is larger, z_{mn}^u is more likely to be a positive ADV. Thus, we normalize the scores and define a new confidence measure ρ for the unlabeled ADVs as,

$$\rho(z_{mn}^u) = \frac{f(z_{mn}^u)}{\max\left(\max_k f(z_{mk}^-), \max_l f(z_{ln}^-)\right)}, \tag{8}$$

On the other hand, with information about the cameras, we can group the unlabeled data according to the camera indexes, i.e.

$$G_{m\cdot} = \{z_{mn}^u = d(x_m^a - x_n^b) | \forall x_n^b\}, G_{\cdot n} = \{z_{mn}^u = d(x_m^a - x_n^b) | \forall x_m^a\} \tag{9}$$

To reduce the proportion of negative matches, we select only one ADV from each $G_{m\cdot}$ or $G_{\cdot n}$ to obtain a set E_1, i.e.

$$E_1 = \{z_{mn'}^u = \arg\max_{z_{mn}^u \in G_{m\cdot}} \rho(z_{mn}^u)\} \cup \{z_{m'n}^u = \arg\max_{z_{mn}^u \in G_{\cdot n}} \rho(z_{mn}^u)\} \tag{10}$$

According to the definition in (10), E_1 contains the best match for each x_m^a under camera a or x_n^b under camera b by the classification function f. Although there may be more than one positive ADVs in each group $G_{m\cdot}$ or $G_{\cdot n}$, the selected one can be representative for others due to the following reasons. Denote two positive ADVs in $G_{m\cdot}$ as $z_{mn_1}^+$ and $z_{mn_2}^+$. According to the definition of difference vector given by (1) and the expanded difference in (4), it has

$$\|z_{mn_1}^+ - z_{mn_2}^+\| \leq \|x_{n_1}^b - x_{n_2}^b\| \tag{11}$$

Since both $z_{mn_1}^+$ and $z_{mn_2}^+$ are positive, the person labels $y_{n_1}^b$ and $y_{n_2}^b$ are equal to y_m^a. This means feature vectors $x_{n_1}^b$ and $x_{n_2}^b$ are extracted from the same person under the same camera view b. Since the variation under the same camera view must be small, the difference between $z_{mn_1}^+$ and $z_{mn_2}^+$ is small according to (11). This implies any positive ADV in a group $G_{m\cdot}$ is representative for others in this group. Similarly, this conclusion is also true for group $G_{\cdot n}$. Thus, it is good enough to select only one positive ADV from each group.

More importantly, we further show that the positive prior in E_1 is much larger than that in all the ADVs. Let c_1 be the rank one accuracy obtained by f, J be the number of persons under both camera views, $J^a(\geq J)$ and $J^b(\geq J)$ be the numbers of persons under cameras a and b, respectively. It has (See Appendix)

$$\tau \approx \frac{J}{J^a J^b}, \tau_1 \geq \frac{Jc_1}{\max(J^a, J^b)}. \text{ If } \max(\frac{1}{J^a}, \frac{1}{J^b}) \ll c_1, \text{ then } \tau \ll \tau_1 \tag{12}$$

where τ is the percentages of the positive data in all the image pairs and τ_1 is the positive prior in E_1. Since the number of persons is usually very large in person re-identification, both $1/J^a$ and $1/J^b$ are very small numbers. On the other hand, using a classification function to obtain the rank one accuracy c_1 should be much better than a random guess with rank one accuracy $1/J^a$ or $1/J^b$. Therefore, the condition in (12) can be satisfied easily. This means the positive prior τ can be increased to τ_1 by only considering rank one matches in E_1. And, it is easier to correctly label a positive image pair from the unlabeled data with higher positive prior.

Since the rank one accuracy c_1 is not very large in person re-identification, there are still many negative ADVs in E_1. Consequently, we select only one potential positive ADV $\hat{z}_{mn}^+$ in E_1 with the highest score in each iteration, i.e.

$$\hat{z}_{mn}^+ = \arg \max_{z_{mn}^u \in E_1} \rho(z_{mn}^u) \tag{13}$$

3.3   Ranking by Regression

Since each positive ADV z_{ij}^+ should be ranked before its corresponding negative ones z_{ik}^- and z_{lj}^+, we learn a weight vector $\boldsymbol{w}$ such that $\boldsymbol{w}^T z_{ij}^+ > \boldsymbol{w}^T z_{ik}^-$ and $\boldsymbol{w}^T z_{ij}^+ > \boldsymbol{w}^T z_{lj}^-$. To preserve the ranking relationship, we set $\boldsymbol{w}^T(z_{ij}^+ - z_{ik}^-) \approx 1$ and $\boldsymbol{w}^T(z_{ij}^+ - z_{lj}^-) \approx 1$ for regression. Then, the optimal weight vector $\boldsymbol{w}$ can be learnt by solving the following least square regression problem,

$$\min_{\boldsymbol{w}} \sum_{i,j,k} \left(\boldsymbol{w}^T(z_{ij}^+ - z_{ik}^-) - 1\right)^2 + \sum_{j,i,l} \left(\boldsymbol{w}^T(z_{ij}^+ - z_{lj}^-) - 1\right)^2 + \mu \boldsymbol{w}^T \boldsymbol{w} \tag{14}$$

where μ is a positive parameter for the regularization term to prevent from overfitting. This optimization problem can be solved by taking the first derivative to zero, and hence the optimal solution $\boldsymbol{w}^*$ is given by

$$\boldsymbol{w}^* = (H + \mu I)^{-1} \boldsymbol{h}, \boldsymbol{h} = \sum_{i,j,k}(z_{ij}^+ - z_{ik}^-) + \sum_{j,i,l}(z_{ij}^+ - z_{lj}^-)$$
$$H = \sum_{i,j,k}(z_{ij}^+ - z_{ik}^-)(z_{ij}^+ - z_{ik}^-)^T + \sum_{j,i,l}(z_{ij}^+ - z_{lj}^-)(z_{ij}^+ - z_{lj}^-)^T \tag{15}$$

where I denotes the unit matrix. According to the solution given by (15), we do not need to save all the positive and negative ADVs. Once a potential positive ADV is selected from the unlabeled data, we can simply update H and $\boldsymbol{h}$, which will be described in the following section. This ensures that the proposed regression based ranking method is computationally efficient.

3.4   Iterative Semi-supervised Ranking

According to the analysis in Sect. 3.1, we follow the self training approach to iteratively label potential positive ADVs and re-train the weight vector $\boldsymbol{w}$.

Algorithm 1. Training procedure of SSR-IPP

Input: Positive ADVs z_{ij}^+, negative ADVs $z_{ik}^-, z_{mk}^-, z_{ln}^-$, unlabeled ADVs z_{mn}^u, parameter μ, number of selected positive ADVs Q, unsupervised classifier g;

1: Compute H, h and w in (15) by z_{ij}^+, z_{ik}^- and z_{lj}^-;
2: Calculate confidence scores for each unlabeled ADV z_{mn}^u by w and g;
3: Construct the rank one matching set E_1;
4: **for** $t = 1, \cdots, Q$ **do**
5:    Calculate confidence scores for each z_{mn}^u in E_1 by w and g;
6:    Select one potential positive ADV $\hat{z}_{mn}^+$ by (13);
7:    Update H, h by (16) and w by (15);
8:    Delete $\hat{z}_{mn}^+$ from E_1;
9: **end for**

Output: Optimal weight vector w^*.

At iteration t, we have calculated H_t, h_t and w_t. With w_t, we can determine the classification function f_t by $f_t(z_{mn}^u) = w_t^T z_{mn}^u$. Since w_t may overfit the training data when the number of positive image pairs is very small, we propose to define f_t by adding an unsupervised classification model g, i.e., $f_t(z_{mn}^u) = w_t^T z_{mn}^u + g(z_{mn}^u)$. Then, we select one potential positive ADV $\hat{z}_{m_t n_t}^+$ in E_1 by (13) and H_t, h_t can be updated by the following equations,

$$
H_{t+1} = H_t + \sum_k (\hat{z}_{m_t n_t}^+ - z_{m_t k}^-)(\hat{z}_{m_t n_t}^+ - z_{m_t k}^-)^T
$$
$$
+ \sum_l (\hat{z}_{m_t n_t}^+ - z_{l n_t}^-)(\hat{z}_{m_t n_t}^+ - z_{l n_t}^-)^T \tag{16}
$$
$$
h_{t+1} = h_t + \sum_k (\hat{z}_{m_t n_t}^+ - z_{m_t k}^-) + \sum_l (\hat{z}_{m_t n_t}^+ - z_{l n_t}^-)
$$

With H_{t+1} and h_{t+1}, we can compute w_{t+1} by (15). After that, $\hat{z}_{m_t n_t}^+$ is deleted from E_1 for the next iteration. Algorithm 1 summarizes the proposed Semi-Supervised Ranking method with Increased Positive Prior (SSR-IPP).

4   Experiments

4.1   Datasets

Three publicly available datasets, namely VIPeR[1] [29], PRID[2] [30] and CUHK[3] [18], are used for evaluation of the proposed method. Example images in these three datasets are shown in Fig. 1(a), (b) and (c), respectively. VIPeR is a

---

[1] http://soe.ucsc.edu/~dgray/VIPeR.v1.0.zip.
[2] https://lrs.icg.tugraz.at/datasets/prid/.
[3] http://www.ee.cuhk.edu.hk/~xgwang/CUHK_identification.html.

re-identification dataset containing 632 person image pairs captured by two cameras outdoor. In this dataset, 632 image pairs are randomly separated into half for training and the other half for testing. PRID dataset consists of person images from two static surveillance cameras. Total 385 persons were captured by camera A, while 749 persons captured by camera B. The first 200 persons appeared in both cameras, and the remainders only appear in one camera. In our experiments, the single-shot version is used, in which at most one image of each person from each camera is available. 100 out of the 200 image pairs are randomly selected as the training set, and the others for testing. CUHK dataset contains five camera pairs. Under each camera view, there are two images for each person. Following the single shot setting in [18], images from camera pair one with 971 persons are used for experiments. On this dataset, 971 persons are randomly split as 485 for training and 486 for testing. For the testing data in VIPeR, PRID or CUHK, the evaluation is performed by searching the 316, 100 or 486 persons in one camera view from another view. These experiments were performed ten times and the average results are reported.

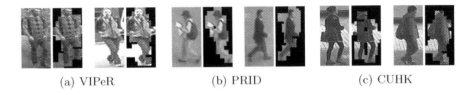

       (a) VIPeR   (b) PRID   (c) CUHK

Fig. 1. Sample images and masked results on three datasets: (a) VIPeR [29], (b) PRID [30] and (c) CUHK [18].

For each image in these datasets, we concatenate two types of features as the input feature vector. The first type of feature is constructed by dividing a person image into six horizontal stripes and compute the RGB, YCbCr, HSV color features and two types of texture features extracted by Schmid and Gabor filters on each stripe as reported in [13,14,17]. For the second type of feature, we perform foreground detection to detect the human pixels by the spatial hierarchy pose estimation method [31] with source code online[4]. Example masked results are shown in Fig. 1(a), (b) and (c) for VIPeR, PRID and CUHK datasets, respectively. Then, the masked person image is divided into 3×1 vertically overlapped boxes and the code[5] in [11] are used to extract color histogram and SIFT features on each box.

4.2 Evaluation of SSR-IPP

In our experiments, we use l_1 distance in the unsupervised classification model g and empirically set $\mu = 1$. Without the time acquisition information in the

---

[4] http://www.cs.cmu.edu/~ILIM/projects/IM/humanpose/humanpose.html.
[5] http://mmlab.ie.cuhk.edu.hk/projects/project_salience_reid/index.html.

PRID, VIPeR and CUHK datasets, negative image pairs from non-overlapping cameras are generated by simulating the synchronization using label information. Ten negative image pairs are randomly generated for each unlabeled person image. We first show the precisions for labeling the positive data, i.e., the number of true positive ADVs divided by the number (Q) of selected potential positive ADVs. The results are shown in Figs. 2(a)–(c) for VIPeR, Figs. 2(d)–(f) for PRID and Figs. 2(g)–(i) for CUHK dataset. For each dataset, we use different numbers ($L = 5, 10, 20$) of labeled positive image pairs to evaluate the performance. Our method by Increasing Positive Prior (IPP) is compared with the direct selection approach given by (7) which selects the ADVs with top classification scores as positive. From Figs. 2(a)–(i), we can see that our method remarkably outperforms the direct selection approach with different numbers (L) of labeled positive image pairs on the three datasets. Thus, our method can achieve better re-identification performance by correctly selecting more (true) positive ADVs for training compared with the direct selection approach.

On the other hand, from Figs. 2(a)–(i), we can see that the positive labeling precision drops when the number (Q) of selected potential positive ADVs increases. This means more ADVs are wrongly labeled when Q is large. However, if Q is too small, we may not have enough labeled data to train a robust model for re-identification. To evaluate the relationship between Q and the re-identification performance, we plot the rank one accuracy for varying Q on the three datasets in Figs. 2(a)–(i), respectively. From these figures, we can see that when Q is large, the rank one accuracy does not drop very much, though the precision for selecting potential positive ADVs drops significantly as shown in Figs. 2(a)–(i). This may be due to that the corresponding negative ADVs are correctly labeled under non-overlapping cameras. Moreover, Figs. 3(a)–(c) show that the rank one accuracy can be increased by training with the potential positive ADVs selected from the unlabeled data. For example, when the number (L) of labeled image pairs is equal to five, the improvement by selecting potential positive ADVs is extremely significant. The rank one accuracies on these three datasets for $L = 5$ and $Q = 20$ are over two times higher than those using only few labeled image pairs for training. These results indicate that it becomes more important to learn from unlabeled data for person re-identification when only a small number of persons are labeled for training.

4.3   Comparison with Existing Methods

In this section, we compare the proposed method with two state-of-the-art distance learning methods for person re-identification, namely Ranked Support Vector Machines (RSVM) [14] and Relative Distance Comparison (RDC) [17]. We have re-implemented these two methods. In our implementation, the parameter C in RSVM is empirically set as 1 for robust performance. According to the results shown in Figs. 3(a)–(c), we set the number of potential positive ADVs as $Q = 20$ on PRID, $Q = 30$ on VIPeR and CUHK datasets.

The CMC curves on VIPeR, PRID and CUHK datasets are shown in Figs. 4(a)–(c), Figs. 4(d)–(f) and Figs. 4(g)–(i), respectively. From these figures,

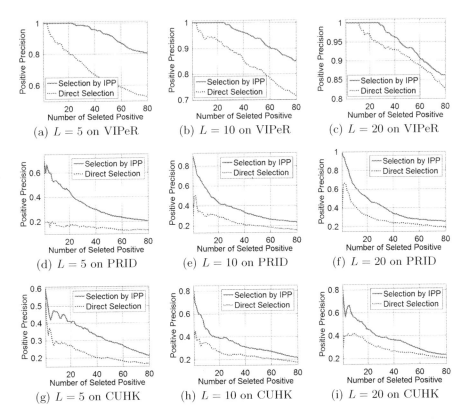

(a) $L = 5$ on VIPeR   (b) $L = 10$ on VIPeR   (c) $L = 20$ on VIPeR

(d) $L = 5$ on PRID   (e) $L = 10$ on PRID   (f) $L = 20$ on PRID

(g) $L = 5$ on CUHK   (h) $L = 10$ on CUHK   (i) $L = 20$ on CUHK

Fig. 2. Precisions for labeling positive ADVs by Increasing Positive Prior (IPP) and Direct Selection with varying numbers (Q) of selected potential positive ADVs on (a)–(c) VIPeR [29], (d)–(f) PRID [30] and (g)–(i) CUHK [18].

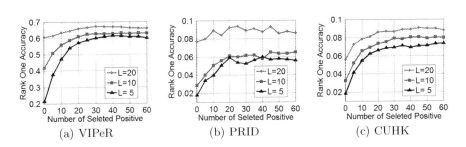

(a) VIPeR   (b) PRID   (c) CUHK

Fig. 3. Rank one accuracy for varying numbers (Q) of selected potential positive ADVs on 3 data sets: (a) VIPeR [29], (b) PRID [30] and (c) CUHK [18].

we can see that the re-identification performance degrades significantly when only few labeled positive image pairs, e.g., $L = 5, 10, 20$, are used for training. When all the training data are labeled, i.e., $L = All$, RSVM and RDC achieve

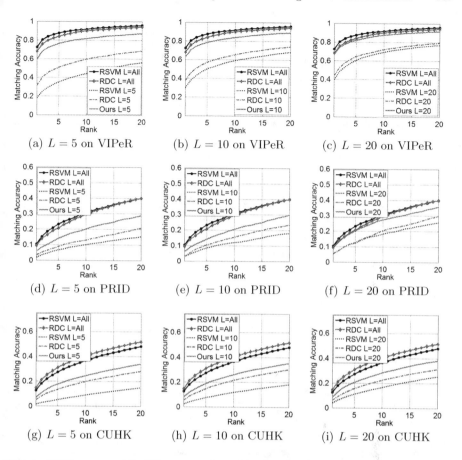

(a) $L = 5$ on VIPeR   (b) $L = 10$ on VIPeR   (c) $L = 20$ on VIPeR

(d) $L = 5$ on PRID   (e) $L = 10$ on PRID   (f) $L = 20$ on PRID

(g) $L = 5$ on CUHK   (h) $L = 10$ on CUHK   (i) $L = 20$ on CUHK

Fig. 4. CMC curves with different numbers ($L = 5, 10, 20$) of labeled image pairs on 3 datasets: (a)–(c) VIPeR [29], (d)–(f) PRID [30] and (g)–(i) CUHK [18].

around 70 % rank one accuracy on VIPeR dataset as shown in Fig. 4(a)[6]. However, when using only five labeled positive image pairs for training, the rank one accuracy degrades to about 20 % by RSVM and 30 % by RDC. This means the degradation of rank one accuracy can be up to about 50 % by RSVM and 40 % by RDC. The reason for these results is, the distance learning methods are over-fitted for the small amount of labeled data. Although both RSVM and RDC have a significant performance degradation, it is interesting to see in Figs. 4(a)–(i) that RDC outperforms RSVM on the three datasets when the

---

[6] Note that the feature used in our experiments is different from those in existing methods. It is very discriminative for VIPeR dataset, so it can achieve 70 % rank one accuracy using 316 matched image pairs for training. Such good performance may be due to the combination of foreground detection and global feature extraction (on a large region of an image) which is very effective for VIPeR dataset. It is interesting to conduct further investigation on this issue, but it is not the focus of this paper.

number of available labels is small. This indicates that RDC has better generalization ability by utilizing the advantages of second-order distance when few labeled data are available for training.

Comparing the proposed method with RSVM and RDC for $L = 5, 10, 20$, our method achieves significantly better ranking performance as shown in Figs. 4 (a)–(i). On VIPeR dataset, the rank one accuracy of our method is above 20 % higher than that of RSVM or RDC when the number of labeled positive image pairs are less than or equal to ten, i.e., $L = 5, 10$. This indicates that our method can significantly improve the performance for re-identification by using unlabeled data. On the other hand, Fig. 4(c) on VIPeR and Fig. 4(f) on PRID show that the CMC curves of our method using only 20 labeled positive image pairs are close to those of RSVM and RDC using all the labeled training data. These results indicate that our method can achieve convincing performance for person re-identification only with few labeled positive image pairs, which helps reduce the expensive cost needed for manual labeling.

5   Conclusion

In this paper, we have developed a novel Semi-Supervised Ranking method with Increased Positive Prior (SSR-IPP) for person re-identification using only few labeled positive image pairs. By analyzing the data distribution properties in person re-identification, we show that the widely used low density separation and graph propagation assumptions are not valid under certain conditions. In this context, we propose to iteratively add the most confident potential positive Absolute Difference Vector (ADV) from the unlabeled data for training. Since it suffers from a severe data imbalance problem in person re-identification, i.e., the number of positive image pairs is much smaller than that of negative ones, it is more likely to select a negative ADV from the unlabeled data. To increase the positive prior, we select the potential positive ADVs from the rank one matching subset in all the unlabeled data. Adding the selected potential positive ADVs to the regression based ranking problem, the confidence measure and weight vector are updated iteratively for the optimal solution.

Experimental results demonstrate that our method significantly outperforms state-of-the-art distance learning methods using only a small number of labeled positive image pairs for training. For example, the rank one accuracy of SSR-IPP is above 20 % higher than that of RSVM or RDC when the number of labeled positive image pairs are less or equal to ten. On the other hand, it is shown that the re-identification performance deteriorates dramatically when the number of labels is very small for training by existing methods. Since our method achieves convincing performance for re-identification with few matched image pairs, it can help reduce the expensive efforts needed for manual labeling. Moreover, our experiments also show that the second-order distance based Relative Distance Comparison (RDC) [17] method has better generalization ability than the first-order distance based Ranking Support Vector Machines (RSVM) [14] when the number of labeled positive image pairs is small. Since the proposed method is based on first-order distance, it is promising to study the development of second-order distance based semi-supervised ranking method for person re-identification.

Acknowledgement. The work is supported in part by ONR-N00014-13-1-0764, NSF-III-1360971, AFOSR-FA9550-13-1-0137, and NSF-Bigdata-1419210.

Appendix: Proof of Equation (12)

Suppose there are N_i^a images for person i under camera a and N_j^b images for person j under b. The number of positive matches for person i in both camera views is $N_i^a N_i^b$. Since the total numbers of images are $\sum_{i=1}^{J^a} N_i^a$ under camera view a and $\sum_{j=1}^{J^b} N_j^b$ under camera view b, the positive prior τ is calculated by

$$\tau = \frac{\sum_{i=1}^{J} N_i^a N_i^b}{\sum_{i=1}^{J^a} N_i^a \sum_{j=1}^{J^b} N_j^b} \tag{17}$$

The total number of image pairs in E_1 is equal to the number of groups $G_{m\cdot}$ and $G_{\cdot n}$, i.e., $\sum_{i=1}^{J^a} N_i^a + \sum_{j=1}^{J^b} N_j^b$. There are $\sum_{i=1}^{J} N_i^a$ groups $G_{m\cdot}$ and $\sum_{j=1}^{J} N_j^b$ groups $G_{\cdot n}$ containing at least one positive ADV. However, the classification function f may wrongly select a negative ADV from $G_{m\cdot}$ or $G_{\cdot n}$ that contains positive ADV(s). Thus, the number of ADVs in E_1 is $(\sum_{i=1}^{J} N_i^a + \sum_{j=1}^{J} N_j^b)c_1$, where c_1 is the rank one accuracy measuring the performance of f. Then, the positive prior τ_1 in E_1 is given by the following equation,

$$\tau_1 = \frac{(\sum_{i=1}^{J} N_i^a + \sum_{j=1}^{J} N_j^b)c_1}{\sum_{i=1}^{J^a} N_i^a + \sum_{j=1}^{J^b} N_j^b} \tag{18}$$

Since it is difficult to compare τ and τ_1 by (17) and (18) directly, we approximate them by assuming $N_i^a \approx \sum_{i'=1}^{J^a} N_{i'}^a / J^a$ and $N_j^b \approx \sum_{j'=1}^{J^b} N_{j'}^b / J^b$. Substituting the approximations of N_i^a and N_j^b into (17) and (18), respectively, τ and τ_1 become

$$\tau = \frac{J}{J^a J^b}, \qquad \tau_1 = \frac{(\frac{J}{J^a}\sum_{i=1}^{J^a} N_i^a + \frac{J}{J^b}\sum_{j=1}^{J^b} N_j^b)c_1}{\sum_{i=1}^{J^a} N_i^a + \sum_{j=1}^{J^b} N_j^b} \geq \frac{Jc_1}{\max(J^a, J^b)} \tag{19}$$

If $\max(1/J^a, 1/J^b) \ll c_1$, multiplying $J^a J^b$ on both sides, we obtain $\max(J^a, J^b) \ll J^a J^b c_1$. Thus, $\tau \ll \tau_1$, which leads to (12).

References

1. Bąk, S., Corvée, E., Brémond, F., Thonnat, M.: Boosted human re-identification using riemannian manifolds. Image Vis. Comput. **30**, 443–452 (2010)

2. Farenzena, M., Bazzani, L., Perina, A., Murino, V., Cristani, M.: Person re-identification by symmetry-driven accumulation of local features. In: CVPR (2010)

3. Bauml, M., Stiefelhagen, R.: Evaluation of local features for person re-identification in image sequences. In: AVSS (2011)

4. Cheng, D.S., Cristani, M., Stoppa, M., Bazzani, L., Murino, V.: Custom pictorial structures for re-identification. In: BMVC (2011)

5. Doretto, G., Sebastian, T., Tu, P., Rittscher, J.: Appearance-based person reidentification in camera networks: problem overview and current approaches. JAIHC **2**, 127–151 (2011)

6. Jungling, K., Arens, M.: View-invariant person re-identification with an implicit shape model. In: AVSS (2011)

7. Bazzani, L., Cristani, M., Perina, A., Murino, V.: Multiple-shot person re-identification by chromatic and epitomic analyses. Pattern Recogn. Lett. **33**, 898–903 (2012)

8. Bąk, S., Charpiat, G., Corvée, E., Brémond, F., Thonnat, M.: Learning to match appearances by correlations in a covariance metric space. In: Fitzgibbon, A., Lazebnik, S., Perona, P., Sato, Y., Schmid, C. (eds.) ECCV 2012, Part III. LNCS, vol. 7574, pp. 806–820. Springer, Heidelberg (2012)

9. Ma, B., Su, Y., Jurie, F.: BiCov: a novel image representation for person re-identification and face verification. In: BMVC (2012)

10. Kviatkovsky, I., Adam, A., Rivlin, E.: Color invariants for person reidentification. TPAMI **35**, 1622–1634 (2013)

11. Zhao, R., Ouyang, W., Wang, X.: Unsupervised salience learning for person re-identification. In: CVPR (2013)

12. Xu, Y., Lin, L., Zheng, W.S., Liu, X.: Human re-identification by matching compositional template with cluster sampling. In: ICCV (2013)

13. Gray, D., Tao, H.: Viewpoint invariant pedestrian recognition with an ensemble of localized features. In: Forsyth, D., Torr, P., Zisserman, A. (eds.) ECCV 2008, Part I. LNCS, vol. 5302, pp. 262–275. Springer, Heidelberg (2008)

14. Prosser, B., Zheng, W.S., Gong, S., Xiang, T.: Person re-identification by support vector ranking. In: BMVC (2010)

15. Avraham, T., Gurvich, I., Lindenbaum, M., Markovitch, S.: Learning implicit transfer for person re-identification. In: Fusiello, A., Murino, V., Cucchiara, R. (eds.) ECCV 2012 Ws/Demos, Part I. LNCS, vol. 7583, pp. 381–390. Springer, Heidelberg (2012)

16. Hirzer, M., Roth, P.M., Köstinger, M., Bischof, H.: Relaxed pairwise learned metric for person re-identification. In: Fitzgibbon, A., Lazebnik, S., Perona, P., Sato, Y., Schmid, C. (eds.) ECCV 2012, Part VI. LNCS, vol. 7577, pp. 780–793. Springer, Heidelberg (2012)

17. Zheng, W.S., Gong, S., Xiang, T.: Reidentification by relative distance comparison. TPAMI **35**, 653–668 (2013)

18. Li, W., Wang, X.: Locally aligned feature transforms across views. In: CVPR (2013)

19. Liu, C., Loy, C.C., Gong, S., Wang, G.: POP: Person re-identification post-rank optimisation. In: ICCV (2013)

20. Zhao, R., Ouyang, W., Wang, X.: Person re-identification by salience matching. In: ICCV (2013)

21. Ma, A.J., Yuen, P.C., Li, J.: Domain transfer support vector ranking for person re-identification without target camera label information. In: ICCV (2013)

22. Chapelle, O., Schölkopf, B., Zien, A., et al.: Semi-supervised Learning, vol. 2. MIT Press, Cambridge (2006)

23. Zhu, X.: Semi-supervised learning literature survey. Computer Science, University of Wisconsin - Madison (2008)
24. Figueira, D., Bazzani, L., Minh, H.Q., Cristani, M., Bernardino, A., Murino, V.: Semi-supervised multi-feature learning for person re-identification. In: AVSS (2013)
25. Bäuml, M., Tapaswi, M., Stiefelhagen, R.: Semi-supervised learning with constraints for person identification in multimedia data. In: CVPR (2013)
26. Iqbal, U., Curcio, I.D.D., Gabbouj, M.: Who is the hero? - semi-supervised person re-identification in videos. In: VISAPP (2014)
27. Amini, M.R., Truong, T.V., Goutte, C.: A boosting algorithm for learning bipartite ranking functions with partially labeled data. In: SIGIR (2008)
28. Hoi, S.C., Jin, R.: Semi-supervised ensemble ranking. In: AAAI (2008)
29. Gray, D., Brennan, S., Tao, H.: Evaluating appearance models for recognition, reacquisition, and tracking. In: IEEE International Workshop on Performance Evaluation for Tracking and Surveillance (2007)
30. Hirzer, M., Beleznai, C., Roth, P.M., Bischof, H.: Person re-identification by descriptive and discriminative classification. In: Heyden, A., Kahl, F. (eds.) SCIA 2011. LNCS, vol. 6688, pp. 91–102. Springer, Heidelberg (2011)
31. Tian, Y., Zitnick, C.L., Narasimhan, S.G.: Exploring the spatial hierarchy of mixture models for human pose estimation. In: Fitzgibbon, A., Lazebnik, S., Perona, P., Sato, Y., Schmid, C. (eds.) ECCV 2012, Part V. LNCS, vol. 7576, pp. 256–269. Springer, Heidelberg (2012)

Robust Visual Tracking with Dual Group Structure

Fu Li, Huchuan Lu$^{(\boxtimes)}$, and Dong Wang

Dalian University of Technology, Dalian, China
lifu.dlut@gmail.com, {lhchuan,wdice}@dlut.edu.cn

Abstract. The "sparse representation"-based tracking framework generally considers the testing candidates and dictionary atoms individually, thus failing to model the structured information within data. In this paper, we present a robust tracking framework by exploiting the *dual group structure* of both candidate samples and dictionary templates, and formulate the sparse representation at group level. The similar samples are encoded simultaneously by a few atom groups, which induces the inter-group sparsity, and also each group enjoys different internal sparsity. In this way, not only the potential commonality shared by the related candidates is taken into account, but also the individual differences between samples are reflected. Then we provide an effective optimization method to solve our formulation by two stages: thresholding and computing with the accelerated proximal gradient method. Finally, we embed the dual group structure model into the particle filter framework for visual tracking. Extensive experimental results demonstrate that our tracker achieves favorable performance against the state-of-the-art tracking methods.

1 Introduction

As one of the most active research topics in recent years, sparse representation (SR) has been widely investigated in numerous practical fields (such as face recognition [1], image restoration [2], object tracking [3] and so on), and achieves quite satisfactory performance. The fundamental assumption of the SR framework is that testing samples from each class reside on a low-dimensional linear subspace which is spanned by the training samples belonging to the given class. Therefore, every testing sample can be approximately represented by a set of training samples (dubbed dictionary) with the sparse constraint.

Tracking can generally be categorized into generative methods (e.g., [4–6]) and discriminative methods (e.g., [7–9]). As a generative tracking model, SR has been extensively studied in the past several years (e.g., [10–12]). In the "sparse representation"-based tracking framework, the samples collected from the first frame and subsequent tracking results are often directly used as the dictionary atoms, and then the ℓ_1 minimization problem attempts to seek for a sparse representation of the testing sample by selecting a few columns of the dictionary. However, treating the dictionary atoms individually suffers several disadvantages [13,14]. Due to the ignorance of the underlying commonality shared by dictionary

© Springer International Publishing Switzerland 2015
D. Cremers et al. (Eds.): ACCV 2014, Part IV, LNCS 9006, pp. 614–629, 2015.
DOI: 10.1007/978-3-319-16817-3_40

atoms, it tends to make selection based on the strength of individual column rather than the strength of groups of similar atoms. Thus, in the SR framework, it is prone to select only one atom from the group and does not care which one is selected.

In the tracking problem, the dictionary enjoys the group property due to the temporal continuity and appearance similarity. For one thing, the tracked object usually undergoes small motions between two consecutive frames. For another, as time proceeds, the target may share similar appearance with that in some previous time. By clustering the dictionary atoms into several groups, we can represent a candidate with a few groups, rather than individual atoms. The active groups include semblable templates with the testing candidate, and representation based on multiple templates contributes to more robust tracking.

Many of current tracking algorithms are based on the Particle Filter (PF) framework, in which hundreds of particles are drawn based on the state of the previous frame and used to depict the appearance of the tracked object. In these methods, the SR method is straightforwardly applied to each testing sample for obtaining the sparse coefficients, in which both dictionary atoms and candidate samples are treated to be individual. Although this manner is simple and easy to be implemented, it is not very satisfactory as it completely ignores the structured information within dictionary atoms and within candidate samples, and it is also computationally expensive by verifying a large number of candidate samples individually. To consider the potential relationships among candidates, Zhang et al. [5] design a SR-based tracker based on the $\ell_{2,1}$-norm, which sparsely codes all candidate samples simultaneously. The regularizer based on $\ell_{2,1}$-norm encourages all samples to share the same sparsity pattern and exploits the underlying relationships among different candidate samples. However, since there always exist obvious differences between candidates, this compulsive constraint may lead to undesirable results. Because of the densely sampling strategy, the appearance of some candidates may be very similar, and therefore we can divide candidate samples into some disjointed groups. To reveal the common characteristics among samples in a group, they are encoded jointly and represented by the same atom groups. In addition, we adopt the ℓ_1 norm to account for the variation between individuals, thereby inducing sparsity within group. Finally, the subgroup with the minimum reconstruction error is selected and the weighted sum over all particles in this selected group is regarded as the final state, which would lead to more robust and stable results than only picking one candidate.

In this paper, we propose a novel tracking formulation exploiting the group structure of both candidate samples and dictionary atoms, which we name *Dual Group Structure*. The structured information within candidate samples considers the potential commonality shared by the related samples, ensuring that data with similar appearance are encoded jointly and bringing large gains in terms of computational efficiency. The structural information within dictionary atoms encourages the grouping effect of coefficients, leading to the selection of a group of atoms which come from the same set rather than an individual atom. Moreover, the sparse-inducing regularizer yields sparsity at both the group and atom level, that is, not only a few groups of atoms are active at a time, but also each group enjoys internal sparsity. In this way, samples from the same class will share group properties, but will not necessarily share the full active sets as they are not identical. The solution to our model can be achieved by using two basic stages: thresholding and computing. Finally, we embed the proposed dual group structure model into the particle filter framework for visual tracking, and adopt challenging image sequences to evaluate the proposed tracker. The experimental results demonstrate the effectiveness of the proposed tracking algorithm in comparison with other competing trackers.

Contributions: The contributions of this work can be summarized into three folds. (1) We exploit the underlying structured information of similar candidates and similar dictionary atoms, and formulate the sparse representation process at the group level. Each sample group is represented by a few atom groups, and inside each atom group only a few members are active at a time. By using this manner, it not only makes full use of the commonality shared by data from the same group, but also takes the differences between individuals into consideration. (2) We provide an efficient optimization procedure by using the Accelerated Proximal Gradient (APG) method. The solution process includes a matrix thresholding and a vector thresholding, naturally yielding to the desired inter-group and intra-group sparsity pattern. (3) We design a generative tracker based on the proposed dual group structure model. Numerous experiments show that the proposed tracking algorithm achieves favorable performance against many state-of-the-art trackers.

2   Related Work

Group Sparse Coding: In recent years, the group property in the SR framework (often called group sparsity) has drawn interesting attentions (such as [15–17] and so on), where dictionary atoms are often divided into several disjointed groups. Given these group memberships, the task is to seek for a solution where a query sample is represented by only a small set of the groups, rather than a few atoms. Yuan and Lin [13] first propose the group lasso criterion for this problem, which exploits the sum of ℓ_2-norm to set most of group coefficients to be exactly zeros. While the group lasso method can provide a sparse set of groups, it fails to consider the sparsity property within each group. To model both sparsity of groups and within each group, Friedman *et al.* [18] present the sparse group lasso by adding an additional ℓ_1-norm regularization term. This model achieves the effect of promoting group selection while at the same time leading to overall sparse feature selection. Based on this theory, several works focus on the practical applications to computer vision. Elhamifar and Vidal [19] cast the face classification problem as a structured sparse recovery problem, the goal of which is to approximate the testing sample by using the minimum number of blocks from the dictionary. Zhang *et al.* [20] utilize the group sparsity properties in feature selection for the image annotation task, which leverages both sparsity and clustering priors to prune the features. Liu *et al.* [21] use a dynamic group sparsity scheme to exploit temporal and spatial relationship for object tracking, which can be solved by a two stage optimization approach. However, all these approaches sparsely code the testing samples individually and do not consider the latent similarities among different samples, thus will causing heavy computational load and the loss of structured information among data.

Simultaneous Sparse Coding: Another line of group coding, dubbed simultaneous sparse coding, offers a solution that involves the potential relation among samples by coding all testing data jointly. Based on the assumption that features or data within a group are expected to share the same sparsity pattern in their representations, a mixed $\ell_{2,1}$-norm is employed to make all the column vectors of the coefficient matrix look alike. Mairal et al. [2] jointly decompose groups of similar patches on the dictionary and combine the non-local means and sparse coding approaches to image restoration within a unified framework. Zhang et al. [5] employ mixed norms to enforce the joint sparsity and learn particle representations together to improve the tracking performance. Chi et al. [16] propose the affine-constrained group sparse coding and extend the sparse representation framework to classification problems with multiple inputs. However, these methods treat the dictionary atoms individually, and thus cannot lead to sparsity in group level. Furthermore, the constraint of forcing these similar yet not identical samples to have the same representations is relatively strong.

Our Work: The proposed formulation takes advantage of the structural constraints of both dictionary atoms and testing samples. On one hand, instead of considering the atoms as singletons, we divide the atoms into groups, with a few of groups active at a time. On the other hand, multiple similar samples are encoded simultaneously, requesting that they all share the same active set. Besides the common characteristics, the sparsity regularizer within each group is added to account for the intrinsic differences between individuals.

3 Problem Formulation

Given a set of observed samples $\mathbf{X} = [\mathbf{x}_1, \mathbf{x}_2, ..., \mathbf{x}_n] \in \mathbb{R}^{m \times n}$, where each column $\mathbf{x}_i$ can be the vectorized image or extracted feature vector, the task is to encode these samples by a dictionary $\mathbf{D} = [\mathbf{d}_1, \mathbf{d}_2, ..., \mathbf{d}_k] \in \mathbb{R}^{m \times k}$ (the column vector $\mathbf{d}_i$ denotes the i-th atom of the dictionary $\mathbf{D}$). By solving some optimization problems, the coefficient matrix $\mathbf{S} = [\mathbf{s}_1, \mathbf{s}_2, ..., \mathbf{s}_n] \in \mathbb{R}^{k \times n}$ can be obtained as the encodings of $\mathbf{X}$, with one column corresponding to one sample. Recently, many sparse-inducing regularizers have been proposed in the literature (e.g., [15,22]), and most of them are based on the sparse-promoting property of the ℓ_1 norm.

In order to achieve group sparsity, we can suppose that the k atoms are divided into $\mathcal{G}$ groups (classes). For ease of notation, we use a matrix $\mathbf{D}^{(g)}$ to represent the set of atoms within the g-th group, and adopt a matrix $\mathbf{S}^{(g)}$ to stand for the corresponding coefficients. Then for each individual sample $\mathbf{x}_i$, the sparse group lasso criterion [18] is formulated as follows:

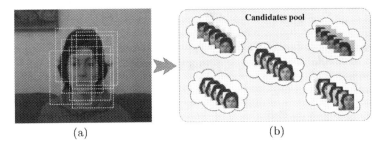

(a)   (b)

Fig. 1. (a) The dense sampling strategy in particle filter framework. (b) The collected candidate samples. We can see they are of strong correlations, and thus can be divided into several groups.

$$\min_{\mathbf{s}_i} \frac{1}{2} \|\mathbf{x}_i - \sum_{g=1}^{\mathcal{G}} \mathbf{D}^{(g)} \mathbf{s}_i^{(g)}\|_2^2 + \lambda_1 \sum_{g=1}^{\mathcal{G}} \|\mathbf{s}_i^{(g)}\|_2 + \lambda_2 \sum_{g=1}^{\mathcal{G}} \|\mathbf{s}_i^{(g)}\|_1, \tag{1}$$

where $\|\cdot\|_2$ and $\|\cdot\|_1$ denote the ℓ_2-norm and ℓ_1-norm respectively, parameters λ_1 and λ_2 control the balance between the two regularization terms.

It can be seen from Eq. (1) that the sparse group lasso method takes the structured information within the dictionary by using an ℓ_2-norm constraint on the coefficients of each group. However, it fails to model the relationships among data samples (i.e., to exploit the structured information of similar samples in $\mathbf{X}$), which is not a good candidate method to solve many vision problems (such as visual tracking). In the "particle filter"-based tracking framework, the candidates are usually densely sampled according to the object's state in the last frame. Thus, these candidate samples are of strong correlations (i.e., have sufficient structured information), as shown in Fig. 1.

In order to exploit the structured information of similar samples in $\mathbf{X}$, we also classify the n data samples into $\mathcal{L}$ groups (classes) based on some criterion. For example, if data is image patch, each group may be the set of patches in a particular image; if instances are human faces, then each group may consist of facial images from one person under different illumination, pose and expression conditions. Likewise, we denote $\mathbf{X}^{(l)}$ as the submatrix correlated to the l-th group and sparsely code one group data jointly. Thus, we can define our objective function as

$$\min_{\mathbf{S}} \frac{1}{2} \|\mathbf{X}^{(l)} - \sum_{g=1}^{\mathcal{G}} \mathbf{D}^{(g)} \mathbf{S}^{(g)}\|_F^2 + \lambda_1 \sum_{g=1}^{\mathcal{G}} \|\mathbf{S}^{(g)}\|_F + \lambda_2 \sum_{g=1}^{\mathcal{G}} \|\mathbf{S}^{(g)}\|_1, \tag{2}$$

where $\|\cdot\|_F$ is the Frobenius norm of matrix. The sum of the F-norm regularizer induces the sparsity in group level, while ℓ_1-norm encourages sparsity in an individual level. It means that samples in $\mathbf{X}^{(l)}$ share group properties as they are from the same class, but will not share the active sets since they are not identical.

We thereby obtain a collaborative sparse model, with the cooperation to identify the class labels by all samples, and the freedom at the individual level inside

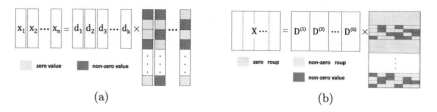

(a)   (b)

Fig. 2. (a) Sparse representation where both testing samples and dictionary atoms are treated to be individual, thus there are no relations among the learned coefficients. (b) Dual group structure model where the coefficient matrix enjoys group sparsity and in-group sparsity. Not only a few of groups are selected, but also in each group, minority of elements admit non-zero values.

the group to adapt to each particular image. The objective function in Eq. (2) is the sum of three convex functions, and thus, the optimization problem (2) is a convex one. In Sect. 3.1, we will provide an effective solution to this problem. The sparsity patterns of SR and our model are illustrated in Fig. 2.

Here, we note that $\sum_{g=1}^{\mathcal{G}} \|\mathbf{S}^{(g)}\|_1 = \sum_{i=1}^{n} \|\mathbf{s}_i\|_1$. When $\lambda_1 = 0$, the grouping effect is neglected, then Eq. (2) reduces to the original sparse representation (lasso) problem [23]. If each individual sample is treated as a group, the optimization problem in Eq. (2) reduces to the sparse group lasso problem [18]. In addition, when $\lambda_2 = 0$ and all dictionary atoms are treated as a single group, the Eq. (2) turns into the multi-task learning problem with the mixed $\ell_{1,1}$-norm [5]. Therefore, we can conclude that all three above-mentioned problems can be viewed as special cases of the proposed formulation.

3.1   Theoretical Calculation

Since Eq. (2) with the ℓ_1-regularization is non-differentiable at zero, the standard unconstrained optimization methods cannot be applied directly. In the following, we develop an optimization method based upon coordinate descent to solve this problem. The formulation can be separable with respect to $\mathbf{S}^{(g)}$, and thus we can update $\mathbf{S}^{(g)}$ individually by fixing other group coefficients. For each subproblem, the solution can be obtained from two stages: thresholding and computing.

Formally, the submatrix $\mathbf{S}^{(g)}$ is obtained by solving the following optimization problem:

$$\mathbf{S}^{(g)} = \arg\min_{\mathbf{Z}} \frac{1}{2}\|\mathbf{R} - \mathbf{DZ}\|_F^2 + \lambda_1\|\mathbf{Z}\|_F + \lambda_2\|\mathbf{Z}\|_1, \qquad (3)$$

where $\mathbf{R} = \mathbf{X}^{(l)} - \sum_{j \neq g} \mathbf{D}^{(j)}\mathbf{S}^{(j)}$ is the residual.

Thresholding: We first check whether the elements of $\mathbf{Z}$ are all zeros, which means the corresponding atom group is not activated. Let $f = \frac{1}{2}\|\mathbf{R} - \mathbf{DZ}\|_F^2$, then the subgradient of the function $\frac{1}{2}\|\mathbf{R} - \mathbf{DZ}\|_F^2 + \lambda_1\|\mathbf{Z}\|_F + \lambda_2\|\mathbf{Z}\|_1$ with respect to each Z_{ij} is:

$$\nabla f + \lambda_1 P_{ij} + \lambda_2 T_{ij}, \quad \forall\, i, j \tag{4}$$

where matrices $\mathbf{P}$ and $\mathbf{T}$ are the subgradient matrices of F-norm and ℓ_1-norm of $\mathbf{Z}$ respectively. The element $P_{ij} = Z_{ij}/\|\mathbf{Z}\|_F$ if $\mathbf{Z}$ is not a null matrix, and otherwise $\mathbf{P}$ is a matrix satisfying $\|\mathbf{P}\|_F \leq 1$. Similarly, the element $T_{ij} = sign(Z_{ij})$ if $Z_{ij} \neq 0$, and $T_{ij} \in [-1, 1]$ if $Z_{ij} = 0$. Moreover, when $\mathbf{Z} = \mathbf{0}$, we can obtain that the first term $\nabla f = -A_{ij}$, where $\mathbf{A} = \mathbf{D}^\top \mathbf{R}$.

To achieve group sparsity, we focus on the case where $\mathbf{Z}$ is a null matrix, then a necessary and sufficient condition for $\mathbf{Z}$ to be zero is that the system of equations,

$$A_{ij} = \lambda_1 P_{ij} + \lambda_2 T_{ij}, \quad \forall\, i, j \tag{5}$$

has a solution with $\|\mathbf{P}\|_F \leq 1$ and $T_{ij} \in [-1, 1]$. With some mathematical manipulations, we can determine this by minimizing the function of $\mathbf{T}$:

$$J(\mathbf{T}) = (1/\lambda_1{}^2) \sum_{i,j} (A_{ij} - \lambda_2 T_{ij})^2 = \sum_{i,j} P_{ij}^2 \tag{6}$$

with respect to $T_{ij} \in [-1, 1]$ and then check if $J(\hat{\mathbf{T}}) \leq 1$. The minimizer is easily seen to be

$$\hat{T}_{ij} = \begin{cases} \frac{A_{ij}}{\lambda_2}, & |\frac{A_{ij}}{\lambda_2}| \leq 1 \\ sign(\frac{A_{ij}}{\lambda_2}), & |\frac{A_{ij}}{\lambda_2}| > 1 \end{cases} \tag{7}$$

and we can compute $J(\hat{\mathbf{T}})$ by Eq. (6). If $J(\hat{\mathbf{T}}) \leq 1$, then we directly set $\mathbf{Z} = \mathbf{0}$ and proceed to solve for the next submatrix.

Computing: Now in the case where $J(\hat{\mathbf{T}}) > 1$, we can see that Eq. (3) is actually the sum of a convex differential function (the first two terms) and a separable penalty, and hence we can employ the APG method to efficiently solve this convex optimization problem. As compared to traditional projected gradient methods, the APG method achieves an $\mathcal{O}(\frac{1}{t^2})$ residual from the optimal solution after t iterations with quadratic convergence [24]. Specifically, APG proceeds the iterative update between the current coefficient matrix $\mathbf{Z}_t$ and an aggregation matrix $\mathbf{V}_t$. Each APG iteration consists of two steps: (1) a generalized gradient mapping step that updates $\mathbf{Z}_t$ with $\mathbf{V}_t$ fixed, where in general an analytic solution is needed to ensure the materialization of APG, and (2) an updating step that promotes $\mathbf{V}_t$ by linearly combining $\mathbf{Z}_{t+1}$ and $\mathbf{Z}_t$.

(1) Gradient Mapping: Given the current estimate $\mathbf{V}_t$, we obtain $\mathbf{Z}_{t+1}$ by solving the following equation:

$$\mathbf{Z}_{t+1} = \arg\min_{\mathbf{Y}} \frac{1}{2} \|\mathbf{Y} - \mathbf{H}\|_F^2 + \tilde{\lambda} \|\mathbf{Y}\|_1, \tag{8}$$

where $\tilde{\lambda} = \eta \lambda_2$ and η is a small step parameter. Denote $g = \frac{1}{2}\|\mathbf{R} - \mathbf{D}\mathbf{V}_t\|_F^2 + \lambda_1 \|\mathbf{V}_t\|_F$, then

$$\begin{aligned} \mathbf{H} &= \mathbf{V}_t - \eta \nabla g_t \\ &= \mathbf{V}_t - \eta \mathbf{D}^\top (\mathbf{D}\mathbf{V}_t - \mathbf{R}) - \eta \lambda_1 \frac{\mathbf{V}_t}{\|\mathbf{V}_t\|_F}. \end{aligned} \tag{9}$$

We decouple Eq. (8) into several disjoint subproblems, one for each row vector $\mathbf{z}^i$:

$$\mathbf{z}^i_{t+1} = \arg\min_{\mathbf{y}^i} \frac{1}{2}\|\mathbf{y}^i - \mathbf{h}^i\|^2_F + \tilde{\lambda}\|\mathbf{y}^i\|_1. \tag{10}$$

Each subproblem is a variant of the projection problem unto the ℓ_1 ball. The optimization can be solved by a soft-thresholding method and the solution is obtained as $\mathbf{z}^i_{t+1} = \mathcal{S}_{\tilde{\lambda}}(\mathbf{h}^i)$, where $\mathcal{S}_{\tilde{\lambda}}$ is the soft-thresholding operator defined as $\mathcal{S}_{\tilde{\lambda}}(a) = sign(a)\max(0, |a| - \tilde{\lambda})$. Note that the $\max(\cdot)$ operator induces the sparsity within group, and samples in the same group enjoy different sparsity patterns.

(2) Updating: We update $\mathbf{V}_t$ as follows:

$$\mathbf{V}_{t+1} = \mathbf{Z}_{t+1} + \alpha_{t+1}(\frac{1}{\alpha_t} - 1)(\mathbf{Z}_{t+1} - \mathbf{Z}_t), \tag{11}$$

where α_t is conventionally set to $\frac{2}{t+3}$. We summarize the algorithm of the APG computing stage in Algorithm 2.

Suppose the number of samples in group g is ρ_g. The computational complexity in thresholding step concentrates on the multiplication of matrices, i.e., the calculation of matrix $\mathbf{A}$, and thus the complexity is $\mathcal{O}(mn\rho_g)$. While in the second stage, the computational complexity is dominated by the gradient computation in Eq. (9) and the soft-thresholding operation in Eq. (10). Similarly, the complexity of Eq. (9) is $\mathcal{O}(mn\rho_g)$, while that of Eq. (10) is $\mathcal{O}(n\rho_g)$. Thus the total complexity of one iteration is $\mathcal{O}((2m+1)n\rho_g)$, linear with respect to the group size ρ_g, therefore the solution can be obtained efficiently.

Our overall algorithm is summarized in Algorithm 1. The convergence is achieved when the relative change in solution falls below a predefined tolerance after several cyclic iterations.

3.2   Noise Handling

In the noisy scenarios, samples are often corrupted by noise or partially occluded. To deal with the unknown corruption, a set of trivial templates are added after the dictionary as in the previous works [1,3]. Then the occluded part is modeled as sparsely additive noises that can take on large values anywhere in the representation.

We employ the identity matrix $\mathbf{I}$ as the trivial atoms, and the corresponding coefficient matrix is denoted as $\mathbf{S}^{(I)}$. The nonzero entries of $\mathbf{S}^{(I)}$ indicate the pixels in sample that are corrupted or occluded. We regard all trivial templates as an atom group and along with other groups solve Eq. (2) to obtain the coefficients. In this way, a set of occluded samples can be represented by both the related dictionary group of the same class and the trivial group.

Algorithm 1. Learning dual group regularized sparse codes

Input: sample matrix $\mathbf{X}$, dictionary $\mathbf{D}$, sample group set $\{1, 2, \ldots, \mathcal{L}\}$, atom group set $\{1, 2, \ldots, \mathcal{G}\}$, regularization parameters λ_1 and λ_2, learning step η
Output: coefficient matrix $\mathbf{S}$

---

1. Initialize $\mathbf{S} = \mathbf{0}$
2. **For** $l = 1$ to $\mathcal{L}$
3.   Initiativly set $g = 1$
4.   Calculate $\mathbf{R} = \mathbf{X}^{(l)} - \sum_{j \neq g} \mathbf{D}^{(j)} \mathbf{S}^{(j)}$, $\mathbf{A} = \mathbf{D}^{\top} \mathbf{R}$
5.   Compute $J(\hat{\mathbf{T}})$ according to Eq. (6) and Eq. (7)
6.   Check whether $J(\hat{\mathbf{T}}) \leq 1$. If so, set $\mathbf{S}^{(g)} = \mathbf{0}$ and proceed to step 7 for the next group directly. Otherwise go to step 6
7.   Compute $\mathbf{S}^{(g)}$ using Algorithm 2
8.   If $g == \mathcal{G}$, reset $g = 1$, else update $g = g + 1$
9.   Iterate the cyclic optimization for $g = 1, 2, \ldots, \mathcal{G}, 1, 2, \ldots$ until convergence
10. **End**
11. **Return** coefficient matrix $\mathbf{S}$

Algorithm 2. learning coefficient with the APG method

Input: residual matrix $\mathbf{R}$, dictionary $\mathbf{D}$, warm start $\mathbf{Z}$, learning steps η and $\tilde{\lambda}$
Output: Coefficient matrix $\mathbf{Z}$.

---

1. Initialize $t = 0$, $\alpha_t = 1$
2. If $\mathbf{Z}$ is null matrix, set $\mathbf{Z}_0 = \mathbf{1}$, else $\mathbf{Z}_0 = \mathbf{Z}$. $\mathbf{V}_0 = \mathbf{Z}_0$.
3. **While** not converged **do:**
4.   Compute $\mathbf{H}$ according to Eq. (9)
5.   Solve the subproblem Eq. (10) to obtain $\mathbf{Z}_{t+1}$
6.   Set $\alpha_{t+1} = \frac{2}{t+3}$.
7.   Update $\mathbf{V}_{t+1}$ by Eq. (11)
8. $t = t + 1$.
9. **End**
10. **Return** coefficient matrix $\mathbf{Z}$

3.3   Visual Tracking

For object tracking task, the tracking results are usually directly used as the dictionary atoms. Since the target object often undergoes various pose changes in the tracking process, the dictionary covers diversity of the appearance variations of the target. Therefore, these dictionary atoms enjoy the group structure of the consecutive tracking results or the similar appearance at different time. We cluster these atoms using K-means method. By sparse group coding, the correct target sample is reconstructed by sparse grouped templates.

When the new frame arrives, large amount of candidates are drawn around the target location in the previous frame. Individually treating them could be computationally expensive. To explore the structural information of positions and features among candidates, we also divide these samples into several disjointed groups according to their coordinates and appearance. Denote

$\phi = [x, y, \mathbf{q}^\top]^\top$ as the extracted feature from a candidate, where x and y are the coordinates, $\mathbf{q}$ is a response vector such as intensity, color or gradients, then the candidates can be clustered by K-means or spectral clustering method. We can also add some weights on the coordinates to adjust their contributions.

For each candidate group $\mathbf{X}^{(l)}$, we compute the corresponding coefficient matrix using Eq. (2), and obtain the reconstruction error only by the best dictionary atom subset:

$$e(l) = \min_g \|\mathbf{X}^{(l)} - \mathbf{D}^{(g)}\mathbf{S}^{(g)}\|_F^2. \tag{12}$$

The best group with the minimum error e is then picked out. The weighted sum over all particles in this group is taken as the final target location, where the weight of each particle is inversely proportional to the reconstruction error. We update the dictionary by replacing the old templates with the new coming tracking results and re-cluster it every five frames. The occlusion handling strategy in [12] is adopted to prevent the blocked part from being updated into the dictionary.

4   Experiments

4.1   Sparsity Pattern

To demonstrate the effectiveness of the proposed method, we first conduct experiments on the ORL face database [25] and examine the sparsity pattern of the learned coefficient matrix. The ORL database contains 400 frontal face images of 40 subjects under different pose and expression conditions. Each face image is scaled to 48×48 pixels and normalized in the preprocessing. A subset with half numbers per individual is collected to form the training set. Images with the same labels are clustered into one atom group and these groups are arranged in the order from label 1 to 40. Note that in the testing stage, the image is not labeled one by one, instead we treat the testing faces of one subject as a whole, and estimate the belonging of this group.

The sparsity patterns of all 40 subjects are illustrated in Fig. 3(a) ordered by the true label, with the red line indicating the group splitting line in each pattern. In the ideal condition, the testing group is represented by only the atom group of the same class, thus resulting in that the non-zero values concentrate on the diagonal line from the overall point of view. For example, in the coefficient relating to the first person, the elements corresponding to the first atom group enjoy most large non-zero values, and thus this atom group admits the minimum reconstruction error and shares the same label with the testing group. Due to the presence of noise, there may exist non-zero entries in other groups. In addition, the convergence curve is shown in Fig. 3(b). We can see that our algorithm could reach convergence smoothly after several iterations without vibrations.

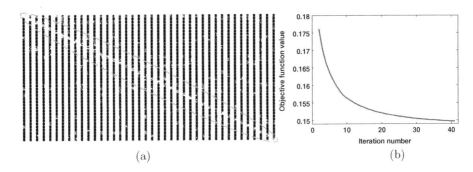

(a)   (b)

Fig. 3. (a) Illustration of the coefficient matrix of all 40 subjects in ORL face database. The white entries indicate the non-zero values while the black ones represent zero elements. (b) Convergence curve.

4.2   Tracking Experiments

In the implementation, each target is initialized manually by a bounding box in the first frame. We resize each image region to 32×32 pixels for post-processing. The parameters λ_1, λ_2 and η are set to 0.01, 0.01 and 0.1 in all experiments. As a trade-off between effectiveness and speed, 600 particles are adopted and our tracker is incrementally updated every 5 frames. The number of atom groups and candidate groups are set to 5 and 10, respectively.

We evaluate the performance of the proposed method on sixteen challenging sequences from [26] and our own. The challenges of these videos include partial occlusion, illumination variation, pose change, deformation and scale change. The proposed tracker is compared with twelve state-of-the-art algorithms including the MIL [7], IVT [27], TLD [28], VTD [29], MTT [5], CT [9], ℓ_1-APG [10], NDLT [30], LSHT [31], SCM [32], STK [8], PBT [33] methods. Both qualitative and quantitative comparative results are presented below.

Table 1. Success rate. The top two results are shown in red and blue fonts respectively.

	MIL	IVT	TLD	VTD	MTT	CT	ℓ_1-APG	NDLT	LSHT	SCM	STK	PBT	OURS
Car4	0.27	1.00	0.86	1.00	0.38	0.27	1.00	1.00	0.27	1.00	0.28	0.39	1.00
David2	0.33	0.88	0.96	0.99	1.00	0.01	1.00	0.96	0.99	0.91	1.00	0.99	0.98
David3	0.35	0.61	0.18	0.53	0.56	0.32	0.05	0.67	0.75	0.58	0.68	0.57	0.98
Faceocc1	0.76	1.00	0.78	0.97	1.00	0.66	1.00	1.00	1.00	1.00	0.96	1.00	1.00
Skater	0.94	0.88	0.48	0.98	1.00	0.95	0.81	0.41	0.16	0.87	0.44	1.00	1.00
Crossing	0.99	0.23	0.52	0.42	0.23	0.99	0.25	0.82	0.44	1.00	0.96	0.99	1.00
Jogging	0.16	0.19	0.86	0.16	0.16	0.15	0.19	0.17	0.15	0.89	0.18	0.17	1.00
Seq1	0.34	0.21	0.94	0.45	0.31	0.23	0.99	0.21	0.94	0.99	0.68	0.45	1.00
Singer1	0.25	0.94	0.46	0.95	0.35	0.25	1.00	0.48	0.25	1.00	0.26	0.23	1.00
Stone	0.28	0.51	0.23	0.62	1.00	0.21	0.83	0.14	0.29	0.95	0.60	0.41	0.97
Leno	0.53	1.00	0.82	1.00	0.98	0.97	1.00	1.00	0.79	0.99	0.78	0.92	1.00
Toystory	0.72	0.94	0.27	0.99	0.39	0.39	0.37	0.37	0.36	0.28	0.38	0.75	1.00
Walking	0.55	0.99	0.39	0.84	0.99	0.53	0.99	0.97	0.55	0.95	0.64	0.55	0.98
Walking2	0.39	0.99	0.34	0.40	0.99	0.39	0.97	0.41	0.39	1.00	0.46	0.42	0.96
Mountainbike	0.58	1.00	0.26	1.00	0.95	0.17	0.83	1.00	0.99	0.98	0.86	1.00	0.97
Dog1	0.65	0.86	0.68	0.71	0.79	0.65	0.99	0.88	0.65	0.85	0.65	0.65	1.00

Table 2. Average center error (in pixels). The best two results are shown in red and blue fonts respectively.

	MIL	IVT	TLD	VTD	MTT	CT	ℓ_1-APG	NDLT	LSHT	SCM	STK	PBT	OURS
Car4	0.27	1.00	0.86	1.00	0.38	0.27	1.00	1.00	0.27	1.00	0.28	0.39	1.00
David2	0.33	0.88	0.96	0.99	1.00	0.01	1.00	0.96	0.99	0.91	1.00	0.99	0.98
David3	0.35	0.61	0.18	0.53	0.56	0.32	0.05	0.67	0.75	0.58	0.68	0.57	0.98
Faceocc1	0.76	1.00	0.78	0.97	1.00	0.66	1.00	1.00	1.00	1.00	0.96	1.00	1.00
Skater	0.94	0.88	0.48	0.98	1.00	0.95	0.81	0.41	0.16	0.87	0.44	1.00	1.00
Crossing	0.99	0.23	0.52	0.42	0.23	0.99	0.25	0.82	0.44	1.00	0.96	0.99	1.00
Jogging	0.16	0.19	0.86	0.16	0.16	0.15	0.19	0.17	0.15	0.89	0.18	0.17	1.00
SeqI	0.34	0.21	0.94	0.45	0.31	0.23	0.99	0.21	0.94	0.99	0.68	0.45	1.00
Singer1	0.25	0.94	0.46	0.95	0.35	0.25	1.00	0.48	0.25	1.00	0.26	0.23	1.00
Stone	0.28	0.51	0.23	0.62	1.00	0.21	0.83	0.14	0.29	0.95	0.60	0.41	0.97
Leno	0.53	1.00	0.82	1.00	0.98	0.97	1.00	1.00	0.79	0.99	0.78	0.92	1.00
Toystory	0.72	0.94	0.27	0.99	0.39	0.39	0.37	0.37	0.36	0.28	0.38	0.75	1.00
Walking	0.55	0.99	0.39	0.84	0.99	0.53	0.99	0.97	0.55	0.95	0.64	0.55	0.98
Walking2	0.39	0.99	0.34	0.40	0.99	0.39	0.97	0.41	0.39	1.00	0.46	0.42	0.96
Mountainbike	0.58	1.00	0.26	1.00	0.95	0.17	0.83	1.00	0.99	0.98	0.86	1.00	0.97
Dog1	0.65	0.86	0.68	0.71	0.79	0.65	0.99	0.88	0.65	0.85	0.65	0.65	1.00

Quantitative Comparison: We first evaluate quantitatively the performance of the trackers mentioned above with the success rate criterion, which is defined as the ratio of the successfully tracked frames. Given the tracking bounding box B_T and the ground truth B_G, if the PASCAL VOC score $\frac{B_T \cap B_G}{B_T \cup B_G}$ is larger than 0.5, then tracking in the frame is regarded as successful. Table 1 presents the success rate results, where a bigger value means better performance. We also utilize the center location error between the tracking results and ground truth to assess these trackers. Table 2 shows the average center error in pixels, where the smaller the value is, the better the tracker performs. From Tables 1 and 2, we can see that our tracker performs favorably against other state-of-the-art methods in terms of both criteria.

Qualitative Comparison

Pose Change: The *Toystory* sequence is challenging for large pose deformation and dusky background. The target toy exhibits different moves and the other one also causes distraction to mislead the tracker. Most of other methods lose the target after frame #147. Since the dictionary in our model captures various target poses and the group structure exploits the temporal information and appearance similarity, our algorithm could track the target successfully throughout the whole sequence. In addition, the weighted sum of all promising candidates contributes to the tracking robustness. In sequences *Skater* and *Dog1*, the appearance of the target changes dramatically due to the pose variation, resulting in great difficulty for tracking. For all that, our tracker is able to catch the target accurately all through. The PAT and SCM methods also do well in some cases as they employ the part-based representations. The target faces in sequences *David2* and *Leno* experience out-of-plane rotation, causing the trackers to fail easily. But our method is able to locate the target all through.

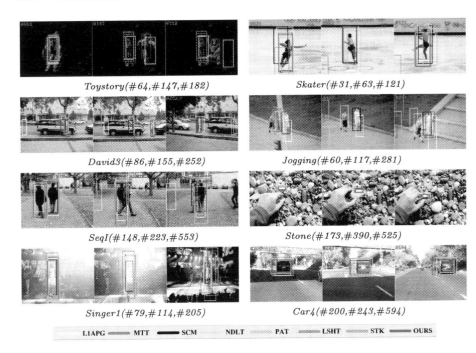

Fig. 4. Sampled tracking results on challenging image sequences. This figure demonstrates the results of seven state-of-the-art tracking methods and the proposed method.

Partial Occlusion: In the *David3*, *Jogging*, *Walking2* and *SeqI* sequences, the target is completely occluded by other similar objects or obstacles, making the tracker easy to drift. We can see that our method performs better than other trackers in these cases, since we introduce the trivial template group to account for the occlusion and use the atom group structure to take advantage of the previous similar appearance information. In sequence *Faceocc1*, the tracked face is blocked by a book from different directions. Because the object undergoes little pose variation, majority of algorithms could track the target generally, yet our method achieves a relatively smaller center error.

Illumination Change and Background Clutter: In sequence *Car4*, the car passes under a bridge which blocks out the light, and in sequence *Crossing*, the human is crossing the sidewalk from the black shadow. While in sequence *Singer1*, the strength of the stage lighting increases all at once. Both the targets in these sequences experience severe illumination change, causing the image pixels to change a lot. Our algorithm is capable of handling this challenge due to the use of dual group structure, and locates the target more stably and accurately than others. The target in the *Stone* sequence is easy to be distracted by other stones of different shapes and colors with cluttered background. Likewise, our method could achieve favorable performance (Fig. 4).

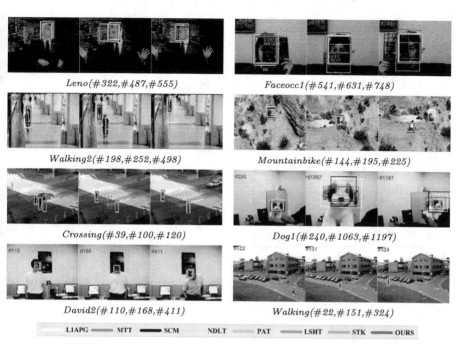

Leno(#322,#487,#555)   Faceocc1(#541,#631,#748)

Walking2(#198,#252,#498)   Mountainbike(#144,#195,#225)

Crossing(#39,#100,#120)   Dog1(#240,#1063,#1197)

David2(#110,#168,#411)   Walking(#22,#151,#324)

L1APG ═══ MTT ═══ SCM   NDLT   PAT ═══ LSHT ═══ STK ═══ OURS

Fig. 5. Sampled tracking results on challenging image sequences. This figure demonstrates the results of seven state-of-the-art tracking methods and the proposed method.

5 Conclusion

We exploit the dual group structure information of both dictionary atoms and testing candidate samples, and formulate the sparse representation at a group level. The commonalities shared by samples and the individual characteristics among data are both taken into account through inter-group sparsity and intra-group sparsity. In this way, the temporal continuity and appearance similarity of tracking results can be made full use of. The objective function is solved efficiently by two stages, thresholding and computing using the accelerated proximal gradient method. Then we devise a generative tracker based on the dual group structure model. Instead of selecting only one best candidate, we estimate the target location with the weighted sum over a set of related particles, which leads to a more stable and robust tracker. Numerous experiments on visual tracking are conducted with a wide variety of challenging factors, including partial occlusion, pose variation, illumination change and background clutter. Experimental results demonstrate that our tracker performs favorably against state-of-the-art methods (Fig. 5).

Acknowledgement. This work was supported by the Joint Foundation of China Education Ministry and China Mobile Communication Corporation under Grant MCM2012 2071, and in part by the Fundamental Research Funds for the Central Universities under Grant DUT14YQ101 and the Natural Science Foundation of China under Grant 61472060.

References

1. Wright, J., Yang, A.Y., Ganesh, A., Sastry, S.S., Ma, Y.: Robust face recognition via sparse representation. IEEE Trans. Pattern Anal. Mach. Intell. **31**, 210–227 (2009)
2. Mairal, J., Bach, F., Ponce, J., Sapiro, G., Zisserman, A.: Non-local sparse models for image restoration. In: ICCV (2009)
3. Mei, X., Ling, H.: Robust visual tracking using ℓ_1 minimization. In: ICCV(2009)
4. Wang, D., Lu, H., Chen, Y.: Incremental MPCA for color object tracking. In: ICPR(2010)
5. Zhang, T., Ghanem, B., Liu, S., Ahuja, N.: Robust visual tracking via multi-task sparse learning. In: CVPR (2012)
6. Zhuang, B., Lu, H., Xiao, Z., Wang, D.: Visual tracking via discriminative sparse similarity map. IEEE Trans. Image Process. **23**, 1872–1881 (2014)
7. Babenko, B., Yang, M.H., Belongie, S.: Visual tracking with online multiple instance learning. In: CVPR (2009)
8. Hare, S., Saffari, A., Torr, P.H.S.: Struck: Structured output tracking with kernels. In: ICCV (2011)
9. Zhang, K., Zhang, L., Yang, M.-H.: Real-time compressive tracking. In: Fitzgibbon, A., Lazebnik, S., Perona, P., Sato, Y., Schmid, C. (eds.) ECCV 2012, Part III. LNCS, vol. 7574, pp. 864–877. Springer, Heidelberg (2012)
10. Bao, C., Wu, Y., Ling, H., Ji, H.: Real time robust l1 tracker using accelerated proximal gradient approach. In: CVPR (2012)
11. Jia, X., Lu, H., Yang, M.: Visual tracking via adaptive structural local sparse appearance model. In: CVPR (2012)
12. Wang, D., Lu, H., Yang, M.H.: Online object tracking with sparse prototypes. IEEE Trans. Image Process. **22**, 314–325 (2013)
13. Yuan, M., Lin, Y.: Model selection and estimation in regression with grouped variables. J. Roy. Stat. Soc., Ser. B **68**, 49–67 (2006)
14. Zou, H., Hastie, T.: Regularization and variable selection via the elastic net. J. Roy. Stat. Soc., Ser. B **67**, 301–320 (2005)
15. Bengio, S., Pereira, F.C.N., Singer, Y., Strelow, D.: Group sparse coding. In: NIPS (2009)
16. Chi, Y.T., Ali, M., Rushdi, M., Ho, J.: Affine-constrained group sparse coding and its application to image-based classifications. In: ICCV (2013)
17. Chi, Y.T., Ali, M., Rajwade, A., Ho, J.: Block and group regularized sparse modeling for dictionary learning. In: CVPR (2013)
18. Friedman, J., Hastie, T., Tibshirani, R.: A note on the group lasso and sparse group lasso. CoRR (2010)
19. Elhamifar, E., Vidal, R.: Structured sparse recovery via convex optimization. CoRR (2011)
20. Zhang, S., Huang, J., Huang, Y., Yu, Y., Li, H., Metaxas, D.N.: Automatic image annotation using group sparsity. In: CVPR (2010)
21. Liu, B., Yang, L., Huang, J., Meer, P., Gong, L., Kulikowski, C.: Robust and fast collaborative tracking with two stage sparse optimization. In: Daniilidis, K., Maragos, P., Paragios, N. (eds.) ECCV 2010, Part IV. LNCS, vol. 6314, pp. 624–637. Springer, Heidelberg (2010)

22. Jenatton, R., Obozinski, G., Bach, F.: Structured sparse principal component analysis. In: AISTATS (2010)
23. Tibshirani, R.: Regression shrinkage and selection via the lasso. J. Roy. Stat. Soc., Ser. B **58**, 267–288 (1994)
24. Nesterov, Y.: Gradient methods for minimizing composite functions. Math. Program. **140**, 125–161 (2013)
25. Samaria, F.S., Harter, A.C.: Parameterisation of a stochastic model for human face identification. In: ACV (1994)
26. Wu, Y., Lim, J., Yang, M.H.: Online object tracking: a benchmark. In: CVPR (2013)
27. Ross, D.A., Lim, J., Lin, R.S., Yang, M.H.: Incremental learning for robust visual tracking. Int. J. Comput. Vision **77**, 125–141 (2008)
28. Kalal, Z., Mikolajczyk, K., Matas, J.: Tracking-learning-detection. IEEE Trans. Pattern Anal. Mach. Intell. **34**, 1409–1422 (2012)
29. Kwon, J., Lee, K.M.: Visual tracking decomposition. In: CVPR (2010)
30. Wang, N., Wang, J., Yeung, D.Y.: Online robust non-negative dictionary learning for visual tracking. In: ICCV (2013)
31. He, S., Yang, Q., Lau, R.W., Wang, J., Yang, M.H.: Visual tracking via locality sensitive histograms. In: CVPR (2013)
32. Zhong, W., Lu, H., Yang, M.: Robust object tracking via sparse collaborative appearance model. IEEE Trans. Image Process. **23**, 2356–2368 (2014)
33. Yao, R., Shi, Q., Shen, C., Zhang, Y., van den Hengel, A.: Part-based visual tracking with online latent structural learning. In: CVPR (2013)

3D Reconstruction of Specular Objects with Occlusion: A Shape-from-Scattering Approach

Yuki Hirofuji[✉], Masaaki Iiyama, Takuya Funatomi, and Michihiko Minoh

Kyoto University, Kyoto, Japan
hirofuji.yuki.56z@st.kyoto-u.ac.jp

Abstract. In this paper, we propose a method to measure specular objects regardless occlusion. The main contribution of this paper is that we have shown that the scattering of incident and specular reflection enable us to measure occluded surfaces. We locate objects in a tank filled with participating media, irradiate a laser beam to the objects, and observe the scattering of incident light and specular reflection. Occluded reflecting points of the laser are estimated from the peak pixel; scattering light that has local maximum intensity. Experimental results with a metallic specular plate demonstrate that our method can estimate the 3D position of occluded reflecting point.

1 Introduction

In a variety of fields, such as CG production and industrial design, it is important to measure the complete three-dimensional (3D) shape of objects. Most 3D shape measurement techniques acquire the shape of an object via reflected light from its surface; therefore, it is difficult to acquire specular objects, whose reflected light is highly directional and hard to observe with these techniques. While some techniques for measuring specular objects have been proposed, they cannot measure occluded surfaces.

In this paper we propose a new approach for measuring the shape of specular objects regardless of occlusion. In our approach, scattered light from a laser beam is used for the measurement. We place the object to be measured in a space filled with a participating medium, irradiate its surface with a laser beam, and observe the scattering in the participating medium as shown in Fig. 1. As the laser beam passes through the medium, some of the light is scattered, and light reflected onto the surface is also partially scattered. In this situation, the path of the incident laser beam and the path of the specular reflection, which would not be observable in a clear air environment, can be observed as scattered light. Using this scattered light, we can estimate the location of the reflection points on the object's surface even when the surface is occluded.

2 Related Work

Most 3D shape measurement techniques such as stereo vision require the observation of reflected light from object surfaces. However, it is difficult to apply these

© Springer International Publishing Switzerland 2015
D. Cremers et al. (Eds.): ACCV 2014, Part IV, LNCS 9006, pp. 630–641, 2015.
DOI: 10.1007/978-3-319-16817-3_41

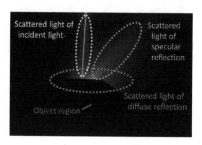

Fig. 1. The scenario for an object located in a tank filled with a participating medium

techniques to measurement of specular objects because the reflected light from their surfaces changes greatly depending on the observing direction. Although several methods [1] for measuring specular objects have been proposed, including specular flow [2], the use of polarization [3], using a known pattern [4], and the shape-from-distortion method [5], none of these can be used to measure occluded shapes. The method proposed by Morris et al. [6] uses specular reflection for measuring shape of objects, and they considered scattering and refraction inside the object. Compared with this method, we assume scattering in participating medium and our method can measure occluded object shapes.

Velten et al. proposed a method that can measure occluded shapes [7]. This method is a time-of-flight (TOF) based measurement technique; that is, it measures the time required for laser light to be reflected off the object and returned to the detector. Their method requires the measured objects to be Lambertian objects; therefore it cannot be applied to measure specular objects. In addition, this method requires expensive femto lasers.

A study related to ours was performed by Hullin et al. [8]. They used fluorescent material for observing laser trails and succeeded in capturing transparent objects that are difficult to measure using most vision-based methods. In their method, scattering of laser trail is used for shape acquisition. However, this method does not consider a case wherein surface is occluded, and cannot also measure specular objects.

Recently, Iiyama et al. proposed a method for acquiring occluded surfaces [9]. This low cost method uses the attenuation of reflected light to estimate the reflection points on occluded shapes; the attenuation is modeled by a $1/r^2$ law for a traveled distance r, and this model is fit to the observed image to estimate the location of the occluded reflection point. The drawback of this method is that it is not robust to image noise. The estimation is highly affected by this noise, because the low intensity pixels, which generally have a low S/N ratio, are necessary for the model fitting. In this paper, we extend this method so that it is robust to image noise. Instead of fitting a $1/r^2$ attenuation model, we use the locations of the scattered light peaks, that is, where a peak is a pixel that has a higher intensity than the pixels around it.

3   Measurement Using Reflection Peaks

3.1   Scattering

Our system configuration is shown in Fig. 2. We placed an object into a tank filled with a participating medium in order to observe the scattered light of a laser beam. A laser unit mounted on a robot arm sent beams toward the object from the upper side of the tank. This robot arm was used for controlling the position of the laser beam.

The incident beams were scattered and were attenuated when they passed through the participating medium, and the beams were then reflected from the object surface. The reflected beams were also scattered and attenuated while passing through the participating medium. The light that was observed by the cameras was primarily comprised of the light scattered in the participating medium. As shown in Fig. 1, the light scattered from the incident light was observed as a bright, bold, line-like region, the light scattered from the specular reflection appeared as a lobe shaped area, and that from the diffuse reflection appeared as a widely spread region. Even when the reflection point on the object's surface was occluded, this scattered light could still be observed.

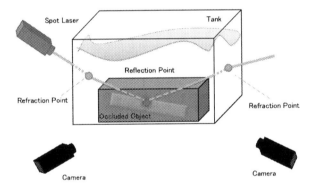

Fig. 2. Our system configuration: A robot arm with a spot laser was located on the upper side of the tank, and the spot laser was directed towards an object located within participating medium. The scattered light was observed with multiple cameras. Reflection point is occluded by other objects and can not be observed by the cameras.

We then estimate the location of the reflection point from this scattering from observed images. Our method uses at least two images taken from different viewpoints for estimating 3D location of single reflection point. It consists on (1) extraction of 2D candidate reflection points, (2) peak pixel detection for calculating the likelihoods, (3) identifying the candidate point with highest likelihood as 2D reflection point, and (4) 3D reflection point estimation.

3.2   Estimation of the Reflection Peaks

When we spot a laser on the object's surface and capture an image, its occluded reflection point on the image exists (1) along the line of the incident light on the images, and (2) in an object region obtained using a background subtraction method. The pixels that fulfill the two conditions are extracted and are designated pixels as "candidate points". Next, we calculate the likelihoods for each candidate point, and identify the candidate point with highest likelihood as the reflection point. The detailed methodology is presented in the following sections.

Candidate Points. To mask the object region, we employ a naive background subtraction method with pre-captured background and foreground images from the room under ambient light conditions. Although we can use more sophisticated methods, the masking in our method does not need to be highly accurate unless the masked region completely covers the entire object region. The remainder of this process will continue to work correctly even if some of the scattering region is contained by the masked region.

We extract the region that corresponded to the incident laser beam and extract the line of the incident light. As described in Sect. 3.1, the incident laser beam is observed as a bright, bold, line-like region, so we binarize the image with a constant threshold and extract the bold line-like region. We start from a high threshold and continuously lower it until the line-like region is extracted from Fig. 3 as shown in Fig. 4 Applying a Hough transform to the extracted region, the line of the incident light is detected. Note that since the extracted region has a rectangular shape, a diagonal of this rectangular region, which does not correspond to the line of the incident light, would also be detected. To avoid this, we apply a thinning operator before applying the Hough transform.

Let O be the object region and S_I be the line of the incident light. The reflecting point exists on the line of the incident light and within the object

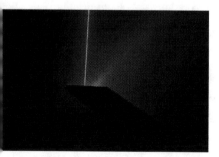

Fig. 3. An observed image. We can observe that the irradiated incident light from upper side is reflected to upper right in this image.

Fig. 4. The image of the extracted incident light from Fig. 3.

region, thus a set of candidate points is defined by $C = S_I \cup O$. We use these candidate points in the following procedure.

Extraction of Peak Pixels. A peak pixel is a pixel that has a higher intensity than the pixels around it, and it is defined as below. Let $r = (r_x, r_y) \in \mathbb{R}^2$ be a pixel and $I(r) \in \mathbb{R}$ be the intensity of a pixel r in an input image. For given a line $l = \{td(\phi) + r_0\}$, an intensity profile along the line l is given by

$$S_{\phi,r_0}(t) = I(td(\phi) + r_0) \tag{1}$$

where $t \in \mathbb{R}$, $d(\phi)$ is the line direction $d(\phi) = (\cos\phi, \sin\phi), 0 \le \phi < 2\pi$, and r_0 is a pixel position $r_0 \in \mathbb{R}^2$. We define a peak pixel to be a pixel that has the local maximum intensity in the intensity profile. For all peaks p, an angle ϕ and a positive value δ that satisfies the following condition exist.

$$S_{\phi,p}(t) \le S_{\phi,p}(0)\ (-\delta \le^\forall t \le \delta), \tag{2}$$

The peak forms a roof edge at $t = 0$ on a line l. Figure 5 presents an example case in which one point on the line of the incident light is a peak of a profile $S_{\phi,r_0}(t)$.

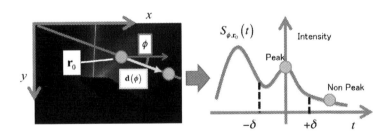

Fig. 5. A profile and the peak pixel. An orange-colored peak pixel on specular reflection has local maximum intensity in $S_{\phi,r_0}(t)$, on the other hand, non peak pixel that is green-colored has NOT local maximum intensity in any direction ϕ (Color figure online).

A reflection point is located on a line of specular reflection; that is, if the peaks are acquired correctly, they will be a strong clue for detection of the reflection points. We extract the peak pixels in regions of the obtained image excluding O.

Ideally, the profile will form a smooth curve and have peaks that are easy to extract, as illustrated the right panel of Fig. 5, however, the profile will actually contain noise. The accuracy of peak detection deteriorates due to the effect of noise and thus "fake" peaks may be extracted. However, the "true" peaks are still detected near the true position because the gradient of the intensity at the true (non-noise) peaks is sufficiently strong in the case where specular reflections exist.

We extract peak pixels along x-axis ($\phi = 0$) and y-axis ($\phi = \pi/2$) instead of a search for ϕ. In the peak pixel extraction along x-axis, for all pixels $\boldsymbol{r}$ in an observed image, we compare $I(\boldsymbol{r})$ and intensity of all pixels around $\boldsymbol{r}$, $D = \{\boldsymbol{r}_t = (r_x + t, r_y)| -\delta \le t \le \delta, \delta > 0\}$ and test whether $\boldsymbol{r}$ satisfies the condition (2). Here, δ is constant through all peak pixel extraction. If $I(\boldsymbol{r})$ has maximum value among all $I(\boldsymbol{r}_t)$, the pixel $\boldsymbol{r}$ is extracted as a peak pixel. The same is true for y-axis. Even if direction of specular reflection is given by ϕ ($\phi \ne 0, \pi/2$) as shown in Fig. 5, pixels on the specular reflection will be extracted as peak pixels, when we only check with respect to $\phi = 0$ and $\pi/2$.

The fragility of the peak detection is also addressed in the likelihood calculation for the candidate points, as described below. We extract the peaks and express them as a binary image $P(\boldsymbol{r})$; the peak pixels are denoted by 1, and the other pixels by 0.

Estimation of the Reflection Point Locations. We estimate the location of the reflection point from $P(\boldsymbol{r})$, the observed image $I(\boldsymbol{r})$ and the candidate points C. In order to determine the reflection point from C, we focus on a half line $l_{\boldsymbol{c},\theta}$ which begins from a candidate point $\boldsymbol{c} \in C$ toward a direction θ. Specular reflection exists on a line that passes through a reflection point, and specular reflection is extracted as peak pixels, thus if $\boldsymbol{c}$ is the reflection point, there must be a half line $l_{\boldsymbol{c},\theta}$ along which the peak pixels exist. Using this idea, we define a likelihood $L(\boldsymbol{c},\theta)$, which is defined as the number of peak pixels weighted by the pixel intensities.

$$L(\boldsymbol{c},\theta) = \int_0^{t_{\max}} P(\boldsymbol{r})I(\boldsymbol{r})dt \qquad (3)$$

$$\boldsymbol{r}(t) = \boldsymbol{c} + t\boldsymbol{d} \qquad (4)$$

$$\boldsymbol{d} = (\cos\theta, \sin\theta), \qquad (5)$$

where $t_{\max}$ is the distance from $\boldsymbol{c}$ to a border of the input image. By assigning a low weight to lower intensity peaks, which are sensitive to noise, we address the fragility of the peak detection. Note that peak pixels which corresponds to the incident light make a line, so we exclude the incident light region before the peak pixel extraction. The likelihood $L(\boldsymbol{c})$ of a possible reflection point is defined by using $L(\boldsymbol{c},\theta)$ as

$$L(\boldsymbol{c}) = \max_{0 \le \theta < 2\pi} \{L(\boldsymbol{c},\theta)\}, \qquad (6)$$

The point $\boldsymbol{c}$ which has the maximum $L(\boldsymbol{c})$ is estimated to be the reflection point $\boldsymbol{e}$. In short,

$$\boldsymbol{e} = \arg\max_{\boldsymbol{c}\in C} \{L(\boldsymbol{c})\}.$$

Figure 6 illustrates the procedure for calculating the likelihood $L(\boldsymbol{c},\theta)$.

3.3   3D Reflection Point Reconstruction

Generally, a point on a camera image corresponds to a 3D view line in the real world. However, due to refraction, in our experimental setup, it corresponds to

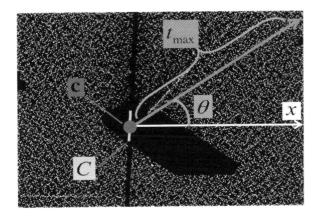

Fig. 6. Calculation of the likelihood

a polyline; therefore, traditional computer-vision based stereo methods cannot be used for determining the reflection point position.

In our method, we reconstruct the 3D position of the reflection point from a single 2D reflection point on a camera image and two position on the line of the incident light of the other camera image. For each camera, we estimate the 2D reflection point, and select one camera Cam_i which detect the 2D reflection point e with the highest likelihood $L(e)$. We calculate the 3D position of e as follows (see Fig. 7).

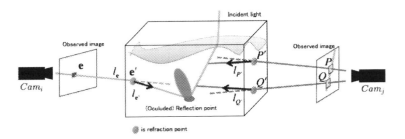

Fig. 7. We estimate a reflection point using camera B and calculated a plane π using camera A; the reflection point is given by the 3D location of the intersection.

Let e be a 2D reflection point on Cam_i image, and P and Q be two position on the line of the incident light on Cam_j image. We first calculate e', P' and Q' which are refraction point of e, P and Q, and view line inside the tank $l_{e'}$, $l_{P'}$ and $l_{Q'}$. $l_{e'}$, $l_{P'}$ and $l_{Q'}$ satisfy,

1. Incident light exists on a plane whose normal vector is $l_{P'} \times l_{Q'}$ and that includes $l_{P'}$ and $l_{Q'}$ in 3D space.
2. A reflection point exists on a line $l_{e'}$.

From 1 and 2, the 3D position of reflection point is obtained as intersection of the plane in 1 and the line in 2.

We obtain the 3D shape of objects by applying the above procedure while changing the position of the laser beam.

4   Experiments

To create a participating medium, about $180\,L$ of water and $1\,mL$ of milk are mixed in a $60\,cm$ cubic tank, and were filtered in order to eliminate dust in the tank. According to Narashimhan et al. [10], in the case where $24\,L$ of water and $15\,mL$ of milk are mixed, the scattering coefficient σ_s is 1.3293×10^{-2} $[mm^{-1}]$. As the scattering coefficient is proportional to density, it is $\sigma_s = 1.1324 \times 10^{-4}$ $[mm^{-1}]$ in our experimental environment; thus, multiple scattering light could be ignored because second scattering coefficient is σ^2. We used four cameras, two of which were placed on one side of the tank and the other two of which were orthogonally located on the other side of the tank as shown in Fig. 8. The cameras were Nikon D7000 single lens reflex cameras, with $4948 \times 3280\,pixels$.

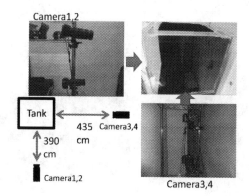

Fig. 8. Locations of the cameras and the tank.

4.1   2D Reflection Point Estimation

We compared the accuracy of the 2D reflection point estimation from our method with that derived using Iiyama et al.'s attenuation-based method. Note that, since it can be difficult to determine ground truth reflection points, we used a metallic plate to facilitate their acquisition (Fig. 9).

In order to determine the ground truth, we used a non-occluded scene for the evaluation as shown in Fig. 10. Masking the object region, we simulated an occluded scene (Fig. 12), and used images that is removed peak pixels on incident light and around object region for further experiments (Fig. 13). We used nine reflection points on the metallic plate. Table 1 lists the errors (in pixels)

Table 1. Average errors for the attenuation-based method and our new method (in pixels).

Estimation	cam1	cam2	cam3	cam4
Attenuation-based method	76.4	147.6	275.4	350.8
Proposed method	11.8	27.3	71.6	62.6

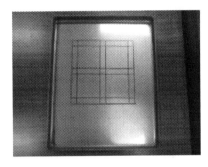

Fig. 9. A metalic plate used in 2D reflection point estimation.

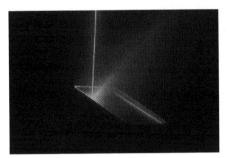   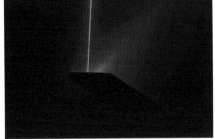

Fig. 10. An observed image.   **Fig. 11.** A masked image by object region O. This image is obtained by Fig. 10. We treat this image as an input image.

in the estimated point locations with respect the correct point locations for the attenuation-based method and our new method. Each error value is averaged over the nine points. In our setup, one pixel is generally equivalent to 0.3 mm.

The average error of our method is about 1/10 obtained when using the attenuation-based method. Figure 14 shows the peak image and detected reflection point with respect to the image shown in Fig. 13. This result demonstrates that our method can measure specular surfaces even if they are occluded.

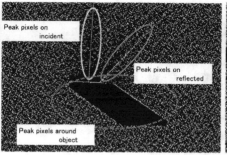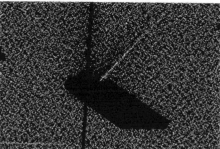

Fig. 12. A binary image extracted peak pixels from Fig. 11. However, this image includes peak pixels on incident light and around object region.

Fig. 13. A final image before performing the weighted Hough transform. Peak pixels on incident light and around object region is removed.

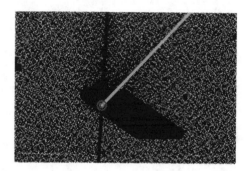

Fig. 14. An estimation result from Fig. 13. A green line shows the direction has highest value in all $L(c, \theta)$, and the center of circles shows the candidate point c (Color figure online).

4.2   3D Reflection Points Estimation

In order to show that our method is able to perform 3D reconstructions, we measured the surface of the mirror shown in Fig. 15. In this experiment, as with the experiment to evaluate the accuracy of our method, we masked the object region and measured pseudo-occluded shapes. The result of the reconstruction, comprised of about 100 reflection points, is shown in Fig. 16. Most the points exist on the same plane; that is, they have been correctly reconstructed.

An estimation failure, which can be observed at the edge of the mirror, was caused by the presence of multiple reflected lights with high intensities. A limitation of our method is that it works under the assumption of existence of specular reflection. In more detail, it cannot correctly measure a shape when multiple reflections are occurring.

A typical failure is shown in Fig. 18, which is the result produced for the ashtray shown in Fig. 17. Figure 18 illustrates a scene in which light was incident

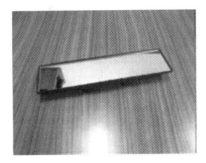

Fig. 15. A measured object, mirror used in 3D reflection points estimation.

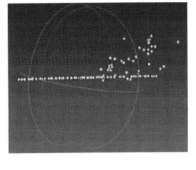

Fig. 16. Reconstruction result of the mirror. This image shows the result from the side. Many points exists on the same plane.

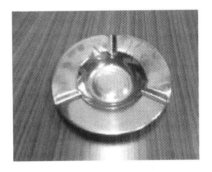

Fig. 17. An ashtray used in 3D reflection points estimation.

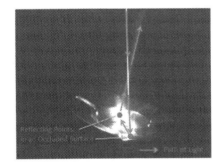

Fig. 18. Multiple reflection.

from above, reflected to the left side of the ashtray surface, and then reflected at the tank many times (outside of the image shown). In this case, multiple reflection occurred inside and outside of the object region, we cannot estimate reflection points in principle under the scene. To find a solution of such multiple reflection is one aspect of our future work.

5   Conclusion

In this paper, we proposed a method that estimates the reflection points of specular objects regardless of occlusion. The peak pixels that have the highest local intensity in the scattered light were used for the estimation. Although the peak pixels are robust to image noise, we enhance their robustness against image noise by applying a weighted Hough transform.

Our method only works when specular reflection is clearly observed. In the case where specular reflection is not observed, this method will instead produce points that are significantly offset from the ground truth. Despite this drawback, our method presents a significant contribution that scattering of specular reflection can provide valuable clues for measuring occluded surfaces.

Improvement of the peak detection is one task planned for our future research. In addition, in our implementation it takes around six minutes to process per one point estimation though we don't parallelize so we must improve processing time. This proposed method and our attenuation-based method could complement each other, and in a future work we will integrate these methods.

Acknowledgement. This work was supported by JSPS KAKENHI Grant Number 26700013.

References

1. Ihrke, I., Kutulakos, K.N., Lensch, H., Magnor, M., Heidrich, W.: State of the art in transparent and specular object reconstruction. In: EUROGRAPHICS 2008 STAR-State of the Art Report, pp. 87–108 (2008)
2. Roth, S., Black, M.J.: Specular flow and the recovery of surface structure. In: Proceedings of IEEE Conference on Computer Vision and Pattern Recognition (CVPR), New York, NY, USA, pp. 1869–1876 (2006)
3. Clark, J., Trucco, E., Wolff, L.B.: Using light polarization in laser scanning. Image Vis. Comput. **15**(1), 107–117 (1997)
4. Kutulakos, K.N., Steger, E.: A theory of refractive and specular 3D shape by light-path triangulation. In: Proceedings of IEEE International Conference on Computer Vision (ICCV), Beijing, China, pp. 1448–1455. (2005)
5. Schultz, H.: Retrieving shape information from multiple images of a specular surface. IEEE Trans. Pattern Anal. Mach. Intell. (PAMI) **16**(2), 195–201 (1994)
6. Morris, N.J.W., Kutulakos, K.N.: Reconstructing the surface of inhomogeneous transparent scenes by scatter-trace photography. In: IEEE 11th International Conference on Computer Vision, ICCV 2007. IEEE (2007)
7. Velten, A., Willwacher, T., Gupta, O., Veeraraghavan, A., Bawendi, M.G., Raskar, R.: Recovering three-dimensional shape around a corner using ultrafast time-of-flight imaging. Nat. Commun. **3**, 745 (2012)
8. Hullin, M.B., Fuchs, M., Ihrke, I., Seidel, H.-P., Lensch, H.P.A.: Fluorescent immersion range scanning. ACM Trans. Graph. **27**(3), Article 87 (2008). Univ British Columbia, Vancouver, BCV5Z IM9, Canada
9. Iiyama, M., Miki, S., Funatomi, T., Minoh, M.: 3D Acqui- sition of Occluded Surfaces from Scattering in Participating Media. In: International Conference on Pattern Recognition (2014)
10. Narasimhan, S.G., Gupta, M., Donner, C., Ramamoorthi, R., Nayar, S.K., Jensen, H.W.: Acquiring scattering properties of participating media by dilution. ACM Trans. Graph **25**(3), 1003–1012 (2006)

2D or Not 2D: Bridging the Gap Between Tracking and Structure from Motion

Karel Lebeda$^{(\boxtimes)}$, Simon Hadfield, and Richard Bowden

University of Surrey, Guildford GU2 7XH, UK
{K.Lebeda,S.Hadfield,R.Bowden}@surrey.ac.uk

Abstract. In this paper, we address the problem of tracking an unknown object in 3D space. Online 2D tracking often fails for strong out-of-plane rotation which results in considerable changes in appearance beyond those that can be represented by online update strategies. However, by modelling and learning the 3D structure of the object explicitly, such effects are mitigated. To address this, a novel approach is presented, combining techniques from the fields of visual tracking, structure from motion (SfM) and simultaneous localisation and mapping (SLAM). This algorithm is referred to as TMAGIC (Tracking, Modelling And Gaussian-process Inference Combined). At every frame, point and line features are tracked in the image plane and are used, together with their 3D correspondences, to estimate the camera pose. These features are also used to model the 3D shape of the object as a Gaussian process. Tracking determines the trajectories of the object in both the image plane and 3D space, but the approach also provides the 3D object shape. The approach is validated on several video-sequences used in the tracking literature, comparing favourably to state-of-the-art trackers for simple scenes (error reduced by 22 %) with clear advantages in the case of strong out-of-plane rotation, where 2D approaches fail (error reduction of 58 %).

1 Introduction

Monocular, model-less, visual tracking aims to estimate the pose of an unknown object in every frame of a video-sequence (or to report its absence), given a bounding box containing the object in the first frame. This is a challenging task since the object appearance often changes significantly during the sequence. Many approaches attempt to learn changes in appearance, some of which come from object pose that cannot be modelled by a simple planar transformation. In this work, we directly address changes caused by a viewpoint variation. Instead of treating it as an "appearance change problem", we model explicitly the 3D information.

Many approaches have been proposed to overcome variations of appearance. Online approaches typically assume that the tracking has thus far succeeded, using this to enrich the representation of the object over time. The object is

---

Electronic supplementary material The online version of this chapter (doi:10.1007/978-3-319-16817-3_42) contains supplementary material, which is available to authorized users.

© Springer International Publishing Switzerland 2015
D. Cremers et al. (Eds.): ACCV 2014, Part IV, LNCS 9006, pp. 642–658, 2015.
DOI: 10.1007/978-3-319-16817-3_42

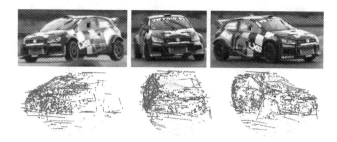

Fig. 1. Out-of-plane rotation change the object appearance significantly, here is a complete change in just 50 frames. First row: original images. Second row: feature cloud and final model returned by the tracker. Notice the bottom and back side of the car, which have not been observed yet, so the point cloud does not reach there and the model is smoothly extrapolated.

usually represented as a 2D patch [1,2], a cloud of 2D points [3,4] or a combination of these [5]. Unfortunately, variations of viewpoint lead to rapid changes in appearance – see Fig. 1 for an example. This causes problems for 2D trackers which do not have sufficient observations to confidently update their object representation.

We take a different approach to this problem. Our proposed tracker explicitly models out-of-plane rotations, which proves beneficial, as they improve the numerical conditioning (wider baseline). The 3D shape of the object is estimated online using techniques developed in the fields of *Structure-from-Motion* (SfM) and *Simultaneous Localisation And Mapping* (SLAM). As such, this work can be seen as a bridge between visual tracking and SfM/SLAM, combining 2D feature tracking and object segmentation with camera pose and 3D point/line estimation, while avoiding the need for initialisation in SLAM [6]. Another difference from SfM/SLAM is object/background segmentation, where only a small portion of the image can be used.

In addition, we present a novel approach to modelling the object 3D shape using a *Gaussian Process* (GP). The model helps us distinguish which parts of the image belong to the projection of the object and which are background, allowing intelligent detection of new features (Sect. 3.1). In addition, the GP shape model (1) provides an initialisation of the 3D positions for newly detected 2D features, (2) mitigates the sparsity of features, (3) the surface normals of the GP indicate which points on the object may be visible to a particular camera and (4) the GP offers a model of the surface for visualisation and subsequent tasks, such as dense reconstruction or robot navigation, etc.

The rest of this work is structured as follows. In Sect. 2 related literature is reviewed. We then describe our tracker in Sect. 3. It is experimentally evaluated in Sect. 4, while Sect. 5 draws conclusions.

2   Related Work

There is a large body of literature in 2D tracking, SfM and SLAM. Here we summarise the most relevant work in each field, as well as recent *state of the art* approaches.

Visual Tracking: One of the most influential works in the field of visual tracking is undoubtedly the Lucas-Kanade tracker (LK) [7]. This technique iteratively matches image patches by linearising the local image gradients and minimising the sum of squared pixel errors. Many current trackers follow and extend this idea by adding an upper layer managing a cloud of LK *tracklets* [4,8]. One recent example is the Local-Global Tracker (LGT) [3] by Cehovin *et al.*, using a coupled-layer visual model. The local layer consists of a set of visual patches, while the global layer maintains a probabilistic model of object features such as colour, shape or motion. The global model is learned from the local patches and in turn it constrains the addition of new patches. FLOTrack (Featureless Objects Tracker) [9] uses a similar two layer approach, however edge features are used instead of conventional points to increase robustness to lack of texture.

Another approach to 2D tracking is *tracking by detection* where tracking is defined as a classification task. Grabner *et al.* [10] employed an *online boosting* method to update the appearance model while minimising error accumulation (drift). Babenko *et al.* [11] use *multiple instance learning*, instead of traditional supervised learning, for a more robust tracker. ℓ_1-norm tracker [12] learns a dictionary from local patches to handle occlusions. Kalal *et al.* combined tracking with detection in their Tracking-Learning-Detection (TLD) [5] framework, where (in)consistency of tracker and detector helps to indicate tracking failure. There are also many successful approaches using *particle filtering* for tracking. One of the most notable is CONDENSATION (Conditional Density Propagation) [13], which brought into the field of visual tracking the use of particles for non-parametric modelling of a pose probability distribution. Ross *et al.* [2] extended particle filtering by introducing *incremental learning* of an object appearance subspace that allowed the model to adapt to changes.

3D monocular tracking typically employs 3D models of the object. These approaches work with a user-supplied or previously learned model of a known object, which is then tracked in the sequence, examples of which are the tracking of the pose of human bodies, or vehicles in traffic scenes [14–17] or general *boxes* [18]. Another body of literature deals with 3D reconstruction of deformable surfaces [19]. However, we will not address these areas further as our focus is on model-less tracking. There have been relatively few attempts at learning 3D tracking models on the fly, but such approaches are fundamental to SfM. An example of a recent model-less 3D tracker is the work of Feng *et al.* [20], who employ SLAM techniques similar to TMAGIC, together with object segmentation. However, they do not attempt to estimate the surface shape beyond just a cloud of points, which allows the more advanced visibility reasoning used in TMAGIC. Another similar approach is the work of Prisacariu *et al.* [21] who uses level-set techniques for object segmentation. Our approach uses both point and line features to increase robustness to lack of texture.

Structure from Motion: *Structure from motion* (SfM) is an area of great interest for the computer vision community. Here, the task is to simultaneously estimate the structure of a scene observed by multiple cameras, and the poses of these cameras. Pictures of the scene can be either ordered in a sequence [22–24] or unordered [25,26]. Great advances have been recently achieved in the size and automation of the SfM process by Snavely *et al.* in their Bundler system [26,27] (based on Bundle Adjustment, BA). Their approach is *sequential*, i.e. starting reconstruction with a smaller number of cameras and then adding progressively more. A different approach has been taken by Gherardi *et al.* [25], who merge smaller reconstructions hierarchically. Pan *et al.* [22] reached real-time speed of SfM in their ProFORMA system for guided scanning of an object. This work is also very related to ours, however the object/background separation allows us to avoid the assumption that the object occupies the majority of the image. A sparse reconstruction can be upgraded to dense as a post-processing step, or alternatively a dense reconstruction can be performed directly [28]. Recently, the approach of Garg *et al.* [29] used variational optimisation from dense point-trajectories to directly estimate dense non-rigid SfM.

Visual SLAM: *Simultaneous localisation and mapping* is an area commonly associated with robotics, with similarities to SfM. The main difference is that SLAM, originally used for navigation of robots, is an online process. Therefore the images are always ordered in a sequence. It further differs in that the reconstructed cloud of features is usually sparse and the reconstructed area larger.

The first monocular vision-based SLAM technique was MonoSLAM by Davison *et al.* [30]. It was later extended to work with straight lines [31,32]. These algorithms (based on the Extended Kalman Filter, EKF) were able to run in real time and typically managed a very low number of features in the point cloud. Recently, there has been a shift from EKF to BA [33,34] and from sparse to dense features [35], ultimately leading to whole-image-alignment works [36,37].

3   Algorithm Description

We seek to track a 3D object throughout a sequence learning a model of appearance on the fly. However, our model differs from most online tracking approaches in that we employ ideas from both SfM and SLAM to form a 3D representation of the model that can cope with out-of-plane rotation. The program and data flow of the TMAGIC tracker is as follows (illustrated in Fig. 2, see the subsequent sections for full descriptions of the individual elements). The tracking loop is performed on every frame. 2D features (points and line segments in the image) are tracked in the new frame (Sect. 3.1), yielding the sets of features currently visible. Using these, the new camera pose can then be estimated (Sect. 3.2), while keeping the corresponding 3D features (points and lines in the real world) fixed. The world coordinate system is not fixed, so we can safely assume that the camera is moving around a stationary object. The tracking loop is repeated until a change in viewpoint necessitates an update of the 3D features, using the modelling subsystem.

The first step of modelling is a Bundle Adjustment (BA, Sect. 3.3). This refines the positions of 3D features and the camera, using the 2D observations. The updated features are subsequently used to retrain the shape model (Sect. 3.4), which can be exploited in two ways. The model defines regions

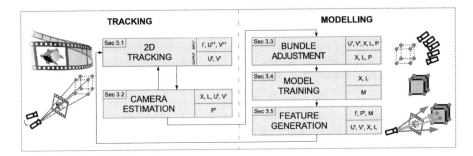

Fig. 2. Overview of the TMAGIC tracker. Symbols on the right side of each element indicate inputs and outputs, as labelled for 2D tracking. While the tracking loop is repeated in every frame, modelling only runs when necessary (according to Eq. (3)).

of the image which are eligible to detect new 2D features. Secondly, it provides an initialisation of the corresponding backprojected 3D features (Sect. 3.5). Features, successfully extracted using the current frame, camera pose and the shape model, enrich the 2D and 3D sets for use in future tracking.

3.1 2D Features and Tracking

The TMAGIC algorithm uses two types of features: points and line segments. The main advantages of point features are that they form readily available unique descriptors (patches), are localised precisely and have intuitive and simple projective properties. On the other hand, line features, which provide complementary information about the image, have different virtues. Lines encode a higher level of structural information [38], e.g. constraining the orientation of the surface. They can be not only texture-based, but also stemming from the shape of the object [9]. Therefore in man-made environments they appear in situations where point features are scarce [31].

The 2D point features $\mathbf{u}_i^t \in \mathcal{U}^t$ are extracted using two techniques: Difference of Gaussians and Hessian Laplace [39]. These features are tracked independently by an LK tracker from frame $\mathtt{I}^{t-1}$ to $\mathtt{I}^t$ ($\mathtt{I}^t$ represents the current frame and derived measurements, such as an intensity gradient). Features, which do not converge are removed from the 2D feature cloud. The tracked features generate a set of correspondences $\{(\mathbf{u}_i^{t-1}, \mathbf{u}_i^t)\}$, which are subsequently verified by LO-RANSAC [40,41]. Outliers to RANSAC, i.e. correspondences inconsistent with a global epipolar geometry model, are removed, as well as their respective 3D features, as these are likely to lie on the background.

The 2D line features $\mathbf{v}_i^t \in \mathcal{V}^t$ are extracted using the LSD [42] approach, a line segment detector with false-positive detection control. Lines are tracked as follows. Firstly, the LSD is executed on $\mathtt{I}^t$ to obtain a set of candidate segments $\mathbf{v}_j'^t \in \mathcal{V}'^t$. Along each of the previous line segments $\mathbf{v}_i^{t-1}$ a number of edge points are then sampled. Each of these is tracked independently, using the *guided edge search* of [9], leading to a new edge point in the current frame. If this new point belongs to a line segment in $\mathcal{V}'^t$, it votes for it. The segment $\mathbf{v}_j'^t$ with the most votes becomes the new feature $\mathbf{v}_i^t$. As there is no way to validate line correspondences w.r.t. an epipolar geometry [43], the features are validated using a threshold on the minimum number of votes (3 out of 5).

3.2 Camera Estimation

The camera with a projection matrix P^t is defined by the rotation R^t and position $\mathbf{C}^t$ of the projection centre in the world coordinate frame, given by the decomposition $\mathsf{P} = \mathsf{KR}\left[\mathsf{I}_{3\times3}\left| - \mathbf{C}\right.\right]$, where K is a calibration matrix of intrinsic camera parameters [43]. For simplicity, we define a general projection function $\mathsf{F_P}$, such that 3D lines are projected as $\mathbf{v}_i^t = \mathsf{F_{P}}(\mathbf{L}_i)$ and 3D points as $\mathbf{u}_i^t = \mathsf{F_{P^t}}(\mathbf{X}_i)$.

Assuming we have a cloud of 3D features (points $\mathbf{X}_i \in \mathcal{X}$ and line segments $\mathbf{L}_i \in \mathcal{L}$, which are defined by their end-points, specified in Sect. 3.3) and their projections $(\mathcal{U}^t, \mathcal{V}^t)$, it is possible to estimate a pose $(\mathsf{R}, \mathbf{C})$ of the camera P^t. We do not attempt to compute the calibration matrix K of the camera exactly, instead we use an estimate based on image dimensions [23]:

$$K = \begin{bmatrix} w + h & 0 & w/2 \\ & w + h & h/2 \\ & & 1 \end{bmatrix} \qquad (1)$$

where w and h are the width and height of the image respectively. This formula would not suffice for cases of strong zoom, wide-angle cameras, or cropped videos (shift of the principal point and narrowed viewing angle). However, Pollefeys et al. [23] show that images obtained by standard cameras are generally well approximated by this formula.

Estimation of calibrated camera pose given 2D to 3D point correspondences is a standard textbook problem, e.g. solved by a P3P (Perspective-3-Points [43]) RANSAC. However, there is no simple generalisation of the P3P problem for lines. Therefore we use an optimisation approach to solve for camera pose:

$$\mathsf{P}^t = \operatorname*{arg\,min}_{\bar{\mathsf{P}}^t} \left(\sum_{i=1}^{|\mathcal{U}^t|} ||\mathbf{u}_i^t - \mathsf{F}_{\bar{\mathsf{P}}^t}(\mathbf{X}_i)||^2 + \sum_{i=1}^{|\mathcal{V}^t|} \left((\tilde{\boldsymbol{\mu}}_{\mathbf{v}_i^t}^\top \tilde{\mathbf{l}}_i^t)^2 + (\tilde{\boldsymbol{\nu}}_{\mathbf{v}_i^t}^\top \tilde{\mathbf{l}}_i^t)^2 \right) \right), \qquad (2)$$

using both point and line features in a unified framework and exploiting the sequential nature of tracking. The error function consists of an error term for each point and line feature (in the first and second summation, respectively). For points, this is just a norm of the projection error. For line features, we define the error terms as orthogonal distances of the end-points of the segment $\mathbf{v}_i^t$ ($\tilde{\boldsymbol{\mu}}_{\mathbf{v}_i^t}, \tilde{\boldsymbol{\nu}}_{\mathbf{v}_i^t}$, in homogeneous coordinates), to the projection of the 3D line $\tilde{\mathbf{l}}_i^t = \mathsf{F}_{\bar{\mathsf{P}}^t}(\mathbf{L}_i)$ (homogeneous, normalised to the unit length of the normal vector). Note that since the line may not be fully visible (and is theoretically infinite), we use only perpendicular distances to cope with the aperture problem [9,31]. This minimisation is initialised at the pose in the previous frame (P^{t-1}). During our experiments, it was found that due to the smooth nature of the derivatives of (2), the basin of convergence for this optimisation is several orders of

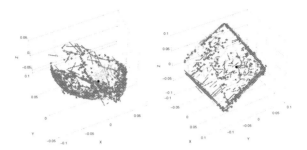

Fig. 3. Examples of 3D feature clouds and GP-learned smooth models. See the supplementary material for more visualisations. Notice the unseen parts of the objects, which are without features and where the model is extrapolated (i.e. the rear side of the car and the "pole" on the left side of the cube).

magnitude larger than typical inter-frame difference. See supplementary material for derivation of the error function Jacobian used.

In the first frame, we choose the world coordinate frame (which is defined only up to a similarity) as follows. The object, initialised as a sphere (see Sect. 3.4 for more details), is centred at the origin and camera centre $\mathbf{C}^1$ is at $(0, 0, 1)^\top$. The rotation $\mathbf{R}^1$ is set such that the origin is projected to the centre of the user-given bounding box and the y axis of the camera coordinate system is parallel to the y-z plane of the world coordinate system (see Fig. 4).

3.3   Bundle Adjustment

After initialisation, 2D tracking is performed until the distance between camera centres exceeds a specified threshold $\theta_{\mathbf{C}}$ [22]:

$$||\mathbf{C}^t - \mathbf{C}^{t'}|| > \theta_{\mathbf{C}} , \qquad (3)$$

where t' is the time of the last BA. When this condition is satisfied, the modelling part of the algorithm is performed. Firstly, the bundle adjustment refines the positions of 3D features $\mathcal{X}, \mathcal{L}$ and cameras $\mathcal{P}$ (for the purposes of BA, we define $\mathcal{P}$ as the set of previous cameras $\mathbf{P}^1, \dots, \mathbf{P}^t$). If speed is an issue, one may limit the BA to take only the last k cameras into account, i.e. to use $\mathcal{P}' = \{\mathbf{P}^i | i \in [\max(1, t-k); t]\}$, however, in our experiments this did not prove necessary (thus we set $k = \infty$). The BA [44] minimises a similar error to (2):

$$\arg\min_{\mathcal{X},\mathcal{L},\mathcal{P}} \sum_{u=1}^{t} \left(\sum_{i=1}^{|\mathcal{U}^u|} ||\mathbf{u}_i^t - \mathbf{F}_{\tilde{\mathbf{P}}^t}(\mathbf{X}_i)||^2 + \sum_{i=1}^{|\mathcal{V}^u|} \left((\tilde{\boldsymbol{\mu}}_{\mathbf{v}_i^t}^\top \tilde{\mathbf{l}}_i^t)^2 + (\tilde{\boldsymbol{\nu}}_{\mathbf{v}_i^t}^\top \tilde{\mathbf{l}}_i^t)^2 + \rho_i^2 \right) \right) , \qquad (4)$$

where the added term ρ_i is a regularisation term, which ensures that the lengths of 3D line segments are close to those observed. Note also that every point from $\mathcal{U}^t$ and $\mathcal{V}^t$ has a correspondence in $\mathcal{X}$ and $\mathcal{L}$ for every t, but not necessarily vice-versa, due to points which are not currently visible.

3.4 Gaussian Process Modelling

As discussed previously, the object shape is modelled as a Gaussian Process [45,46]. This allows us to infer a fully dense 3D model from the finite collection of discrete observations $\mathcal{X}$ and $\mathcal{L}$. Using the GP in this manner can be seen as estimating a distribution over an infinite number of possible shapes. The expectation of such a distribution (the most probable shape) can be used to model the object, while the variance at any point represents confidence.

The obtained model is non parametric, i.e. it can fit to any type of object without needing reparameterisation. The probabilistic nature of the model prevents overfitting through an implicit "Occam's-razor" effect, that favours models which are both simple and which explain the observations well.

In TMAGIC, we use a parameterisation of the shape as follows. The observed 3D points (point features $\mathcal{X}$ and end-points[1] of line features $\mathcal{L}$) are first re-expressed as a vector from the centre of mass of the object ($\mathbf{Y}_i \in \mathcal{Y}$). We then use these as training points, where the unit-length normalised vectors $\hat{\mathbf{Y}}_i = \mathbf{Y}_i/||\mathbf{Y}_i||$ represent the independent variable and the radii $r_{\hat{\mathbf{Y}}_i} = ||\mathbf{Y}_i||$ the dependent variable. As it does not suffer from a singularity in any direction, we found this parameterisation superior to alternatives such as spherical coordinates (predicting a radius from azimuth and elevation), despite the higher dimensionality. This representation prevents us from modelling complicated shapes (e.g. extreme concavities), however it proves sufficient in our experiments.

Without loss of generality, we can assume that the centre of mass of the training points coincides with the origin of the world coordinate system. In this case, for a query direction $\hat{\mathbf{Q}}$ (where $||\hat{\mathbf{Q}}|| = 1$), the resulting 3D point $\mathbf{Q}$ is predicted as [45]:

$$
\mathbf{Q} = \hat{\mathbf{Q}} \left[\mathrm{K}(\hat{\mathcal{y}},\hat{\mathbf{Q}})^\top \, \mathrm{K}(\hat{\mathcal{y}},\hat{\mathcal{y}})^{-1} \, \mathbf{r}_{\hat{\mathcal{y}}} \right.
$$
$$
\left. \pm \mathrm{K}(\hat{\mathcal{y}},\hat{\mathbf{Q}})^\top \, \mathrm{K}(\hat{\mathcal{y}},\hat{\mathcal{y}})^{-1} \, \mathrm{K}(\hat{\mathcal{y}},\hat{\mathbf{Q}}) \right] , \tag{5}
$$

or more succinctly as $\mathbf{Q} = \hat{\mathbf{Q}} \left(r_{\hat{\mathbf{Q}}} \pm \sigma_{\hat{\mathbf{Q}}} \right)$, where $r_{\hat{\mathbf{Q}}}$ is the predicted radius and $\sigma_{\hat{\mathbf{Q}}}$ is the confidence. K is the kernel function of the GP, relating to the surface properties of the modelled object, and may be any positive definite two-parameter function. This function is learned during tracking, such that the likelihood of the training data is maximised. The notation $\mathbf{r}_{\hat{\mathcal{y}}}$ represents a vector of norms of all vectors in the training set $\mathcal{Y}$, i.e. $\mathbf{r}_{\hat{\mathcal{y}};i} = r_{\hat{\mathbf{Y}}_i} = ||\mathbf{Y}_i||$.

Intuitively, Eq. (5) shows that the predicted radius at any point is defined by the training radii while accounting for the spatial relationships between the data points. The variance relates to these spatial relationships. The influence of any particular element of the training data is quantified by $\mathrm{K}(\hat{\mathcal{y}},\hat{\mathbf{Q}})$, while $\mathrm{K}(\hat{\mathcal{y}},\hat{\mathcal{y}})^{-1}$ removes any correlation within the training data.

We tried several alternative approaches for the surface shape modelling, such as mesh-based or modelling as a parametric probability distribution. However,

---

[1] It is possible to sample more points along line features which have high confidence.

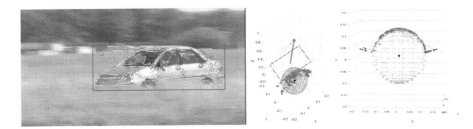

Fig. 4. State of the proposed TMAGIC tracker after the first frame. Left: a bounding box, $\mathcal{U}^1$ and $\mathcal{V}^1$. Right: $\mathcal{X}, \mathcal{L}$, initial model M (the blue sphere) and P^1 (magenta). For the camera, the visualisation shows the projection centre $\mathbf{C}$, principal direction and image plane. The upper left corner of the image plane is indicated by the dashed line (Colour figure online).

none had the properties required. The benefits of the GP include the ability to model a wide range of shapes without prior knowledge (non-parametric), no overfitting, good theoretical foundation and its probabilistic nature, giving confidence estimates across the object.

3.5   Feature Generation

For camera pose estimation (Sect. 3.2), we assumed that the 3D feature clouds $\mathcal{X}$ and $\mathcal{L}$ are known. In this section, we address the issue of feature generation and localisation. The assumption is made that a shape model of the object is given.

In the first frame I^1, initial sets of 2D features $\mathcal{U}^1$ and $\mathcal{V}^1$ are generated inside a user-supplied bounding box. When generating a 3D feature $\mathbf{X}_i$ for a new 2D point $\mathbf{u}_i^t$ (in the case of line features, both end-points must lie on the surface), the process is as follows. Firstly, the corresponding ray $\mathbf{Z}$ (parameterised by $\bar{\alpha}$) from the camera centre is generated:

$$\mathbf{Z}(\bar{\alpha}) = \mathbf{C} + \bar{\alpha}(\mathsf{KR})^{-1}\tilde{\mathbf{u}}_i^t \qquad (\bar{\alpha} > 0) , \tag{6}$$

where $\tilde{\mathbf{u}}_i^t$ is a homogeneous representation of $\mathbf{u}_i^t$. Then a search for an intersection between the ray and the shape is performed:

$$\mathbf{X}_i = \mathbf{Z}(\alpha) , \tag{7}$$

$$\alpha = \underset{\bar{\alpha}>0}{\arg\min}\,\bar{\alpha} \qquad \text{s.t.} \|\mathbf{Z}(\bar{\alpha})\| = r_{\hat{\mathbf{Z}}(\bar{\alpha})} . \tag{8}$$

If the minimisation of (8) has no solution, it means that the ray does not intersect the *mean surface* given by the GP (from the distribution of possible surfaces). The use of the mean surface corresponds to a threshold such that there is an equal probability of false positives (a detection on the background was added to the feature set) and false negatives (a point on the object surface was rejected). If there is prior knowledge about the respective robustness of other components available, this can be exploited by adding the appropriate factor (multiple of $\sigma_{\hat{\mathbf{Z}}(\bar{\alpha})}$) to $r_{\hat{\mathbf{Z}}(\bar{\alpha})}$ in (8).

Thus far, the process has been the same both for initialisation in the first frame and for adding new features after model retraining in the subsequent frames. However, there are several differences. Firstly, if a ray does not intersect the surface during the generation of new features in frame $f > 1$, it is not used (features are detected over the whole image). However, in the first frame, all the 2D features will lie inside the user-specified bounding box. In this case, we reconstruct them such that they minimise the distance to the surface (even when they do not intersect), leading to the fringe seen in Fig. 4:

$$\alpha = \arg\min_{\bar{\alpha} > 0}(\|\mathbf{Z}(\bar{\alpha})\| - r_{\hat{\mathbf{Z}}(\bar{\alpha})})^2 . \tag{9}$$

Generation of new features in $f > 1$ has one further condition. Since adding new features increases the time complexity of all other computations, new features are added only into uncertain regions of the object (with variance greater than a specified threshold, $\sigma_{\hat{\mathbf{Z}}(\alpha)} > \theta_\sigma$).

As previously mentioned, some of the 3D features may be temporarily occluded, i.e. without 2D correspondences. Surface normals, given by the shape model, provide us with one tool to determine which parts of the object are (not) visible from a particular direction. TMAGIC uses this information in two complementary ways. Firstly, if a 3D feature is deemed not visible, but it has 2D correspondence (e.g. adheres to an object contour), it can be removed. On the other hand, if a 3D feature has no 2D correspondence, but is on a surface which is seen by $\mathbf{P}^t$ under an angle close to normal, the 2D feature can be redetected. This is performed by projecting it into $\mathbf{I}^t$ by $\mathbf{P}^t$ and then tracking it in 2D using a stored appearance patch. *Loop closures* (as termed in the SLAM literature) are thus possible when a number of previously seen features are redetected.

4   Experimental Evaluation

In all experiments, the parameters were fixed as follows: $\theta_\mathbf{C} = 10\,\%$, $\theta_\sigma = 0.5\,\%$, relative to the scene size. Our proof-of-concept implementation currently runs in seconds per frame. However, there are possibilities for trivial technical improvements and for parallelisation, allowing real-time application.

Synthetic Data: Firstly, we show results on a synthetic sequence CUBE1 (Fig. 5). This has been rendered to have the following properties. It contains a cube, rotating with speed $1°$/frame. Some of the sides are rich in texture, some are weakly textured. From the point of view of our tracker, the camera circles around the fixed cube with a perfect circular trajectory (see Fig. 6). However, since the world coordinate frame is defined only up to a similarity transform and can be moved freely during the BA, it is not possible to measure quality of a tracker directly w.r.t. this expected position (i.e. no absolute ground truth is possible). Therefore we fit a 3D circle to the points and measure the error as

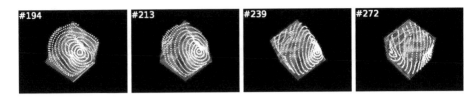

Fig. 5. Selected frames from the CUBE1 sequence. Notice, how TMAGIC learns the new face of the cube. #194: unknown shape, the surface is smoothed over. #213: first features detected, shape roughly estimated. #239: more features identified, shape refined. #272: Final state, model in agreement with the object.

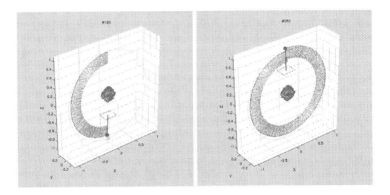

Fig. 6. The 3D scene in $t = 180$ and 360. The camera and features are shown in the same way as in Fig. 4, the camera trajectory (centres and principal directions for each previous frame) is shown in black. Ground-truth trajectory is in yellow. The details of the model can be seen in Fig. 3 (Colour figure online).

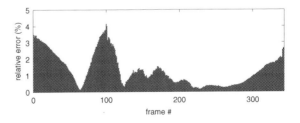

Fig. 7. Deviation of the trajectory from a perfect circle (least-squares fitted). Errors are relative to the radius of the circle. The trajectories at the beginning and end of the sequence did not meet (due to accumulated error prior to loop closure), thus the deviation from the fitted ground truth is distributed between the two. The peak around frame #100 is due to a temporary inaccuracy during the transition between sides of the cube, when the continuously visible side is lacking visual features. However, TMAGIC recovers once sufficient visual evidence has been accumulated.

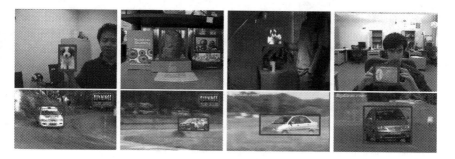

Fig. 8. First frames from the test sequences. From top and left: DOG, FISH, SYLVESTER, TWININGS, RALLY-LANCER, RALLY-VW, TOPGEAR1 and TOPGEAR2. The initial bounding boxes are overlaid.

an orthogonal distance from this circle. Figure 7 shows and explains the results. If we assume the camera orbits at a distance of 1 m, the mean camera pose error is 1.3 cm. This indicates a very close approximation to the circular trajectory. Despite being based on sparse data, the learned shape model represents the cubic shape (of side equal to approximately 17 cm) accurately, having mean reconstruction error 3.4 mm. See supplementary material for the input video and results.

To compare our method with currently used reconstruction approaches, we processed this sequence (with no background to account for) with VisualSfM [47,48] and Bundler [27,49]. While Bundler surprisingly failed, reconstructing 2 separate cubes, VisualSFM performs worse than TMAGIC with a comparable reconstruction error of 2.8 mm, but 72 % larger camera trajectory error of 2.3 cm.

Real Data: The performance of TMAGIC was further analysed on several sequences, used in previous 2D visual tracking publications. These sequences contain visible out-of-plane rotation in all cases. Additionally, we use several new sequences of drifting cars, which have, besides strong motion blur, significant out-of-plane rotation as a challenge. The first frames are shown in Fig. 8.

We compared our tracker with several state of the art tracking algorithms in Table 1: LGT [3], TLD [5] and FoT [8]. The FoT (Flock of Trackers) tracker is similar to our approach, in that it employs a group of independently tracked features with a higher management layer, however in 2D only. The next columns show the effect of the different stages of TMAGIC on performance. 3D tracking (**T**) assumes a fixed 3D model (sphere) and feature locations, added reconstruction (**TMIC**) allows updating of the feature clouds and a primitive object inference (a rigid sphere fit). Finally, TMAGIC gives performance for the full system. The performance metric was *localisation error*, i.e. the distance of the centre of the bounding box to the ground-truth centre. The results are visualised in Fig. 9 and the mean values tabulated in Table 1. Additionally, we show mean overlap of the tracked and ground-truth bounding boxes.

Table 1. Tracking results: mean localisation error/mean overlap. Bold numbers indicate the best result, underlined numbers the second best. See the text for discussion.

	LGT	TLD	FoT	T	T-MIC	TMAGIC
Dog [50]	19.3/20	12.3/56	**4.7**/63	13.9/<u>65</u>	<u>9.3</u>/**71**	12.1/46
Fish [2]	15.6/20	8.8/<u>72</u>	9.2/**75**	<u>8.0</u>/68	10.4/65	**5.6**/69
Sylvester [2]	**13.1**/16	18.0/**58**	18.0/**58**	37.3/42	35.3/9	<u>17.8</u>/<u>48</u>
Twinings [11]	22.5/18	<u>13.2</u>/38	15.5/<u>44</u>	42.9/31	16.2/29	**9.1**/**53**
Rally-Lancer	145.8/19	333.5/13	734.5/13	127.8/<u>43</u>	<u>121.3</u>/42	**94.3**/**53**
Rally-VW	<u>91.3</u>/21	152.5/<u>48</u>	196.9/39	149.4/39	148.3/39	**47.6**/**62**
TopGear1	**16.3**/<u>49</u>	65.1/34	80.4/41	<u>39.0</u>/<u>49</u>	44.5/43	40.0/**56**
TopGear2	84.3/37	104.3/21	117.9/29	<u>48.4</u>/<u>51</u>	84.1/31	**34.7**/**59**

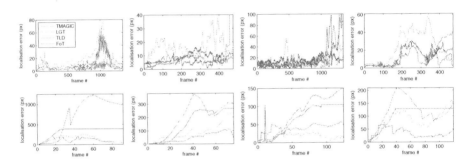

Fig. 9. Visualisation of results of the quantitative performance analysis. From top and left: Dog, Fish, Sylvester, Twinings, Rally-Lancer, Rally-VW, TopGear1 and TopGear2.

On the Dog sequence, the TMAGIC and TLD trackers perform similarly, and LGT slightly worse. All these trackers experience difficulties at about frame #1000, where the dog is partially occluded by the image border. This is however not a problem for FoT, which estimates the position accurately even under such strong occlusion. The Fish sequence is relatively easy, with all the trackers reaching low errors and TMAGIC being the best one. On the Sylvester scene, TMAGIC as well as FoT track consistently well until the end. Both LGT and TLD have similar momentary failures (frames #450 and #1100, respectively) but both are able to recover. For LGT, the duration of the problematic part of the sequence is shorter and the error is smaller, rendering it the best tracker for this sequence. The Twinings sequence contains full rotation and was originally created to measure trackers' robustness to out-of-plane rotation [11]. Unsurprisingly, TMAGIC significantly outperforms the state of the art on this sequence. The average localisation error reduction for all these scenes is 22 %.

The cars sequences are chosen because they contain rigid 3D objects under strong out-of-plane rotation (around 180°) with significant camera motion.

Therefore the TLD and FoT trackers, which are trying to track a plane only (one side of the car) instead of the 3D object, fail. As the cars rotate, the tracked parts are no longer usable and TLD reports this (the horizontal sections in Fig. 9). FoT is incapable of reporting object disappearance and it attempts to continue tracking, exacerbating the situation. The LGT tracker, which has a less rigid model of the object, is sometimes capable of tracking after the cars start to rotate, if the rotation is slow enough for the 2D shape model to adapt. The TMAGIC tracker is also able to adapt as the object rotates, and explicitly modelling the car in 3D improves robustness by allowing us to intelligently detect new features. While 2D trackers attempt to mitigate the effects of out-of-plane rotation, TMAGIC actively exploits it. This gives it a significant edge, resulting in the localisation error being reduced by 58 % on average. Notice that the errors in the RALLY sequences are generally higher, due to the higher resolution. The resulting model for the RALLY-VW sequence is visualised in Figs. 1 and 3. The car is modelled accurately, except for missing elements at the rear of the vehicle, which have not been observed during the sequence.

The last three columns of Table 1 show the effect of the different stages of TMAGIC on performance. Firstly, we compare FoT with T (2D and 3D trackers based on the same principle). FoT performs better on sequences without rotation (higher accuracy of the solution) and the advantage of 3D tracking becomes apparent with stronger out-of-plane rotations (decreasing the error up to five-fold). The next step is performing refinement of the 3D features and fitting a naïve spherical model (T→TMIC). However, the effect of this procedure on the performance of tracking in the image plane is imperceptible, despite the improved plausibility of the feature cloud. The final stage is training a more complex shape model using the feature cloud (TMIC→TMAGIC). This yields the most significant improvement (average error reduction of 50 %), rendering TMAGIC by far the best of the evaluated trackers in cases of out-of-plane rotations. In the case of TOPGEAR1, mostly the front part of the car is being modelled, shifting the centre of the bounding box forward and therefore adversely affecting the final results.[2]

5   Conclusion

The experiments show that the TMAGIC (Tracking, Modelling And Gaussian-Process Inference Combined) tracker is able to track standard sequences, used in many previous publications, with a comparable performance to the state of the art. However, by explicitly modelling the 3D object, it handles out-of-plane rotations significantly better and can also track in cases of full rotation. TMAGIC consistently outperforms simpler variants (TMIC etc.), especially in scenarios when the object/background segmentation is vital. This shows the benefit of the shape model, used for filtering features and initialisation of their 3D positions.

---

[2] See http://cvssp.org/Personal/KarelLebeda/TMAGIC/ for the sequences and more results.

TMAGIC works under the assumption that the object is rigid. TMAGIC is robust to small shape variations (e.g. a face), but is not capable of tracking articulated objects, e.g. a walking person, and extension to non-rigid object tracking is the subject of future work. One possible approach would be storing multiple models to span the area of possible shapes. This can also help with redetection to recover from drift. Another limitation would be full occlusions in long-term tracking. An additional redetection stage (as in TLD and other long-term trackers) could fix this, but is beyond the scope of this paper. Fast motion may also cause failure in the underlying 2D tracking. However, the algorithm is robust to low textured objects through the use of line features (taken from texture-less tracking literature).

TMAGIC tracks a single object. A naive multi-object extension, running it multiple times in parallel, would be trivial since TMAGIC doesn't require any pre-learning and the object properties are estimated online. Advanced correlation or occlusion reasoning would be an interesting field for future research.

Acknowledgement. This work was supported by the EPSRC grant "Learning to Recognise Dynamic Visual Content from Broadcast Footage" (EP/I011811/1).

References

1. Hare, S., Saffari, A., Torr, P.H.S.: Struck: structured output tracking with kernels. In: ICCV (2011)
2. Ross, D., Lim, J., Lin, R.S., Yang, M.H.: Incremental learning for robust visual tracking. IJCV **77**, 125–141 (2008)
3. Cehovin, L., Kristan, M., Leonardis, A.: Robust visual tracking using an adaptive coupled-layer visual model. PAMI **35**, 941–953 (2013)
4. Kolsch, M., Turk, M.: Fast 2D hand tracking with flocks of features and multi-cue integration. In: CVPRW (2004)
5. Kalal, Z., Mikolajczyk, K., Matas, J.: Tracking-learning-detection. PAMI **34**, 1409–1422 (2012)
6. Mulloni, A., Ramachandran, M., Reitmayr, G., Wagner, D., Grasset, R., Diaz, S.: User friendly SLAM initialization. In: ISMAR (2013)
7. Lucas, B., Kanade, T.: An iterative image registration technique with an application to stereo vision. In: IJCAI (1981)
8. Matas, J., Vojir, T.: Robustifying the flock of trackers. In: CVWW (2011)
9. Lebeda, K., Matas, J., Bowden, R.: Tracking the untrackable: how to track when your object is featureless. In: Park II, J., Kim, J. (eds.) ACCV 2012. LNCS, vol. 7729, pp. 347–359. Springer, Heidelberg (2012)
10. Grabner, H., Leistner, C., Bischof, H.: Semi-supervised on-line boosting for robust tracking. In: Forsyth, D., Torr, P., Zisserman, A. (eds.) ECCV 2008, Part I. LNCS, vol. 5302, pp. 234–247. Springer, Heidelberg (2008)
11. Babenko, B., Yang, M.H., Belongie, S.: Robust object tracking with online multiple instance learning. PAMI **33**, 1619–1632 (2011)
12. Xing, J., Gao, J., Li, B., Hu, W., Yan, S.: Robust object tracking with online multi-lifespan dictionary learning. In: ICCV (2013)
13. Isard, M., Blake, A.: CONDENSATION - conditional density propagation for visual tracking. IJCV **29**, 5–28 (1998)

14. Prisacariu, V.A., Segal, A.V., Reid, I.: Simultaneous monocular 2D segmentation, 3D pose recovery and 3d reconstruction. In: Lee, K.M., Matsushita, Y., Rehg, J.M., Hu, Z. (eds.) ACCV 2012, Part I. LNCS, vol. 7724, pp. 593–606. Springer, Heidelberg (2013)
15. Dame, A., Prisacariu, V., Ren, C., Reid, I.: Dense reconstruction using 3D object shape priors. In: CVPR (2013)
16. Sigal, L., Isard, M., Haussecker, H., Black, M.: Loose-limbed people: estimating 3D human pose and motion using non-parametric belief propagation. IJCV **98**, 15–48 (2012)
17. Wojek, C., Walk, S., Roth, S., Schindler, K., Schiele, B.: Monocular visual scene understanding: understanding multi-object traffic scenes. PAMI (2013)
18. Kim, K., Lepetit, V., Woo, W.: Keyframe-based modeling and tracking of multiple 3D objects. In: ISMAR (2010)
19. Varol, A., Shaji, A., Salzmann, M., Fua, P.: Monocular 3D reconstruction of locally textured surfaces. PAMI **34**, 1118–1130 (2012)
20. Feng, Y., Wu, Y., Fan, L.: On-line object reconstruction and tracking for 3D interaction. In: ICME (2012)
21. Prisacariu, V.A., Kahler, O., Murray, D.W., Reid, I.D.: Simultaneous 3D tracking and reconstruction on a mobile phone. In: ISMAR (2013)
22. Pan, Q., Reitmayr, G., Drummond, T.: ProFORMA: probabilistic feature-based on-line rapid model acquisition. In: BMVC (2009)
23. Pollefeys, M., Van Gool, L., Vergauwen, M., Verbiest, F., Cornelis, K., Tops, J., Koch, R.: Visual modeling with a hand-held camera. IJCV **59**, 207–232, (2004)
24. Tanskanen, P., Kolev, K., Meier, L., Camposeco, F., Saurer, O., Pollefeys, M.: Live metric 3D reconstruction on mobile phones. In: ICCV (2013)
25. Gherardi, R., Farenzena, M., Fusiello, A.: Improving the efficiency of hierarchical structure-and-motion. In: CVPR (2010)
26. Agarwal, S., Snavely, N., Simon, I., Seitz, S.M., Szeliski, R.: Building Rome in a day. In: ICCV (2009)
27. Snavely, N., Seitz, S.M., Szeliski, R.: Modeling the world from internet photo collections. IJCV **80**, 189–210 (2007)
28. Furukawa, Y., Ponce, J.: Accurate, dense, and robust multi-view stereopsis. PAMI **32**, 1362–1376 (2010)
29. Garg, R., Roussos, A., Agapito, L.: Dense variational reconstruction of non-rigid surfaces from monocular video. In: CVPR (2013)
30. Davison, A.J., Reid, I., Molton, N., Stasse, O.: MonoSLAM: Real-time single camera SLAM. PAMI **29**, 1052–1067 (2007)
31. Smith, P., Reid, I., Davison, A.J.: Real-time monocular slam with straight lines. In: BMVC (2006)
32. Hirose, K., Saito, H.: Fast line description for line-based slam. In: BMVC (2012)
33. Holmes, S.A., Murray, D.W.: Monocular SLAM with conditionally independent split mapping. PAMI **35**, 1451–1463 (2013)
34. Strasdat, H., Montiel, J.M.M., Davison, A.: Real-time monocular SLAM: why filter? In: ICRA (2010)
35. Klein, G., Murray, D.: Parallel tracking and mapping for small AR workspaces. In: ISMAR (2007)
36. Newcombe, R.A., Davison, A.J.: Live dense reconstruction with a single moving camera. In: CVPR (2010)
37. Newcombe, R.A., Lovegrove, S., Davison, A.: DTAM: dense tracking and mapping in real-time. In: ICCV (2011)

38. Zhang, L.: Line primitives and their applications in geometric computer vision. Ph.D. thesis, Department of Computer Science, Kiel University (2013)
39. Vedaldi, A., Fulkerson, B.: VLFeat: an open and portable library of computer vision algorithms (2008). http://www.vlfeat.org/
40. Lebeda, K., Matas, J., Chum, O.: Fixing the locally optimized RANSAC. In: BMVC (2012)
41. Chum, O., Matas, J.: Matching with PROSAC - PROgressive SAmple Consensus. In: CVPR (2005)
42. von Gioi, R., Jakubowicz, J., Morel, J.M., Randall, G.: LSD: a fast line segment detector with a false detection control. PAMI 32, 722–732 (2010)
43. Hartley, R.I., Zisserman, A.: Multiple View Geometry in Computer Vision, 2nd edn. Cambridge University Press, Cambridge (2004)
44. Agarwal, S., Mierle, K., Others: Ceres solver. http://code.google.com/p/ceres-solver/
45. Rasmussen, C.E., Williams, C.K.I.: Gaussian Processes for Machine Learning. MIT Press, Cambridge (2006)
46. Hensman, J., Fusi, N., Andrade, R., Durrande, N., Saul, A., Zwiessele, M., Lawrence, N.D.: GPy library. http://github.com/SheffieldML/GPy
47. Wu, C., Agarwal, S., Curless, B., Seitz, S.M.: Multicore bundle adjustment. In: CVPR (2011)
48. Wu, C.: Towards linear-time incremental structure from motion. In: 3DV (2013)
49. Snavely, N., Seitz, S.M., Szeliski, R.: Photo tourism: exploring image collections in 3D. In: SIGGRAPH (2006)
50. Chen, M., Pang, S.K., Cham, T.J., Goh, A.: Visual tracking with generative template model based on riemannian manifold of covariances. In: ICIF (2011)

Clouds in the Cloud

Dmitry Veikherman$^{(\boxtimes)}$, Amit Aides, Yoav Y. Schechner,
and Aviad Levis

Department of Electrical Engineering, Technion - Israel Institute of Technology,
Haifa, Israel
agate@tx.technion.ac.il

Abstract. Light-field imaging can be scaled up to a very large area, to
map the Earth's atmosphere in 3D. Multiview spaceborne instruments
suffer low spatio-temporal-angular resolution, and are very expensive and
unscalable. We develop sky light-field imaging, by a wide, scalable network
of wide-angle cameras looking upwards, which upload their data to the
cloud. This new type of imaging-system poses *new computational vision
and photography problems*, some of which generalize prior monocular tasks.
These include radiometric self-calibration across a network, overcoming
flare by a network, and background estimation. On the other hand, network redundancy offers *solutions* to these problems, which we derive.
Based on such solutions, the light-field network enables unprecedented
ways to measure nature. We demonstrate this experimentally by 3D recovery of clouds, in high spatio-temporal resolution. It is achieved by space
carving of the volumetric distribution of semi-transparent clouds. Such
sensing can complement satellite imagery, be useful to meteorology, make
aerosol tomography realizable, and give new, powerful tools to atmospheric and avian wildlife scientists.

1 Introduction

Plenoptic, light-field and integral imaging [1,6,8,12,23,29,35] sample the directional and spatial distribution of radiance. This imaging mode has been used in
small-scale setups. However, it can be scaled up to map the Earth's atmosphere
in 3D. Sampling the atmospheric radiance spatio-angularly is achieved by a few
spaceborne and airborne instruments, including the Multiangle Imaging Spec-
troRadiometer (MISR) [18,21], the Airborne Multiangle SpectroPolarimetric
Imager (AirMSPI) [19,20] and POLDER [10,14,39]. These architectures have
crude resolution spatially (up to kilometers per pixel), angularly (≈9 angles per
view) [47], or temporally (orbit takes several days to return to the same terres-
trial spot). Furthermore, spaceborne instruments are extremely expensive and
unscalable. We develop a complementing approach: the atmospheric light-field
is captured from below, by wide-angle cameras looking upwards. This approach
is a *scalable sensor network*, that captures images simultaneously over a very
large area, densely.

Electronic supplementary material The online version of this chapter (doi:10.
1007/978-3-319-16817-3_43) contains supplementary material, which is available to
authorized users.

© Springer International Publishing Switzerland 2015
D. Cremers et al. (Eds.): ACCV 2014, Part IV, LNCS 9006, pp. 659–674, 2015.
DOI: 10.1007/978-3-319-16817-3_43

Creating and exploiting such a network poses several requirements: low-cost units, communications, and tailored computational photography algorithms. The first two requirements are met thanks to wireless infrastructure, low-cost cameras and *cloud computing* services. Hence, we can deploy solar-powered cameras wherever communication reaches. By wireless, they upload their sky-images to the "cloud", from which the light-field data can be analyzed. However, this new type of imaging-system gives rise to new problems and algorithms, part of which we deal with in this paper. In a sense, the network generalizes some problems that had been posed for monocular setups a decade ago. On the other hand, network redundancy offers *solutions* to these problems.

The computational photography problems include radiometric self-calibration across a network of cameras, background estimation, and overcoming saturation and flare by a network. We demonstrate this in real field experiments by building a small version Sky-Technion Array of Sensors (STARS). Such a network enables unprecedented 3D imaging of cloud fields, in high spatio-temporal resolution. This approach can complement multi-angular satellite imagery. It can make aerosol tomography [2,5] realizable, offer new ways to study weather phenomena and avian wildlife, and aid electric power management [40].

2   Background

2.1   Monocular Radiometric Self-calibration

A large network should use low-cost camera units. Such cameras often have spatial and temporal radiometric inconsistencies. For example, spatial gain (e.g., by vignetting [27,36]) is often modeled by a function $M(\mathbf{x})$, where $\mathbf{x} = (x, y)$ is a camera pixel. The image irradiance at time t is $\tilde{I}_t(\mathbf{x}) = M(\mathbf{x})I_t(O)$, where $I_t(O)$ is the pixel irradiance when $M = 1$, for observed object O. For a single camera, consistent readouts can be obtained in the field by self-calibration. The strongest methods rely on redundant images, taken at modulated settings. Correspondence is established between modulated readouts, e.g. by aligning a pan sequence. Assuming brightness constancy, corresponding measurements yield constraints. Aggregating constraints over different pixels and frames recovers parameters of radiometric inconsistencies. This recovery makes monocular pixel readout spatially consistent. Section 4 expands this principle to a camera-array.

2.2   Avoiding Blooming, Lens-Flare in a Single Camera

In wide-angle sky-views, the sun is liable to frequently shine directly into the lens, creating blooming. Moreover, sun-rays create an additive, spatially varying lens-flare. Reducing flare was suggested [30,42,43,48] using either a specialized detector array for nearby objects, or camera rotation during capture of a static scene. Both ways complicate the need for simple, low-cost units and operation.

Sky-observing wide-field cameras often have a *dynamic sun blocker*: an opaque object raised above the camera optics, blocking the Sun from view. There are various configurations, but all of them *move*, as the Sun direction changes during

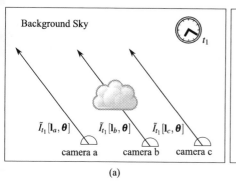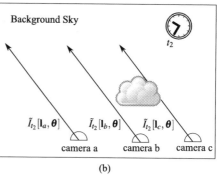

(a)   (b)

Fig. 1. Regional stationarity: in a wide region, objects at infinity and the background sky should have the same color, for a common view angle θ, e.g., $[l_a, \theta]$ vs. $[l_c, \theta]$ at t_1. Nearby objects (clouds) result in pixel differences, e.g., $[l_b, \theta]$ vs. $[l_c, \theta]$ at t_1. Nevertheless, the statistics (spatio-temporal variations and correlations) are stationary across viewpoints. This enables statistical processing across viewpoints and time. Residual measured bias is attributed to slight inter-camera radiometric inconsistencies.

the day and across the year. Motorized solutions [41] that need to work year-around significantly complicate such camera units, making them very expensive. Section 7 explains that a large camera network inherently bypasses the problem, without a need to constantly move a Sun blocker.

2.3 Current 3D Cloud Mapping

Existing research and operational sky-imaging systems[1] are few, relying on high quality components [3,9,16,28,37,46]. Due to their complexity and costs, they were only used to estimate *cloud-base* over narrow regions right above a narrow-baseline camera pair. Satellite-based estimation of 3D *cloud-tops* has been proposed by MISR [45]. It takes several minutes for MISR to capture multiple viewpoints of a region, during which the clouds generally move. Weather radars sense *raindrops*, which are much larger than cloud-drops and ice crystals.

3 Regional Stationarity in a Camera Network

A network of sky-observing cameras is spread over a region. The location vector of camera c is l_c. Any image pixel $\mathbf{x}$ of camera c is back-projected to a ray at direction-angle vector (zenith, azimuth) θ in a global coordinate system. The data is the radiance measured per location, direction and time, $\tilde{I}_t[l_c, \theta(\mathbf{x})]$. An interesting assumption that can be made is *regional stationarity*. In a region containing the cameras, the chance of a cloud, clear sky, or haziness affecting $\tilde{I}_t[l_c, \theta]$ is *independent* of c. Thus, inter-camera image variations due to atmospheric conditions are *random and unbiased*. This is illustrated in Fig. 1.

---

[1] There are also ground viewing webcams that happen to see sky parts [13,26] and weather cameras that are too sparse to be integrated for recovery.

Some monocular algorithms tend to rely on gathering statistics over time, thus assuming temporal stationarity. Nevertheless, *simultaneous* images captured by *different camera nodes* are generally different from each other. Due to regional stationarity, a change of viewpoint has an effect similar to change in time: a cloud in $\tilde{I}_t[\mathbf{l}_c, \boldsymbol{\theta}]$ is often not in $\tilde{I}_t[\mathbf{l}_{c'}, \boldsymbol{\theta}]$. Consequently, monocular algorithms can be extended to statistics gathered over both time and viewpoint (as done underwater in [4]). Regional stationarity is supported by meteorological research [7,33]. Stationarity breaks down across large topographic discontinuities: a mountain ridge, coast line. These locations are known, and hence can be handled or avoided in stationarity-based analysis.

4   Self-calibration in a Camera Network

Internal geometric and radiometric camera characteristics (including distortions, radiometric response) are calibrated in the lab using established monocular methods. However, once a camera is placed in the field, unknown parameters are introduced. External sources in the vicinity of a camera may create a weak lens glare, that *offsets* radiometric readings, in way that varies both spatially and across viewpoints. Moreover, residual *gain* variations may be between different cameras, despite lab calibration. This may be exacerbated in the field by dirt accumulation on lenses. Similarly to Sect. 2.1, the solution relies on redundant measurements at corresponding points.

For correspondence, geometric calibration [44] is necessary. The internal parameters Ψ_c of camera c are pre-calibrated in the lab. In the field, the location vector $\mathbf{l}_c$ is known by GPS but the orientation (yaw, pitch and roll angle vector $\boldsymbol{\Theta}_c$) is loosely set. The orientation is calibrated by automatically detecting and tracking extra-terrestrial (XT) objects (Moon, planets, Sun) [32,44], across night or day,[2] at pixel $\mathbf{x}_{\text{measured}}^{\text{XT}}(t)$. Using astronomical charts, an XT object is known[3] to be at angle vector (zenith, azimuth) $\boldsymbol{\theta}^{\text{XT}}(t)$ relative to a global coordinate system. Given camera orientation $\boldsymbol{\Theta}_c$, a projection Π converts a ray direction $\boldsymbol{\theta}^{\text{XT}}(t)$ to pixel $\Pi(\boldsymbol{\theta}^{\text{XT}}(t); \boldsymbol{\Theta}_c, \Psi_c)$.

During the course of a day or night, the number of frames N^{frames} is $\mathcal{O}(100)$, leading to a simple optimization formulation:

$$\hat{\boldsymbol{\Theta}}_c = \arg\min_{\boldsymbol{\Theta}_c} \sum_{t=1}^{N^{\text{frames}}} \| \Pi(\boldsymbol{\theta}^{\text{XT}}(t); \boldsymbol{\Theta}_c, \Psi_c) - \mathbf{x}_{\text{measured}}^{\text{XT}}(t) \|^2. \tag{1}$$

We solved it using exhaustive search or gradient descent from null initialization, with the same results. The orientation calibration is illustrated in Fig. 2.

Based on $\hat{\boldsymbol{\Theta}}_c$, all captured images $\tilde{I}_{c,t}(\mathbf{x})$ taken by camera c are aligned to the global coordinate system: the backprojected ray has direction vector

$$\boldsymbol{\theta}(\mathbf{x}) = \Pi^{-1}(\mathbf{x}; \hat{\boldsymbol{\Theta}}_c, \Psi_c). \tag{2}$$

---

[2] Manual tracking of a special flight and long exposures at night were used in [44].

[3] Higher than $20°$ above the horizon [11], errors caused by atmospheric refraction are smaller than $0.05°$, much less than the angular size of each of our pixels, $0.18°$.

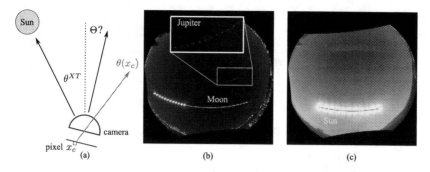

Fig. 2. (a) To estimate the camera yaw-pitch-roll angle vector $\boldsymbol{\Theta}_c$, we rely on image locations of extra-terrestrial objects, whose direction vector $\boldsymbol{\theta}^{\mathrm{XT}}(t)$ is known $\forall t$. (b) Photo-montage of night sky images. It shows the Moon at different times, the expected trajectory based on the estimated $\boldsymbol{\Theta}_c$, and a close-up on the corresponding sampled images of Jupiter. (c) Photo-montage of the daylight sky. It shows the Sun at different hours, the expected trajectory based on the estimated $\boldsymbol{\Theta}_c$ and lens-flares.

Inter-camera Relative Radiometric Self-calibration. Consider a *fixed* view direction $\boldsymbol{\theta}$ observed by several cameras. The set $\{\tilde{I}_t[\mathbf{l}_c, \boldsymbol{\theta}]\}_c$ corresponds to readouts of parallel rays, back-projected from all cameras in the network. Values in this set generally differ from each other: $\tilde{I}_t[\mathbf{l}_c, \boldsymbol{\theta}] \neq \tilde{I}_t[\mathbf{l}_{c'}, \boldsymbol{\theta}]$. There are two causes for this difference:

1. Different camera locations mean different observed objects. Momentarily, camera c may observe a cloud while c' observes a clear sky, or vice versa. Camera c' may momentarily observe a somewhat denser haze volume than c, etc.
2. Slight inter-camera radiometric inconsistencies, which we need to estimate.

Cause 1 is usually dominant. We need to overcome it, in order to analyze cause 2. Here we rely on the regional stationarity described in Sect. 3. Per camera c and view angle $\boldsymbol{\theta}$, bias is due to cause (2). We easily detect and characterize the bias by capturing *statistics over time*.

We performed experiments, with a small field-deployed network (STARS), detailed in Sect. 5. Figure 3a shows radiometric inconsistency between cameras a and b. Figure 3b is a scatter-plot of $\tilde{I}_t[\mathbf{l}_a, \boldsymbol{\theta}]$ vs. $\tilde{I}_t[\mathbf{l}_b, \boldsymbol{\theta}]$, $\forall t, \boldsymbol{\theta}$, for the red-channel. From such plots, we hypothesized that camera a has a slight offset vs. b. We thus estimated, per color channel, the map of radiometric offset (across pixels, or ray-directions). A temporal median was used:

$$\hat{o}_{b-a}(\boldsymbol{\theta}) = \mathrm{median}_t\{\tilde{I}_t[\mathbf{l}_b, \boldsymbol{\theta}] - \tilde{I}_t[\mathbf{l}_a, \boldsymbol{\theta}]\}. \tag{3}$$

The map $\hat{o}_{b-a}(\boldsymbol{\theta})$ was then spatially smoothed and used to correct $\tilde{I}_t[\mathbf{l}_a, \boldsymbol{\theta}]$. As shown in Fig. 3d, the results have much better inter-camera consistency. A similar process was applied to other cameras, but they had negligible radiometric offsets with respect to camera b. The spatially varying offset in camera a was later found to be due to a nearby light source.

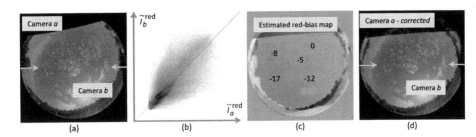

Fig. 3. [a] Splitting the field of view to upper/lower halves, to pixels corresponding respectively to either $\tilde{I}_t[\mathbf{1}_a, \boldsymbol{\theta}]$ or $\tilde{I}_t[\mathbf{1}_b, \boldsymbol{\theta}]$. In the line between the marked arrows, radiometric inconsistency shows-up as a seam across which colors slightly change (**please view on a color computer screen**). [b] Scatter-plot of $\tilde{I}_t[\mathbf{1}_a, \boldsymbol{\theta}]$ vs. $\tilde{I}_t[\mathbf{1}_b, \boldsymbol{\theta}]$, $\forall t, \boldsymbol{\theta}$, red-channel. [c] The estimated offset map $\hat{o}_{b-a}(\boldsymbol{\theta})$, red channel. It is derived based on a set of images taken during several hours. [d] Splitting the field of view in half, to *corrected* pixels from either $\hat{I}_t[\mathbf{1}_a, \boldsymbol{\theta}]$ or $\hat{I}_t[\mathbf{1}_b, \boldsymbol{\theta}]$: inconsistencies in the line between the marked arrows are greatly diminished (Color figure online).

A similar process detects slight variations of gain (vignetting). Suppose there is no offset. In analogy to Eq. (3), the gain in b is higher than in a by a factor

$$\hat{M}_{b/a}(\boldsymbol{\theta}) = \mathrm{median}_t\{\tilde{I}_t[\mathbf{1}_b, \boldsymbol{\theta}]/\tilde{I}_t[\mathbf{1}_a, \boldsymbol{\theta}]\}. \tag{4}$$

This way, all the network is radiometrically aligned to a single master camera. After radiometric corrections, the light-field samples are denoted $\hat{I}_t[\mathbf{1}_b, \boldsymbol{\theta}]$.

5   More Details About the Experimental Setup

Before proceeding with mathematical problems and solutions, we give more details about a small version STARS network. Each of the five nodes is built from a basic component set. Its core is a Raspberry-Pi computer and a 5 MP Raspberry-Pi camera, whose gain, response and white-balance can be fixed, avoiding temporal radiometric variations. We manually mounted small fisheye lenses. Due to this coarse lens-to-chip alignment, each camera has a different peripheral dead-region, creating a missing part in the view-field and distinct vignetting (Fig. 4). As we explain, a network as-a-whole can inherently overcome these issues. Every 30 s, synchronously, all units automatically transmit image data to the internet (cloud-service). Each unit is solar powered. STARS operated for weeks from rooftops at the Technion, uploading data [17].

6   Network-Assisted Background Estimation

In monocular settings, change-detection algorithms use temporal filtering to characterize the background: foreground dynamic objects are at *different locations at different times* and are thus pruned. In our case this translates to stating

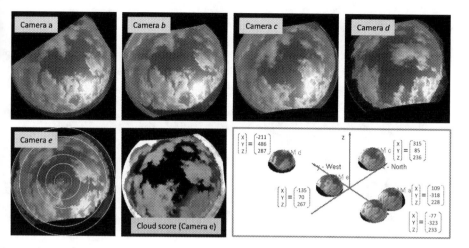

Fig. 4. Images taken simultaneously by a 5-node STARS network. They are geometrically aligned to the zenith and north, and resampled to *polar azimuthal equidistant* projection in this global system. Equidistant zenith angle circles are overlayed on $\tilde{I}_t[\mathbf{l}_e, \boldsymbol{\theta}]$ (camera e). Each camera had dead-regions, due to rough lens alignment. Corresponding to the frame in camera e, a *cloud score* map (Eq. 8) has high values in cloud-pixels, diminishing outside them. [Bottom-right] The 3D setup of the small STARS, laterally spread over hundreds of meters, at somewhat different altitudes (Color figure online).

that a cloud in $\tilde{I}_t[\mathbf{l}_c, \boldsymbol{\theta}]$ is often not in $\tilde{I}_{t'}[\mathbf{l}_c, \boldsymbol{\theta}]$, when $t' \neq t$. However, if clouds move slowly, while illumination gradually changes, temporal filtering may be insufficient. This is illustrated in Fig. 5.

A light-field network enhances this principle, with more effective pruning-per-time. Recall regional stationarity (Sect. 3). A change of viewpoint has an effect similar to change in time: a cloud in $\tilde{I}_t[\mathbf{l}_c, \boldsymbol{\theta}]$ is often not in $\tilde{I}_t[\mathbf{l}_{c'}, \boldsymbol{\theta}]$. Consequently, background sky values are obtained by data filtering over *both* time and viewpoint. This network-based principle can enhance arbitrary background estimation algorithms, which would otherwise be monocular. We demonstrate this using a simplistic, basic criterion. In broad daylight, clouds are brighter than the sky [24]. Hence, an estimator for the sky background can be, for example

$$\text{SKY}(\boldsymbol{\theta}) = \arg\min_{t,c} \tilde{I}_t[\mathbf{l}_c, \boldsymbol{\theta}] \qquad (5)$$

where $t \in [1 \dots N^{\text{frames}}]$ and $c \in [1 \dots N^{\text{views}}]$. This is illustrated in Fig. 5.

7 Bypassing the Sun Through a Camera Network

As Sect. 2.2 explains, in existing full sky-imagers, effects of direct sunlight are often mitigated by a small dynamic sun-blocker, which complicates the system and its cost, while having a blind-region. The network offers a different solution, which can be radical, yet simple. On each camera, the sun-blocker is *static*, and

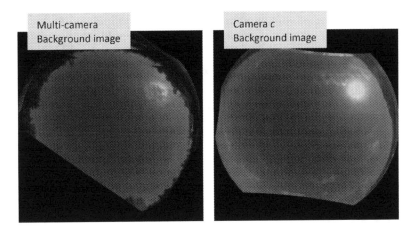

Fig. 5. [Left] Estimation of the sky background, using Eq. (5) based on five temporal instances and five viewpoints. [Right] Estimation of the sky background, using five temporal instances, but just a single viewpoint, resulting in more residual clouds.

has no moving part. The blocker can be large, covering the entire range of directions the Sun may occupy during the year or part of it. In this configuration, each camera unit has a large blind area (See Fig. 6). Nevertheless, the entire *network has no blind spot*, when viewing the atmosphere. This remarkable property is a result of network-redundancy, as we explain.

A static year-round sun blocker on camera c permanently obstructs a set Γ_c of atmospheric voxels. These voxels, however, are generally visible at several other cameras, e.g., those indexed e, f, g in Fig. 6. Hence, a sufficiently wide network has no 3D blind spot, despite permanent sun-blocking. Voxels that are not obstructed in any view are better constrained than voxels in Γ_c.

We now quantify the implication of this approach to the network extent, referring to the northern hemisphere without loss of generality. Nearly all weather phenomena are under the tropopause, whose altitude H above sea level is typically 17 km at the equator, and decreasing with latitude. The solar seasonal angle amplitude is $\beta \approx 23.5^o$. At latitude γ, thus, a permanent sun blocker spans zenith angles in the range $\gamma \pm \beta$. Earth is divided here to three region classes:

- In the tropics, the sky directly above a camera is blocked. Consider a small area $\mathcal{A}$, e.g., 1 km wide. According to Fig. 6c, the sky above $\mathcal{A}$ can efficiently be observed without a blind spot by cameras to its *south*. The network needs units extending to distance $D = H \tan(\beta - \gamma) + \epsilon$ from $\mathcal{A}$, where ϵ is a small distance, sufficient for triangulation at H. At the equator $D \approx 7.4$ km. It can be shown that if $\mathcal{A}$ is wider than $2H[\tan(\beta - \gamma) + \tan(\beta + \gamma)]$, the network can triangulate all the sky above it.
- As latitude increases towards the tropic circles, D decreases to zero. Thus the network can observe and triangulate all the sky right above it, anywhere outside the tropics, in the mid-latitudes.

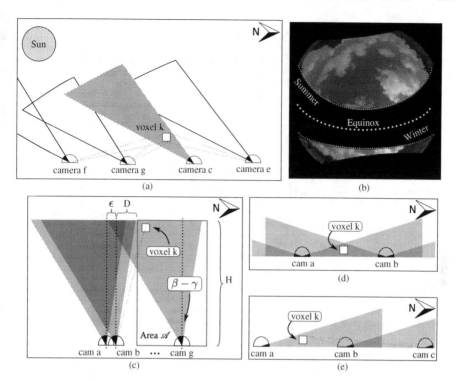

Fig. 6. [a] Camera c has a blind-region, covering Sun directions at l_c. The blind region corresponds to set Γ_c of atmospheric voxels not sensed by camera c. The network as a whole still has coverage of voxels $k \in \Gamma_c$, as they are observed by cameras e, f, g. [b] Simulation of a whole sky image (polar azimuthal equidistant projection), blocking all solar directions during the year, at a mid-latitude. [c] In the topics, the network must have nodes at distance D outside surveyed area $\mathcal{A}$, if $\mathcal{A}$ is narrow. The distance D depends on the latitude γ, while $\beta \approx 23.5°$. [d] In the arctic, the blind region is adjacent to the horizon, in all azimuth angles. Fixed blocking of the Sun over $360°$ blocks low-altitude voxel k. [e] Arctic cameras fitted with a fixed north-facing sun blocker create a network that operates 12 h a day. An adjacent camera at each node has a fixed south-facing sun blocker, for imaging during complementing hours.

- In the arctic and antarctic summer, the Sun can appear in all azimuth angles over the day. A single 24-hour fixed sun-blocker blocks the horizon. So as shown in Fig. 6d, voxel k is not observed. One solution would be to mount two cameras, side by side, in each network node. Each camera in a node has a fixed sun blocker, covering half of the azimuth angles. One camera operates in the *polar daytime* (local 6AM to 6PM), as it has a south-oriented fixed blocker. The other camera operates in the complementing time (Fig. 6e), having a north-oriented fixed blocker. This way, the network never has a blind spot.

8   3D Clouds by a Camera Network

One application is estimation of the 3D cloud field above the network domain, and beyond. This can be done by the following steps: (A) Per time t, give a cloud score s to each ray $[\mathbf{l}_c, \boldsymbol{\theta}]$, as we explain below. (B) Perform a fuzzy version of space carving [25,31].

We first describe a simple method to implement (B). The set of all sampled light-field rays is $\mathcal{R}$, where $|\mathcal{R}| = N^{\text{rays}}$. A ray is indexed by r, and it corresponds to a specific $[\mathbf{l}_c, \boldsymbol{\theta}]$. Voxel k projects to a subset of the rays $\rho_k \subset \mathcal{R}$, that reach ν_k viewpoints. Suppose a ray $r \in \mathcal{R}$ has a cloud-score $s(r) \in [0,1]$, where $s = 0$ means there is definitely no cloud on the ray, while $s = 1$ means there is confidently a cloud there. Per voxel k, define a back-projected score

$$B_k = \left[\prod_{r \in \rho_k} s(r) \right]^{1/|\rho_k|} \quad \text{if } \nu_k \geq 2 . \tag{6}$$

This score is null, if k is not observed by at least two viewpoints. This score is null also if $s(r) = 0$ for any $r \in \rho_k$. If all $r \in \rho_k$ have same score s, then $B_k = s$. Equation (6) carves-out voxels that contradict support for clouds.

Different cloud regions have signature appearances. Ignoring this would allow erroneous matching of, say, a darker cloud-bottom to a bright sun-lit side of a cloud. Thus, photometric and appearance consistency across viewpoints is incorporated (the photo-hull concept in space-carving [31]). From the images, a feature vector $\mathbf{v}(r,t)$ is extracted for any measured ray r. We used SIFT descriptors [38] and the radiance in each color channel. Element q of $\mathbf{v}(r,t)$ is $v_q(r,t)$. The values of this element, for all rays that intersect voxel k, is $\mathcal{V}_q(k,t) \equiv \{v_q(r,t)\}_{r \in \rho_k}$. Across viewpoints, the measured variance in this set is $\text{VAR}[\mathcal{V}_q(k,t)]$. Define an appearance consistency score [49] as

$$P_k = \exp\left(-\Sigma_q\{\text{VAR}[\mathcal{V}_q(k,t)]\}/\sigma^2 \right) , \tag{7}$$

where σ^2 is a scale parameter. The total cloud-score of a voxel is $T_k = B_k P_k$. The resulting 3D field $\{T_k\}$ is a volumetric estimate of cloud occupancy. It is biased to yield clouds larger than they really are: high-altitude voxels occluded by the cloud-base from all viewpoints are interpreted as being cloudy, since for them T_k is high. This is a realization of a basic ambiguity: if a voxel is occluded from all viewpoints, then there is no way of telling if it is cloudy or not, unless auxiliary or prior knowledge is available. Incorporating a visibility prior favors smaller clouds that explain the data. If voxel k is completely occluded by other cloudy voxels, then it can be pruned (carved) out. Voxel k can maintain its T_k if there are at least two camera viewpoints from which k is not occluded by other cloudy voxels. Pruning is achieved by sweeping [31] the field $\{T_k\}$ iteratively. The pruned 3D cloud occupancy field is denoted $\{\tilde{T}_k\}$. We can maintain the non-binary (fuzzy) nature or $\{\tilde{T}_k\}$. This way, it possesses the inherent semi-transparency and subtle ambiguity of clouds.

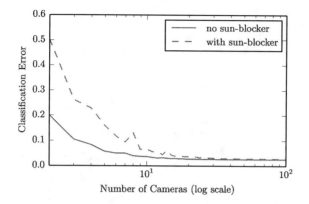

Fig. 7. Classification error rate vs. N^{views}, without or with a sun blocker.

Basic Cloud Score. In the literature there are various functions [40] for a basic cloud score (step A). A ratio of image readout at the red/blue color channels, $\tilde{I}^{\text{red}}/\tilde{I}^{\text{blue}}$, is widely used [44,50]. Overall, we found it effective in broad daylight: clouds are grey (unit red-blue ratio), and the cloudless sky is significantly biased to blue. Thus, for demonstrations in this paper, the cloud-score we used per ray (pixel) is

$$
s(r) = \begin{cases} \dfrac{6[\tilde{I}^{\text{red}}(r)/\tilde{I}^{\text{blue}}(r)-0.8]}{0.2+\tilde{I}^{\text{red}}(r)/\tilde{I}^{\text{blue}}(r)} & \text{if } \tilde{I}^{\text{red}}(r)/\tilde{I}^{\text{blue}}(r) > 0.8 \\ 0 & \text{otherwise} \end{cases} . \tag{8}
$$

Here $s \in [0,1]$, where either bound is achieved at gray clouds or blue sky, respectively. An example of applying this operator on an image is shown in Fig. 4.

Simulations. Quantitative assessments used atmospheric-science simulators. An atmosphere over $8 \times 8\,\text{km}$ was produced using off-the-shelf large eddy simulation (LES), creating clouds between heights of $500\,\text{m}$–$1500\,\text{m}$. Lighting conditions were consistent with Copenhagen. Radiative transfer using the discrete ordinate spherical-harmonic method (SHDOM) [22] rendered images taken by 100 cameras in a $2.5 \times 2.5\,\text{km}^2$ domain. Recovery simulations used random subsets of the network, where the whole network is either with or without a sun blocker. In the LES, a voxel is occupied by cloud if its water-mass parameter is not null. In the recovery, voxel k is classified as cloud if $T_k > 0.01$. We measured the classification error rate, across all voxels. The results are plotted in Fig. 7. As expected of space carving, results improve fast from 2 to 10 cameras (Fluctuations are within the random sampling standard deviation). Even with a sun blocker, the algorithm is able to reconstruct the cloud formation, but, more cameras are needed in order to compensate for the limited view of each camera.

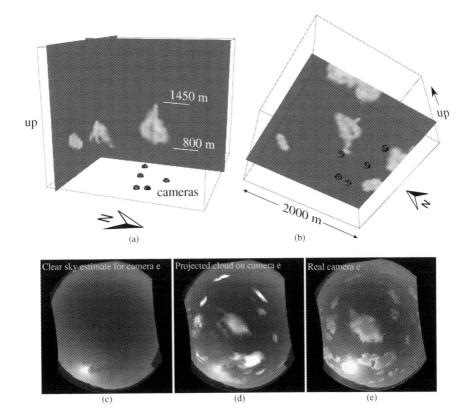

Fig. 8. 3D cumulus cloud recovery results. (a,b) Cross-sections of the recovered cloud-occupancy field $\{\tilde{T}_k\}$. The domain of the clouds is much larger than STARS. Cloud altitude is above sea-level. (c) Estimated sky-background image. Based on four view-points (indexed a, b, c, d), the 3D volumetric cloud-occupancy field $\{\tilde{T}_k\}$ was derived. The field $\{\tilde{T}_k\}$ was projected to viewpoint e, and overlayed on the estimated sky-background image. The resulting synthetic cloud-score image $J[l_e, \boldsymbol{\theta}]$ is shown in (d). This can be compared to the real captured image $\hat{I}_t[l_e, \boldsymbol{\theta}]$, shown in (e).

Cloud Reconstruction Experiment. We applied the approach on various captured scenes.[4] One scene had cumulus clouds. Cross-sections of the recovered 3D cloud-occupancy field $\{\tilde{T}_k\}$ are shown in Fig. 8. The lateral domain of the clouds is much larger than STARS. Accounting for the altitude of STARS above sea-level, the clouds mainly reside between 800 m to 1450m above sea-level. We used two indicators to validate the results. First, a balloon-based radiosonde measured the vertical humidity profile in Beit-Dagan. It is on a similar coastal strip, and roughly used by forecasters for our Technion location. It indicated a layer of high humidity that can yield clouds in the range $[770, 1881]$ m above sea-level, consistent with our clouds.

---

[4] Sun blocker was not used here, since saturation and blooming do not impair cloud shape reconstruction.

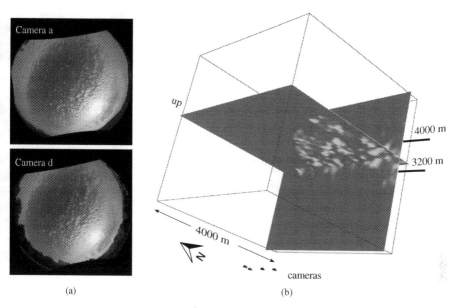

(a)   (b)

Fig. 9. 3D altocumulus cloud recovery results. (a,b) Sample frames. (c,d) Cross-sections of the recovered cloud-occupancy field $\{\tilde{T}_k\}$. Cloud altitude is above sea-level.

Second, we cross-validated 3D recovery *with a missing field of view*. We used four cameras (indexed a, b, c, d) out of five, for 3D estimation. Camera e was ignored. Then, we projected the estimated 3D cloud distribution into viewpoint e, and compared to the ground truth. The rendered image is created as follows. *Ray casting* [34] of field $\{\tilde{T}_k\}$ is performed on a ray corresponding to $[\mathbf{l}_e, \boldsymbol{\theta}]$. Ray-casting aggregates $\{\tilde{T}_k\}$ on all voxels intersected by the ray. The result is a cloud-score image $w[\mathbf{l}_e, \boldsymbol{\theta}]$. To visualize $w[\mathbf{l}_e, \boldsymbol{\theta}]$, we used it as α-map to the estimated sky-background image (Eq. 5). The α-map is

$$\alpha[\mathbf{l}_e, \boldsymbol{\theta}] = \begin{cases} 2w[\mathbf{l}_e, \boldsymbol{\theta}] & \text{if } 2w[\mathbf{l}_e, \boldsymbol{\theta}] < 1 \\ 1 & \text{otherwise} \end{cases}. \tag{9}$$

The rendered image is then $J[\mathbf{l}_e, \boldsymbol{\theta}] = \alpha[\mathbf{l}_e, \boldsymbol{\theta}] + (1 - \alpha[\mathbf{l}_e, \boldsymbol{\theta}])\text{SKY}(\boldsymbol{\theta})$. This image does not pretend to properly render clouds in their true shades and effect on the sky. It simply served to visualize the result (Fig. 8d), compared to the true corresponding image $\hat{I}_t[\mathbf{l}_e, \boldsymbol{\theta}]$, in Fig. 8e. Like sun-blocking, this rendering exploits network redundancy. Even if a viewpoint is blocked, much of its information can be derived using other viewpoints compounded with 3D recovery.

Another scene had a layer of altocumulus clouds. Figure 9 shows sample frames from this scene, and a cross-section of the recovered 3D cloud-occupancy field $\{\tilde{T}_k\}$. Accounting for the altitude of STARS, these estimated clouds mainly reside on a horizontal layer at $\approx 3450 \pm 500\,\text{m}$ above sea-level. Here, the radiosonde indicated a layer of high humidity that can yield clouds in height range $[3072, 4180]\,\text{m}$ above sea-level. This is in strong agreement with our results.

9   Discussion

Scaling light-field imaging hugely to sense the sky, would use a large network of camera nodes, each having a wide field of view, deployed over a wide area. Such a network can reach anywhere communication exists. This sensing approach offers significant advantages over existing technologies (experimental and operational) of atmospheric sensing, particularly 3D imaging, and doing so in high spatio-temporal resolution. This sensing approach poses new questions for computer vision and computational photography. These include network-based extensions to monocular tasks including network-based radiometric calibration and background estimation. Network redundancy offers the ability of by-passing saturation or blind spots, as those created by the sun, without moving parts.

To enable a massive network, each node should have very low-cost. To demonstrate this can work, units in the small STARS used very basic components and coarse alignment. This concept can spawn more interesting research. In the direction of the sun blocker, other sensors can be incorporated. Night-time operation is an interesting challenge. Furthermore, such a light-field system can be used for studying airborne animals (birds, bats [15], locust), in 3D time-lapses.

Acknowledgments. We are grateful to Pinhas Alpert, Daniel Rosenfeld, Orit Altaratz-Stollar, Nir Stav, Raanan Fattal, Arnon Karnieli, David Diner and Anthony Davis for useful discussions. We thank Mark Shenin and Technion building superintendents for experiment assistance. We thank Johanan Erez, Ina Talmon, Tamar Galateanu and Dani Yagodin for technical support. Yoav Schechner is a Lanadu Fellow - supported by the Taub Foundation. His research is supported in part by the Israel Science Foundation (ISF Grant 1467/12) and the Asher Space Research Institute. This work was conducted in the Ollendorff Minerva Center. Minerva is funded through the BMBF.

References

1. Adelson, E., Wang, J.: Single lens stereo with a plenoptic camera. IEEE Trans. PAMI **14**, 99–106 (1992)
2. Aides, A., Schechner, Y.Y., Holodovsky, V., Garay, M.J., Davis, A.B.: Multi sky-view 3D aerosol distribution recovery. Opt. Express **21**, 25820–25833 (2013)
3. Allmen, M.C., Kegelmeyer Jr, P.: The computation of cloud base height from paired whole-sky imaging cameras. Mach. Vis. Appl. **9**, 160–165 (1997)
4. Alterman, M., Schechner, Y.Y., Swirski, Y.: Triangulation in random refractive distortions. In: Proceedings of the IEEE ICCP, pp. 1–10 (2013)
5. Alterman, M., Schechner, Y.Y., Vo, M., Narasimhan, S.G.: Passive tomography of turbulence strength. In: Fleet, D., Pajdla, T., Schiele, B., Tuytelaars, T. (eds.) ECCV 2014, Part IV. LNCS, vol. 8692, pp. 47–60. Springer, Heidelberg (2014)
6. Alterman, M., Swirski, Y., Schechner, Y.Y.: STELLA MARIS: stellar marine refractive imaging sensor. In: Proceedings of the IEEE ICCP, pp. 1–10 (2014)
7. Atkinson, B.W.: Meso-Scale Atmospheric Circulations. Academic Press, New York (1989)
8. Basha, T., Avidan, S., Hornung, A., Matusik, W.: Structure and motion from scene registration. In: Proceedings of the IEEE CVPR, pp. 1426–1433 (2012)

9. Baumgarten, G., Fiedler, J., Fricke, K.H., Gerding, M., Hervig, M., Hoffmann, P., Müller, N., Pautet, P.D., Rapp, M., Robert, C., Rusch, D., von Savigny, C., Singer, W.: The noctilucent cloud (NLC) display during the ECOMA/MASS sounding. Ann. Geophys. **27**, 953–965 (2009)

10. Baxter, B., Hooper, B.A., Williams, J.Z., Dugan, J.P.: Polarimetric remote sensing of ocean waves. In: Proceedings of MTS/IEEE OCEANS, pp. 1–5 (2009)

11. Bennett, G.G.: The calculation of astronomical refraction in marine navigation. J. Navig. **35**, 255–259 (1982)

12. Bishop, T.E., Zanetti, S., Favaro, P.: Light field superresolution. Proc. IEEE ICCP **129**, 1–9 (2009)

13. Bradley, E.S., Toomey, M.P., Still, C.J., Roberts, D.A.: Multi-scale sensor fusion with an online application: integrating GOES, MODIS, and webcam imagery for environmental monitoring. IEEE Sel. Top. Appl. Earth Obs. Remote Sen. **3**, 497–506 (2010)

14. Brdon, E.M., Bréon, F.M.: An analytical model for the cloud-free atmosphere/ocean system reflectance. Remote Sens. Environ. **43**, 179–192 (1993)

15. Breslav, M., Fuller, N., Sclaroff, S., Betke, M.: 3D Pose estimation of bats in the wild. In: Proceedings of the IEEE WACV (2014)

16. Cazorla, A., Olmo, F.J., Aladosarboledas, L., Alados-Arboledas, L.: Using a sky imager for aerosol characterization. Atmos. Environ. **42**, 2739–2745 (2008)

17. Clouds in the Cloud webpage and data link. http://webee.technion.ac.il/people/yoav/research/clouds_inthe_cloud.html

18. Diner, D.J., Beckert, J.C., Reilly, T.H., Bruegge, C.J., Conel, J.E., Kahn, R.A., Martonchik, J.V., Ackerman, T.P., Davies, R., Gerstl, S.A.: Multi-angle imaging spectro-radiometer (MISR) instrument description and experiment overview. IEEE Trans. Geosci. Remote Sens. **36**, 1072–1087 (1998)

19. Diner, D.J., Davis, A., Hancock, B., Gutt, G., Chipman, R.A., Cairns, B.: Dual-photoelastic-modulator-based polarimetric imaging remote sensing. Appl. Opt. **46**, 8428–8445 (2007)

20. Diner, D.J., Davis, A., Hancock, B., Geier, S., Rheingans, B., Jovanovic, V., Bull, M., Rider, D.M., Chipman, R.A., Mahler, A.B., McClain, S.C.: First results from a dual photoelastic-modulator-based polarimetric camera. Appl. Opt. **49**, 2929 (2010)

21. Diner, D.J., Martonchik, J.V.: Atmospheric transmittance from spacecraft using multiple view angle imagery. Appl. Opt. **24**, 3503–3511 (1985)

22. Evans, K.F.: The spherical harmonics discrete ordinate method for three-dimensional atmospheric radiative transfer. J. Atmos. Sci. **55**, 429–446 (1998)

23. Horstmeyer, R., Euliss, G., Athale, R., Levoy, M.: Flexible multimodal camera using a light field architecture. In: Proceedings of the IEEE ICCP, pp. 1–8 (2009)

24. Hosek, L., Wilkie, A.: An analytic model for full spectral sky-dome radiance. ACM TOG **31**, 95:1–95:9 (2012)

25. Ihrke, I., Magnor, M.: Image-based tomographic reconstruction of flames. In: Proceedings of the ACM SIGGRAPH, pp. 365–373 (2004)

26. Jacobs, N., King, J., Bowers, D., Souvenir, R.: Estimating cloud maps from outdoor image sequences. In: Proceedings of the IEEE WACV (2014)

27. Kang, S.B., Weiss, R.: Can we calibrate a camera using an image of a flat, texture-less lambertian surface? In: Vernon, D. (ed.) ECCV 2000. LNCS, vol. 1843, pp. 640–653. Springer, Heidelberg (2000)

28. Kassianov, E., Long, C., Christy, J.: Cloud-base-height estimation from paired ground-based hemispherical observations. J. Appl. Meteorol. **44**, 1221–1233 (2005)

29. Kim, J., Lanman, D., Mukaigawa, Y., Raskar, R.: Descattering transmission via angular filtering. In: Daniilidis, K., Maragos, P., Paragios, N. (eds.) ECCV 2010, Part I. LNCS, vol. 6311, pp. 86–99. Springer, Heidelberg (2010)
30. Koreban, F., Schechner, Y.Y.: Geometry by deflaring. In: Proceedings of the IEEE ICCP, pp. 1–8 (2009)
31. Kutulakos, K., Seitz, S.: A theory of shape by space carving. IJCV **38**, 199–218 (2000)
32. Lalonde, J.F., Narasimhan, S., Efros, A.: What do the sun and the sky tell us about the camera? IJCV **88**, 24–51 (2010)
33. Lensky, I., Rosenfeld, D.: The time-space exchangeability of satellite retrieved relations between cloud top temperature and particle effective radius. Atmos. Chem. Phys. **6**, 2887–2894 (2006)
34. Levoy, M.: Efficient ray tracing of volume data. ACM TOG **9**, 245–261 (1990)
35. Levoy, M., Ng, R., Adams, A., Footer, M., Horowitz, M.: Light field microscopy. ACM TOG **25**, 924–934 (2006)
36. Litvinov, A., Schechner, Y.Y.: Addressing radiometric nonidealities: a unified framework. In: Proceedings of the IEEE CVPR, vol. 2, pp. 52–59 (2005)
37. Long, C.N., Sabburg, J.M., Calbo, J., Pages, D., Calbó, J., Pagès, D.: Retrieving cloud characteristics from ground-based daytime color all-sky images. J. Atmos. Oceanic Technol. **23**, 633–652 (2006)
38. Lowe, D.G.: Distinctive image features from scale-invariant keypoints. IJCV **60**, 91–110 (2004)
39. Mol, B.V., Ruddick, K., van Mol, B., Ruddick, K.: The compact high resolution imaging spectrometer (CHRIS): the future of hyperspectral satellite sensors. In: Proceedings of Airborne Imaging Spectroscopy Workshop on Imagery of Oostende Coastal and Inland Waters (2004)
40. Peng, Z., Yoo, S., Yu, D., Huang, D., Kalb, P., Heiser, J.: 3D cloud detection and tracking for solar forecast using multiple sky imagers. In: Proceedings of the ACM Symposium Applied Computing, pp. 512–517 (2014)
41. Pust, N.J., Shaw, J.A.: Digital all-sky polarization imaging of partly cloudy skies. Appl. Opt. **47**, H190–H198 (2008)
42. Raskar, R., Agrawal, A., Wilson, C.A., Veeraraghavan, A.: Glare aware photography. ACM TOG **27**, 56:1–56:10 (2008)
43. Rouf, M., Mantiuk, R., Heidrich, W., Trentacoste, M., Lau, C.: Glare encoding of high dynamic range images. In: Proceedings of the IEEE CVPR, pp. 289–296 (2011)
44. Seiz, G., Baltsavias, E., Gruen, A.A.: Cloud mapping from the ground: use of photogrammetric methods. Photogram. Eng. Remote Sens. **68**, 941–951 (2002)
45. Seiz, G., Davies, R.: Reconstruction of cloud geometry from multi-view satellite images. Remote Sens. Environ. **100**, 143–149 (2006)
46. Seiz, G., Shields, J., Feister, U., Baltsavias, E.P., Gruen, A.: Cloud mapping with ground-based photogrammetric cameras. Int. J. Remote Sens. **28**, 2001–2032 (2007)
47. Schechner, Y.Y., Diner, D., Martonchik, J.: Spaceborne underwater imaging. In: Proceedings of the IEEE ICCP, pp. 1–8 (2011)
48. Talvala, E.V., Adams, A., Horowitz, M., Levoy, M.: Veiling glare in high dynamic range imaging. ACM TOG **26**, 37:1–37:9 (2007)
49. Veikherman, D., Aides, A., Schechner, Y.Y., Levis, A.: Clouds in the cloud: supplementary material for Proceedings of ACCV (2014)
50. Yamashita, M.: Cloud cover estimation using multitemporal hemisphere imageries. In: Proceedings of the XXth Congress of the Society for Photogrammetry and Remote Sensing, pp. 818–821 (2004)

Fast Segmentation of Sparse 3D Point Trajectories Using Group Theoretical Invariants

Vasileios Zografos$^{(\boxtimes)}$, Reiner Lenz, Erik Ringaby, Michael Felsberg, and Klas Nordberg

Computer Vision Laboratory, Linköping University, Linköping, Sweden
{vasileios.zografos,reiner.lenz,erik.ringaby,
michael.felsberg,klas.nordberg}@liu.se

Abstract. We present a novel approach for segmenting different motions from 3D trajectories. Our approach uses the theory of transformation groups to derive a set of invariants of 3D points located on the same rigid object. These invariants are inexpensive to calculate, involving primarily QR factorizations of small matrices. The invariants are easily converted into a set of robust motion affinities and with the use of a local sampling scheme and spectral clustering, they can be incorporated into a highly efficient motion segmentation algorithm. We have also captured a new multi-object 3D motion dataset, on which we have evaluated our approach, and compared against state-of-the-art competing methods from literature. Our results show that our approach outperforms all methods while being robust to perspective distortions and degenerate configurations.

1 Introduction

Motion is a powerful low-level cue, which when correctly disambiguated can significantly aid many computer vision problems, such as object segmentation, video post-processing, visual surveillance, robotic and autonomous vehicle navigation and activity recognition. Thus in the last few years a number of approaches have tried to solve the sparse motion segmentation problem. Namely, grouping point trajectories where each group is associated with a distinct 3D motion. 3D Motion segmentation can be performed directly in 2D. Assume the measured 2D coordinates of a point as:

$$\tilde{x} = \frac{sX}{Z} + o_1 + \varepsilon_1, \qquad \tilde{y} = \frac{sY}{Z} + o_2 + \varepsilon_2, \qquad (1)$$

where $\mathbf{x} = [X, Y, Z, 1]^T$ are its 3D homogeneous coordinates relative to the camera coordinate system, Z is the depth, s, o_1, o_2 the intrinsic camera parameters and $[\varepsilon_1, \varepsilon_2]$ the tracking noise. We can rewrite (1) for point $p = 1...P$ and frame $f = 1...F$ as:

$$\mathbf{w}_p^f = \begin{pmatrix} \tilde{x}_p^f \\ \tilde{y}_p^f \end{pmatrix} = \frac{1}{Z_p^f} \left(s \begin{pmatrix} \mathbf{c}_1 \\ \mathbf{c}_2 \end{pmatrix} + \begin{pmatrix} o_1 \\ o_2 \end{pmatrix} \mathbf{c}_3 \right) \mathbf{x}_p, \qquad (2)$$

with $\mathbf{c}_k = [r_{k1}\, r_{k2}\, r_{k3}\, t_k]$ being the elements of the rigid transformation of the 3D points $\mathbf{x}_p$, now expressed relative to the world coordinate system. The vectors

© Springer International Publishing Switzerland 2015
D. Cremers et al. (Eds.): ACCV 2014, Part IV, LNCS 9006, pp. 675–691, 2015.
DOI: 10.1007/978-3-319-16817-3_44

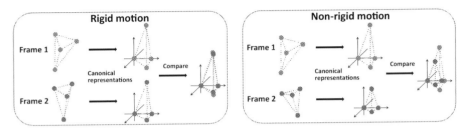

Fig. 1. Overview of our method. Given a set of rigid points (e.g. 4) in 2 frames, we can find a canonical representation, which allows us to compare the points between frames. For rigid motions (left example), the canonical representations will be near-identical. For non-rigid motions (right example), the canonical representations will differ considerably.

$\mathbf{w}_p^f$ are aggregated into a $2F \times P$ data matrix $\mathbf{W} = [\mathbf{w}_p^f]$ for all points and all image frames.

The traditional approach to 3D motion segmentation from 2D uses an affine camera model assumption, in which Z_p^f is constant and as a consequence, $\mathbf{W}$ factorizes into a motion component and a 3D shape component [1]. This result implies that each trajectory lies in a 4D subspace and as such motion segmentation may be solved as the equivalent task of subspace clustering [2]. Notable solutions are the SSC method [3], which describes each point by a sparse set of points from the same subspace; the LRR method [4], which tries to recover a low-rank representation of the data points; LSR by [5], which exploits the data sample correlation and groups points that have high correlation together; the SC approach [6], which looks at the cosine angle between pairs of points as the clustering criterion; or the more recent DiSC method [7], which uses an ensemble of quadratic classifiers each trained from unlabelled data. The main advantage of working with 2D data is that 2D point trajectories may be easily obtained from a single camera. However, using only 2D trajectories to segment 3D motions can be problematic due to ambiguities and potential degeneracies in the motions from the lack of associated depth information. Also, because of the affine camera model employed, 2D methods are prone to failure when they are faced with strong perspective distortions.

With the arrival of new and inexpensive RGB-D sensors (structured light and ToF cameras) it is possible to obtain depth, and thus 3D trajectories, from a single device. Three-dimensional data is not so much affected by degeneracies or perspective distortions, and as a result motion segmentation should be more accurate if carried out directly in 3D. If depth is available it may be incorporated into the final solution in different ways. The first way is the *depth scaling* approach: Given a depth measurement $\tilde{Z} = Z + \delta$ for every point in the scene, where δ is the depth noise, we may instead use the fully projective camera model. Multiplying the depth onto the image coordinates in (1), in homogeneous form, gives us:

$$\mathbf{w}_p^f = \begin{pmatrix} \tilde{Z}_p^f \cdot \tilde{x}_p^f \\ \tilde{Z}_p^f \cdot \tilde{y}_p^f \\ \tilde{Z}_p^f \end{pmatrix} = \left(s \begin{pmatrix} \mathbf{c}_1 \\ \mathbf{c}_2 \end{pmatrix} + \begin{pmatrix} o_1 \\ o_2 \end{pmatrix} \mathbf{c}_3 \right) \mathbf{x}_p. \tag{3}$$

As with (2), the depth scaled version (3) allows us to construct a $3F \times P$ data matrix $\mathbf{W}_\mathcal{P}$ that has columns which lie in a 4D subspace. This means that both (2) and (3), can be solved in an identical manner via subspace clustering. Note that where $\mathbf{W}$ and $\mathbf{W}_\mathcal{P}$ differ is in the way that they are affected by noise. $\mathbf{W}$ is only perturbed by the tracking noise $[\varepsilon_1, \varepsilon_2]$, whereas $\mathbf{W}_\mathcal{P}$ is perturbed by the multiplicative effects of both the tracking noise and the depth noise δ. As a result, if there is considerable noise in the depth measurements, then using $\mathbf{W}_\mathcal{P}$ may produce inferior segmentation results.

The second way is by extracting 3D trajectories and using motion segmentation methods that can work with three-dimensional data. Recent techniques for extracting very accurate 3D trajectories from depth sensors include the work by [8] that uses a particle filter and that by [9] that tracks surface patches inside a Lucas-Kanade framework. The simplest and fastest, albeit less precise, way of extracting the 3D trajectories is directly from the combination of 2D and depth measurements. Similarly to (3), given a tracked point from (1) and its depth measurement $\tilde{Z}$, the 3D position of the point can be estimated as

$$\tilde{X} = \frac{\tilde{Z}(\tilde{x} - o_1)}{s} = X + \frac{\delta X}{Z} + \frac{\varepsilon_1 Z}{s} + \frac{\varepsilon_1 \delta}{s},$$
$$\tilde{Y} = \frac{\tilde{Z}(\tilde{y} - o_2)}{s} = Y + \frac{\delta Y}{Z} + \frac{\varepsilon_2 Z}{s} + \frac{\varepsilon_2 \delta}{s}. \tag{4}$$

The estimates $[\tilde{X}, \tilde{Y}, \tilde{Z}]$ are calculated in the camera coordinate system instead of the world coordinate system, which would require estimation of the camera pose. However, since we are only interested here in the relative positions between points, and those do not change from camera to world coordinates, it suffices to use the representation in (4).

The literature on motion segmentation from 3D is rather limited mainly because obtaining 3D trajectories has not always been an easy task. An early example is the work by [10], where they use the variance of the Euclidean distance between pairs of points as the motion similarity (affinity) criterion. Once the authors have constructed a pairwise affinity matrix for all the 3D points in the scene, they obtain the motion segmentation solution by using spectral clustering [11]. More recently, in [12] the authors also use the variance of the Euclidean distance, but instead they recover the final motion clusters using a maximal cliques algorithm. In [13], similarly to [12], the authors build a graph from the interest points in the 2D image. The edges of the graph are pruned using a 3D velocity similarity criterion and additional refinement techniques. In their work on both monocular and stereoscopic vision for driving assistance systems [14], the authors segment motions either by checking a number of geometric constraints (for the monocular case) or by calculating the velocity of 3D points (for the stereoscopic case). Both cases are limited in that they require estimation of the camera's ego-motion beforehand. In [15] the authors obtain dense 3D trajectories from a Time-of-Flight (ToF) camera and segment motions using 3D velocity and distance. Finally in [16] the authors present an algorithm for segmenting motions in 3D SLAM applications, which employs various motion grouping criteria based on pairwise distances. However, their method is only presented for 2 frames at a time and extension to longer sequences is not so straight forward due to the problem of label switching between two-frame windows.

As of late, new methods have appeared for object segmentation from motion and depth, which use additional information beyond 3D geometry, such as image intensity. For example the EM-style method by [17] that switches between segmentation and motion estimation, or the semi-supervised object segmentation from RGB-D by [18] or that by [19]. However related they might appear, these methods solve different, higher-level problems (dense object segmentation vs sparse motion segmentation). In addition, they are not generic solutions but are tied to specific sensors. For these reasons they are not explored further in this paper.

Our method (see Fig. 1) is a novel approach, which works directly with 3D trajectories and uses the theory of transformation groups to define a set of invariants of points located on the same rigid object at different frames. These invariants can be readily converted into a set of robust motion affinities between the points. Because calculation of the invariants is based primarily on QR factorizations of relatively small matrices and can be applied to all points simultaneously, the method is also very fast. Coupled with a localised sampling step and spectral clustering for recovering the final clusters, our method provides a very accurate solution to the problem of 3D motion segmentation from sparse 3D point trajectories. We have tested our approach on real and synthetic sequences of 3D motions and compared against state-of-the-art methods. The results show that our method outperforms all existing methods, especially in sequences that exhibit strong perspective effects and degenerate configurations. Our key contributions are:

- A fast and highly accurate algorithm for segmenting 3D trajectories,
- A framework for simultaneous calculation of group-theoretical motion invariants on sets of 3D points,
- A multi-object dataset for evaluating sparse 3D motion segmentation algorithms,
- Comprehensive evaluation of state-of-the-art motion segmentation approaches on real and synthetic data.

2   Background Theory and Method

Consider two 3D points located on different rigid objects, with the objects moving independently in two frames (see Ex. 1 in Fig. 2). The Euclidean distance between the points is not invariant but changes over time. In other words, non-zero variance in the pairwise distance suggests that the points lie on different moving objects. However, the opposite is not always true. For example, the objects might have a relative motion that does not change the distance between

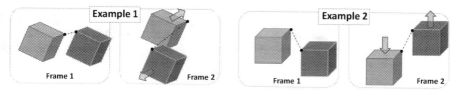

Fig. 2. Example 1 showing that the 3D distance between two points changes if the points lie on different moving objects. Example 2 showing that under certain configurations the distance might stay the same yet the two points lie on different moving objects.

the points (see Ex. 2 in Fig. 2). As such, non-varying Euclidean distance is a necessary but not a sufficient condition for determining relative motion between two points. Despite this inherent weakness, the Euclidean distance invariant can be used for motion segmentation [10,12], and given enough pairwise point samples and image frames, the impact of these ambiguous configurations may be effectively reduced. However, since the number of frames is finite, there is a limitation as to how much we can moderate the effects of ambiguities by using more images.

Our hypothesis is that we can use more invariants, say of N points, to make motion segmentation even more robust to ambiguous and degenerate configurations. Take for example $N = 4$ points that define a tetrahedron in 3D space. There are 6 geometric invariants that uniquely determine a rigid tetrahedron. One such choice is the 6 pairwise lengths of the tetrahedron. Thus if we sample 4 points, we should have 6 different values that we could test for invariance. Even though still not sufficient, this plurality of invariants reduces considerably the likelihood of obtaining a tetrahedron that maintains all its geometric properties unchanged under non-rigid motion. The problem with calculating the geometric invariants from the example above at every frame, is that it can quickly become a very expensive task, especially given a large number of points and long frame sequences. In addition, if we want to use more than 4 points at a time, the number of invariants as well as their associated computational costs increase considerably. For example, the pairwise lengths between N points form an overcomplete set of *dependent* invariants that grows quadratically with increasing N. For this reason, we have used the elements of group theory to define a framework for motion segmentation using invariants, that is *general*: extending to any number $N \geq 2$ of points; *simple*: defining geometric invariants in a straightforward way; and *fast*: where the invariants can be calculated by factorizations of small matrices.

2.1   Group Theoretical Invariants

The use of group invariants is a well studied subject in computer vision (cf. the overview article [20]), with particular focus on shape matching and object recognition. There are many ways to construct such invariants, for example the approach described by [21] using Lie theory and PDEs, or the method by [22]. While we follow along the same lines, in this paper we apply the theory of group invariants to the mostly unexplored problem of 3D motion segmentation. We use the fact that transformation groups split the space on which they operate into equivalence classes and for each such equivalence class we select one unique representative. The parameters of this representative element are by definition invariant under the group action. This approach for extracting the invariants is simpler than [21,23] and only involves QR factorizations.

The main idea that we will exploit here, is that in general we may recover a canonical representation of a collection of N 3D points by some unique alignment with the coordinate axes, so that the effects of the rigid transformation (i.e. from the motion of the points) can be removed. In that canonical representation, the N points can be compared along the frames without the temporal effects of their motion. If the points come from the same rigid object then their canonical coordinates should be near-identical (invariant) over all frames F (see Fig. 1 left). If the points do not come from the same rigid object, then there would be other influences outside the rigid transformation group that will not be removed by the alignment procedure and will show up as variation in their canonical coordinates and thus changes in the invariants (see Fig. 1 right).

G-invariant: We define the 3D coordinates of a point as the vector $\mathbf{x}$, a collection of N such vectors as the $3 \times N$ matrix $\mathbf{X}$ and the set of all matrices as $\mathcal{X}$. Next we introduce the special Euclidean transformation group SE(3) as the *set* of all element pairs $g = (\mathbf{R}, \mathbf{t})$, where $\mathbf{R}$ is a 3D rotation matrix and $\mathbf{t}$ is a 3D translation vector. We can operate on matrices $\mathbf{X}$ by transforming all points simultaneously as $g \cdot \mathbf{X}$, and define the *orbit* of an element $\mathbf{X}$ under the group SE(3) as the set

$$\mathcal{O}_{\mathbf{X}}^{\text{SE}(3)} := \{ g \cdot \mathbf{X} \mid g \in \text{SE}(3) \}. \tag{5}$$

A *G-invariant* may be defined as the function $\mathcal{F} : \mathcal{X} \to \mathbb{R}$, which has *constant* values $\alpha_{\mathbf{X}}$ on the orbit $\mathcal{O}_{\mathbf{X}}^{\text{SE}(3)}$. This is written as

$$\mathcal{F}(g \cdot \mathbf{X}) := \alpha_{\mathbf{X}} \text{ for all } g \in \text{SE}(3). \tag{6}$$

We may generate a complete set of independent G-invariants by starting from an arbitrary but fixed element $\mathbf{X}$ on an orbit, and then constructing a *unique* element $g_{\mathbf{X}} \in \text{SE}(3)$ such that $g_{\mathbf{X}} \cdot \mathbf{X} = \mathbf{X}_o$. We call $\mathbf{X}_o$ the *canonical* element on the orbit with $g_{\mathbf{X}_o} = [\mathbf{I}, \mathbf{0}]$ being the identity element in SE(3), $\mathbf{0}$ the zero vector and $\mathbf{I}$ the identity matrix.

The construction[1] of the unique element is carried out by the following steps:

1. *Given* $\mathbf{X}$, *select* $t = -\mathbf{x}_1$, *where* $\mathbf{x}_1$ *is the first column in* $\mathbf{X}$, *and subtract it from all other columns in the matrix:*

$$(\mathbf{I}, -\mathbf{x}_1)\mathbf{X} = [\mathbf{0}, \hat{\mathbf{X}}], \tag{7}$$

where $\hat{\mathbf{X}}$ *are the translated last three columns of* $\mathbf{X}$.

---

[1] For ease of exposition, we will consider here that $N = 4$, but the following construct is similar for any $N \geq 2$.

2. *Using the QR factorization, $\hat{\mathbf{X}}$ is decomposed as $\hat{\mathbf{X}} = \mathbf{RV}$, where $\mathbf{R}$ is a rotation matrix (by enforcing a determinant of 1) and*

$$\mathbf{V} = (\mathbf{v}_1, \mathbf{v}_2, \mathbf{v}_3) = \begin{pmatrix} a\ b\ d \\ 0\ c\ e \\ 0\ 0\ f \end{pmatrix} \tag{8}$$

is a 3×3 upper triangular matrix.

3. *Finally define the second part of the transformation by $(\mathbf{R}^T, 0)$ and obtain:*

$$\begin{aligned} g \cdot \mathbf{X} &= (\mathbf{R}^T, \mathbf{0})\,(\mathbf{I}, -\mathbf{x}_1)\,\mathbf{X} \\ &= (\mathbf{R}^T, \mathbf{0})[\mathbf{0}, \hat{\mathbf{X}}] = [\mathbf{0}, \mathbf{V}]. \end{aligned} \tag{9}$$

Due to the uniqueness of the translation and the QR factorization it follows that $g_{[\mathbf{0},\mathbf{V}]} = [\mathbf{I}, \mathbf{0}]$. Each column in $[\mathbf{0}, \mathbf{V}]$ now contains the canonical coordinates of the transformed points from $\mathbf{X}$. This process is shown in Fig. 3. A geometrical interpretation of the above is that the first three columns of $\mathbf{X}$ represent the corners of a base triangle. The ordering of the columns is arbitrary and we may eliminate the effects of permutations by a fixed ordering of the columns in $\mathbf{X}$ according to falling norms and some basic rule to break ties. Geometrically, this means we choose the point nearest to the origin of the original coordinate system as the starting corner of the base triangle. Then we sort out the remaining three points such that the lengths of the corresponding sides of the triangle are increasing.

Following the above construction, we have many choices for defining G-invariant functions $\mathcal{F}$. In particular, we wish to detect large variations in $\mathbf{V}$, over the F frames in the sequence. Large variations in the elements of $\mathbf{V}$ will most likely indicate that the original 4 points in $\mathbf{X}$ do not come from the same rigid object. We could of course look at the variance of the 6 nonzero elements in $\mathbf{V}$ from (8) and calculate 6 invariants. However since the 3 columns $\mathbf{v}_1, \mathbf{v}_2, \mathbf{v}_3$ of $\mathbf{V}$ represent the canonical coordinates of the last three 3D points in $\mathbf{X}$ (the canonical coordinates of the first point are always 0 by construction in (9)), a geometrically inspired and more robust set of G-invariants are the median centered ℓ^2-norms of the columns of $\mathbf{V}$:

$$\mathcal{F}_n(g \cdot \mathbf{X}) = \frac{1}{F} \sum_f \left\| \mathbf{v}_n^f - \boldsymbol{\mu}_n \right\|_2, \tag{10}$$

with $n = 1, ..., 3$, $f = 1, ..., F$, $\mathbf{v}_n^f$ the nth column of $\mathbf{V}$ at frame f, and $\boldsymbol{\mu}_n$ being the marginal median of $\mathbf{v}_n$ over the frames. In the absence of noise, (10) will be zero for all the points that lie on the same object. Furthermore due to the geometric nature of the ℓ^2-norm, the 3 resulting scalar G-invariants from (10), will behave in a more predictable way in the presence of noise than the individual elements of $\mathbf{V}$. This is the reason why it is preferable to consider *functions* of the 6 elements and obtain only 3 robust G-invariants, rather than use the 6 elements directly and obtain 6 non-robust G-invariants. It should be noted that by constructing the robust G-invariants via (10), we no longer obtain a complete

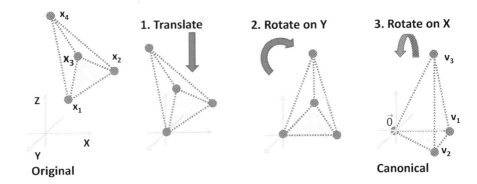

Fig. 3. Calculation of the canonical representation of a set of points. First the points are translated to the origin using the first vertex of a chosen base triangle (shaded), and then a combined rotation is recovered that aligns the base triangle with the axes.

set of invariants, but rather the robust G-invariants now span a 3-dimensional subspace in $\mathbb{R}^6$. From the robust invariants in (10) we may construct a motion affinity measure (explained in the next section) and form the basis of our motion segmentation algorithm.

3   The Motion Segmentation Algorithm

Our motion segmentation algorithm follows the typical pipeline which involves constructing a pairwise motion affinity matrix for all the points in the scene, and then using spectral clustering [11] for recovering the motion clusters. The construction of the affinity matrix is preceded by an efficient local sampling step, designed to exploit the property of "common fate" in proximal data, and thereby improve the segmentation results. Once again, for ease of understanding we present the algorithm for $N = 4$ points, but the algorithm has a similar extension to any $N>2$.

3.1   The Motion Affinity

In the previous section we have presented the construction of the G-invariants for $N = 4$ number of points (i.e. a 4-tuple). In order to utilize these invariants for motion segmentation, we need to apply them to all the 3D points in the scene and extract a motion relationship between them. In other words, given a $3F \times P$ data matrix $\mathbf{W}$ of P 3D points in F frames, what we want is to use the G-invariants for obtaining a $P \times P$ *pairwise* motion affinity matrix between all the 3D points. The pairwise affinity matrix can be used as input to a clustering algorithm (e.g. [11]) and obtain the final clusters.

Since (10) represents a direct relationship between a 4-tuple we may only say something about 4 points at a time and not about only 2 points (pairwise). Consider the set S_1 of all possible 4-tuples of P points. Sampling all the elements of S_1 and deriving a relationship between pairs of points would be practically infeasible. Instead, we can use the technique by [24], which allows us to sample a small number C from the set S_2 of 3-tuples, with $C \ll |S_2| < |S_1|$, and create the $P \times C$ *4-way* affinity matrix $\mathbf{E}$. The pairwise affinity matrix may be then approximated as $\mathbf{A} \approx \mathbf{E}\mathbf{E}^T$. The 4-way affinity matrix $\mathbf{E}$ may be calculated, one column $\mathbf{e}_c$ at a time, by first sampling a 3-tuple and then calculating the 4-way affinity between that and every other scene point in turn. The 4-way affinity is defined as:

$$\mathbf{e}_c(p) = \exp\left(-d_c(p)/\sigma_c\right), \quad c = 1, \ldots, C, \tag{11}$$

where from (10) we have

$$d_c(p) = \mathcal{F}_n(g \cdot \mathbf{X}_{p,c}), \quad p = 1, \ldots, P, \tag{12}$$

with $\mathbf{X}_{p,c} = [\mathbf{W}(f, S_2(c)), \mathbf{W}(f, p)]$ being the 4 points. σ_c is a kernel parameter defined as the ρth percentile of each column $\mathbf{e}_c$. This way of choosing σ_c allows for both local scaling of the kernel in each column and a kernel parameter which adapts to the range of the data.

Completing one column of $\mathbf{E}$ requires P-3 evaluations of (10) (and thus QR factorizations) for the calculation of the G-invariants. However, we may reduce the computations considerably by exploiting the incremental construction of the G-invariants and noting that for each of the P-3 evaluations, the initially sampled 3-tuple $\mathbf{W}(f, S_2(c))$ remains fixed. We may therefore pre-calculate the first two columns $\mathbf{v}_1, \mathbf{v}_2$ of $\mathbf{V}$ in (9) from the fixed 3-tuple, using the exact same steps described in Sect. 2.1. The last column $\mathbf{v}_3$ of $\mathbf{V}$ may be obtained simultaneously for all the 3D scene points $\mathbf{W}(f, :)$ by a matrix multiplication with the rotation matrix $\mathbf{R}^T$ estimated from the QR factorization of the 3-tuple. This incremental construction allows us to go from $C \times (P-3)$ QR factorizations per frame required to construct $\mathbf{E}$, to C QR factorizations and C matrix multiplications per frame, which is considerably faster.

3.2 Local Sampling

Since we are only sampling a small number C of 3-tuples for approximating the pairwise affinity matrix $\mathbf{A}$, it is important to increase the probability that each 3-tuple comes from the same rigid object. Otherwise, there will be a large variance in the canonical coordinates of the points due to non-rigid motion and the 4-way affinity in (11) will always be low, irrespective of the 4th point used. In [24] the authors proposed randomly sampling the 3-tuples. However, this requires a large number C of samples to ensure that enough columns of $\mathbf{E}$ contain points from the same object. An iterative technique was suggested by [25], which involves random sampling, obtaining an initial motion segmentation solution and then repeating the process by sampling from the identified motion clusters. We propose a better sampling scheme, which exploits the locality property in the data. That is, points on the same object generally lie in close proximity to other points from the same object. Local sampling has a much higher likelihood of obtaining 3-tuples that are rigid and as a result can produce good results with far fewer number of samples. To acquire C local 3-tuples points we start by randomly sampling C points. For each point, we then sample the 2-nearest neighbours in 3D Euclidean distance. The advantage of the local sampling technique can be seen in Fig. 4 and the complete motion segmentation method is formulated in Algorithm 1.

Algorithm 1: Motion Segmentation algorithm

1   **Input**: data matrix $\mathbf{W}$, # of samples C, # of motions m ; **Output**: motion labels $\mathbf{Y}$
2   Local sampling of C number of 3-tuples from S_2
3   **for** *sample* $c = 1 : C$ **do**
4   **for** *frame* $f = 1 : F$ **do**
5   Let $\mathbf{X} = \mathbf{W}(f, S_2(c))$ and $\mathbf{t} = \mathbf{X}(:, 1)$
6   Translate as $\hat{\mathbf{X}} = \mathbf{X} - \mathbf{t}$ and $\mathbf{W}_1 = \mathbf{W}(f, :) - \mathbf{t}$
7   QR factorize $\hat{\mathbf{X}} = \mathbf{RV}$
8   Transform ALL points $\mathbf{W}_2(f, :) = \mathbf{R}^T \mathbf{W}_1$
9   Calculate $d_c(p) = \frac{1}{F} \sum_f \left\| \mathbf{W}_2(f, p) - \boldsymbol{\mu}_p \right\|_2$ from (12)
10   Calculate $\mathbf{E}$ column as $e_c(p) = \exp\left(-d_c(p)/\sigma_c\right)$ from (11)
11 $\mathbf{Y}$ = spectral clustering on $\mathbf{A} = \mathbf{EE}^T$ with m clusters

---

3.3   Generalization to Any $N \geq 2$

The construction of the G-invariants and Algorithm 1 have been described for $N = 4$ points, but have similar constructions for any number $N \geq 2$ points. For $N = 3$ points the construction is identical, leading to a unique QR factorization, 2 unique robust G-invariants from (10), and the formation of a 3-way affinity matrix $\mathbf{E}$ from (11). For $N > 4$, we first calculate the G-invariants for 4 arbitrary but fixed points as in Sect. 2.1 and then compute the canonical coordinates of the remaining points based on the estimated QR factorization. We obtain $3*(N\text{-}2)$ nonzero elements in $\mathbf{V}$ from (8), resulting in $N - 1$ robust G-invariants that grow linearly with N. For the special case of $N = 2$, the QR factorization is no longer unique but the resulting G-invariants still are. Furthermore, $\mathbf{V}$ is now a column vector and (10) leads to a single G-invariant. This G-invariant is a robust form of the Euclidean distance variance between the two points. This is very closely related to the motion affinity used by [10,12] and in fact both published methods can be considered as a special case of our framework for $N = 2$. Finally when $N = 2$, Algorithm 1 simplifies to a direct calculation of the pairwise affinity matrix $\mathbf{A}$ without the need for local sampling.

4   Experiments

We present the results from our experiments on real and synthetic data. We have compared our method against compatible state-of-the-art approaches from literature that use sparse point trajectories only, and where computer code was

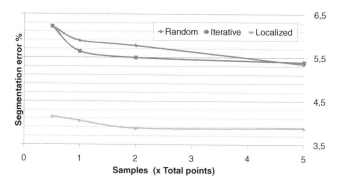

Fig. 4. Effect of different sampling schemes on the segmentation error of the real dataset from Sect. 4, as a function of the number C of N-tuples sampled.

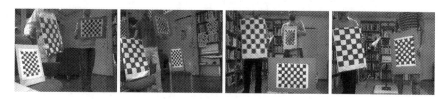

Fig. 5. Samples from our captured real dataset with superimposed tracked feature points on multiple moving objects.

available. Specifically, the 2D motion segmentation methods SC [6], SSC [3], DiSC [7], LSR [5] and LRR [4] and the 3D method by [10,12] denoted here as Euc3D. Furthermore, all 2D methods were extended by scaling with the depth measurements (depth scaling approach $\mathbf{W}_\mathcal{P}$ from (3)), and are denoted here as $SC_\mathcal{P}$, $SSC_\mathcal{P}$, $DiSC_\mathcal{P}$, $LSR_\mathcal{P}$ and $LRR_\mathcal{P}$ respectively. All competing methods were tuned either as suggested by their corresponding authors or to the best of our ability. Our method's parameters were set to: $N = 10$, $C = 2P$ where P is the number of points in the scene, and $\rho = 15$ as the percentile of σ_c from (11). All algorithms were given the number of motions m, and their parameters were kept fixed across all experiments.

Unfortunately there is no publicly available 3D trajectory dataset with multiple motions. To our knowledge there are two dynamic RGB-D datasets in literature, both requiring extraction of 3D trajectories, but none of which were suitable for our tests. The first [26], contains very few sequences where only two articulated objects are moving and over a very limited range. The second [27], consists of multiple objects moving in front of a static camera, but due to the heavy motion blur and limited presence of the objects in the scene, it has not been possible to extract any useful trajectories. We have therefore captured our own 3D dataset and have used it to evaluate the different methods. This new dataset contains 460 sequences of 10 frames each, with 2–5 moving objects and with on average 390 tracked points per sequence. The sequences have been captured with a Kinect sensor, and 3D trajectories were extracted using the simple approach from (4). We have pre-processed the data in the following ways: first we have used the cross-checking scheme by [28] to only retain complete trajectories and reject those with gross tracking errors. Second, we have discarded any points with missing or ambiguous depth measurements. Such points are usually located on depth discontinuity boundaries, and are therefore easily identified by means of an edge detector in the depth image. Note that despite this preprocessing, the dataset still contains many challenging 3D trajectories due to the considerable amount of noise, particularly in the depth measurements. Labelled examples from the dataset are illustrated in Fig. 5.

The results from running all methods on the 3D dataset are summarised in terms of the segmentation error in Table 1, for the different types of motions. As expected all methods start with a low error for 2 motions (with the exception of LRR and Euc3D) and deteriorate at different rates as the number of motions (and hence the 3D trajectories) increase. We see that only our method has remained consistently accurate with a low error, and obtains the overall best result for the complete set of 460 sequences. Second best is DiSC but at a much higher computational cost. Unsurprisingly, the other competing 3D method (Euc3D) shows quite poor results, which is evidence that a single invariant between two points is not robust enough, and one has to consider multiple invariants. Regarding the depth scaled versions of the 2D methods, they are systematically much worse than when using the 2D trajectories alone. This is expected and can be attributed to two factors: the considerable amount of noise

Table 1. Results from the real dataset. Each column shows the mean segmentation error of each method over the sequences, while the last column shows the execution speed of each algorithm (all tests ran on the same computer). The stochastic methods (DiSC, LSR, LRR, Our) have been executed 100 times and their averaged results are displayed here.

Method	2 motions 15 seq.	3 motions 215 seq.	4 motions 220 seq.	5 motions 10 seq.	Total 460 seq.	Time
	\multicolumn{5}{} Average segmentation error					
SC [6]	0.04%	6.21%	8.42%	8.52%	7.12%	0.64 sec
SC$_\mathcal{P}$	0.89%	15.62%	16.73%	22.11%	15.81%	—"—
SSC [3]	0.27%	**5.38%**	5.01%	27.51%	5.52%	113.10 sec
SSC$_\mathcal{P}$	0.61%	7.99%	8.19%	36.33%	8.47%	—"—
DiSC [7]	0.13%	6.66%	2.55%	8.08%	4.51%	9.53 sec
DiSC$_\mathcal{P}$	1.03%	24.81%	28.36%	17.57%	25.57%	—"—
LSR [5]	0.25%	7.21%	8.1%	18.5%	7.66%	0.09 sec
LSR$_\mathcal{P}$	14.63%	32.30%	36.22%	28.08%	33.51%	—"—
LRR [4]	2.92%	7.57%	10.17%	18.77%	8.91%	0.58 sec
LRR$_\mathcal{P}$	21.96%	49.56%	61.18%	61.55%	54.48%	—"—
Euc3D [10, 12]	1.20%	7.29%	9.51%	16.04%	8.34%	0.28 sec
Our	**0.01%**	5.59%	**2.49%**	**4.98%**	**3.92%**	0.34 sec

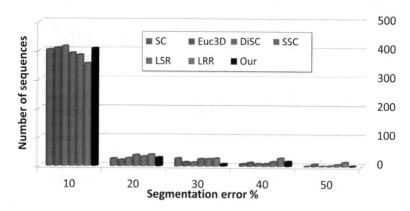

Fig. 6. Segmentation error histograms showing the detailed performance of each algorithm on the real dataset.

in the depth measurements, and the multiplicative effect of the tracking and depth noise already explained in Sect. 1. The performance of each algorithm is further illustrated in the histograms in Fig. 6. It is evident that our method together with DiSC and SSC have very similar performance in terms of the cumulative segmentation errors that they obtain, with most sequences from the dataset in the range of 0–10%, and with very few sequences in the range 20–50%. This is not the case for methods such as LRR, LSR and Euc3D, since they segment considerably more sequences with a high error in the range 20–50%.

In terms of speed (last column of Table 1), LSR is the fastest method, albeit rather inaccurate, with Euc3D following closely with around 20 ms more computational time on average. Our method is the third fastest at 0.34 s but achieves more than double the accuracy of Euc3D and LSR. Notice that the next two most accurate methods (DiSC and SSC) are 40–400 times slower by comparison. In summary, only our approach is both fast and accurate enough to provide a viable solution to the motion segmentation problem, while being largely unaffected by the additional depth error in the 3D trajectories.

We have also performed an extra set of experiments on synthetic 3D trajectories in order to further evaluate the performance of each algorithm against: different *types* of motions, increasing *number of objects*, increasing *noise* and decreasing *trajectory length*. Each test was executed 100 times with randomized placement and motion of the objects. Figure 7 (upper left) shows the segmentation results for general 3D motions, motions with strong perspective distortions and degenerate motions (i.e. all points located on 3D planes undergoing rotations and translations parallel to the image plane). We see that for general 3D motions, all methods perform equally well. However, for perspective and degenerate motions, the majority of algorithms fail, particularly the 2D methods that assume an affine camera model. Only our method and DiSC are able to deal with the challenging projective and degenerate motions. In Fig. 7 (upper right), we see the segmentation error vs an increasing number of objects. Our method

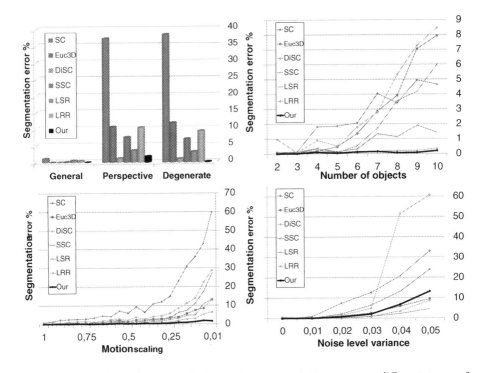

Fig. 7. Results from the synthetic dataset of segmentation error vs different types of motions (upper left), increasing number of objects (upper right), decreasing trajectory length (lower left) and increasing noise (lower right). Our method is displayed in bold.

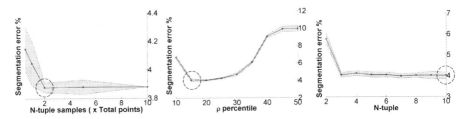

Fig. 8. Average segmentation error % versus different parameter values (solid line). Each test was executed 10 different times and the standard deviation is shown in the shaded regions. The chosen parameters for the main tests in Table 1 are indicated by the circles.

is largely unaffected by the number of objects, something which is also reflected in Table 1. DiSC is the only other method that has similar accuracy in this experiment. In Fig. 7 (lower left), we show segmentation error vs trajectory length, that is, motions becoming increasingly smaller with each experiment. Smaller motions should be more difficult to disambiguate. We observe that our method is once again the most accurate, and not really degrading much by the decreasing trajectories. Figure 7 (lower right) shows segmentation error vs noise, scaled independently in both 2D and depth. Notice how LRR breaks down due to its sensitive numerical nature. Our method is not the most robust but shows good very good performance in relation to the majority of competitors. Although geometric in nature, our method has the random element in choosing the N point samples and their ordering in the F frames. We believe that we may further improve the robustness to noise by incorporating an explicit error model, which can describe the joint perturbations of 3D points, in order to select more stable base triangles for the canonical representation.

Lastly, we examine the performance of our method against different parameter settings. All the experiments have been run on the real dataset, where each parameter was changed in turn while the rest of the parameters were kept fixed. There are three parameters that are used in our algorithm: the N-tuple **sample size** parameter C, the **size** N of the N-tuple, and the **percentile** parameter ρ for the kernel size σ_c. We see that the performance of the method is very stable and with low error (i.e. wide valleys) across a large region of the parameter space. This illustrates that our method can perform well without the need for extensive tuning (Fig. 8).

5   Conclusion

We have presented a novel method for segmenting different motions from sparse 3D trajectories. Our approach uses the theory of transformation groups to derive a set of invariants of points located on the same rigid object. Because we exploit the particular structure of the problem, these invariants can be quickly calculated using a QR factorization and readily converted to a set of robust motion affinities for clustering motion trajectories together. We have evaluated our motion segmentation method using synthetic data and a new, real dataset that we have captured specifically for this work. In our comparisons against state-of-the-art motion segmentation methods, we have found that our method is more accurate than the competitors, while also being very fast. We expect that our method will perform even better if a more advanced 3D trajectory extraction algorithm is used, like [8,9], that does not induce so much noise in the resulting 3D coordinates. In light of these results it is our conclusion that our original hypotheses that (i) *motion segmentation in 3D is more accurate than in 2D*, as well as that (ii) *additional invariants lead to more robust motion segmentation*, hold. The combined good performance, fast execution speed, and stability under increasing data complexity, establish our method as a very attractive and viable solution to the problem of motion segmentation of sparse 3D trajectories.

Acknowledgements. This work has been supported by Vinnova through a grant for the project iQmatic, by SSF through a grant for the project VPS, by VR through a grant for the project ETT, and through the Strategic Areas for ICT research CADICS and ELLIIT.

References

1. Costeira, J.P., Kanade, T.: A multibody factorization method for independently moving objects. IJCV **29**(3), 159–179 (1998)
2. Vidal, R.: Subspace clustering. IEEE Sig. Process. Mag. **28**(3), 52–68 (2011)
3. Elhamifar, E., Vidal, R.: Sparse subspace clustering. In: CVPR (2009)
4. Liu, G., Lin, Z., and Yu, Y.: Robust subspace segmentation by low-rank representation. In: ICML (2010)
5. Lu, C.-Y., Min, H., Zhao, Z.-Q., Zhu, L., Huang, D.-S., Yan, S.: Robust and efficient subspace segmentation via least squares regression. In: Fitzgibbon, A., Lazebnik, S., Perona, P., Sato, Y., Schmid, C. (eds.) ECCV 2012, Part VII. LNCS, vol. 7578, pp. 347–360. Springer, Heidelberg (2012)
6. Lauer, F., Schnörr, C.: Spectral clustering of linear subspaces for motion segmentation. In: ICCV (2009)
7. Zografos, V., Ellis, L., Mester, R.: Discriminative subspace clustering. In: CVPR (2013)
8. Hadfield, S., Bowden, R.: Kinecting the dots: Particle based scene flow from depth sensors. In: ICCV, pp. 2290–2295 (2011)
9. Quiroga, J., Devernay, F., Crowley, J.: Scene flow by tracking in intensity and depth data. In: CVPR Workshops (2012)
10. Mateus, D., Horaud, R.: Spectral methods for 3-D motion segmentation of sparse scene-flow. In: WMVC (2007)
11. Ng, A.Y., Jordan, M.I., Weiss, Y.: On spectral clustering: Analysis and an algorithm. In: NIPS, pp. 849–856 (2001)
12. Perera, S., Barnes, N.: Maximal cliques based rigid body motion segmentation with a RGB-D camera. In: Lee, K.M., Matsushita, Y., Rehg, J.M., Hu, Z. (eds.) ACCV 2012, Part II. LNCS, vol. 7725, pp. 120–133. Springer, Heidelberg (2013)
13. Lenz, P., Ziegler, J., Geiger, A., Roser, M.: Sparse scene flow segmentation for moving object detection in urban environments. In: Intelligent Vehicles Symposium, pp. 926–932 (2011)
14. Klappstein, J., Vaudrey, T., Rabe, C., Wedel, A., Klette, R.: Moving object segmentation using optical flow and depth information. In: Wada, T., Huang, F., Lin, S. (eds.) PSIVT 2009. LNCS, vol. 5414, pp. 611–623. Springer, Heidelberg (2009)
15. Ghuffar, S., Brosch, N., Pfeifer, N., Gelautz, M.: Motion segmentation in videos from time of flight cameras. In: IWSSIP (2012)
16. Wang, Y., Huang, S.: An effient motion segmentation algorithm for multibody RGB-D SLAM. In: Proceedings of Australasian Conference on Robotics and Automation (2013)
17. Stuckler, J., Behnke, S.: Efficient dense 3D rigid-body motion segmentation in RGB-D video. In: BMVC (2013)
18. Teichman, A., Lussier, J., Thrun, S.: Learning to segment and track in RGBD. IEEE Trans. Autom. Sci. Eng. **10**(4), 841–852 (2013)
19. Herbst, E., Ren, X., Fox, D.: Object segmentation from motion with dense feature matching. In: Workshop on Semantic Perception, Mapping and Exploration (ICRA) (2012)
20. Weiss, I.: Geometric invariants and object recognition. Inter **10**(3), 201–231 (1993)
21. Gool, L.V., Moons, T., Pauwels, E., Oosterlinck, A.: Vision and Lie's approach to invariance. Image Vis. Comput. **13**(4), 259–277 (1995)

22. Schulz-Mirbach, H.: Anwendung von Invarianzprinzipien zur Merkmalgewinnung in der Mustererkennung, ser. Fortschritt-Berichte VDI : Reihe 10, Informatik, Kommunikation; Nr. 372. VDI-Verl. Dusseldorf (1995) isBN 3-18-337210-X
23. Schulz-Mirbach, H.: Invariant features for gray scale images. In: DAGM (1995)
24. Govindu, V.M.: A tensor decomposition for geometric grouping and segmentation. In: CVPR, vol. 1, pp. 1150–1157 (2005)
25. Chen, G., Lerman, G.: Spectral curvature clustering (SCC). IJCV **81**(3), 317–330 (2009)
26. Sturm, J., Engelhard, N., Endres, F., Burgard, W., Cremers, D.: A benchmark for the evaluation of RGB-D SLAM systems. In: IROS (2012)
27. Spinello, L., Arras, K.O.: People detection in RGB-D data. In: IROS (2011)
28. Baker, S., Scharstein, D., Lewis, J.P., Roth, S., Black, M.J., Szeliski, R.: A database and evaluation methodology for optical flow. In: ICCV (2007)

Superpixels for Video Content Using a Contour-Based EM Optimization

Matthias Reso[1]([☒]), Jörn Jachalsky[2], Bodo Rosenhahn[1],
and Jörn Ostermann[1]

[1] Leibniz Universität Hannover, Hannover, Germany
reso@tnt.uni-hannover.de
[2] Technicolor Research and Innovation, Hannover, Germany
joern.jachalsky@technicolor.com

Abstract. A wide variety of computer vision applications rely on super-pixel or supervoxel algorithms as a preprocessing step. This underlines the overall importance that these algorithms have gained in the recent years. However, most methods show a lack of temporal consistency or fail in producing temporally stable segmentations. In this paper, we propose a novel, contour-based approach that generates temporally consistent superpixels for video content. It can be expressed in an expectation-maximization framework and utilizes an efficient label propagation built on backward optical flow in order to encourage the preservation of super-pixel shapes and their spatial constellation over time. Using established benchmark suites, we show the superior performance of our approach compared to state of the art supervoxel and superpixel algorithms for video content.

1 Introduction

In [1] superpixels were introduced as new image primitives grouping spatially coherent pixels that share the same low-level features as e.g. color or texture into small segments of approximately same size and shape. Over the last decade, superpixel algorithms have become a common preprocessing step for a variety of computer vision applications. These applications include e.g. video segmen-tation [2,3], tracking [4], multi-view object segmentation [5], scene flow [6], 3D layout estimation of indoor scenes [7], interactive scene modeling [8], image pars-ing [9], and semantic segmentation [10,11]. Using such an over-segmentation has two major benefits. First, the number of image primitives is significantly reduced. Second, superpixels provide a spatial support for the extraction of region-based features [12].

More recently, the idea of superpixels was extended from the domain of still images to the domain of video sequences. In general, all related approaches can be classified as generating either supervoxels (e.g. [13–15]) or superpixels that are temporally consistent (e.g. [16–19]). As noted in [18], superpixels with tem-poral consistency and supervoxels can be converted into the other class if certain constraints are met. While over-segmentation algorithms for still images should

© Springer International Publishing Switzerland 2015
D. Cremers et al. (Eds.): ACCV 2014, Part IV, LNCS 9006, pp. 692–707, 2015.
DOI: 10.1007/978-3-319-16817-3_45

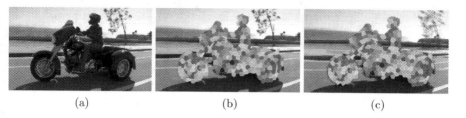

(a)   (b)   (c)

Fig. 1. Example of a superpixel segmentation providing temporal consistency and a steady spatial constellation of the superpixels over time. Despite the movement and the jiggling camera shot the superpixels stay at their initial positions on the motorcycle over several frames. (a) Original frame; (b) A full superpixel segmentation of the video was performed and a subset of superpixels was manually selected in one frame and colored for visualization; (c) Subset with the same superpixels after several frames. Same color as in (b) means temporal connectedness.

capture main object boundaries, the methods for video content should additionally capture the temporal connections between regions in successive frames. In order to achieve a consistent labeling, that can be leveraged for applications like tracking or video segmentation, it is also important for the segments to reflect the motion of the image regions they represent. Thus, a segment should not change its shape if the corresponding image region does not change its shape and the spatial constellation of the segments should stay constant over time as long as the corresponding regions do not change positions (See Fig. 1 for an example). In the following, we briefly describe oversegmentation approaches for video content that aim at compact and spatially coherent regions of approximately the same size and shape that are also consistent over time. An early example, which is not explicitly labeled as superpixel or supervoxel approach but shares a similar idea, can be found in [20].

In [14] a first supervoxel approach was published that covers the video volume with overlapping cubes, whereas each cube corresponds to one label. The volume of the cubes determines the maximum volume of the supervoxels to be generated. The longer the cubes are, the higher the temporal consistency can be. The assignment of each voxel to one label is done using energy minimization techniques. In [15] not only the SLIC superpixel approach is described but also its extension to supervoxels. Thereby, it introduces a temporal distance term penalizing supervoxels with a long duration.

Other approaches like [13, 16–18, 21] aim at supervoxel and superpixel representations with extended temporal duration. In [13] an approach for hierarchical video segmentation is proposed that is based on the graph-based image segmentation approach introduced in [22], which is first applied on pixel-level and then iteratively on region-level in order to create a hierarchical segmentation. Streaming capabilities were added to [13] in [21] by applying a Markov assumption on the video stream. Both, [13, 21] generate supervoxel segmentations, which—if converted to a superpixel representation—show a lack of temporal stability as the shapes of the segments change extensively from frame to frame.

A first approach towards temporal superpixels was introduced in [19] using optical flow information to initialize the seeds for the superpixels in each new frame. Using these seeds, the superpixels are grown only on frame level. While achieving a more temporally stable superpixel segmentation it fails to explicitly handle structural changes in the video sequences. A strategy for creation or splitting as well as termination of superpixels, which provides the capability to handle structural changes in the video scene, was first introduced by [16]. The approach utilizes a generative probabilistic model for superpixels in video sequences. Moreover, the flow is explicitly modeled between the frames in order to propagate the superpixels. In [17] an online video superpixel algorithm based on [23] was introduced. It uses hill climbing for the optimization and considers a hierarchy of blocks at different sizes. The results of the intermediate block level are used to initialize new frames. The superpixel approach presented in [18] uses a global color subspace and multiple spatial subspaces to cluster the pixels in an observation window that comprises multiple frames and is shifted along the video volume. In order to initialize new frames the spatial centers of the superpixels are propagated into a new frame similarly to [19].

Although [16] provides a mostly temporally stable segmentation it falls behind the more recent approaches of [17,18] with respect to the duration of the spatio-temporal segments. However, the latter two algorithms—each to some extent—fail to produce segmentations with a steady spatial constellation of the superpixels over time. Hence, in this work we introduce a novel method for superpixels on video content. We utilize the main ideas of [18] to maximize the length of the spatio-temporal segments and introduce new techniques to generate a temporally more stable segmentation. The key contributions of this paper are the following: *(i)* we propose a fully contour-based approach for superpixels on video sequences, which is expressed in an expectation-maximization (EM) framework, and generates superpixels that are spatially coherent and temporally consistent. *(ii)* We utilize an efficient label propagation using backward optical flow in order to encourage the preservation of superpixel shapes when appropriate. Finally, *(iii)* we present superior results comparing our approach against the state of the art using the established benchmark suites [24,25].

The remainder of the work is organized as follows: In Sect. 2, we discuss the details of our approach and present in Sect. 3 the experimental results comparing it to the state of the art using the established benchmark suites. Section 4 concludes this paper.

2   Superpixels for Video Content

Our algorithm is based on an analysis of the approach proposed in [18], entitled *Temporally Consistent Superpixel* (TCS). Thus, before we discuss our algorithm in Sect. 2.2, we will shortly summarize the main ideas of TCS.

2.1 Temporally Consistent Superpixels in a Nutshell

In general, TCS performs an energy-minimizing clustering using a multi-dimensional feature space. For the clustering, the feature-space is separated into a global color subspace and multiple local spatial subspaces.

More specifically, the energy-minimizing framework used in TCS clusters pixels based on their five dimensional feature vector $\begin{bmatrix} l & a & b & x & y \end{bmatrix}$. Each vector contains the three color values $\begin{bmatrix} l & a & b \end{bmatrix}$ in CIELAB-color space and the pixel coordinates $\begin{bmatrix} x & y \end{bmatrix}$. In order to capture the temporal connections between superpixels in successive frames, the clustering is performed over an observation window spanning K frames. The separated feature space is realized in the following way. Each cluster center represents one temporal superpixel. A cluster center consists of one color center for the complete observation window and multiple spatial centers with one for each observed frame.[1]

While processing the video volume the observation window is shifted in steps of one frame along the timeline. After each step an optimal set of cluster centers Θ_{opt} is obtained. The mapping of the pixels inside the observation window to these cluster centers is denoted as σ_{opt}. An energy function (1) is defined, which sums up the energies necessary to assign a pixel at position x, y in frame k to a cluster center $\theta \in \Theta_{opt}$. This assignment or mapping is here denoted by $\sigma_{x,y,k}$.

$$E_{total} = \sum_{k} \sum_{x,y} (1 - \alpha) E_c(x, y, k, \sigma_{x,y,k}) + \alpha E_s(x, y, k, \sigma_{x,y,k}) \qquad (1)$$

The energy needed for an assignment is the weighted sum of a color dependent energy $E_c(x, y, k, \sigma_{x,y,k})$ and a spatial energy $E_s(x, y, k, \sigma_{x,y,k})$. Both energy terms are proportional to the Euclidean distance in color space and image plane, respectively. The trade-off between color-sensitivity and spatial compactness is controlled by a weighting factor α, which has a range between 0 (fully color-sensitive) and 1 (fully compact). Thereby, $\alpha = 1$ leads to Voronoi cells. The energy function is minimized using an iterative optimization scheme, which can be viewed as an EM approach.

In the expectation-step (E-step) of iteration $l+1$ a new estimation of the optimal mapping, here denoted as $\hat{\sigma}_{x,y,k}^{l+1}$, is determined, which minimizes (1) based on the estimation of the optimal set of cluster centers $\hat{\Theta}_{opt}^{l}$ calculated in the maximization-step (M-step) of iteration l.

After that, the estimation of the optimal set of cluster centers $\hat{\Theta}_{opt}^{l+1}$ is updated in the M-step of iteration $l+1$ given the updated mapping by calculating the mean color and mean spatial values of the assigned pixels. The alternation of the two steps continues until the energy (1) drops below a specific bound or a fixed number of iterations is performed. In the hybrid clustering proposed for TCS, only the $K_F < K$ most future frames in the observation window are reassigned during the optimization. For the remaining $K - K_F$ frames the determined mapping is kept in order to preserve the color clustering found.

---

[1] The underlying assumption is that a temporal superpixel should share the same color in successive frames but not necessarily the same position.

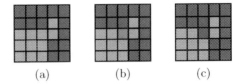

(a)   (b)   (c)

Fig. 2. The three subfigures exemplarily show pixels between two superpixels (green and blue). If the centered pixel (colored orange in (b)) changes its assignment, the two pixels on its right lose connection to the green superpixel and thus they would be split-off from the main mass (as shown exemplarily in (c)). Therefore, no assignment change is performed in situations like these (Color figure online).

While shifting the observation window new frames entering the window need to be initialized. In TCS this is done by projecting each spatial center of the most future frame into the new frame in the direction of the weighted average of the dense optical flow calculated over the corresponding superpixel.

2.2 Superpixels for Video Content Using a Contour-Based EM Optimization

Revisiting the ideas of TCS, we made the following two observations: *(a)* In order to achieve a higher run-time performance the initial energy-minimizing clustering and the contour-based post processing are separated steps. Thereby, the shape of the superpixels can change completely in each iteration. *(b)* New frames added to the observation window are initialized by propagating only the spatial centers of the preceding frame into the new frame. As a consequence, the shape information obtained in the frames before is discarded. These observations lead to our two proposals.

Firstly, we employ the optimization scheme, proposed by [26] for still images, to optimize the energy function (1). This means that only pixels at a contour of a superpixel, so called contour pixels, can change their assignment to a cluster. A contour pixel at position x, y has at least one pixel in its 4-connected neighborhood $\mathcal{N}_{x,y}^4$, which is assigned to a different cluster, i.e. a temporal superpixel, or is unassigned. The occurrence of unassigned pixels and their handling is described in detail below. Moreover, the assignment of a contour pixel can only be changed to one of the clusters of the pixels in $\mathcal{N}_{x,y}^4$ as proposed by [26]. The E-step of the optimization can be expressed as

$$\hat{\sigma}_{x,y,k}^{l+1} = \underset{\hat{\sigma}_{\tilde{x},\tilde{y},k}^{l}:\tilde{x},\tilde{y}\in(\mathcal{N}_{x,y}^4\cup x,y)}{\operatorname{argmin}} (1-\alpha)E_c(x,y,k,\hat{\sigma}_{\tilde{x},\tilde{y},k}^{l})+\alpha E_s(x,y,k,\hat{\sigma}_{\tilde{x},\tilde{y},k}^{l}) \,\forall x,y\in\mathcal{C}_k^l$$

$$(2)$$

where $\mathcal{C}_k^l$ is the set of contour pixels after iteration step l in frame k. The optimization is done for the K_F most future frames in the observation window. The M-step remains unmodified. The optimization can be terminated if there are no further assignment changes for the contour pixels or if a maximum number of iterations has been reached.

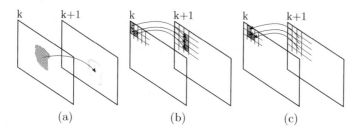

(a)   (b)   (c)

Fig. 3. Possible variations of superpixel label propagation to new frames: (a) The whole superpixel is shifted by the mean optical forward flow, (b) each label is propagated using a dense optical forward flow and (c) for each pixel in the new frame the label is looked up at a position determined by the optical backward flow. For case (c) no collisions can occur as for each pixel position only one label is looked up in the previous frame. Gaps cannot occur as the optical backward flow vector are cropped when pointing outside the valid image area.

In addition to the description above, there are two constraints. (a) An assignment change is only done if the spatial coherency of the superpixels is guaranteed. This constraint prevents that fragments of a temporal superpixel are split-off during the optimization, as shown in Fig. 2 (See [27] for more details on this constraint). (b) A newly proposed constraint affects unassigned contour pixels. These are assigned to a cluster of one of its adjacent pixels based on (2). As a consequence, the additional post-processing step required in TCS [18] to ensure the spatial coherency is not necessary and can be omitted.

Secondly, we propose to transfer the whole shape of the superpixels to the new frame to be initialized leveraging optical flow information unlike the approach described in [17]. This helps to preserve the shape information as well as the superpixel constellation obtained in previous frames. There are several ways to realize such an initialization of the new frames. One could be the shift of the complete superpixel label using the mean optical flow as depicted in Fig. 3a. An alternative would be the usage of a dense optical flow predicted for each pixel of the superpixel. Thus, the superpixel label is propagated into the new frame as shown in Fig. 3b.

These two options have the following drawback: If two superpixels propagated into the new frame overlap, it is necessary to detect collisions. In addition, it is possible that there are unassigned parts in the frame that need to be initialized if e.g. adjacent superpixels are moved away from each other, resulting in a gap between the superpixels. Both cases are illustrated in Fig. 4 and occur in the same manner propagating the labels by a dense optical forward flow.

To prevent these problems, we propose to use a dense optical backward flow, which is computed from the frame entering the observation window $k + 1$ to the preceding frame k in the window. The initial mapping of pixels to cluster centers of the new frame $k + 1$ denoted as $\hat{\sigma}^{init}_{x,y,k+1}$ can be deduced from the mapping for frame k (after L iteration steps) as follows:

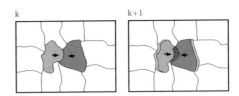

Fig. 4. Problems that can occur when propagating whole superpixels by mean optical flow from frame k to frame $k+1$: Moving adjacent superpixels in opposite directions produces gaps (cyan) while a movement toward each other leads to overlapping areas (dark blue). This also occurs in the same manner propagating the labels by a dense optical forward flow (Color figure online).

$$\hat{\sigma}^{init}_{x,y,k+1} = \hat{\sigma}^{L}_{x+u,y+v,k},\tag{3}$$

where u and v are the optical backward flow components, which are rounded to the nearest integer for the horizontal and vertical direction. Additionally, the components are clipped if pointing outside of the valid image area.

By using this approach no collisions have to be detected as for each pixel position only one label is determined eliminating the possibility of collisions. Gaps do not occur as the optical backward vectors are cropped if pointing outside the valid image area. The only issue left, which also exists for the both cases using optical forward flow, is that the propagated superpixels can be fragmented, i.e. they are not spatially coherent. In that case, the largest fragment is determined and the others are set to unassigned. These are handled in the E-step of the optimization, as they are part of the contour pixels. The first frame to be segmented is initialized with non-overlapping rectangles of equal size.

In [18] a heuristic was introduced to encounter structural changes in the video volume, which are e.g. occlusions, disocclusions, and objects approaching the camera as well as zooming. The decision to split or terminate a temporal superpixel was made based on a linear growth assumption of the superpixel size. Additionally, a separate balancing step was performed to keep the number of superpixels per frame constant. We replaced these two steps with a single one by introducing an upper and lower bound for the superpixel size. Superpixels that are larger than the upper bound are split. The ones that are smaller than the lower bound are terminated. These bounds are coupled to the number of superpixels initially specified by the user. Thus, the user defines a minimum and maximum number of superpixels per frame N_{min} and N_{max}, respectively. Based on that, the upper and lower bound A_{low} and A_{up} are set as follows

$$A_{low} = \frac{|P|}{N_{max}} \quad \text{and} \quad A_{up} = \frac{|P|}{N_{min}}\tag{4}$$

where $|P|$ is the number of pixels per frame. In our implementation we specified a number of superpixels N and set N_{min} and N_{max} to $\frac{1}{2}N$ and $2N$.

3   Experimental Results

In this section, we evaluate the quantitative performance of the proposed approach using standard benchmark metrics. Additionally, we present qualitative
results and compare the approach to state of the art supervoxel and superpixel
approaches for video content. For the experiments we set α to 0.96, the window
size K to 15 and performed $L = 5$ EM-iterations.[2] We used the datasets provided by [28,29]. The first dataset provides 40 training and 60 test sequences of
up to 121 frames. A multi-label ground truth segmentation is made available by
[30] including four segmentations for every twentieth frame. We use the half-HD
version of the dataset and show the results for the test sequences. The second dataset provides 8 video sequences of around 80 frames including a single
multi-label ground truth segmentation for every frame. The results are shown
as mean values calculated over each dataset separately. To create them we use
version 3.0 of LIBSVX originally published in [24] as well as the code provided
by [25]. Our current MATLAB implementation processes 3 to 4 video frames (in
an HD-ready resolution) per minute including the optical flow calculation and
$N = 3000$ superpixels. Thereby, it should be noted that the current version is
only moderately optimized with respect to the runtime-performance.

3.1   Metrics and Baseline

As the quality of the spatio-temporal segmentation is as important as the quality
of the segmentation on frame level, we considered the following set of supervoxel
and superpixel benchmark metrics that we will review briefly below. For a more
thorough explanation please refer to [21,24,31,32]. The first four metrics are
tailored to the evaluation of supervoxel and video segmentation algorithms and
indicate the quality of the spatio-temporal segmentation. The last two metrics
are suitable for evaluating the image segmentation quality on frame level.

3D Undersegmentation Error (*UE*): This metric proposed by [24] counts
the number of voxels *bleeding out* of the ground truth segmentation volume. For
a given segmentation with non-overlapping segments $s_1, s_2, ..., s_M$ and a ground
truth segment g_n the 3D undersegmentation error is calculated as follows

$$UE(g_n) = \frac{\left[\sum_{(s_m | s_m \cap g_n \neq \emptyset)} |s_m|\right] - |g_n|}{|g_n|}. \tag{5}$$

Here $|s_m|$ denotes the number of voxels of the segment. The error is then averaged
over all ground truth segments.

3D Segmentation Accuracy (*SA*): Also proposed in [24] the 3D segmentation
accuracy denotes the fraction of the video volume that can be reproduced by
the segmentation's overlap with the ground truth segments if for each segment

---

[2] The changes after 5 iterations are only marginal. It should be noted that the boundary can move more than 1 pixel per iteration.

only the overlap with a single ground truth segment is counted. Therefore, the segments are assigned to the ground truth segment, for which it has the maximum overlap with, and then just the overlap of the segments with its assigned ground truth segment is counted:

$$SA = \frac{1}{N} \sum_{n=1}^{N} \frac{\sum_{o \in O_n}(|s_o \cap g_n|)}{|g_n|} \quad (6)$$

N is the number of ground truth segments and O_n is the set of segments s_o assigned to g_n.

Average Temporal Length: This metric was introduced in [21] for measuring the ability to track regions over time by calculating the mean duration of the spatio-temporal segments. This metric always has to be evaluated in conjunction with a metric like 3D segmentation accuracy or 3D undersegmentation error as a long temporal segment duration is only valuable together with a high quality spatio-temporal segmentation.

Explained Variation (EV): This metric was proposed in [31] and indicates how well the original information can be represented with a given over-segmentation as a representation of lower detail.

2D Boundary Recall (BR): The 2D boundary recall measures the fraction of the boundary annotated in the ground truth that is covered by a superpixel boundary. A ground truth boundary pixel is counted as covered if a superpixel boundary is within the pixel-distance ϵ, which is set to 1 for our experiments.

Variance of Area (VoA): In [32] the variance of area was proposed as a metric for the homogeneity of superpixel sizes and is calculated for a frame k as follows

$$VoA(k) = \mathrm{var}\left(\frac{A_{m,k}}{\bar{A}_k}\right). \quad (7)$$

$A_{m,k}$ is the area of a superpixel in frame k belonging to a supervoxel m and $\bar{A}_k$ is the mean superpixel area in frame k.

In [16] the 3D benchmark metrics like UE and SA are plotted over the average number of superpixels per frame arguing that different video length and content require in general a different number of supervoxels. We will plot only the BR and VoA over the average number of superpixels per frame as otherwise the temporal consistency of the spatio-temporal segmentation is not taken into consideration at all in the 3D metrics. We think it is reasonable to plot the metrics over the number of supervoxels as long as the number of frames in the sequences used is not deviating too much.

3.2   Quantitative Evaluation

The baseline (BL) for the following experiments is [18] with the slight modification that for the optical flow [33] is used instead of [34]. First we successively

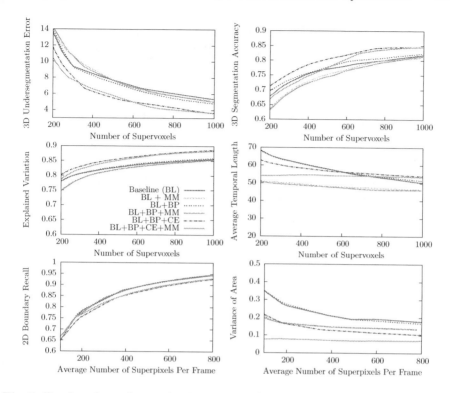

Fig. 5. Benchmark results on the dataset from [29] for the baseline implementation and our contributions. Please note that the 2D boundary recall and the variance of area are plotted over the average number of superpixels per frame and not over the number of supervoxels as in the other diagrams.

show the impact of our contributions that were added to the baseline version: the contour-based optimization scheme in an EM framework (CE), label propagation for initialization using the optical backward flow (BP) as well as the simplified handling of structural changes, i.e. the splitting and termination of superpixels based on a minimal and maximal number of superpixels (MM). As the contour-based optimization requires label propagation, the results for CE alone cannot be presented, only in combination with the optical backward flow propagation (BP). For each contribution, we performed several segmentations of the video sequences provided by [29] using a range of desired superpixels per frame (resulting in different numbers of supervoxels) and used the aforementioned metrics to evaluate the segmentations. The results are shown in Fig. 5.

It is evident that MM and BP alone and their combination (MM+BP) have virtually no effect on the UE, SA, EV and BR compared to the baseline (BL). Only a slight degradation for small numbers of supervoxels for UE, SA and EV can be noticed. In addition, MM reduces the average temporal length while at the same time VoA is improved. This can be explained with the fact that the baseline (BL) allows for smaller superpixels. Again, BP alone achieves nearly identical

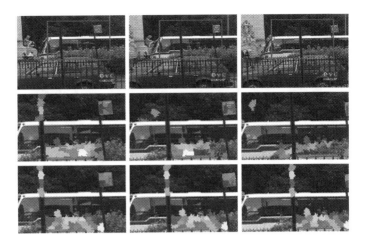

Fig. 6. Example for a challenging segmentation task with low contrast and high motion. Top row shows the original sequence with a marked area magnified in the rows below. For the two lower rows a full segmentation was performed with the baseline approach (BL, middle) and the proposed approach (BL+BP+CE+MM, bottom). Only a subset of superpixels is shown, which was manually selected and colored. Same color means temporal connectedness. In the middle row the superpixels are torn away by the motion introduced by the camera panning, while they keep their position and constellation for the proposed approach (Color figure online).

results as the baseline for the average temporal length as well as *VoA*. The improvements are achieved with the introduction of CE. Nearly for all metrics improved results are obtained, especially for higher numbers of supervoxels. Only the *BR* is slightly impaired. This highlights the positive impact of the contour-based optimization approach that it can achieve in combination with the efficient label propagation using optical backward flow.

3.3   Qualitative Evaluation

Temporal superpixels should cover corresponding image regions over time. Hence, their spatial constellation should not change if they cover a nearly rigidly moving object. Although this seems to be an easy task to accomplish, Fig. 6 shows an example of a scene likely to be found in natural video sequences were previous approaches fail. The top row shows the original sequence. The region of interest including low contrast (street light, trees) and high motion (bus, flowers) is marked with a red rectangle and cropped in the rows below. The marked superpixels in the middle row are taken from the segmentation produced by the baseline approach (BL) from Sect. 3.2. The superpixels in the lower row were taken from a segmentation with our proposed approach (BL+BP+CE+MM). It can be seen that, while both approaches use the same optical flow algorithm, the baseline approach has an issue with keeping the superpixels to their initial positions. Even in the area with higher contrast (flowers) the superpixels change

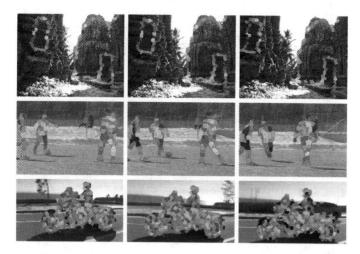

Fig. 7. Results generated by our algorithm showing the segmentation quality and temporal stability. For each sequence a full superpixel segmentation was performed and a subset of superpixels was manually selected in one frame (**not** necessarily in the first frame). Same color means temporal connectedness.

their position from frame to frame in an unpredictable way. In the bottom row, showing the result of our proposed approach, the superpixels stick to their original positions. While this is only a single example picked out for illustration, this behavior can be observed in other sequences and is also common for supervoxel methods. It should also be noted that present established benchmark metrics do not capture these kinds of errors as the jumping superpixels often stay within the same ground truth label and therefore do not have a negative impact on metrics like undersegmentation error or segmentation accuracy.

In Fig. 7 additional qualitative results are shown. The upper row of images shows equally spaced frames from a subsequence spanning 40 frames of an unsteady hand camera shot. Despite the shaking camera, the superpixel formations stick close to their initial positions. The second row illustrates the performance of our approach for non-rigid motion. The sequence shown in the third row spans 69 frames of a sequence with high motion blur noticeable e.g. in the second image. It should be noted that the last two images reveal the limits of the approach as some superpixels are misled and switch to the car that is overtaken by the motorcycle.

3.4 Comparison to State of the Art Algorithms

In this section we compare our final approach to four state of the art algorithms producing supervoxels or temporally consistent superpixels. We compare our approach to *StreamGBH* published in [21], which is the only representative of the class of supervoxel algorithms. Furthermore, we compare it against

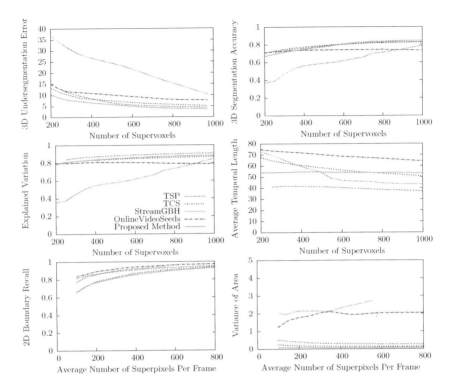

Fig. 8. Benchmark results for the dataset from [29] for state of the art supervoxel and superpixel algorithms for video content. Please note that the 2D boundary recall and the variance of area are plotted over the average number of superpixels per frame. Higher values are better except for the 3D undersegmentation error and variance of area.

the superpixel approaches *Temporally Consistent Superpixel* (TCS) [18], *Temporal Superpixels* (TSP) [16] and *OnlineVideoSeeds* [17]. For StreamGBH, TSP, and OnlineVideoSeeds, the source code of the algorithms was publicly available. We used the sources from the authors' websites to produce the following results. For TCS, we used the original version that was the basis for [18]. Whenever possible, the parameters were set as mentioned in the authors' publications or documentations. For the dataset [29], the benchmarks results are depicted in Fig. 8 and for the dataset [28] with ground truth segmentations from [30] results are shown in Fig. 9.

For [29] our algorithm performs best in *UE* and *VoA* and is also slightly better in *SA* for higher numbers of supervoxels while performing worst in *BR* with comparable results to TCS (see Fig. 8). On the second dataset, which is much larger and more diverse, our method performs best in *SA*, *EV* as well as *VoA* and for higher numbers of supervoxels also in *UE* (see Fig. 9). The unusual behavior of OnlineVideoSeeds for *UE* may have its roots in the code provided by the authors. The number of histogram bins is hard coded for several fixed

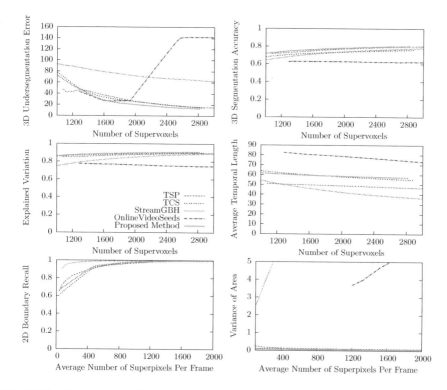

Fig. 9. Results generated for the dataset provided by [28] including scenes with diverse types of camera motion, motion blurring and non-rigid-motion. Please note the different abscissa. Higher values are better except for the 3D undersegmentation error and variance of area.

numbers of superpixels, which may not work well on the dataset provided by [28], as it is has a higher resolution and is more complex than [29]. In the *VoA* diagram of Fig. 9 the graphs of StreamGBH and OnlineVideoSeeds rise approximately linearly to a *VoA* of 18.4 and 7.9, respectively, for 2000 superpixels per frame.

4   Conclusion

We presented a novel, contour-based approach to generate temporally consistent superpixels for video content. It is based on an EM framework performing the optimization only on the pixels at the superpixel boundaries and leverages the optical backward flow for the propagation of superpixel labels for the initialization of new frames. In combination both contributions help to preserve superpixel shapes over multiple frames leading to a steady and accurate superpixel constellation. The evaluation on standard benchmarks shows that our approach outperforms or produces comparable results to state of the art supervoxel and temporal superpixel approaches, even on datasets with different kinds of camera movement, non-rigid motion, and motion blur.

References

1. Ren, X., Malik, J.: Learning a classification model for segmentation. In: ICCV, pp. 10–17 (2003)
2. Lezama, J., Alahari, K., Sivic, J., Laptev, I.: Track to the future: spatio-temporal video segmentation with long-range motion cues. In: CVPR, pp. 3369–3376 (2011)
3. Galasso, F., Cipolla, R., Schiele, B.: Video segmentation with superpixels. In: Lee, K.M., Matsushita, Y., Rehg, J.M., Hu, Z. (eds.) ACCV 2012, Part I. LNCS, vol. 7724, pp. 760–774. Springer, Heidelberg (2013)
4. Wang, S., Lu, H., Yang, F., Yang, M.H.: Superpixel tracking. In: ICCV, pp. 1323–1330 (2011)
5. Djelouah, A., Franco, J.S., Boyer, E., Le Clerc, F., Pérez, P.: Multi-view object segmentation in space and time. In: ICCV, pp. 2640–2647 (2013)
6. Vogel, C., Schindler, K., Roth, S.: Piecewise rigid scene flow. In: ICCV, pp. 1377–1384 (2013)
7. Zhang, J., Kan, C., Schwing, A.G., Urtasun, R.: Estimating the 3D layout of indoor scenes and its clutter from depth sensors. In: ICCV, pp. 1273–1280 (2013)
8. van den Hengel, A., Dick, A., Thormählen, T., Ward, B., Torr, P.H.S.: VideoTrace. ACM TOG **26**, 86 (2007)
9. Tighe, J., Lazebnik, S.: Superparsing. IJCV **101**, 329–349 (2012)
10. Roig, G., Boix, X., Nijs, R.D., Ramos, S., Kuhnlenz, K., Gool, L.V.: Active MAP inference in CRFs for efficient semantic segmentation. In: ICCV, pp. 2312–2319 (2013)
11. Jain, A., Chatterjee, S., Vidal, R.: Coarse-to-fine semantic video segmentation using supervoxel trees. In: ICCV, pp. 1865–1872 (2013)
12. Hoiem, D., Efros, A.A., Hebert, M.: Geometric context from a single image. In: ICCV, pp. 654–661 (2005)
13. Grundmann, M., Kwatra, V., Han, M., Essa, I.: Efficient hierarchical graph-based video segmentation. In: CVPR, pp. 2141–2148 (2010)
14. Veksler, O., Boykov, Y., Mehrani, P.: Superpixels and supervoxels in an energy optimization framework. In: Daniilidis, K., Maragos, P., Paragios, N. (eds.) ECCV 2010, Part V. LNCS, vol. 6315, pp. 211–224. Springer, Heidelberg (2010)
15. Achanta, R., Shaji, A., Smith, K., Lucchi, A., Fua, P., Susstrunk, S.: SLIC superpixels compared to state-of-the-art superpixel methods. TPAMI **34**, 2274–2282 (2012)
16. Chang, J., Wei, D., Fisher, J.W.: A video representation using temporal superpixels. In: CVPR, pp. 2051–2058 (2013)
17. Van den Bergh, M., Roig, G., Boix, X., Manen, S., Van Gool, L.: Online video seeds for temporal window objectness. In: ICCV, pp. 377–384 (2013)
18. Reso, M., Jachalsky, J., Rosenhahn, B., Ostermann, J.: Temporally consistent superpixels. In: ICCV, pp. 385–392 (2013)
19. Levinshtein, A., Sminchisescu, C., Dickinson, S.: Spatiotemporal closure. In: Kimmel, R., Klette, R., Sugimoto, A. (eds.) ACCV 2010, Part I. LNCS, vol. 6492, pp. 369–382. Springer, Heidelberg (2011)
20. Zitnick, C.L., Jojic, N., Kang, S.B.: Consistent segmentation for optical flow estimation. In: ICCV, pp. 1308–1315 (2005)
21. Xu, C., Xiong, C., Corso, J.J.: Streaming hierarchical video segmentation. In: Fitzgibbon, A., Lazebnik, S., Perona, P., Sato, Y., Schmid, C. (eds.) ECCV 2012, Part VI. LNCS, vol. 7577, pp. 626–639. Springer, Heidelberg (2012)

22. Felzenszwalb, P.F., Huttenlocher, D.P.: Efficient graph-based image segmentation. IJCV **59**, 167–181 (2004)
23. Van den Bergh, M., Boix, X., Roig, G., de Capitani, B., Van Gool, L.: SEEDS: superpixels extracted via energy-driven sampling. In: Fitzgibbon, A., Lazebnik, S., Perona, P., Sato, Y., Schmid, C. (eds.) ECCV 2012, Part VII. LNCS, vol. 7578, pp. 13–26. Springer, Heidelberg (2012)
24. Xu, C., Corso, J.J.: Evaluation of super-voxel methods for early video processing. In: CVPR, pp. 1202–1209 (2012)
25. Arbeláez, P., Maire, M., Fowlkes, C., Malik, J.: Contour detection and hierarchical image segmentation. TPAMI **33**, 898–916 (2011)
26. Schick, A., Fischer, M., Stiefelhagen, R.: Measuring and evaluating the compactness of superpixels. In: ICPR, pp. 930–934 (2012)
27. Schick, A., Fischer, M., Stiefelhagen, R.: An evaluation of the compactness of superpixels. Pattern Recogn. Lett. **43**, 71–80 (2014)
28. Sundberg, P., Brox, T., Maire, M., Arbelaez, P., Malik, J.: Occlusion boundary detection and figure/ground assignment from optical flow. In: CVPR, pp. 2233–2240 (2011)
29. Chen, A., Corso, J.J.: Propagating multi-class pixel labels throughout video frames. In: WNYIPW, pp. 14–17 (2010)
30. Galasso, F., Nagaraja, N.S., Cárdenas, T.J., Brox, T., Schiele, B.: A unified video segmentation benchmark: annotation, metrics and analysis. In: ICCV, pp. 3527–3534 (2013)
31. Moore, A.P., Prince, S., Warrell, J., Mohammed, U., Jones, G.: Superpixel lattices. In: CVPR, pp. 1–8 (2008)
32. Perbet, F., Maki, A.: Homogeneous superpixels from random walks. In: MVA, pp. 26–30 (2011)
33. Liu, C.: Beyond pixels: exploring new representations and applications for motion analysis. Ph.D. thesis, Massachusetts Institute of Technology (2009)
34. Horn, B.K.P., Schunck, B.G.: Determining optical flow. AI **17**, 185–203 (1981)

Transformed Principal Gradient Orientation for Robust and Precise Batch Face Alignment

Weihong Deng$^{(\boxtimes)}$, Jiani Hu, Liu Liu, and Jun Guo

Beijing University of Posts and Telecommunications, Beijing, China
whdeng@bupt.edu.cn

Abstract. This paper addresses the problem of simultaneously aligning a batch of linearly correlated images despite large misalignment, severe illumination and occlusion. Our algorithm assumes that the gradient orientation of images, if correctly aligned, can be robustly represented by an underlying transformed principal gradient orientation (TPGO) subspace. With such a linear representation prior, the proposed method connects PGO subspace learning, gradient orientation reconstruction, and batch alignment in a unified framework with an efficient alternating optimization solution. Besides inherent robustness from the gradient orientation and the low-rank structure, TPGO maintains the pixel-accurate registration precision and the efficient optimization of Lucas & Kanade framework. Experimental results show TPGO based batch alignment is more precise and robust than the state-of-the-art methods such as RASL and SIFT feature base Congealing. Moreover, integrated with a SIFT based pre-alignment procedure, TPGO is able to align a large number of images of multiple objects with large deviation, illumination, and occlusion in the precision that surpasses the handcrafted alignments (provided by the standard database distributions), in term of our face recognition experiments on the Extended Yale B, AR and FERET databases.

1 Introduction

Batch Image alignment is an interesting task of automatic batch alignment of an ensemble of misaligned images to a fixed canonical template in an unsupervised manner. As the dramatic increase in the amount of visual data available, the image congealing technique has numerous applications in object detection, tracking, recognition, and retrieval. For instances, previous works on face recognition has proven that the recognition performance highly depend on the preciseness of the image alignment [1–4]. Two basic assumptions underlying most algorithms are that (1) images are subjected to randomly selected transformation of known nature, such as translation, similarity or affine, and that (2) images reside in a low dimensional subspace approximately after aligned to a fixed canonical template, e.g. faces [5,6], handwritten digits, etc. Clearly, the fundamental issue on batch image alignment is the multivariate similarity measures of an image ensemble, and the associated optimization methods.

Electronic supplementary material The online version of this chapter (doi:10. 1007/978-3-319-16817-3_46) contains supplementary material, which is available to authorized users.

© Springer International Publishing Switzerland 2015
D. Cremers et al. (Eds.): ACCV 2014, Part IV, LNCS 9006, pp. 708–723, 2015.
DOI: 10.1007/978-3-319-16817-3_46

The pioneer work of Learned-Miler [7], named *congealing*, constructed the multivariate similarity measure as a sum of entropies of pixel values at each pixel location in the whole image ensemble. To address the nonlinearity of entropy function, an sequential parameter update based optimization strategy is employed. In this congealing framework, clustered SIFT feature based entropy was also proposed to address the complex variations such as illumination and local deformation involved in the image ensemble [8]. To remedy the difficulty in the nonlinear optimization of congealing method, Cox et al. [9] proposed a least-square congealing method by employing the sum of squared distances between pairs of images to measure the similarity of the image ensemble. An inverse-compositional strategy was further proposed to address the "irrecoverable lost" problem caused by applying a single warp to a stack of images, which makes LS-Congealing applicable to align a large number of images. Both congealing methods ideally assume the matrix of aligned images will have exactly rank one, which may not be realistic for images with complex variations.

The other family of algorithms have been proposed to address the robust alignment problem by taking the advantage of the low-dimensional subspace structure. The early work of Frey and Jojic [10] used an EM algorithm to fit a low dimensional linear model, subject to domain transformation drawn from a know group. Schweitzer [11] proposed a more practical iterative procedure that jointly optimize the eigenspace model and the transformation parameters. Baker et al. used a similar technique to construct the active appearance model [12]. The Robust Parameterized Component Analysis (RPCA) algorithm used the robust fitting function to reduce the influence of occlusion and corruption. Vadaldi et al. [13] proposed a straightforward measure based on the dimension of subspace spanned by the aligned image, i.e. the rank of the image data matrix, but this measure may be sensitive to small corruption or occlusion of the images. To address this problem, Peng et al. [14] formulated a more robust measure by considering both the dimension of the subspace and the L1 norm of residuals from the subspace, and propose an influential method named RASL.

A major limitation of current batch alignment techniques is that their robustness is not enough to address the severe illumination and occlusion in the realistic images. Recent advance in image representation [15] have shown that it is indeed possible to invariantly represent facial images despite significant changes of illumination and occlusion, using the low-rank principal subspace of image gradient orientation. Inspired by this breakthrough work [15], this paper proposes a new algorithm to **achieve enhanced robustness by taking advantage of both the illumination/occlusion invariance and the low rank property of the aligned image gradient orientation**. Specifically, the contributions of this paper are as follows.

(1) **A new batch alignment algorithm called Transformed principal gradient orientation (TPGO)** is proposed for robustly aligning linear corrected images, despite uncontrolled lighting and large occlusions. Our algorithm assumes that the gradient orientation of unaligned image, if correctly aligned, can be robustly represented by a linear combination of the bases of an underlying

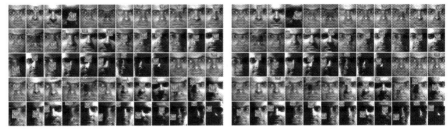

(a) Unaligned images with severe illumi-   (b) Aligned images via TPGO
nation and occlusion

Fig. 1. Batch image alignment via TPGO. (a) A full set of 60 images of the first person on the Extended Yale B database [16] with severe illuminations, simulated occlusions, and random transformations. For this challenging image ensemble, TPGO produces precise alignment within one pixel accuracy in the recovered eye centers, as shown in (b).

low dimensional Transformed principal gradient orientation (TPGO) subspace. With such a linear representation prior, the proposed method connects PGO subspace learning, gradient orientation reconstruction, and batch alignment in a unified framework with an efficient alternative optimization solution. Besides inherent robustness from image gradient orientation [15], the "joint TPGO Subspace learning and batch Alignment" algorithm maintains the pixel-accurate registration precision (Fig. 1) and the efficient optimization of Lucas & Kanade framework [17], under the challenging variations of illuminations and occlusions. The effectiveness of the proposed TPGO is shown in term of the better alignment accuracy and robustness against two state-of-the-art batch alignment methods, namely SIFT-congealing [8] and RASL [14].

(2) **A coarse-to-fine batch alignment approach** is proposed to handle the task with large-misalignment and real-world illumination and occlusion. We observe that the real-world occlusions tend to largely deviate the bounding box of object detector, and makes the subsequent alignment algorithms cannot converge. Our approach applies a SIFT based pre-alignment procedure to coarsely align the images, before the fine alignment via TPGO. Experimental results on the 1000 images of 100 subjects from AR database show that our fully automatic batch alignment results (combined with VJ face detector) can reduce the recognition errors by a half, when compared to the manually aligned images distributed by the AR database.

(3) **TPGO is demonstrated be beneficial to fully automatic face recognition applications** where a TPGO subspace is first learned from the training images, and then the gallery images and probe images are aligned to the subspace so that they can be well compared. Recognition experiment on the FERET database with 1196 persons demonstrates that TPGO based alignment is more precise than SIFT-Congealing and Deformable sparse recovery method [18], as well as the manually labeled eye-coordinate based alignment, which is widely used as ground-truth alignment for this popular database.

2 Transformed Principal Gradient Orientation (TPGO)

In this section, we introduce a robust batch alignment approach named Transformed Principal Gradient Orientation (TPGO). The novelty of TPGO comes from the fact that it exploiting both the illumination/occlusion-invariant descriptor and the low rank structure of aligned images, and, at the same time, maintains the preciseness of alignment and the elegance of the optimization.

2.1 Problem Formulation

Image Gradient Orientations: For an image of p pixels, we denote the image gradient at pixel i along the horizontal and vertical direction as $g_{i,x}$ and $g_{i,y}$ with $i = 1, \ldots, p$. Hence, the gradient orientation (angle) can be computed by $\phi_i = \arctan(g_{i,y}/g_{i,x}) \in [0, 2\pi)$, where $i = 1, \ldots, p$. In this way, the gradient orientation of each image I^i can be represented by a p dimensional complex vector $\Phi^i = [\phi_1^i, \ldots, \phi_p^i]^T \in \mathcal{R}^p$. Alternatively, one can map the gradient orientation from an angle to a complex number $\phi_k \rightarrow z_k = e^{j\phi_k}$, $k = 1, \ldots, p$. In this sense, the gradient orientation of each image I^i can be represented by a p dimensional complex vector $z^i = [e^{j\phi_1}, \ldots, e^{j\phi_p}]^T \in \mathcal{C}^p$.

Gradient Orientation Distance: For two images I^i and I^j, the local distance of the gradient orientations at pixel k is naturally defined as a cosine function of the angle difference, i.e. $d^2(\phi_k^i, \phi_k^j) \triangleq [1 - cos(\phi_k^i - \phi_k^j)]$, which can be further formulated by the square distance between corresponding complex numbers, i.e. $d^2(\phi_k^i, \phi_k^j) = \frac{1}{2}\|e^{j\phi_k^i} - e^{j\phi_k^j}\|^2$. Therefore, the gradient orientation distance between two images I^i and I^j, the sum of the distances at each pixel, can be naturally formulated by the corresponding complex vectors, i.e.

$$d^2(\phi^i, \phi^j) = \frac{1}{2}\|z^i - z^j\|^2 \tag{1}$$

Besides its well-known invariance to illumination, the gradient orientation based distance is also robust to the occlusion of the images because the sum of distance computed from the occluded portion tends to be zero [15].

Principal Gradient Orientation (PGO) Subspace: Given a set of N images $\{I^i\}_{i=1}^N$, we compute the corresponding set of gradient orientation $\{z^i\}_{i=1}^N$. We look for a set of $K < p$ orthonormal bases $U = [u_1 \cdots u_K] \in \mathcal{C}^{p \times K}$ with the goal of minimizing the sum of the distances from subspace

$$U^* = \arg \min_{U_K} = \|Z - U_K U_K^H Z\|_F^2, \ s.t. \ U^H U = I \tag{2}$$

where $Z = [z^1 \cdots z^N] \in \mathcal{C}^{p \times N}$. The solution can be efficiently given by the K left singular vectors of Z corresponding to the K largest singular values. Recently, this subspace learning method has been successfully applied to the illumination- and occlusion- robust object recognition [15].

Transformed PGO Subspace: Given an ensemble of unaligned images, we assume that the gradient orientation of unaligned image, if correctly aligned, can be robustly represented by a linear combination of the bases of an underlying low dimensional Transformed principal gradient orientation (TPGO) subspace. The term "Transformed" indicates that the underlying TPGO subspace would characterize the intrinsic structure of the aligned object that is invariant to the transformations of the specific images.

For the simplicity of formulation, we use $z^i[\mathbf{p}^i]$ to denote the gradient orientation vector of the aligned image $I^i\left(\mathbf{W}(\mathbf{x};\mathbf{p}^i)\right)$, T^i to denote the reconstructed template gradient vector of $z^i[\mathbf{p}^i]$, which is represented as a function $T^i(U,\mathbf{p}^i)$ of the subspace U and transformation parameter $\mathbf{p}^i$ itself. The objective function of TPGO is naturally formulated as follows.

$$E\left(U,\{T^i\}_{i=1}^N,\{\mathbf{p}^i\}_{i=1}^N\right) = \sum_{i=1}^N \left\|z^i[\mathbf{p}^i] - T^i(U,\mathbf{p}^i)]\right\|^2 \tag{3}$$

2.2   Optimization Procedure

The proposed model (3) involves multiple variables and is hard to minimize directly. We adopt the alternating minimization scheme which reduces the original problem into several simpler subproblems. Specifically, we address the subproblems for each of the three variables in an alternating manner and present an overall efficient optimization problem. At each step, our algorithm reduces the objective function value, and finally converge to a local minima. To start, we initialize the alignment parameter $\mathbf{p}^i = 0$.

PGO Subspace Estimation: Optimizing U_K. Given the current transformation parameter $\mathbf{p}^i$ for each image, we want to update the bases of the underlying PGO subspace. We compute the corresponding set of gradient orientation $\{z^i[\mathbf{p}^i]\}_{i=1}^N$. We look for a set of $K << p$ orthonormal bases $U = [u_1 \cdots u_K] \in \mathcal{C}^{p \times K}$ with the goal of minimizing the sum of the distances from subspace

$$U^* = \arg\min_{U_K} = \|Z[\mathbf{p}] - U_K U_K^H Z[\mathbf{p}]\|_F^2, \ s.t. \ U^H U = I \tag{4}$$

where $Z[\mathbf{p}] = \left[z^1[\mathbf{p}^1] \cdots z^N[\mathbf{p}^N]\right] \in \mathcal{C}^{p \times N}$. The solution can be efficiently given by the K left singular vectors of $Z[\mathbf{p}]$ corresponding to the K largest singular values.

Latent Template Reconstruction: Optimizing T^i. With the underlying PGO subspace U_K and transformation parameter $\mathbf{p}^i$, we can reconstruct a latent template to be regarded as a virtual target for alignment. First, the current warped gradient orientation vector is projected onto the PGO subspace to obtain the reconstructed gradient as follows.

$$g^{i,t} = U_K U_K^H z^i[\mathbf{p}^i] \tag{5}$$

A normalization procedure is then applied to compute the template of gradient orientation

$$T_k^i = g_{k,x}^{i,t}/\|g_k^{i,t}\| + jg_{k,y}^{i,t}/\|g_k^{i,t}\| \tag{6}$$

Image-to-Template Alignment: Optimizing $\mathbf{p}^i$. With the reconstructed template T^i, the minimization of the objective function (3) is decomposed to N subproblems on the maximization of the coherence between the warped gradient orientation vector and the corresponding template for each image, i.e.

$$\max_{\mathbf{p}^i} \sum_{k \in \mathbb{P}} z_{k,x}^i [\mathbf{p}^i] T_{k,x}^i + z_{k,y}^i [\mathbf{p}^i] T_{k,y}^i \tag{7}$$

In light of the inverse-compositional gradient correlation algorithm [19], the transformation parameters are updated by

$$\mathbf{W}(\mathbf{x}; \mathbf{p}^i) \leftarrow \mathbf{W}(\mathbf{x}; \mathbf{p}^i) \circ \mathbf{W}(\mathbf{x}; \Delta\mathbf{p}^i) \tag{8}$$

where $\circ$ denotes composition, and

$$\Delta\mathbf{p}^i = \lambda \left(J^T J \right)^{-1} J^T S_{\Delta\phi} \tag{9}$$

where J is a $p \times n$ Jacobian matrix whose k-th row has n element corresponding to the $1 \times n$ vector

$$J_k = \frac{T_{k,x}^i \frac{\partial g_{k,y}^{i,t}}{\partial p} + T_{k,y}^i \frac{\partial g_{k,x}^{i,t}}{\partial p}}{\sqrt{(g_{k,x}^{i,t})^2 + (g_{k,y}^{i,t})^2}} \tag{10}$$

and

$$\begin{bmatrix} \frac{\partial g_{k,x}^{i,t}}{\partial p} \\ \frac{\partial g_{k,y}^{i,t}}{\partial p} \end{bmatrix} = \begin{bmatrix} g_{k,xx}^{i,t} & g_{k,xy}^{i,t} \\ g_{k,yx}^{i,t} & g_{t,yy}^{i,t} \end{bmatrix} \frac{\partial W}{\partial \mathbf{p}} \bigg|_{\mathbf{p}=0} \tag{11}$$

$S_{\Delta\phi}$ is a $N \times 1$ vector whose k-th element is equal to $\sin \left(\phi_k^i [\mathbf{p}^i] - \phi_k^{i,t} \right)$.

2.3   Algorithm and Implementation Details

The overall algorithm optimizes the PGO bases U, latent gradient orientation template T^i, and alignment parameters $\mathbf{p}^i$ alternatively. Algorithm 1 describes the procedures of our Joint TPGO Subspace learning and Batch Alignment algorithm

There are two loops in Algorithm 1. For each image, the inner loop aims to aligning it to the current subspace. In each inner loop, since the reconstructed template may not be accurate, we only update the transformation parameters once to avoid divergency. In contrast, the outer loop updates the subspace for more precise alignment.

2.4   Application to Fully Automatic Face Recognition

It should be noted that the proposed TPGO method is readily applicable to fully automatic face recognition. Specifically, In the training stage, Algorithm 1 can be applied on a training image ensemble (or the gallery ensemble) to obtain a

Algorithm 1. Joint TPGO Subspace learning and Batch Alignment algorithm

Input: An ensemble of unaligned image gradient orientation $\{z^i\}_{i=1}^N$,
Output: TPGO subspace bases U_K, transformation parameter $\{\mathbf{p}^i\}_{i=1}^N$
1: **Initalization:** transformation parameter $\mathbf{p} = 0$
2: **for** $l_O = 1, 2, \ldots, L_O$ **do**
3:     **Subspace Estimation:** update the PGO subspace U_K by minimizing Eq. (4)
4:     **for** $i = 1, 2, \ldots, N$ **do**
5:         **for** $l_I = 1, 2, \ldots, L_I$ **do**
6:             **Template Reconstruction:** update the latent template T^i using Eq. (6)
7:             **Image-to-Template Alignment:** update the transformation parameters
                $\mathbf{p}^i$ (once) by (8)
8:         **end for**
9:     **end for**
10: **end for**

PGO subspace, which defines a fixed canonical template for image comparison. Then, in the test stage, the gallery image and probe image could be aligned to the PGO subspace so that they can be suitable compared. In this stage, as the PGO subspace is settle, the image can be aligned to the subspace by iteratively performing "template reconstruction" and "Image-to-Template Alignment" in Algorithm 1.

Compared with the commonly used eye-coordinate based alignment, a advantage of this procedure is its full automation, which means no human labeling work involved in both training and testing stages. In addition, pixel-accurate alignment could be achieved by TPGO based alignment, but the error induced by eye localization is usually larger than one pixel, even for the human labeler. Therefore, it is possible that TPGO-based alignment could be better than eye-coordinate based alignment for recognition. We would test this possibility in our final experiment on the FERET database.

3   SIFT Feature-Based Generic Face Pre-alignment

In practice, severe illumination and occlusion not only affect the object appearance, but also largely deviate the bounding box of the object detector, which makes alignment algorithms more difficult to converge. For instance, we find that the scale of the bounding boxes of the commonly used Voila-Jones face detector is much larger for the face with sunglasses. These large initialized deviations are often outside the region of attraction for most batch alignment methods, especially when the images are with occlusion. To address this limitation, we proposed a SIFT feature based generic face pre-alignment approach[1].

Inspired by the similar shape of the common face, our approach relies on a generic facial SIFT feature database which is constructed by extracting the

---

[1] Due to the space limit, the implementation details of the SIFT feature based prealignment is described in the supplementary material.

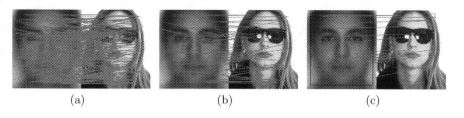

(a)   (b)   (c)

Fig. 2. (a) The feature match pairs using Lowe's match algorithm, each red line connecting the left to right represents a estimated match point pairs, to simplify, we just show the location relationship of matched pairs without the scale and orientation of key points. We use a mean image to visualize the feature database from multiple images; (b) Match point pairs after eliminating most of outliers by our normalization method (Step 2). (c) The outliers are further reduced by RANSAC, and the transformation from the black rectangle to the blue rectangle is the similarity transformation we calculate to roughly align the image (Color figure online).

SIFT feature points from a large set of aligned facial images. In our experiment, we have used 200 manually aligned faces from diverse sources. This generic feature database provides a prior distribution of the feature location of the human face. Given a novel input image, we first apply the Lowe's matching algorithm to obtain a large number of matching point pairs between the input image and the generic database. Then, we eliminate a large proportion of the mismatching point pairs by adding a set of normalization constraints on the geometric information. Finally, based on the remaining matching point pair, we robustly estimate a similarity transformation (from the generic faces to the input face) by RANSAC algorithm. The implementation details is described in the supplementary material (Fig. 2).

4   Experiments

In this section, we demonstrate the efficacy of TPGO on batch alignment tasks despite severe lighting variation and occlusion, by comparing its performance with SIFT-Congealing and RASL. We test algorithms on a large number of realistic and challenging images taken from the Extended Yale B (EYB) database [16], the AR database [20], and FERET database [21]. EYB database contains full set of illumination images for human faces and AR database involves different lighting conditions and real-world large occlusions caused by accessories such as sunglasses and scarf. The FERET database contains a large number of subjects with diverse variations. Therefore, they are ideal for evaluating the robustness of batch alignment algorithms.

For comparison purpose, we also implemented three state-of-the-art methods: (1) SIFT-Congealing [8]: a robust alignment approach to complex images by minimizing the sum of entropies of the dense SIFT features; (2) RASL [14]: robust alignment via sparse and low-rank decomposition; (For the first two algorithms, we preserve all the default settings of the publicly available codes). For

Table 1. Mean error of the registered eye centers using different batch alignment algorithms under different initialized error. The notation $\downarrow$ characterizes the proportion of the error reduced by batch alignment.

Init	1.92 ± 0.88	2.80 ± 1.17	4.03 ± 1.25
SIFT-Congealing	1.84 ± 1.15 ($\downarrow 4\%$)	1.78 ± 1.78 ($\downarrow 36\%$)	2.32 ± 1.51 ($\downarrow 42\%$)
RASL	1.21 ± 1.67 ($\downarrow 37\%$)	1.43 ± 1.97 ($\downarrow 49\%$)	1.53 ± 1.89 ($\downarrow 62\%$)
TPGO	0.68 ± 0.44 ($\downarrow 65\%$)	0.76 ± 0.49 ($\downarrow 73\%$)	1.39 ± 0.82 ($\downarrow 66\%$)

TPGO, the subspace dimension is set to 5 for EYB, and 15 for AR and FERET. The number of outer iterations is set to 10. For the l_O-th outer iteration, the number of inner iterations is set to $L_I = \max(5, 15 - l_O)$.

4.1   Aligning Images with Severe Illuminations and Occlusion

The experiment involves the full set of 60 images of the first person on the EYB database (See Fig. 1). First, all the images are first aligned by two (manually labelled) eye centers. Then, we perturbed the two points of eye centers using a Gaussian noise of standard deviation σ. Finally, using the similarity warp which the original and perturbed points defined, we generate the similarity distorted image. Specifically, we generate three sets of permuted images with $\sigma = \{3, 4, 5\}$, in which the mean of the eye mislocation[2] of the eye centers are 1.92, 2.80, and 4.03 pixels, respectively. The performance of batch alignment algorithm is evaluated by the mean, as well as the standard deviation, of the eye mislocation in the aligned images. If the mean error is reduced after batch alignment, the algorithm is considered convergent.

The comparative batch alignment performance of the three algorithms is enumerated in Table 1 and one can see from the Table that, in all three test cases, TPGO performs better than RASL, followed by SIFT-Congealing. In addition, the standard deviation of the eye mislocation become larger after the batch alignment by RASL and SIFT-Congealing. These results indicate that (1) local invariance of SIFT feature makes it not hard to perform pixel-accurate alignment; and (2) TPGO, which exploits both the illumination invariance and the low-rank structure of images, performs significantly stabler than RASL, which just considers the low-rank structure.

We further tests the robustness of the algorithms by adding synthetical occlusions to the illuminated images. On the three sets of images used in previous experiment, 10 %, 20 %, and 30 % pixel occlusions are synthesized, respectively, before the image permutation. The results are listed in Table 2. As expected, all tested methods become worse when the occlusion proportion because larger.

---

[2] In an image ensemble, mean location is calculated as the averaged coordinate of the (left or right) eye centers in all images. The mean of the eye mislocation is defined as the average value of all the distances between each eye center and its corresponding mean location.

Table 2. Mean error of the registered eye centers using different batch alignment algorithms under different initialized error and occlusion proportion. The notation ↓ characterizes the proportion of the error reduced by batch alignment.

Init	1.92 ± 0.88	2.80 ± 1.17	4.03 ± 1.25
10 % Occlusion			
SIFT-Congealing	1.90 ± 1.11 ($\downarrow 1\%$)	2.14 ± 1.63 ($\downarrow 24\%$)	2.65 ± 2.10 ($\downarrow 34\%$)
RASL	1.61 ± 2.30 ($\downarrow 16\%$)	1.68 ± 1.77 ($\downarrow 40\%$)	1.97 ± 2.22 ($\downarrow 51\%$)
TPGO	0.68 ± 0.50 ($\downarrow 65\%$)	0.87 ± 1.17 ($\downarrow 69\%$)	1.69 ± 1.50 ($\downarrow 58\%$)
20 % Occlusion			
SIFT-Congealing	2.27 ± 1.52 ($\uparrow 18\%$)	2.60 ± 2.16 ($\downarrow 7\%$)	3.66 ± 2.70 ($\downarrow 9\%$)
RASL	1.62 ± 1.67 ($\downarrow 16\%$)	2.15 ± 2.16 ($\downarrow 23\%$)	2.45 ± 2.58 ($\downarrow 39\%$)
TPGO	0.89 ± 0.53 ($\downarrow 54\%$)	1.24 ± 1.36 ($\downarrow 56\%$)	2.16 ± 1.51 ($\downarrow 46\%$)
30 % Occlusion			
SIFT-Congealing	3.11 ± 1.91 ($\uparrow 62\%$)	3.17 ± 2.14 ($\uparrow 13\%$)	3.72 ± 2.36 ($\downarrow 8\%$)
RASL	2.24 ± 2.07 ($\uparrow 17\%$)	2.58 ± 2.41 ($\downarrow 8\%$)	2.99 ± 2.43 ($\downarrow 26\%$)
TPGO	1.28 ± 0.89 ($\downarrow 33\%$)	1.65 ± 1.54 ($\downarrow 41\%$)	2.73 ± 1.66 ($\downarrow 32\%$)

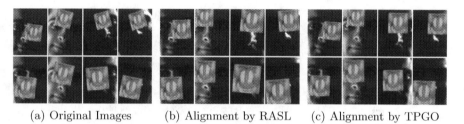

(a) Original Images   (b) Alignment by RASL   (c) Alignment by TPGO

Fig. 3. The alignment results of very challenging images with large misalignment, severe illumination and occlusion.

The mean and standard deviation of the proposed TPGO are smallest un all test cases. Under all nine test cases with occlusion, TPGO is the only method that can converge (reduce the mean error after batch alignment) all the time. Figure 3 shows some alignment results that TPGO converges to reasonable results but RASL and SIFT-Congealing fails, as the illumination and occlusion become severer.

4.2 Aligning 1000 Images of 100 Subjects with Real-World Illuminations and Occlusions

This experiment involves a large number of facial images from the AR database. Unlike the synthetically occluded images in previous experiment, these images exhibit real-world large occlusions caused by sunglasses and scarves, in additional to lighting changes. Specifically, 1000 images of 100 subject from the

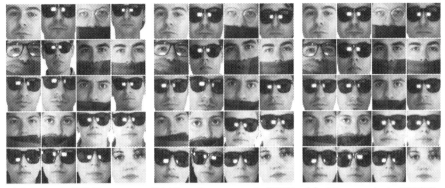

(a) Init via VJ Detector   (b) Pre-alignment via SIFT   (c) Alignment via TPGO

Fig. 4. Example images of the batch image alignment on the AR database.

Section 1 of AR database are selected, with the conditions on natural light, left-side light, right-side light, both-side light, wearing sunglasses, sunglasses plus left-side light, sunglasses plus right-side light, wearing scarves, scarves plus left-side light, scarves plus right-side light, respectively (See Table 3 for examples).

We obtain an initial estimate of the transformation in each image using the VJ detector of OpenCV, followed by a SIFT feature based pre-alignment procedure[3]. After that, we align the images to an 80×80 canonical frame using the three tested batch alignment methods. Finally, since there is no ground truth for this data set, we evaluate the preciseness of batch image alignment methods in term of the comparative recognition accuracy on their aligned image ensembles.

For each subject, the image with natural light is used as gallery, and the rest 9 images are used as probes. For the simplicity, whitened cosine similarity based nearest neighbor classifier is used for recognition. We have tested this classifier with LBP, Gabor, and HOG features, and find the LBP feature produce best results for all kinds of aligned images. Specifically, the $LBP_{8,2}^{U2}$ operator [23] is adopted in 10×10 pixel cell, for each cell accumulating a local histogram of 59 uniform patterns over the pixels of the cell. The combined histogram entries form the representation, resulting in a 3776 $(8 \times 8 \times 59)$ dimensional feature vector.

Table 3 enumerates the comparative recognition accuracy on differently aligned ensembles. One can see from the table that (1) the cropped facial images via VJ detector receive a low recognition accuracy, especially for the images wearing sunglasses. This is because, as shown in Fig. 4(a), the sunglasses largely deviate the scale and translation of the bounding box, when compared with the

---

[3] None of the tested algorithms can align the images with sunglasses precisely without the SIFT based pre-alignment, because the initial transformation estimate of the off-the-shelf detector is largely biased by the occlusions. The detailed implementation of the pre-alignment procedure is described in the supplementary material.

Table 3. Evaluation of preciseness of batch image alignment methods in term of the comparative recognition accuracy (%) on their aligned image ensembles of the 1000 images from AR database. The natural image of each subject is used for template and the others are used as probes. The notation ↓ characterizes the proportion of the recognition error reduced by the batch alignment method.

Alignment										Total
VJ-Detector	98	97	73	15	9	6	79	68	53	55.3
Pre-align	96	99	77	85	67	56	89	66	53	76.4
	↑100%	↓67%	↓15%	↓82%	↓64%	↓53%	↓48%	↑6%	↓0%	↓47%
Pre-align+	100	99	92	93	75	62	85	63	46	79.4
SIFT-Congealing	↓100%	↓67%	↓70%	↓92%	↓73%	↓60%	↓29%	↑16%	↑15%	↓54%
Pre-align+	100	100	94	94	72	74	95	87	75	87.9
RASL	↓100%	↓100%	↓78%	↓93%	↓69%	↓72%	↓76%	↓59%	↓47%	↓73%
Pre-align+	100	100	95	99	89	84	98	89	85	93.2
TPGO	↓100%	↓100%	↓81%	↓99%	↓88%	↓83%	↓90%	↓66%	↓68%	↓85%
Handcrafts [22]	99	98	90	97	82	71	94	85	64	86.7

non-occluded images. (2) Our pre-alignment procedure is effective to correct the deviated detection of the occluded images, resulting in a notable improvement on recognition accuracy, as shown in Fig. 4(b). (3) All the three fine-alignment algorithms provide further improved accuracy based on the pre-alignment results. In particular, TPGO produces the highest accuracy on all the nine testing conditions. Some example of TPGO-aligned images are shown in Fig. 4(c).

Due to the difficulty in aligning the occluded images, AR database has provided a standard distribution of aligned images by the handcrafted approach described in [22]. To compare our automatic alignment with the manual alignment, the manually aligned images are first cropped to include similar facial region with our alignment, and then interpolated to the same size of 80×80 pixels. As listed in Table 3, TPGO produces the higher accuracy than the handcrafted approach on all the nine testing conditions, and the overall error rate is reduced by over a half (from 13.5% to 6.8%). This result suggests that TPGO could potentially be very helpful for improving the performance of current object clustering or recognition systems despite large object occlusion.

Speed and scalability of TPGO. For this large-scale task, using 64-bit Matlab platform on a PC with Dual Core 2.93 GHz Pentium CPU and 4 GB memory, our implementation of TPGO requires less than 8 min to align the 1000 images of size 80×80, whereas RASL requires over 3 h. This impressive computational efficiency is a direct result of using correlation of gradient orientation, instead of L1-norm of pixel intensity, for robust optimization.

4.3 Fully Automatic Face Recognition

In this section, we evaluate the effectiveness of TPGO on fully automatic face recognition using 3307 facial images of 1196 subjects from the gray-level FERET database, which is a standard testbed for face recognition technologies [21]. The tested images display diversity across gender, ethnicity, and age, and were acquired without any restrictions imposed on expression, illumination and accessories for examples). Specifically, the experiment follows the standard data partitions of the FERET database:

- *gallery training set* contains 1,196 images of 1,196 people.
- *fb probe set* contains 1,195 images taken with an alternative facial expression.
- *fc probe set* contains 194 images taken under different lighting conditions.
- *dup1 probe set* contains 722 images taken in a different time.
- *dup2 probe set* contains 234 images taken at least a year later, which is a subset of the dup1 set.

Our algorithm starts with facial images detected by the common face detectors. Viola and Jones face detector[4], which outputs a square bounding box indicating the predicated center of the face and its scale, is applied for its stable performance and high speed. Given a detected face image of the width w, we crop the face according to the eye locations[5] of $(0.305w, 0.385w)$ and $(0.695w, 0.385w)$ using the CSU face identification evaluation system [24]. The cropped and scaled face images of a standard size 150×130, which subsequently is referred to as "*detected faces*". These detected faces are used for the initialization of TPGO learning. Since the detection deviation of the FERET images is small, the pre-alignment is not involved in this experiment.

It is well-known that sparse Representation-based Classification[6] (SRC) [25] is sensitive to the pixel-level misalignment of image, we therefore use it to evaluate the precision of alignment for automatic recognition. To solve the misalignment problem in SRC, a Deformable Sparse Recovery and Classification (DSRC) [18] have used tools from sparse representation to address the alignment problem. For the simplicity, TPGO and SIFT-Congealing[7] first build an appearance model from the batch alignment of the gallery set, and than align the probe images to the model for recognition.

For comparison purpose, we also apply SRC to the eye-aligned faces and the detected faces. For a fair comparison, all the aligned faces are all downsampled to 75×65 to be compatible with those used in [18]. The face recognition performance of SRC using the five alignment methods is tabulated in Table 4, which shows that the best performance on three of the four probe sets is achieved

---

[4] We use the OpenCV implementation of the Viola and Jones's face detector. Since there is only one face in each image, we reduce the false alarms by reserving the bounding box of the maximum size in each image. The detector missed only six faces out of all the 3307 images involved in our experiments, and we have manually completed these six bounding boxes.

[5] They are roughly the averaged locations of the two eyes of the typical bounding faces determined by the VJ face detector.

[6] The Homotopy method is applied to solve the ℓ^1-minimization problem with the regularization parameter $\lambda = 0.003$.

[7] RASL has not been tested since it is not directly applicable to align unseen images for automatic recognition.

Table 4. Comparative FERET recognition rates on differently aligned faces using SRC

Alignment	fb	fc	dup1	dup2
Human labeled Eye-aligned faces + SRC	83.2	74.2	46.1	30.8
Detected faces + SRC	73.5	38.7	34.5	33.3
DSRC [18]	**95.2**	28.4	46.1	20.3
SIFT-Congealing + SRC	82.0	73.2	55.3	42.3
TPGO-aligned faces + SRC	87.9	**82.4**	**61.2**	**50.0**

using TPGO-based faces. DSRC performs better than TPGO+SRC only when expression variation (fb set) is presented. In contrast, using TPGO-aligned faces achieves substantially improved accuracy (about 6 % to 18 %) than other alignment methods on the fc, dup1, and dup2 probe sets. This suggests that TPGO constructs an unified appearance model that is more robust against the complex variations of the facial appearance.

5 Conclusions

We have presented an image alignment method that can simultaneously align multiple images by exploiting both the illumination/occlusion invariance and the low rank property of the aligned image gradient orientation. Our approach is based on recent advances in image representation of gradient orientation that come with theoretical guarantees. The proposed algorithm consists of solving an efficient alternating optimization. This allows us to simultaneously align hundreds or even thousands of images on a typical PC in matter of minutes. We have shown the efficacy of our method with extensive experiments on images taken under laboratory conditions and on natural images of various types taken under a wide range of real-world conditions.

Experimental results show TPGO based batch alignment is more precise and robust than the state-of-the-art methods such as RASL and SIFT feature base Congealing. Furthermore, integrated with our proposed SIFT based pre-alignment procedure, TPGO is able to align a large number of images of multiple objects with large deviation, illumination, and occlusion in the precision that surpasses the handcrafted alignment, in term of our face recognition experiments on the AR and FERET databases.

Acknowledgement. This work was partially sponsored by National Natural Science Foundation of China (NSFC) under Grant No. 61375031, No. 61471048, and No. 61273217. This work was also supported by the Fundamental Research Funds for the Central Universities, Beijing Higher Education Young Elite Teacher Project, and the Program for New Century Excellent Talents in University.

References

1. Deng, W., Hu, J., Guo, J., Cai, W., Feng, D.: Robust, accurate and efficient face recognition from a single training image: a uniform pursuit approach. Pattern Recogn. **43**(5), 1748–1762 (2010)
2. Deng, W., Hu, J., Lu, J., Guo, J.: Transform-invariant PCA: a unified approach to fully automatic face alignment, representation, and recognition. IEEE Trans. Pattern Anal. Mach. Intell. **36**(6), 1275–1284 (2014)
3. Deng, W., Hu, J., Guo, J.: Extended SRC: undersampled face recognition via intraclass variant dictionary. IEEE Trans. Pattern Anal. Mach. Intell. **34**(9), 1864–1870 (2012)
4. Deng, W., Hu, J., Zhou, X., Guo, J.: Equidistant prototypes embedding for single sample based face recognition with generic learning and incremental learning. Pattern Recogn. **47**(12), 3738–3749 (2014)
5. Deng, W., Hu, J., Guo, J., Zhang, H., Zhang, C.: Comments on "globally maximizing, locally minimizing: unsupervised discriminant projection with applications to face and palm biometrics". IEEE Trans. Pattern Anal. Mach. Intell. **30**(8), 1503–1504 (2008)
6. Deng, W., Liu, Y., Hu, J., Guo, J.: The small sample size problem of ICA: a comparative study and analysis. Pattern Recogn. **45**(12), 4438–4450 (2012)
7. Learned-Miller, E.G.: Data driven image models through continuous joint alignment. J. IEEE Trans. Pattern Anal. Mach. Intell. **28**(2), 236–250 (2006)
8. Huang, G.B., Jain, V., Learned-Miller, E.: Unsupervised joint alignment of complex images. In: IEEE 11th International Conference on Computer Vision, 2007, ICCV 2007, pp. 1–8. IEEE (2007)
9. Cox, M., Sridharan, S., Lucey, S., Cohn, J.: Least squares congealing for unsupervised alignment of images. In: IEEE Conference on Computer Vision and Pattern Recognition, 2008, CVPR 2008, pp. 1–8. IEEE (2008)
10. Frey, B.J., Jojic, N.: Transformed component analysis: joint estimation of spatial transformations and image components. In: The Proceedings of the Seventh IEEE International Conference on Computer Vision, 1999, vol. 2, pp. 1190–1196. IEEE (1999)
11. Schweitzer, H.: Optimal eigenfeature selection by optimal image registration. In: IEEE Computer Society Conference on Computer Vision and Pattern Recognition, 1999, vol. 1. IEEE (1999)
12. Baker, S., Matthews, I., Schneider, J.: Automatic construction of active appearance models as an image coding problem. IEEE Trans. Pattern Anal. Machine Intell. **26**(10), 1380–1384 (2004)
13. Vedaldi, A., Guidi, G., Soatto, S.: Joint data alignment up to (lossy) transformations. In: IEEE Conference on Computer Vision and Pattern Recognition, 2008, CVPR 2008, pp. 1–8. IEEE (2008)
14. Peng, Y., Ganesh, A., Wright, J., Xu, W., Ma, Y.: RASL: robust alignment by sparse and low-rank decomposition for linearly correlated images. In: 2010 IEEE Conference on Computer Vision and Pattern Recognition (CVPR), pp. 763–770. IEEE (2010)
15. Tzimiropoulos, G., Zafeiriou, S., Pantic, M.: Subspace learning from image gradient orientations. IEEE Trans. Pattern Anal. Machine Intell. **34**(12), 2454–2466 (2012)
16. Georghiades, A., Belhumeur, P., Kriegman, D.: From few to many: illumination cone models for face recognition under variable lighting and pose. IEEE Trans. Pattern Anal. Machine Intell. **23**(6), 643–660 (2001)

17. Baker, S., Matthews, I.: Lucas-kanade 20 years on: a unifying framework. Int. J. Comput. Vision **56**(3), 221–255 (2004)
18. Wagner, A., Wright, J., Ganesh, A., Zhou, Z., Mobahi, H., Ma, Y.: Toward a practical face recognition system: robust alignment and illumination by sparse representation. IEEE Trans. Pattern Anal. Mach. Intell. **34**(2), 372–386 (2012)
19. Tzimiropoulos, G., Zafeiriou, S., Pantic, M.: Robust and efficient parametric face alignment. In: 2011 IEEE International Conference on Computer Vision (ICCV), pp. 1847–1854. IEEE (2011)
20. Martinez, A.M., Benavente, R.: The AR face database. CVC Technical report #24, June 1998
21. Phillips, P.J., Moon, H., Rizvi, P., Rauss, P.: The feret evaluation method for face recognition algorithms. IEEE Trans. Pattern Anal. Mach. Intell. **22**, 0162–8828 (2000)
22. Martínez, A.M.: Recognizing imprecisely localized, partially occluded, and expression variant faces from a single sample per class. IEEE Trans. Pattern Anal. Mach. Intell. **24**(6), 748–763 (2002)
23. Ahonen, T., Hadid, A., Pietikinen, M.: Face description with local binary patterns: application to face recognition. IEEE Trans. Pattern Anal. Mach. Intell. **28**(12), 2037–2041 (2006)
24. Bolme, D.S., Beveridge, J.R., Teixeira, M., Draper, B.A.: The CSU face identification evaluation system: its purpose, features, and structure. In: Crowley, J.L., Piater, J.H., Vincze, M., Paletta, L. (eds.) ICVS 2003. LNCS, vol. 2626, pp. 304–313. Springer, Heidelberg (2003)
25. Wright, J., Yang, A., Ganesh, A., Sastry, S., Ma, Y.: Robust face recognition via sparse representation. IEEE Trans. Pattern Anal. Machine Intell. **31**(2), 210–227 (2009)

Author Index

Printed in the United States
By Bookmasters